Transforming Ehlers-Danlos Syndrome

STÉPHANE DAENS ET AL.

Transforming
Ehlers-Danlos Syndrome

A Global Vision of the Disease
The Epigenetic Revolution
Emergencies

First Edition, 2022
English version

In collaboration with the GERSED Belgium members
and thirty international specialists

First edition, English

ISBN 979-8-775-73660-6

The GERSED Belgium

244, Ninoofsesteenweg
1700 Dilbeek, Belgium
www.gersedbelgique.com

Care has been taken to confirm the accuracy of the information presented and to describe generally accepted practices. However, the author and co-authors are not responsible for errors or omissions or for any consequences from application of the information in this book and make no warranty, expressed or implied, with respect to the contents of the publication.

The author and co-authors have exerted every effort to ensure that drug selection and dosage set forth in this text are in accordance with current recommendations and practice at the time of publication. However, in view of ongoing research, changes in government regulations, and the constant flow of information relating to drug therapy and drug reactions, the reader is urged to check the package insert for each drug for any change in indications and dosage and for added warnings and precautions. This is particularly important when the recommended agent is a new or infrequently employed drug.

Some drugs and medical advices presented in this publication have Food and Drug Administration (FDA) clearance for limited use in restricted research settings. It is the responsibility of the health care provider to ascertain the FDA status of each drug or device planned for use in their clinical practice.

"You are still just a little boy to me, just like a hundred thousand other little boys. Moreover, I do not need you. Furthermore, you do not need me either. I am only a fox to you, like a hundred thousand foxes. However, if you tame me, we will need each other. You will be, for me, unique in the world. I will be for you unique in the world..."

Antoine de Saint-Exupéry
The Little Prince (1943)

Testimony of Sylvain, 41 years old

The essential thing in a war is to know your opponents, but the game was rigged from the start.

A childhood like any other that is what I thought…

Tired of hearing "stop complaining", I soon became convinced that I was too soft. So I became rough.

I wanted to show that I could be what was expected of me. At first, I succeeded, while at the same time inflicting much violence on my body.

Medical certainties, dozens of diagnoses, hundreds of medications, thousands of days of professional absence.

And then one day, a hypothesis: "Maybe I am a zebra."

I look, I match, I am diagnosed.

I feel like I have been in apnea for 40 years, and I am breathing for the first time.

On paper, the announcement of a disease, a genetic defect, should make me morose. Now it was the other way around.

My tears stay inside, but now I know why.

If we do not know the value of pain, we do not know the value of joy, of gentleness.

Take care of yourself,

Sylvain B.

Diagnosed in December 2018 at age 40.

Acknowledgments

To my beloved and darling Mummy, who gave me everything, sacrificing a lot of herself. Well, I certainly do not tell you this often enough, so: I love you, Mom!

To my late Father, the great architect who left when I was a child, I hope he would have been proud of his son.

To Professor Claude Hamonet, dear Master and Friend. Thank you for changing my life and vision of Medicine. Thank you for your enthusiasm, so communicative, and the perseverance showed, beyond all limits, to make this disease (Ehlers-Danlos Syndrome) known and recognized.

To the collaborators and precious advisers of this book: Doctor Isabelle Dubois-Brock (main co-author), Professor Claude Hamonet, Professor Daniel Frédy, Doctor Trinh Hermanns-Lê, Mr. Olivier Hougrand, Professor Jaime F. Bravo, Professor Stephen W. Porges, Doctor Katja Kovacic, Doctor Jacek Kolacz, Mr. David Leroy, Mr. Dominique Ouhab, Doctor Michael P. Healy, Professor David Levine, Professor Michel Vervoort, Professor Andràs Pàldi, Doctor Daniel Grossin, Doctor Pradeep Chopra, Doctor Norman Marcus, Professor Anne Maitland, Doctor Jessica Pizano, Doctor Georges Verougstraete, Doctor Georges Obeid, Doctor Kambyse Samii, Doctor Richard Amoretti, Doctor Emmanuel Tran-Ngoc, Doctor Michel Horgue, Professor Antonio Bulbena-Vilarrasa, Professor Carolina Baeza-Velasco, Professor Andrea Bulbena-Cabré, Mrs. Dominique Weil.

To Mr. Yannick Atambona (Certified Healthcare Interpreter and Translator) for his translation from the original French text.

I am thankful for your devotion that made this book see the daylight.

Thanks to my mentor in Rheumatology: Professor Anne Peretz.

Thanks to my close and precious friends, who have carried and supported me for many years and who have encouraged me in the writing of this book: Richard L., Patricia H., Anne G. and Pascal J.,

Viviane L. and Alain K., Michel and Myriam V.-I., Frédéric P. and Patricia D., Tamara S., Pierre L., Isabelle D.- B. and to the artist RAAL for his exceptional iconographic contribution. I indeed forget some.

Thanks to the meticulous proofreaders of this book: Dr. Isabelle Dubois-Brock, Mr. Yannick Atambona, Mr. Richard Lambert & Mrs. Soizic Hendriks.

To the family doctors, specialists, and paramedics who have made a tremendous effort to learn about the disease over the years.

To all the patients who have shown exceptional courage and resilience facing this disease. Moreover, going through misunderstanding and abuse from some caregivers.

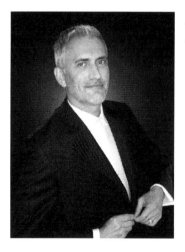

Dr. Stéphane Daens (main author)
Belgium, December 2021.

"It is only with the heart that one can see rightly, what is essential is invisible to the eye."

Antoine de Saint-Exupéry
The Little Prince (1943)

"Every EDS patient knows that one of the hardest parts of our day is the moment we open our eyes and waken into the reality of our bodies."

Michael Bihovsky (1986-)
Composer, actor, singer, songwriter

Errors: every attempt has been made to reduce errors in this text. Such is the nature of human existence, however, that mistakes are unavoidable. In the interests of improving future editions, the authors would be grateful to have their mistakes pointed out. Email: transformingedsb@gmail.com

Sylvie's testimony

After 20 years of medical wandering, we would finally put a name on my condition...

After being labeled with Fibromyalgia, called a hypochondriac, and persecuted with the phrase: "it is psychological! "...

I was finally recognized as a patient suffering from Ehlers-Danlos Syndrome...

This disease is little known to the medical profession, but has symptoms that should have alerted many specialists!

It is an obstacle course that has often made me doubt or give up, but I am so proud of it.

Furthermore, It made individual members of my family aware and get diagnosed themselves, avoiding years of the medical wandering I suffered from!

For that, thank you for putting the name EDS to this, because each EDS is unique!

Beautiful day,

Sylvie L.

Preface by Professor Claude Hamonet

Specialist in Physical Medicine and Rehabilitation

Doctor in Social Anthropology
Professor at Paris-Est-Créteil University
Ehlers-Danlos consultations, Paris, France
Honorary President of GERSED Belgium
Co-Author

"Transforming Ehlers-Danlos Syndrome" is the work of a doctor who has extensive experience of this disease whose modalities of expression are so variable and so multiple that one of his patients wrote, "Thanks for putting a name on my EDS because each EDS is unique! "

This conglomerate of symptoms confuses both patients and doctors, making diagnosis and dialogue difficult. First, because the patients have proprioceptive disorders, causing difficulties in locating and describing their functional impairments. There is chronic pain above all. Many are emotional and anxious about the physician not understanding them, not believing them, or not taking them seriously. In the US this is known as "White Coat Syndrome." On the other side are the doctors, who are more and more trained in a medicine divided by organs and anchored on data from paraclinical examinations. They are bewildered by the contrast between the richness of symptoms and the paucity of current sophisticated imagery and biology.

Belgium has a particular advantage here, having demonstrated that transmission electron microscopy could provide proof where genetic biology fails.

Stéphane Daens, with great humanity, delivers in his book a considerable amount of information about the disorder and its pathophysiology. He drew them both from his personal experience, with his patients, and from ever increasing international data on a disease that has emerged from oblivion over the last twenty years.

He has collaborated with other doctors mobilized around Ehlers-Danlos Syndrome, particularly within the Ehlers-Danlos Syndrome Study and Research Group (GERSED), of which he chairs the Belgian association. Some of them participate in chapters of this work.

It is necessary to underline the effort made to connect the aspects of clinical trials and biological modifications, to better identify the disease and its pathophysiological mechanisms. This is complex, and underlines the enormous work carried out by Stéphane Daens.

This book is not only the current compilation of what we know about Ehlers-Danlos; it is also a practical treatise for the practitioner and the patient, especially in situations that seem unusual to those who are not familiar with the disorder's pathology. For example, cases of pseudoparalysis are invariably confused with the diagnosis of hysteria with psychiatrization.

This book will likely surprise those who did not know, or poorly understood, Ehlers-Danlos Syndrome. It will now enable them to avoid erroneous diagnostic orientations, which we encounter daily in our specialized consultations, such as: Fibromyalgia, asthma, ankylosing spondylitis, rheumatoid arthritis, Goujerot-Sjögren, Raynaud, Marfan, multiple sclerosis, Lupus, myopathies, epilepsy (dystonia attacks), autism, Asperger and above all, "it is in the (patient's) head."

An essential contribution of Doctor Daens is legal and judicial: this book can prevent the wrongful removal of children with Ehlers-Danlos under the false accusation of abuse, citing physical violence (bruises) or Münchhausen by proxy.

This book will help stop a medical error from turning into a miscarriage of justice.

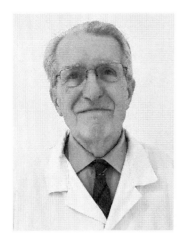

Professor Claude Hamonet
First edition, French version.

"It is a sad thing to think that nature speaks
and that mankind does not listen."
Victor Hugo (1802-1885)

"Imagination was given to man to compensate
him for what he is not, and a sense of humor
was provided to console him for what he his."
Oscar Wilde (1854-1900)

13

Preface by Professor Michel Vervoort

Zoology, Molecular Biology, Developmental Genetics

University Professor at the University of Paris, France
Head of the "Stem Cells, Development and Evolution" at
the Jacques Monod Institute (CNRS / Université de Paris)
Honorary Member of the *Institut Universitaire de France*
Honorary President of GERSED Belgium
Co-Author

Ehlers-Danlos Syndrome (EDS) is a complex disease that can be extremely debilitating for people suffering from it. Still little (and poorly) known to many doctors, this disease's diagnosis is often delayed, sometimes by several years, leading to physical suffering and intolerable psychological effects in many patients with EDS. Although still often categorized as a rare disease, its prevalence in the population is far from low; without doubt, it is a relatively common disease from 0.5 to 3.5%. It is a genetic disease, hereditary, but whose exact causes and transmission are still imperfectly known.

In this context, the book "Transforming Ehlers-Danlos Syndrome" constitutes an essential work to understand EDS better and help doctors and patients to understand this disease better in all its complexity. The author of the book, Doctor Stéphane Daens, a Belgian rheumatologist trained with Professor Claude Hamonet, the pioneer in diagnosing and treating EDS in France, devoted his time several years to this disease and to his patients who are affected. This commitment against EDS and his patients' day after day in his practice continues within the Ehlers-Danlos Syndrome Study and Research Group (GERSED) Belgium (of which Stéphane Daens is the president). Moreover, it finds a form result in this book.

"Transforming Ehlers-Danlos Syndrome" is indeed both an exhaustive summary of the state of knowledge concerning this disease and a practical manual for use by physicians and their patients. The work of synthesis, research, and reflection produced by Stéphane Daens, partly in collaboration with colleagues involved, like him, in the fight against this disease, is colossal and remarkable. I would especially like to mention the chapter on EDS's genetic causes, because it is within my competence range. Stéphane Daens synthesizes current knowledge and offers innovative hypotheses, particularly on the disease's potentially epigenetic character.

The passion that drives Stéphane Daens shines through the text, along with his dedication to treating EDS affected patients. From time to time, it also points to anger in front of attitudes and decisions, especially at the health organization level, complicating patients' lives and management already heavily impacted by the disease. May the decision-makers of these health policies take the time to read this work! Doctors, patients, and anyone interested in EDS will find all they have always wanted to know about this disease (and even more!) in this book, along with ample food for thought to furnish long winter evenings or other seasons. Read and enjoy!

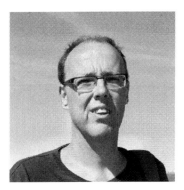

Professor Michel Vervoort
First edition, French version.

Preface by Professor Anne Maitland

Specialist in Internal Medicine, Allergy and Immunology

Fellow of the American College of Allergy, Asthma and Immunology
Member of the American Academy of Allergy, Asthma and Immunology
Mount Sinai Hospital, New York, USA
Comprehensive Allergy and Asthma Care, Tarrytown, NY, USA
Honorary President of GERSED Belgium
Co-Author

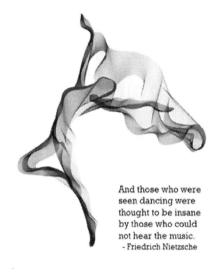

And those who were seen dancing were thought to be insane by those who could not hear the music.
- Friedrich Nietzsche

For some people, there are illnesses that can be quickly sorted out at a minute clinic.

For many, at times, a few words of assurance, a prescription or an injection will do.

Others, the cure is time, as their ailment fades with rest, water and a nutritious meal.

But nowadays, nearly one out of two of us are plagued by silent killer conditions and illnesses that will slowly sap our vitality, if not detected early and treated. Numerous studies, shedding light on commonly known disorders, such as cancer, diabetes, and asthma, and less known syndromes, such as immunodeficiencies and now COVID, have shown the benefits of early detection and tailored medical intervention. As Benjamin Franklin once said, an ounce of prevention is worth a pound of cure.

"Within all of their noses' reach, they may agree,
what lies beyond, they cannot see."

Johann Wolfgang von Goethe, Faust Pt 1 and 2, 2003

But what if your doctor does not know to look for a condition that was inherited or acquired, along one's arduous journey on mother Earth? Or what if the child does not have the words to describe lingering, vague symptoms, such as fatigue, pain, heightened sensitivity to environmental stimuli? Or the adult that had never learned that some signs warrant mention to their doctor, which means diversion of time and money for a doctor's appointment? The fate of these patients, with overlooked or unseen conditions, was captured by "one of the bonafide superheroes of early modern medicine" in 1926. As the scientific method ushered in the golden age of medicine of the early 20th century, Francis Peabody described the medical odyssey that fell upon most patients "characterized by the presence of symptoms that cannot be accounted for by organic disease". These patients, who comprise a sizeable number of any physician's practice, often referred to as having "nothing the matter" with them:

"Medically speaking, they are not serious cases as regards prospective death, but they are often extremely serious as regards prospective life. Their symptoms will rarely prove fatal, but their lives will be long and miserable, and they may end by nearly exhausting their families and friends. Death is not the worst thing in the world, and to help a man to a happy and useful career may be more of a service than the saving of life."

Francis Peabody, The Care of the Patient (Peabody, 1927)

Such is the fate of too many children and adults with inherited connective tissue disorders, such as Ehlers-Danlos Syndrome (EDS) and Hypermobile Spectrum Disorder (HSD). Equipped with connective tissue that served their ancestors well, in a different time and space, children and adults with EDS and HSD are now at risk for a triad of ailments: symptomatic connective tissue disorders, dysregulation of the immune system and autonomic dysfunction.

The human race has come to dominate its environment so completely that any analysis of the increase or appearance of a disease has to take changes in our lifestyle into account. In the case of [emerging diseases], changes in our environment, diet, water quality, and personal behavior over the last 150 years have played a dominant role in the specificity of these diseases, as well as in prevalence and severity.

Thomas A. E. Platts-Mills, MD, PhD, FRS, The Allergy Epidemics (Platts-Mills, 2015)

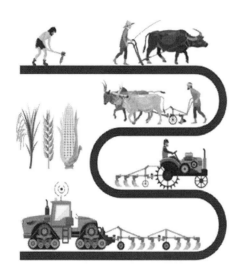

Before modernization of our communities – within the structures we live in, the foodstuffs we consume, our modes of transportation, the clothing we wear - the skills and talents of children and adults with EDS/HSD were on display in the classroom, on the stage, as well as on the playing fields and gymnasiums. Consider how hypermobile joints lend to the display of grace and power of a ballerina or gymnast or swimmer; the soft velvety skin lends to enduring beauty of actors and models, as the seasons pass; or the heightened senses allow one to see or feel changes in the immediate surroundings, before anyone else in the room.

As the places where we sleep, work, study and play, the food we consume, and the air we breathe has been transformed, a growing number of patients, with inherited pliability of their connective tissue network, started to exhibit ailments, beyond that originally recognized by Drs. Tschernogobow, Ehlers and Danlos and then the geneticists and rheumatologists of the mid-20th century (*Hamonet & Brock, 2016*). Along with generalized joint hypermobility, children and adults also may have blood vessels that twist and kink, epithelial or mucosal linings that elongate and fold over each other, or ligaments that stretch and allow joints to slip in and out of place. If these events come and go, in the wrong place, tissue injury ensues. This is followed by activation of nearby immune and nerve pathways, leading to signs and symptoms, depending on the site of injury: headache disorders, fatigue, sleep disturbance, anxiety, gastrointestinal complaints, body aches, brain fog, and exercise intolerance are not uncommon among children and adults, whose bendy bodies have been increasingly challenged by the fast-paced routines and elements of modern living. As captured by Charles Dickens to the Dalai Lama, "the paradox of our age" is "we spend more, but we have less; bigger houses, but smaller families; more conveniences, but less time; more medicines, but less healthiness…" (*Conversation agent, 2016*)

Those with inherited connective tissue disorders are the canaries of the mines: one of the first to be challenged and more likely to become ill, by mass produced foods, clothing, and the building structures, where we live, work, study and play.

"Medical education, however, is less likely to suffer from such stagnation, for whenever the lay public stops criticizing the type of modern doctor, the medical profession itself may be counted on to stir up the stagnant pool and cleanse it of its sedimentary deposit."

Francis Peabody, The Care of the Patient, JAMA 1927

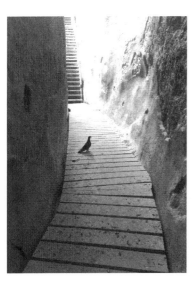

Even though connective tissue is the largest system in the human body, most symptomatic EDS patients report a decade or more of symptoms, before receiving a name or diagnosis that could lead to effective, tailored care. What is the hold up? Look no further than our healthcare systems. Our modern health care is an impressive plant, which has with thousands of commercially available tests; sophisticated surgical procedures; pathogen free operating theaters; a robust, innovative pharmaceutical industry; and, in some communities, a health care provider to every 500 residents in a community. However, little is taught about disorders of connective tissues to medical professionals, beyond classic autoimmune disorders; and, a patient may have minutes to describe their chief complaint, so that a medication, a test, a procedure or a referral to another healthcare provider is provided (*Ross, 2007*). So a patient, who shows no objective, organic pathology, from

19

standard testing – no detectable auto-antibodies, no gross changes on biopsies, no abnormalities on radiology exams, when lying or standing still - often are deemed "nothing the matter with them", given a script to treat anxiety, and often labeled with one of the Scarlett letters of medicine – "C" for conversion disorder, "F" for factitious disorder, "H" for hypochondriasis, or "M" for Münchhausen". The not so implicit bias of health care systems against patients, with vague complaints such pain or fatigue and "normal tests", was on display recently. After a flurry of complaints from educated healthcare consumers, patients using Twitter, an internal Medicine Board Review question had to be withdrawn and an apology issued by the authors of this question, due to accusations of misogyny in medicine (*Cassidy, 2018*). It is not as though patients with CTDs cannot develop psychiatric disorders. However, too often these psychiatric diagnoses trump further investigation and treatment of patients with hEDS/HSD, who consider themselves "hiding" in pain and fatigue, in plain sight of too many health care providers.

Time, sympathy and understanding must be lavishly dispensed, but the reward is to be found in that personal bond which forms the greatest satisfaction of the practice of medicine. One of the essential qualities of the clinician is interest in humanity, for the secret of the care of the patient is in caring for the patient.

Francis Peabody, 1927 (Peabody, 1927)

To bypass the seemingly vast sea of unawareness of EDS/HSD and the disorders, which frequently travel with these inherited connective tissue disorders, patients and their practitioners must be willing and able to learn from those who have already charted this uneven, often unforgiving healthcare landscape.

Here is a new bible for EDS patients, that serves as a beacon, lighting the way for those in pain, often despair, and hiding in plain sight of the modern, biomedical community.

The authors of "Transforming EDS" are physicians and scientists, who bring nearly 30 years of clinical experience, in the diagnosis and comprehensive management of EDS/HSD patients (*Hamonet & Brock, 2016*) (*Brissot, Amoretti, Ducret, & Hamonet, 2020*).

Learning of their multi-discipline team efforts has lifted the blinders of my miseducation, in the hallways of some of the most pre-eminent medical centers in the country; and, to improve the most valuable asset in life - health, here is to a multidisciplinary effort, to foster partnerships across clinical specialties and national lines to do as we promised- to help and do no harm.

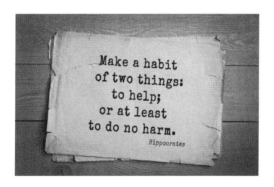

References

Brissot, R., Amoretti, R., Ducret, L., & Hamonet, C. (2020). *Ehlers-Danlos and respiratory function. Clinical data on a cohort of 5,700 patients: oxygen therapy and physical rehabilitation medicine (P.R.M.). J Neuroscience and Neurological Surgery*, 1-6. Retrieved from http://claude.hamonet.free.fr/shared/eds-and-respiratory-function.pdf

Cassidy, E. (2018, July 26). *Twitter Calls Out Practice Exam Question for 'Medical Misogyny'*. Retrieved from https://sports.yahoo.com/: https://sports.yahoo.com/twitter-calls-practice-exam-apos-170944079.html

Castori, M. (2012). *Ehlers-Danlos syndrome, hypermobility type: an underdiagnosed hereditary connective tissue disorder with mucocutaneous, articular, and systemic manifestations. Dermatology*, 1-22. doi: doi: 10.5402/2012/751768. Epub 2012 Nov 22.

Conversation agent. (2016). *The Paradox of our Age*. Retrieved from conversationagent.com: https://www.conversationagent.com/2015/12/the-paradox-of-our-age.html

Gazit, Y., Jacob, G., & Grahame, R. (2016). *Ehlers-Danlos Syndrome-Hypermobility Type: A Much Neglected Multisystemic Disorder. Rambam Maimonides Med J, 7(4), 1-10.*

Goethe, J. W. (2003). *Faust Pt 1 and 2 poetry in translation. Retrieved from poetryintranslation.com: https://www.poetryintranslation.com/klineasfaust.php*

Hamonet, C., & Brock, I. (2016, November 3). *Webinar: "A French Perspective on Ehlers Danlos". Retrieved from https://www.youtube.com/watch?v=Ril8-DcT-lo*

Peabody, F. W. (1927). *The care of the patient. J Amer Med Association, 88(12), 877-882.*

Platts-Mills, T. A. (2015). *The allergy epidemics: 1870-2010. J Allergy Clin Immunol, 136, 3-13.*

Ross, M. A. (2007). *Physicians and patients, then and now. BC Medical Journal, 429-435. Retrieved from https://bcmj.org/premise/physicians-and-patients-then-and-now*

Time magazine. (1969, February 2). *The Plight of the US Patient. Time Magazine, pp. 1-14. Retrieved January 16, 2014.*

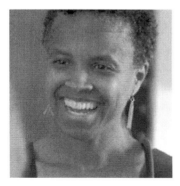 Professor Anne Maitland

Preface by Professor Stephen W. Porges

Neuroscience

Distinguished University Scientist, Kinsey Institute, Indiana University
Professor of Psychiatry, University of North Carolina, USA
Professor Emeritus, University of Illinois & Maryland
Honorary President of GERSED Belgium
Co-Author

It is an honor and pleasure to write a preface for Dr. Daens' volume, *Transforming Ehlers-Danlos Syndrome*. The volume provides an expansive review of cutting-edge research documenting the disparate symptoms associated with EDS. In this comprehensive clinically oriented volume, expert clinical researchers effectively disentangle the plausible mechanisms underlying EDS. These clinical researchers share their compassionate attempt to identify common themes associated with the diagnosis and describe treatment strategies that are helpful in reducing the burden of pain and dysfunction.

Dr. Daens provides a long-needed resource that has the potential to inform medical practice that the symptoms associated with EDS are "real" and not psychogenic. The volume provides a broad tapestry of the clinical complexity of EDS and the history of inaccurate diagnoses and inappropriate treatments, which have led to suffering and uncertainty for many patients. The chapters, written by expert researchers in EDS, discuss symptoms associated with various subtypes, plausible underlying mechanisms, and optimistic management strategies that will enhance quality of life for those who are diagnosed with EDS.

Too many patients have been victimized by medicine in which uninformed physicians miss the defining symptoms of EDS and have inappropriately assumed their patients were feigning symptoms. Through well documented clinical research, the chapters provide a prospective that EDS and the various subtypes of EDS have predictable symptom profiles. This information provides the physician with a new insight into the patient's experience that will move the physician-patient interaction towards helpful management of symptoms and a reduction of the patient's uncertainty.

The specific chapters that Dr. Daens has written highlight his personal journey with EDS. He describes his own diagnosis and the potential impact of his own personal trauma as a triggering event leading from vulnerability to disease. His experiences contribute to his deep personal and passionate commitment to develop a better understanding of the disorder and to contribute to compassionate treatments of EDS. Moreover, his experience highlights the frequently observed relationship between a trauma experience and the diagnosis. This observation suggests that there may be a larger subset of individuals with a vulnerability to being diagnosed as EDS, but currently are not diagnosed or express severe symptoms. The observation also provides a clue that severity of symptoms might be a function of an interaction between a threat reaction to the trauma and a pre-existing (genetic or epigenetic) vulnerability due to the disease.

It is only during the past decade that I have become aware of EDS. For several decades my research as a scientist has focused on the neural regulation of the autonomic nervous system and how the autonomic nervous system provides a "neural platform" for our emotional, cognitive, physiological, and behavioral reactivity. Little did I know that this background would provide an important lens that would contribute to a reconceptualization of EDS. Being invited into the world of EDS was an unexpected opportunity. My personal journey in this community is the product of my interactions with two dedicated physician scientists who are committed to understanding and treating patients with EDS. Working with them has provided me with opportunities to contribute to reorganizing the apparent disparate array of symptoms into a more predictable and understandable narrative.

I was introduced to EDS about 8 years ago, when Dr. Bulbena, an author in this book, contacted me. He was studying prevalence of anxiety symptoms in EDS. He wanted to apply a scale that I developed to assess autonomic reactivity in his research with EDS. The scale, known as the Body Perception

Questionnaire (BPQ), uses subjective methods to estimate autonomic reactivity. I was intrigued with Dr. Bulbena's interest in the link between anxiety and EDS. As a psychiatrist, he was interested in anxiety and other mental health comorbidities of EDS. As a neuroscientist, my interest focused on the neural mechanisms that supported anxiety. I viewed anxiety as an emergent property of a dysregulated autonomic nervous system (i.e., dysautonomia). From my perspective (e.g., Polyvagal Theory) autonomic state provided a "neural platform" for anxiety and other features of emotional reactivity. I speculated that the autonomic regulation of an EDS patient would hypothetically be associated with a destabilized autonomic nervous system characterized by blunted neural regulation of the calming and homeostatic functions via the vagus and increased sympathetic excitation. Such an autonomic profile would support defensive strategies including fight and flight behaviors. The BPQ had subscales designed to capture the reactivity of the autonomic nervous system to enable inference regarding neural pathways, vagal or sympathetic, influencing autonomic state. The BPQ data supported this speculation (*Bulbena-Cabré et al., 2017*).

The BPQ data suggested that anxiety and other mental health morbidities frequently observed in EDS were psychological manifestations of an autonomic nervous system locked in a state of chronic threat. From my theoretical perspective the prevalence of anxiety and emotional instability observed in EDS was a clue that these mental health vulnerabilities would have an autonomic substrate.

As I read the chapters in the book, I realized that this speculation was consistent with the clinical observations of dysautonomia. However, to adequately test the hypothesis, the questionnaire data from the BPQ needed convergent objective measures of autonomic regulation. Fortuitously, this opportunity followed when I met Dr. Kovacic (see this volume).

Dr. Kovacic is an extremely talented and inquisitive clinician-researcher who directs an active pediatric gastroenterology clinic. She was conducting research on the effectiveness of noninvasive vagal nerve stimulation on functional abdominal disorders in adolescents. Her mode of vagal stimulation applied electrical stimulation to the vagal afferents on the ear. She wanted to investigate whether reduction in abdominal pain was paralleled by a valid indicator of vagal regulation of the heart and whether the patient's autonomic profile prior to intervention was related to whether the vagal stimulation would effectively reduce pain.

Since she was interested in learning methods to accurately monitor vagal regulation of the heart, she contacted me, and we initiated a fruitful collaboration. In our shared journey we learned that in her clinic approximately about half the patients with functional abdominal disorders had Beighton scores of 4 or greater and about a third had Beighton scores of 5 or greater. Many of the patients with high Beighton scores did not have an EDS diagnosis. We learned that the patients, who had noticeable pain reduction during vagal stimulation, were characterized by an atypical decoupling between a measure of cardiac vagal tone (respiratory sinus arrhythmia) extracted from the beat-to-beat heart rate variability. The metric we used is a functional measure of vagal efficiency. This metric evaluates the dynamic parallel changes between heart rate and cardiac vagal tone (measured via the respiratory sinus arrhythmia component of heart rate variability). Functionally, the low vagal efficiency reflects a decoupled feedback system, and the decoupled system may optimize the effectiveness of exogeneous vagal stimulation. Conceptually, the decoupled feedback system might result in the endogenous circuit not competing with the exogenous stimulation. Conceptually, the stimulator would function more like a prosthetic source of vagal information that would not be competing with the ineffective endogenous feedback circuit. In support of this model, once the stimulator was turned off pain returned.

Most relevant to understanding EDS, we observed a strong relationship between high Beighton scores and low vagal efficiency (*Kolacz et al., 2021*). The vagal efficiency metric appears to be providing a robust metric of dysautonomia, a feature that is mentioned in most chapters in this volume. The vagal efficiency metric is relatively easy to assess and in conjunction with measures of joint hypermobility might help refine the diagnosis of hEDS. In our other research we have observed vagal efficiency to degrade with alcohol (*Reed, Porges, Newlin, 1999*), prematurity (*Porges et al. 2019*), trauma history, and the multisystem shutdown that precedes death (*Williamson et al., 2010*).

Through the lens of the Polyvagal Theory, consistent the views of expressed in several of the chapters in this book, many of the features of EDS can be viewed as being dependent clinical features of dysautonomia. Dysautonomia is the clinical manifestation of an autonomic nervous system that is poorly regulated. Through the lens of the Polyvagal Theory, the destabilized autonomic nervous system described by low vagal efficiency would provide the neural platform for many of the behavioral, psychological, and medical symptoms observed in patients with EDS.

Our initial documentation of a link between low vagal efficiency and severity of joint hypermobility provides another potential explanatory narrative. In this narrative, the observed poorly regulated autonomic nervous system is not a symptom of EDS but a component of a neural reaction that is locked in a chronic state to support threat. This state would be supported by the sympathetic activation without access to calming influence of a vagal circuit. In the terminology of the Polyvagal Theory, the dynamic regulation of the calming vagal brake is unavailable resulting in an autonomic state that would promote anxiety and dysregulated emotions.

However, our research suggests that the prevalence of low vagal efficiency in EDS identifies has an optimistic portal for treatment. It appears that a low vagal efficiency provides a portal that enables exogeneous vagal nerve stimulation to be effective in reducing functional abdominal pain. Given the prevalence of dysautonomia in EDS, it is possible that with the reduction in functional abdominal pain other autonomic dependent processes related to mental and physical health might also be improved.

In reading this volume, I have gained an appreciation for the progress that has been made in understanding and treating EDS.

This volume provides an accessible portfolio of the pioneering work of clinical researchers at the forefront of research on EDS. These clinical researchers are actively reframing our understanding of the mechanisms underlying EDS and are developing and testing innovative treatments that will optimize the quality of life for their patients.

Bulbena-Cabré, A., Pailhez, G., Cabrera, A., Baeza-Velasco, C., Porges, S., & Bulbena, A. (2017). Body perception in a sample of nonclinical youngsters with joint hypermobility. Ansiedad y Estrés, 23(2-3), 99-103.

Kolacz J, Kovacic K, Lewis GF, Sood MR, Aziz Q, Roath OR, Porges SW (2021). Cardiac autonomic regulation and joint hypermobility in adolescents with functional abdominal pain disorders. Neurogastroenterol Motil. Doi: 10.1111/nmo.14165

Porges, S. W., Davila, M. I., Lewis, G. F., Kolacz, J., Okonmah-Obazee, S., Hane, A. A., ... & Welch, M. G. (2019). Autonomic regulation of preterm infants is enhanced by Family Nurture Intervention. Developmental psychobiology, 61(6), 942-952.

Reed, S. F., Porges, S. W., & Newlin, D. B. (1999). Effect of alcohol on vagal regulation of cardiovascular function: contributions of the polyvagal theory to the psychophysiology of alcohol. Experimental and clinical psychopharmacology, 7(4), 484.

Williamson, J. B., Lewis, G., Grippo, A. J., Lamb, D., Harden, E., Handleman, M., ... & Porges, S. W. (2010). Autonomic predictors of recovery following surgery: a comparative study. Autonomic Neuroscience, 156(1-2), 60-66.

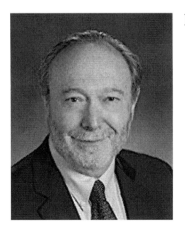 Professor Stephen W. Porges

SUMMARY

FIRST PART:
Ehlers-Danlos Syndrome
History, Signs, and Symptoms

SECOND PART:

Genetic and Epigenetic Postulates

THIRD PART:

The Mechanisms of Pain
Specific Treatments for EDS
Manage Emergency Situations in EDS

List of Abbreviations

ALA	Alpha Lipoic Acid
AMPA	Amino-Methyl-Phosphonic Acid
AN	Author's Note
ANA	Anti-Nuclear Antibodies
ANCA	Anti-Neutrophil Cytoplasmic Antibodies
ANS	Autonomous Nervous System
Anti-CCP	Cyclic Citrullinated Peptide Antibodies
ASCA	Anti-Saccharomyces Cerevisiae Antibodies
ASD	Autistic Spectrum Disorder
BID	Bis in die, i.e. twice a day
BNDF	Brain-Derived Neurotrophic Factors
CBD	Cannabidiol
CBG	Cannabigerol
CFS	Chronic Fatigue Syndrome
CGRP	Calcitonin Gene Related Peptide
CNS	Central Nervous System
CRP	C-Reactive Protein
CRPS	Complex Regional Pain Syndrome
csEDS	Common Systemic EDS
DNA	Deoxyribonucleic acid
DRG	Dorsal Root Ganglion
DVT	Deep vein thrombosis
EDS	Ehlers-Danlos Syndrome
ESR	Erythrocyte Sedimentation Rate
FBN	Fibrillin
FMS	Fibromyalgia Syndrome
G-HSD	Generalized HSD
G-JHS	Generalized JHS
GABA	Gamma Amino-Butyric Acid
H-HSD	Historical HSD
hEDS	Hypermobile EDS
HSD	Hypermobile Spectrum Disorder
IgA	Immunoglobulin Type A
IgE	Immunoglobulin Type E
IgG	Immunoglobulin Type G
IgM	Immunoglobulin Type M
IL	Interleukin
JHS	Joint Hypermobility Syndrome
KA	Kainate
L-HSD	Localized HSD

L-JHS	Localized JHS
LPS	Lipopolysaccharide (endotoxin)
MCA	Mast Cell Activation
MCA/EDS	MCA related to EDS
MCAD	Mast Cell Activation Disorder
MCAS	Mast Cell activation Syndrome
MCD	Mast Cell Disorder
MVP	Mitral Valve Prolapse
NAC	N-Acetylcysteine
NF-kB	Nuclear Factor - kappa B
NK1	Neurokinin-1
NLD	Naltrexone Low Dose
NMDA	N-Methyl-D-Aspartate
PCS	Postural Control System
PDS	Proprioceptive Dysfunction Syndrome
P-HSD	Peripheral HSD
P-JHS	Peripheral JHS
PDS	Proprioceptive Deficiency Syndrome
PEA	Palmitoylethanolamide
RNA	Ribonucleic acid
RSD	Reflex Sympathetic Dystrophy
SEMDJL2	Spondyloepimetaphyseal Dysplasia with Joint Laxity 2
SIP	Sympathetically Independent Pain
SMDK	Spondylo-Metaphyseal Dysplasia Koslowski type
SMP	Sympathetically Maintained Pain
SR	Sedimentation rate
TEM	Transmission Electron Microscopy
THC	Tetrahydrocannabinol
TID	Ter in die, i.e. three times a day
TLR	Toll Like Receptor
TNF	Tumor Necrosis Factor
trkB	Tropomyosin receptor kinase B
Trps	Tender points
TRVP4	Transient Receptor Potential Cation Channel Subfamily V member genes
UPS	Upright Postural System
VAS	Visual Analogic Scale

Introduction to the First Edition

*E*hlers-Danlos, a medical term, among thousands learned in five minutes during my seven years of study in the Faculty of Medicine. Five minutes are barely sufficient to remember its name and a few medical characteristics that have become obsolete: "These are circus people with hyper-stretchable skin, contortionists!".

Three years of specialization in Internal Medicine followed, and not a word on this syndrome. It was never mentioned during our seminars or at the *Grand Tour* of Internal Medicine, weekly gatherings during which clinical cases were presented and discussed. The same occurred during my two years of specialization in Rheumatology, *"Ehlers Danlos Syndrome? It is not clinically significant, and it is a curiosity. It does not cause any pain, apart from inevitable dislocations or sprains, and it is sporadic! "*.

Either way, the years passed. At the age of 35 I had completed my six year residency and rose to be the Deputy Head of the Clinic of Rheumatology at a University Hospital in Brussels. I mainly take care of the diagnosis and monitoring of patients with rheumatoid arthritis, ankylosing spondylitis, spondyloarthropathies linked to inflammatory bowel diseases, psoriatic arthritis, disseminated lupus erythematosus, and rare cases of systemic scleroderma.

Curious about everything, after my medical studies I sought training in acupuncture, ultrasound evaluation of the musculoskeletal system, infiltration techniques under ultrasound location, diagnostic mini-arthroscopy (with synovial biopsies), peripheral neurophysiology examinations and electromyography, in bone densitometry and radiation protection.

I like to think that curiosity, along with an open mind and the constant questioning of one's knowledge, is one of the keys to evolving and feeling fulfilled in the profession as a physician.

However, I never thought of becoming an actor in the renewal of my knowledge about Ehlers-Danlos Syndrome.

In 2014, I was attacked by seven individuals: one homophobic act, among others. I suffered a concussion and took two weeks of sick leave. The weeks go by, but this pain in my head does not go away. Fatigue becomes a burden, dragging at me day by day. Days are getting longer. Minutes seem like hours. Then pain, clumsiness, acid reflux, and dizziness!

I cannot stand it anymore. I cannot even take part in my Aïkido class, a Japanese martial art that I have been practicing for over 30 years.

Fortunately, I was consulting in a private structure, parallel to my hospital practice, in which worked a professor emeritus of rheumatology, Daniel Manicourt, a pioneer of Ehlers-Danlos Syndrome in Belgium.

After noticing that I was in *bad shape*, he asked me a few questions; he examined me and announced, "I think you have EDS!"

"A what? ", I replied.

"EDS. Ehlers-Danlos Syndrome! "

"Really? But this disease is rare, isn't it? "

"Oh no! I think the best thing is that you read the website of a French teacher I know well, Claude Hamonet. He is a world specialist in this disease. We will talk about it next week."

I spent the whole weekend reading this website. I make moon eyes, I am amazed at what I read! Maybe there are so many patients I misdiagnosed! Why were we not taught about this disease during our studies? I wander between amazement and sadness.

I tell Daniel M. about my readings the following Wednesday, and he suggests: "If you wish, I will put you in touch with

Professor Hamonet. You can go to Paris and follow his consultations."

"Okay, I am interested, that would be great! "

A few weeks pass, and I go to Paris to the ELLAsanté Center where Professor Hamonet works. Welcoming, warm-hearted, and generous, he then teaches me, without restriction, as days go by, during multiple meetings.

What should I to do seeing so much ignorance and mistreatment by medical professionals? What should be done in front of desperate patients? How can I help? I was diagnosed relatively quickly, compared to the years and years of medical wandering that most of these women and men undergo. You have to move, Stéphane! You must adapt your work schedule to this strange disease!

Also, why not spend the rest of your career helping those who, like you, are suffering? Go ahead, says my Jiminy!

A few years later, here I am writing a second book about Ehlers-Danlos Syndrome.

What is it about?

I felt a sudden necessity to make this complex and multifaceted hereditary disease known to as many caregivers and patients as possible. EDS is a disease in which pain and chronic fatigue form a deep-rooted foundation. It is a disease that evolves in crises and generates difficult situations of disability. People who suffer from this disease are ignored, put into psychiatry, mistreated, or poorly treated. No other disease has been so rejected and ignored by Medicine, even though it was introduced to the world almost 130 years ago! An attempt was made to classify these patients in the remaining boxes. Then, in the 1980s, came Fibromyalgia.

There is an urgent need for information and training so we no longer misinform and ignore!

We are currently estimating 1 to 4% of the general population has EDS. I.e., more than 300,000 people in Belgium, more than a million in France, and up to 225 million people worldwide. EDS is no longer a rare or orphan disease. Many treatments exist (supplements, orthoses, compression garments, sequential oxygen therapy, specific drugs, and more) to relieve and help the vast majority of EDS patients.

So, I took up the pen with the help and participation of thirty international experts. A geneticist, an epigeneticist, several paramedics, and many doctors, promptly responded.

I am thankful for that.

I wanted to make the book accessible to all, both caregivers and patients. Medical terms are explained in every step. At the end of reading this book, which I wanted to punctuated with poignant testimonies from individual patients, I dare to hope that the reader will have *tamed* the disease, and will inevitably recognize it when he or she encounters it.

In the first part of the book, the disease's history, and its signs and symptoms are introduced. In the second part of the book, there are clues of EDS transmission from parents to children and how it evolves throughout life. In the third part, the most disabling symptoms which are often disconcerting because of their singular clinical presentations, and their specific management are detailed.

By Dr. Stéphane Daens.

Let us all get to grips with this Ehlers-Danlos Syndrome together.

Testimonial of Glenn, 41 years old

"It is one of those days again,

One of those days where even the great reaper turns around.

Where the Pain, which has gradually set in,

Keeps you from moving forward.

Like paralyzed, with frozen limbs,

Vulnerable as a newborn baby.

This evil that gnaws inside,

Makes us unusual people.

Soldiers, fighters, survivors, we smile and move on,

No matter how many obstacles get in our way.

Dislocations, scars, bruises,

We do not care about any of these,

Even when we are misunderstood by many of our people,

And rejected by some."

Glenn F., 41, Belgium

First Part

EHLERS-DANLOS SYNDROME:

History, Signs, and Symptoms

CHAPTER I

EDS, a Thwarted Story - International Diagnostic Criteria: Critical and Discussion

By Dr. Stéphane Daens

A Story with Twists and Turns

Two dermatologists gave the name Ehlers-Danlos Syndrome (EDS). First, named Edvard Lauritz Ehlers (1863-1937), son of Copenhagen mayor, was well-known for his engagement in the fight against leprosy and syphilis. In front of the Danish Society of Dermatology and Syphiligraphy, he described on December 15, 1900, the case of a 21-year-old law student. That clinical case abundantly exhibited the EDS problem's complexity: skin alterations, proprioception disorders, and dysautonomia. He entitled his paper: *"Cutis laxa, internal bleeding skin predispositions, several joints loosening (diagnosis case)."* His patient's skin presented with a certain fragility, frequent hematomas, moderately stretchy, iterative joint dislocations, subluxations, and keratosis pilaris. Also, he observed suggestive signs of dysautonomia with a pseudo-Raynaud's syndrome and increased sweating. The same patient also walked in a way that can be considered ataxic and timid.

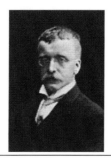

Edvard Lauritz EHLERS

43

This description of Edvard Ehlers[1] followed that of the Russian Alexandr Nicolaevich Chernogubow (or Tchernogobow)[2], who, in 1892, reported two cases to the Moscow Society of Dermatology and Venereology: a 17-year-old man and a 50-year-old woman. His descriptions turned out to be remarkly close to the description of Ehlers' case. In Russia, still today, EDS is called Chernogubow Syndrome.

In 1900, Malcolm Morris (1849-1924) presented a 14-year-old boy to the Old Dermatological Society of London: "*Loose skin with numerous cutaneous nodules*"; he had hyper-stretchy skin, hypermobile finger joints, and a tendency to bruise.

In 1907, Paul Cohn's turn was to report a case to the IXth Congress of the German Dermatological Societies[3].

Henri-Alexandre Danlos (1844-1912) was a French dermatologist and physicist. He was the first to introduce radium needles into skin cancers and lupus erythematosus, inspired by Marie Curie's work. In 1908, he described, with Lucien-Marie Pautrier (1876-1959), a "*Case of cutis laxa with tumors by chronic contusion of the elbows and knees*" to the French Society of Dermatology and Syphiligraphy of Paris[4]. These two authors reviewed the case presented previously, on May 3, 1906, by François Henri Hallopeau (1842-1919) and Macé de Lépinay: "*On a case of tuberous xanthoma with juvenile tumors offering the characteristics of diabetic xanthoma.*"

---

[1] Ehlers E. Cutis laxa, Neigung zu Haemorrhagien in der Haut, Lockerung mehrerer Artikulationen, Dermat. Ztschr. 1901;8:173-174.
[2] Chernogubow N. A. Über einen Fall von Cutis laxa. (Presentation at the first meeting of Moscow Dermatologic and Venerologic Society, Nov 13, 1891.) Monatshefte für praktische Dermatologie, Hamburg. 1892;14: 76.
[3] Cohn P. Demonstration eines Patienten mit Gummihaut (Cutis laxa) und eigentümlichen zirkumskripten Hautveränderungen, braunroten, eindrückbaren Erhebungen, Verhandl. Deutsch, dermat. Gesellsch. 1907;9:415-420
[4] Danlos A. Un cas de cutis laxa avec tumeurs par contusion chronique des coudes et des genoux (xanthome juvénile pseudo-diabétique de MM Hallopeau et Macé de Lépinay) Bull. Soc. Fr. Dermatol. Syphiligr. 1908;19,70-72.

H.-A. Danlos insisted, unfortunately, one could say at present, on two signs known today to be inconstant: *abnormal thinness* and *extraordinary elasticity* of the skin. Since then, these two characteristics have been misleading a good number of colleagues. Most doctors expect an impressive stretchability of the skin whereas, most often, it is only moderate, and sometimes even normal. By stubbornly seeking this skin elasticity, many patients with the disease are neglected. Moreover, it seems that the clinic and the histological data of the Danlos case are closer to a case of *pseudo-xanthoma elasticum*, a sporadic connective tissue disease but independent of EDS.

Achille Miget (1901-1934) reinforced the connection between Ehlers and Danlos during his medical thesis, defended in Paris in 1933[5]. Schulmann and Levy Coblentz had already mentioned this eponymous name earlier in 1932[6] to describe this *new disease*: the Ehlers-Danlos Syndrome. In 1936, it was supported by the English dermatologist Frederick Parkes Weber (1863-1962), who proposed the same name for a case he reported[7].

After being abandoned by Dermatology, Rheumatology (Rodney Grahame) and Genetics (Peter Beighton) took over the work of describing and classifying the disease. The classification of Ehlers-Danlos Syndrome was initially done in 11 subtypes (Berlin, 1988), then in six (Villefranche, 1997), and finally in 13 (New York Consortium, 2016). Recently, a fourteenth subtype seems to have been classified.

As a rheumatologist-internist, doing only EDS consultations, four subtypes are the most frequent:

♦ The hypermobile form (the old type III), in more than 95% of my patients.

---

[5] Miget A. *Le syndrome d'Ehlers-Danlos,* Thèse Médecine Paris, 1933.
[6] Schulmann E, Lévy-Coblentz G. Hyperélasticité cutanée (cutis laxa) et laxité articulaire avec fragilité anormale de la peau et tumeurs molluscoïdes post-traumatiques (syndrome de Danlos). Bull. Soc. Fr. Dermatol. Syphiligr. 1932;39,1252-1256.
[7] Weber FP. Ehlers-Danlos Syndrome. Proc R Soc Med. 1936 Nov;30(1):30-1.

- The classical form (the old types I and II), in less than 1% of my patients.
- The vascular form (the old type IV) in 1 to 2 cases per 1000 patients. This last variant is often described as frightening: it can cause repeated aneurysms and severe internal organ ruptures.
- I also meet in consultation some families of the kyphoscoliotic type (the old type VI B).

It is also necessary to consider potential mixed forms.

Clinical case:

I remember a young man, 15 years old, who suffered from articular pains and instabilities, myalgias, abdominal pains, frontal headaches, and intense fatigue with sleep disorders. He presents with irregular dentition and an ogival palate (high and narrow); his sclerae were bluish. The skin could be stretched over 3 cm at the neck and 4 cm at the forearm. Beighton's score was only 4 out of 9 due to musculotendinous contractures around the elbows and knees; these are common in this disease, especially in children and adolescents, thus distorting the expected higher score. The ankles, shoulders, and hips were also hypermobile, as were other fingers of the hands. The feet were typical of the Lelièvre type (false hollow foot), and there were piezogenic papules (small fatty herniation) on the heels and the feet's inner surfaces. There was discrete dorsal kyphoscoliosis and lumbar scoliosis.

Although dry in the lower limbs with a keratosis pilaris, the skin was soft and velvety in the trunk and upper limbs (in my practice, the skin is dry on the legs in more than 90% of cases). There were striae distensae (stretch marks) on the trunk, inner thighs, and roots of the arms. There were multiple atrophic scars, no papery scars. The most impressive was a dermographism with maculopapular, erythematous, and very itchy lesions, diffusely distributed over the trunk, shoulders, and root of the limbs superiors (Darier's sign). These lesions are experienced as intense burns. This sensation, as well as the redness, were worse after showering, with an urge to rest and lie down after. This is so common in EDS accompanied by Mast Cell Activation Disorder (MCAD) that Dr. Daniel Grossin and I called it "the sign of the shower".

Cardiopulmonary exams are commonplace, as well as cardiac transthoracic ultrasound, and CT scan of the thoracoabdominal aorta. Clinical signs and symptoms met the new international classification (2017) criteria for hypermobile-type EDS (hEDS). The patient's mother, as well as her sister and brothers, exhibited the same hEDS phenotype. His father had no complaints. Also, none of them met the 2010 criteria, revised in Ghent, for Marfan syndrome (neither the thumb sign of Steinberg, nor Walker's wrist sign, and the wingspan was less at 1.05 times its size).

The skin biopsy (photos below) confirmed, by transmission electron microscopy, compatibility with hEDS: collagen bundles, which include fibrils of different diameters, variable interfibrillar spaces, deposits of granulofilamentous material within the collagen bundles, fibrils in the shape of small flowers ("flower-like fibrils," arrows on the left photo) whose diameter is close to adjacent normal fibrils. The number of mast cells does not appear to be increased in this biopsy. There is also an moth-eaten aspect (arrow on the picture on the right) of elastic fibers, as found in Marfan syndrome.

Intrigued by this aspect of elastic fibers, a blood test was taken to find a mutation of fibrillin-1 (FBN-1), typical of Marfan disease. The same fibrillin-1 mutation was found in this young patient and his father (the c6778G>A variant, p.Glu2260Lys in the state heterozygous on exon 56 of FBN-1 gene). This mutation is not known, to this day, to give forms of Marfan. Maybe this is a discovery that does not give, a priori, anything significant clinically but which, on the other hand, causes ultrastructural changes to skin biopsy.

The boy was, therefore, a possible mixture, a patchwork of the two parents, at least genetically and histologically.

The severe skin lesions of this patient made us quickly think of a MCAD. Treatment with Levocetirizine (5 mg twice daily) combined with Ranitidine (300 mg daily) as well as Montelukast (10 mg per day) and vitamin C (1000 mg per day) was started. After two weeks, the patient saw almost all of the skin lesions, pruritus, and the sign of the shower disappear; thus, considerably improving his quality of life. He was able to resume classes and, finally, regain a social life.

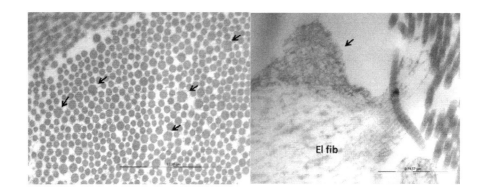

El fib

The Paris Criteria were presented in 2017 at the National Academy of Medicine in Paris[8]. They are based on a 62-item Somato-Sensory Clinical Scale (ECSS-62), rated from 0 to 4 on a Likert scale, and supported by the computerized statistical modeling tool. The authors were able to establish, for the first time, the probability of a diagnosis of hEDS against a control group consisting of patients from general medicine and occupational medicine. These will be detailed in Chapter IV.

The order of things and the classifications come to us first from Aristotle (384-322 B.C.) and, later, from botanists such as François Boissier de Sauvages de Lacroix (1706-1767). The latter will initiate the nosology of diseases based on the classification of plants and living beings.

Edvard Lauritz Ehlers was an excellent clinician who had already sensed the difficulty of labeling his syndrome would encounter. He wrote this remarkable sentence: *"Defining diseases based on their etiology is much more important than trying to label rare diseases, trying to classify."*

Ehlers-Danlos Syndrome (EDS) is the most common inherited connective tissue disorder. Its mode of transmission is believed to vary according to the subtypes, but for the most common form, known as hypermobile EDS (hEDS), there is no genetic test

---

[8] Hamonet C, Brock I, Pommeret S et al. Ehlers-Danlos Syndrome (EDS) type III (hypermobile): validation of a Somato-Sensory Clinical Scale (ECSS-62), concerning 626 cases. Bull Acad Natle Méd. 2017;201(2). Session of February 28, 2017).

available at present. The mutations would mainly be located on genes involved in the synthesis of collagens or the development of their three-dimensional shape. Human tissue contains at least 28 different collagens, and tissues often contain a mixture of several types.

The Collagens

They are structural proteins, glycoproteins. Their name comes from the Greek κολλα (colla): producer of glue. More than 4000 years ago, the Egyptians used them as a real glue to fix pieces of wood in cabinet making. Collagens, which account for a quarter of mammals' protein mass, are the most abundant animal kingdom proteins. They account for up to 80% of the weight of connective tissue. Collagens adopt a fibrillar form and are indispensable for our healing process.

Their fundamental element is tropocollagen, a glycoprotein 280 nanometers long by 1.5 nanometers in diameter. A glycoprotein is mainly composed of amino acids, but it also contains small attached sugars (galactose and glucose). The amino acids that make up collagen(s) are mainly glycines (for 33% of the total), but also prolines, 5-hydroxylysines, and 4-hydroxyprolines (for 25% of the total). Glycines are repeated throughout the molecule, and, quite singularly for a protein, glycine is repeated every three amino acids (Gly - X - Y). We often find the triplet Glycine - Proline - Hydroxyproline (Gly - Pro - Hyp). These repetitions are quite particular to collagens and are not generally found in other proteins in the human body. They are essential to understand where mutations in EDS reside.

Sugars (or carbohydrates) are always bound to hydroxylysines. The hydrogen bonds between the glycines and hydroxyprolines ensure the three alpha left helixes (denoted A) into a right superhelix. The tropocollagen thus resembles a scoubidou in which the three chains, respectively called alpha 1 (denoted A1), alpha 2 (denoted A2), and alpha 3 (denoted A3), intertwine.

In the food industry, cosmetics or photography, it is made into gelatin when the three strands of tropocollagens are hydrolyzed. Covalent bonds and hydrogen bridges, located between hydroxylysines and hydroxyprolines, are cut here, resulting in the separation of the three strands.

Less frequently, mutations in EDS affect glycosaminoglycans' synthesis, connective tissue molecules composed of a central protein and lateral sugar chains. Sometimes, mutations affect fibronectin, tenascin X, and more.

Prevalence of Ehlers-Danlos Syndrome

The mode of transmission of hEDS is reported in the literature as autosomal dominant, with variable penetrance (one in two children is affected by the disease if only one of the two parents is a carrier). I am not sure about this mode of transmission. I will explain this later in the chapter on genetics and epigenetics.

Unfortunately, many doctors still consider EDS as a rare disease (defined as less than 1 case in 2000) and an orphan disease (for which there is no known treatment). We will see later in this book that all these data are out of date and intellectually subject to controversies, not to say being inconceivable.

Girls and boys are equally carriers (male : female ratio is 1 : 1) but women are more frequently and more severely symptomatic than men. The cause of this gender disparity is still unknown. Perhaps, it involves the role of sex hormones and their circulating rate variations? A role of epigenetics? Is EDS a genetic disease with a parental imprint or a gendered genetic disease? (see further).

In our experience, more than 85% of patients who consult spontaneously are women in an age group between 35 and 45 years old. Before an EDS diagnosis, the wandering from doctor to doctor, looking for an answer, is mind-blowing. Shameless machismo, well concealed by many doctors, has the consequence that the mean diagnostic latency in women is more than twenty years; that is seven years more than for men, despite the latter being generally less symptomatic. So, in a collective (un-) conscience, women would be seen more as liars and hysterics. Let us not forget that the word hysterical comes from the Latin *Uterus*, which means the mother's womb. Patients with EDS are often not listened to or believed by some doctors, and they regularly hear themselves say, "This is in your head!" or "These are your hormones!" This kind of talk is devastating and can ultimately worsen the symptoms of the illness, both stress and distress of these patients are significant.

The prevalence of EDS would be related to hypermobility (or hyperlaxity) in a given population. There would be between 10 and 15% of hypermobile individuals in the Caucasian population, of which 10% could develop symptoms related to EDS throughout their lifetime, which represents 0.75 to 2% of the general population (*Hakim and Sahota, 2006*[9]; *Hamonet et al., 2015*[10]). Patients become symptomatic more or less quickly and more or less young; and the disease can only then begin to manifest itself in their third decade of age.

According to *Mulvey et al. (2013)*[11], in a study bringing together 12,853 participants, 3.4% of the population had joint hypermobility (JH) and evocative signs of hEDS. By projection, it would concern around 330,000 people in Belgium, one and a half million in France, two million in the United Kingdom, 10 million in the USA, 17 million in Europe, and 225 million people worldwide (*Tinkle et al., 2017*[12]). It is based on an equal prevalence in all ethnicities, which is unlikely to be the case. Based on this, EDS is a common disease![13] We must stop disinformation widely used by the medical profession.

---

[9] Hakim AJ, Sahota A. Joint hypermobility and skin elasticity: the hereditary disorders of connective tissue. Clin Dermatol. 2006;24:521-533.

[10] Hamonet C, Gompel A, Mazaltarine G, et al. Ehlers-Danlos syndrome or disease? J Syndrome. 2015;2:5.

[11] Mulvey MR, Macfarlane GJ, Beasley M, et al. Modest association of joint hypermobility with disabling and limiting musculoskeletal pain: results from a large-scale general population-based survey. Arthritis Care and Research. 2013;65(8):1325-1333. doi: 10.1002/acr.21979

[12] Tinkle B, Castori M, Berglund B, Cohen H, Grahame R, Kazkaz H, Levy H, 2017. Hypermobile Ehlers Danlos syndrome (a.k.a. Ehlers-Danlos syndrome type III and Ehlers-Danlos syndrome hypermobile Type): clinical description and natural history. Am J Med Genet Part C Semin Med Genet 9999C:1-22.

[13] Morris SL, O'Sullivan PB, Murray KJ, et al. Hypermobility and musculoskeletal pain in adolescents. J Pediatr. 2016;16:31044-31047

Therefore, the prevalence of EDS could be higher in other populations or other ethnicities in which hypermobility is more prevalent. In South Africa, Peter Beighton (1973) had already argued that the Melano-African population was laxer than the Indian population, and that the latter were laxer than the Caucasian population (the white Africans). In Latin America, up to 40% of the population show hyperlaxity and more than 5% EDS. In Chile, J.F. Bravo and C. Wolff[14] found a prevalence of joint hypermobility up to 39%. In Spain, 25% of patients consulting rheumatology are hyperlaxes (*Gumà M and Olivé A et al., 2001*)[15], and for Rodney Grahame[16][17] (the United Kingdom, 2009), up to 45% of patients referred in rheumatology met the Brighton criteria to be diagnosed as symptomatic hypermobile.

In hot countries, patients would suffer less joint pain, perhaps thanks to the favorable climate, but, on the other hand, the high temperature would cause more symptoms related to a disturbance of the autonomic nervous system: dizziness, cardiac arrhythmias, orthostatic hypotension, presyncope discomfort, fatigue, headache, memory and concentration disorders, and more.

There is often a trigger in this disease such as: parental violence, rape, physical or psychological trauma (separation, bereavement, the grief of love, and more), a road accident, a cerebral concussion, sudden hormonal variations (as in the first and last periods or after delivery). The trigger often occurs at a distance from the onset of clinical symptoms or their aggravation: a few days, a few weeks, or a few months later. The potential role of epigenetics and its placement after the trigger is

---

[14] Bravo J, Wolff C. Clinical study of hereditary disorders of connective tissues in a Chilean population. Joint hypermobility syndrome and vascular Ehlers-Danlos Syndrome. Arthritis Rheum. 2006;54:515-523.
[15] Gumà M, Olivé A, Holgado S et al. Una estimacion de la laxitud en la consulta externa. Rev Esp Reumatol. 2001;28 :298-300.
[16] Grahame R. Joint hypermobility syndrome pain. Curr Pain Headache Rep. 2009;13(6):427-433. Review.
[17] Hakim A, Grahame R. Joint hypermobility. Best Pract Res Clin Rheumatol. 2003;17:989-1004.

interesting here and will be developed later in the chapter dedicated to genetics and epigenetics.

The alterations associated with EDS also affect the connective tissue of the skin and fascia, muscles and tendons, ligaments, intervertebral discs, and various menisci, mucous membranes in the broad sense, support internal organs' structures, sense organs and the wall of blood vessels.

The brain and nerves are most often spared, except in central sensitization of Pain, or in specific MRI manifestations (see below). It is an important notion when we meet a multitude of patients to whom, for decades sometimes, it has been repeated: *"Everything you tell me, it is in your head! "*.

EDS is a peripheral disease, not a central disease that initially affects the brain. Usually, anything can be achieved in the EDS except the brain. He is a good brain, maybe even better, but tired.

The brain is tired, yes, but it responds well to data that it receives. The brain must process more peripheral information due to hypersensoriality and dysproprioception (the afferent messages). These afferents are often wrong or approximate. Indeed, the particular fragility of fabrics, which include and hold the sensors in place, often results in inappropriate stimulation. In the corollary, the brain responds to the side of the plate (efferent messages), while the sensors and the nerve pathways are perfectly normal.

It is an entirely different conception, not only for doctors but also for patients who finally tell us: *"I knew I was not crazy, doctor."*

Personal Reviews of the New York Criteria

Warning: I have applied, and still apply, carefully, the New York Criteria since March 2017, the month of release of said criteria in the *American Journal of Medical Genetics*. Apply them does not mean that we are not entitled to criticize and bring personal light to it, based on experience, to improve and refine these criteria. It is a right and even a duty as a doctor. I, therefore, offer you grounds for reflection.

The criteria for hypermobile EDS are described in the article by *Malfait F, Francomano C, Byers P et al.* entitled: *"The international classification of the Ehlers-Danlos syndromes." Am J Med Genet, part C: Semin Med Genet, 2017;175C:8-26, pages 16 to 19.*

I will discuss, here, only the part of the article on the so-called *Hypermobile EDS*, because I consider this form as the basis of the *Global Vision of EDS*, as I will explain later in my first postulate (see the second part of this book).

I called this basic form the *Common Systemic form* or *csEDS*.

In this first postulate, I consider that most of the other forms of EDS described in this same article are specific variants of the Common Systemic form by adding one or more mutations, possibly known, to its unknown genotype.

csEDS is an intuitively *Polygenic Disease* and, after all, related to a *Complex Genetic Disease*.

Therefore, these *additional mutations* could bring out *a particular phenotype* that can potentially be in the foreground, induce visceral or arterial complications, and require special care. These particular genome mutations (which is the set of genes in DNA) would therefore affect the final phenotype (i.e. the patient, the final product) depending on whether they affect collagens present more particularly in the wall of arterial vessels (such as COL3A1 in the vascular variant or vEDS), in supporting tissues and skin (such as COL5 A1 & COL5 A2 in the classical variant, or cEDS) or other molecules, such as glycosaminoglycans, in the so-called spondylodysplastic variants or spEDS (via mutations in β-galactosyltransferases).

Reviews of Part I of the New York Criteria (hEDS)

Part I of the New York Criteria is based on the score of Beighton and joint hypermobility.

Professor Peter Beighton is a South African internist and clinical geneticist of British origin, born in 1934 in Lancashire, England. He had a brilliant academic career at the University of Cape

Town and had many awards for his work. His research was largely on inherited disorders of the skeleton and connective disorders. He established, among other things, an articular hypermobility scale done in a nine-point scoring system. This became the second classification of EDS, from his observation of 100 patients, in 5 distinct forms: gravis, mitis, hypermobile, ecchymotic, and the X-linked syndrome.

The Beighton's score assesses the *joint hypermobility* of a patient. It was described in a well-known article: *P. Beighton, L. Solomon, C.L. Soskolne. Articular mobility in an African population. Ann Rheum Dis. 1973;32:413-418.* In his article, Peter Beighton (and his colleagues) assessed articular hypermobility in a population of 1,081 subjects of all ages, belonging to the Tswana village of Phokeng, located at the foot of Magaliesburg Mountains in the western Transvaal, about 97 km from Johannesburg. Hypermobility was assessed in nine points.

The joints targeted by this score are as follows:

➢ Elbows at more than 10° extension: 2 points - One point per arm.
➢ The knees at more than 10° recurvatum: 2 points - One point per leg.
➢ The possibility of touching the forearm with the thumbs in front: 2 points - One point per thumb.
➢ The extension of the fifth finger of the hands at least 90°: 2 points - One point per hand.
➢ The possibility of touching the ground (while standing, legs extended) with both hands flat: 1 point.

Peter Beighton also assessed the influence of age, gender, joint complaints (arthralgia), and somatotype[18] on hypermobility.

---

[18] By evaluating the correlation between joint mobility, weight index (height in inches divided by the square root of the weight in pounds), and the second metacarpal length.

Photos from P. Beighton et al.'s article

(Ann Rheum Dis. 1973;32:413-418)

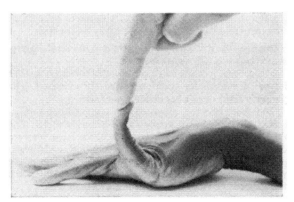

FIG. 1   *Hyperextension of the fifth finger. In this particular illustration, the extension angle does not reach the required 90°*

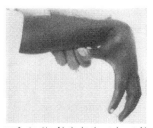

FIG. 2   *Apposition of the thumb to the ventral aspect of the forearm*

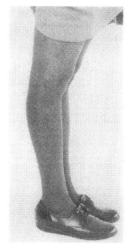

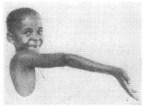

FIG. 3   *Hyperextension of the elbow joint beyond 10°*

FIG. 4   *Hyperextension of the knee joint beyond 10°*

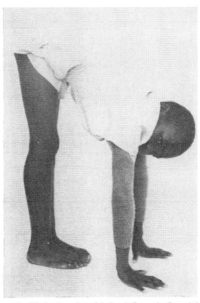

FIG. 5 *Placing the palms of the hands flat on the floor while maintaining the knees in full extension*

The Findings of P. Beighton et al.

➢ Women are more hypermobile than men. Beighton also points out in his text that these data support the data from the *Ellis and Bundick (1956)*[19] study of *American Negroes* (see my parenthesis below).

➢ Joint mobility decreases with age, rapidly in childhood and more slowly in adulthood.

➢ Passive hyperextension of the 5th finger is closely related to an individual's overall hypermobility, regardless of age and sex.

➢ Joint mobility decreased on the dominant side (joints are less mobile on the right side in right-handed people and on the left side in left-handed people).

➢ Joint complaints are positively correlated with joint hyperlaxity. The joint complaints were assessed according to a brief questionnaire and probably altered by the language barrier:

---

[19] Ellis FE, Bundick WR. Cutaneous elasticity and hyperelasticity. AMA Arch Derm. 1956;74(1):22-32.

    o   *Any pains in the hands or feet?*
    o   *Any other joint pains?*
    o   *Any backache?*
    o   *Any other pains in the limbs?*

➢ Tall, thin subjects tended to be more loose-jointed than those with a short, stocky physique.

Parenthesis regarding hearsay:

Some say this score is racist or that P. Beighton's article was imbued with the Apartheid regime in South Africa.

I wanted to know more about these allegations.

Regarding the population used in *Beighton et al.*, the population chosen was Melano-African and from a rural village. On the one hand, they could rightly be criticized for not having compared White African subjects in the same study. On the other hand, why were the terms *negro* or *relatively sophisticated* population used to refer to these Melano-African subjects? These are thorny, disturbing questions that some colleagues advised against using in this book, saying they should be avoided. Others encouraged me to do so. I decided to talk about it, even if it meant being castigated. However, I have tried to weigh the pros and cons. Medicine is reading, studying, learning, listening, knowing, reflecting, criticizing, questioning, and proposing new avenues (sometimes by challenging preconceived ideas and established dogmas).

Can one be shocked and rebel against certain writings in which women and men are referred to as *negroes* in a segregationist political regime? At that time, and in this country in particular, was it customary to do so? Was it the rule established and imposed by a political regime and local culture?

Arguments for these allegations:

The article states: "*The population, although living in a rural environment, were relatively sophisticated and readily cooperated in the investigation.*"

It is legitimate to ask why the term *relatively sophisticated* was used? Were the others *savages*? Furthermore, why were they so *easily cooperative* (secondary benefits, methods of persuasion)?

On several occasions in this article, the pejorative term *negro* has been used to describe this Melano-African population during the Apartheid period:

- "*For instance, Negroes and Indians have been shown to have a greater range of movements than Caucasians of the same age and sex (Harris and Joseph, 1949[20]).*"

- And further on, he differentiates between Indigenous and White South Africans: "*Similarly, in an investigation in Cape Town, Indians were found to be more loose-jointed than indigenous Xhosa et Hlubi, who in turn had a greater degree of joint laxity than white South African (Schweitzer, 1970).*"

A quick search on the *PubMed medical bibliography* site, for the years 1974 and after, will find titles of articles such as:

- *George PM, Ebanks GE, Nobbe CE. Role perception and performance of lower class black men and women of Barbados and their contraceptive behavior. Soc Cult. 1974;5(2):161-176.*

- *Pompe van Meerdervoort HF. Congenital dislocation of the hip in black patients. S Afr Med J. 1974;48(59):2436-2440.*

- *Myers BW, Cheatum DE. Ankylosing spondylitis in a black women. Association with HL-A W-27. JAMA. 1975;20;231(3):278-279.*

- *Pompe van Meerdervoort HF. Congenital musculoskeletal malformation in South African Blacks: a study of incidence. S Afr Med J. 1976;50(46):1853-1855.*

However, Peter Beighton had written some articles that mention the term *negro*, and those can be found on the same pages online:

- *Beighton P, Solomon L, Soskolne CL et al. Serum uric acid concentrations in a urbanized South African Negro population. Ann Rheum Dis. 1974;33(5):442-445.*

- *Beighton P, Solomon L, Valkenburg HA. Rheumatoid arthritis in a rural South African Negro population. Ann Rheum Dis. 1975;34(2):136-141.*

---

[20] Harris H, Joseph J. Variation in extension of the metacarpophalangeal and interphalangeal joint of the thumb. J Bone Joint Surg Br. 1949;31B(4):547-59, illust.

- *Solomon L, Beighton P, Lawrence JS. Rheumatic disorders in the South African Negro. Part II. Osteo-arthrosis. S Afr Med J. 1975;49(42):1737-1740.*

- *Solomon L, Beighton P, Lawrence JS. Osteoarthrosis in rural South African Negro population. Ann Rheum Dis. 1976;35(3):274-278.*

- And even later in 1984: *Viljoen DL, Beighton P. The split-hand and split-foot anomaly in a central African Negro population. Am J Med Genet. 1984;19(3):545-552.*

I have a lot of respect for the doctor and the scientist Peter Beighton. He wrote many articles on high-quality scientists.

Most of my peers say that negro was a term not pejorative for the time or a synonym of black people, although it was also a time of claiming *Negro art*. Nevertheless, we can only note that most authors used the term black people simultaneously.

Apartheid (a word derived from Afrikaans, meaning separation or set aside) was abolished on June 30, 1991. It was a policy known as *separate development*, affecting populations according to racial or ethnic criteria, in specific geographic areas. It was established in 1948, in South Africa, by the National Party.

In 1973, when the article was released, it had been ten years since J.F. Kennedy had been assassinated (Dallas, November 22, 1963). President Frederik de Klerk was elected in August 1989. The future President Nelson Mandela was released from prison on February 11, 1990 (after 27 years of abusive imprisonment).

Argument against these allegations:

In 2014/2015, Professor Peter Beighton was nominated, at the age of 80, for the *NSTF-BHP Billiton Awards*. This price rewards contribution to Science, Engineering, Technology and Innovation in South Africa. In this article, we talk about the significant involvement of Peter Beighton to help and supervise young scientists from *disadvantaged communities*.

Conclusion:

I think that the politics of the years 1960-1980 in South Africa pushed for segregation and that the term negro was, unfortunately, used. It is more of a particular ethological context at a particular time than a deliberate act of racism by Peter Beighton and his co-authors. However, being a scientist, he could have chosen case and control groups' scientific wording, and not fall into the common or popular use of derogative wording stigmatizing a chosen group of people. One odd observation that deserves to be questioned, is whether a selection bias was committed by choosing a specific group of people. In my opinion, further study on the evaluation of the hypermobility score including more joints, needs to be done.

End of the parenthesis.

In response to this study by *Beighton et al. (1973)*, Professor Rodney Grahame replied that he had tested mobility with 295 children in London[21]. He confirmed that the evaluation of the 5th finger (little finger) was an important part, but the other joint tests offered were not sensitive enough in his sample. Grahame found no difference between women and men, nor between right-handed and left-handed people.

My criticisms of the Beighton's score itself:

➤ Oddly, this score does not include large joints of the human body, such as shoulders, hips, ankles, kneecaps, and more. However, it is precisely these last joints that patients complain about the most often.

➤ One may wonder why Beighton did not explore a population of white Africans in Cape Town or Johannesburg rather than a Melano-African population from a village at the foot of the mountains. Was it simpler and easier to use (both literally and figuratively) an indigenous population?

➤ The location of the selected joints is more than strange for a rheumatologist, even if, in a previous article, *Cedric Carter and John Wilkinson (1964)* [22] had already used some: fingers' hyperextension of the hands, the thumbs on the wrists,

---

[21] Silverman S, Constine L, Harvey W et al. Survey of joint mobility and in vivo skin elasticity in London schoolchildren. Ann Rheum Dis. 1975;34:177.
[22] Carter C, Wilkinson J. Persistent joint laxity and congenital dislocation of the hip. Journal of Bone and Joint Surgery. 1964;46B(1):40-45.

hyperextension of the elbows, knees recurvatum and hyperflexion of the dorsal feet.

➢ As a rheumatologist and familiar with EDS, the score of Beighton appears to be imperfect in practice:

♦ There are four points out of nine which concern the hands, where osteoarthritis and successive trauma, as well as possible musculotendinous retractions, can impair mobility (what was already mentioned before: *Ridge and Wright in 1966*[23]; *Schweitzer et al. in 1970*[24,25]).

♦ There are two points on the knees, which can also disappear in the event of trauma (skiing, football, and more), surgery, muscle contractures, excessive flexor retractions (especially in children).

♦ It is the same at the elbows, where we meet regularly hyperalgesic tendonitis limiting the movements and sometimes even young patients in flessum because of the retractions.

♦ Back pain, frequent in this disease, and lower limb flexor retractions limit potentially the last point. Many patients have unfortunately benefited from a lumbar arthrodesis, which decreases the movements of the spine.

Another important message in EDS :

• There is often retraction of the flexor muscles at the upper and lower limbs, but not of the extensor muscles. As proof, we can put the patient in the prone position and easily apply the heels to his buttocks.

[23] Ridge MD, Wright V. Rheological analysis of connective tissue. A bio-engineering analysis of the skin. Ann Rheum Dis. 1966;25(6):509-15.
[24] Schweitzer G. Laxity of metacarpophalangeal joints of fingers and interphalangeal joint of the thumb: a comparative inter-racial study. S Afr Med J. 1970;44(9):246-9.
[25] Schweitzer G, Sophangisa E. Contracture of proximal interphalangeal joints of the fingers associated with pes valgus. S Afr Med J. 1970;44(13):389-91.

- Children and men are the most affected by these retractions contributing to the Beighton's score being *abnormally or falsely* lower than in women.

Pictures from Carter et Wilkinson's article (1964)

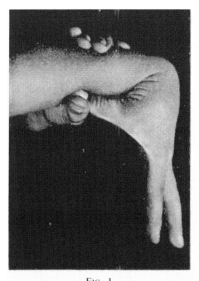 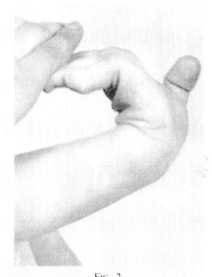

FIG. 1   FIG. 2

Figure 1—Passive apposition of the thumb to the flexor aspect of the forearm. Figure 2—Passive hyperextension of the fingers so that they lie parallel with the extensor aspect of the forearm.

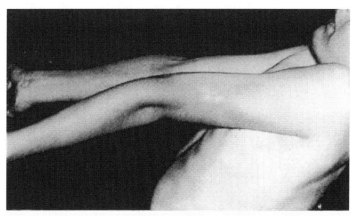

FIG. 3
Hyperextension of the elbow.

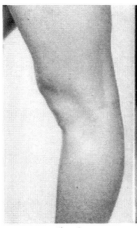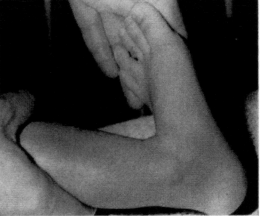

FIG. 4
Hyperextension of the knee.

FIG. 5
Increased dorsiflexion of the ankle and eversion of the foot.

According to the New York International Criteria (2017):

➢ Between puberty and the age of 50, Beighton's score must be equal to or greater than 5/9.

➢ For pre-pubertal age, Beighton's score must be equal to or greater than 6/9.

➢ After age 50, it is sufficient at 4/9.

If one point of Beighton's score is missing, one point can be added to the score obtained if one obtains at least 2 points from Professor Rodney Grahame's 5-part Historical Questionnaire (5pHQ).

See: *Hakim AJ, Grahame R. A simple questionnaire to detect hypermobility: an adjunct to the assessment of patients with diffuse musculoskeletal pain. Int J Clin Pract. 2003;57(3):163-166.*

N.B.: Analysis demonstrated that a positive answer to any two question in the five-part questionnaire gave the highest combined sensitivity (84%) and specificity (80%) for detecting hypermobility.

5-Part Historical Questionnaire

> ➢ Were you able to put your hands flat on the floor without bending your knees?
>
> ➢ Were you able to bend your thumbs to touch your forearms?
>
> ➢ As a child, did you entertain your friends by twisting your body in strange positions or could you do the splits?
>
> ➢ As a child or teenager, did your shoulder or knee dislocate more than once?
>
> ➢ Do you consider yourself to be disarticulated with hyperlaxity joints?

In the same article by *Malfait et al. (2017)*, it is also stated that one point could be added if the patient's other joints, not included in the Beighton's score, are hypermobile:

"For patients with lower Beighton scores, the assessment of other joints is often considered, including temporo-mandibular joint, shoulder, hip, foot, wrist, ankle, and other digits. Increased ankle and wrist dorsiflexion, increased internal and external hip rotation, and pes planus have been correlated with Beighton's score (Smits-Engelsman B et al., 2011)".

And,

"Therefore, like any clinical tool, there is some subjectivity and this is a guideline not to replace the judgement of the experienced clinician".

In my opinion, it is essential to test the other joints not included in the Beighton's score, not only if the score is too low.

The regular and pathological angles are strangely not noted there, I quote them to you (the acceptable upper limit): the ankles (pro-supination 15°/35°), the big toes (max 90° of extension, in the Bulbena's score), the hips (lower limbs in extension) in internal rotation (max 35°) and external rotation (max 45°), the hips (thighs and legs flexed) in internal rotation (max 45°) and external rotation (max 60°), the shoulders in abduction (max 85°; Cypel test: the sensitivity and specificity of the test, at an amplitude of more than 90°, are respectively 92.5% and 96.4%[26]) and in external rotation (max 85°). The other fingers require attention: metacarpophalangeal (maximum 70° of extension), the presence of an angle in extension at the proximal interphalangeal joints (this angle is ordinarily non-existent, i.e. 0°) and the distal interphalangeal joints (maximum 30° of extension).

Delbarre Grossemy I. Goniométrie. Manuel d'évaluation des amplitudes articulaires des membres et du rachis. Éditions Elsevier Masson SAS, 2008. ISBN : 978-2-294-02162-6.

Cleland J, Koppenhaver S. Examen clinique de l'appareil locomoteur. Éditions Elsevier Masson SAS, 2007 & 2012. ISBN : 978-2-294-71427-6.

I also consider the frequent subluxations of the ulnar styloid that form a protuberance on the dorsal and internal face of the wrists (the *Hamonet's sign*), the anterior flexion of the wrists (maximum 90°), and the flatfeet (in practice, these are often *hollow and sometimes false Lelièvre's flatfeet*).

To appreciate the shoulder's abduction, I modified the Cypel test, practiced with the patient seated and the doctor standing next to him. Since I am almost 190 cm tall, patients are generally smaller than me, and my back does not resist to this passive shoulder abduction maneuver, according to Cypel. So, I decided to establish a *modified Cypel test* where the patient lies on his back; I stand behind him and block the scapula's movement with one of my two hands. On the other hand, I hold the patient's elbow and perform passive abduction of the glenohumeral joint. If the angle exceeds 95°, I consider the shoulder to be hypermobile (in fact, the joint is subluxated). Theoretically, the head of the humerus hits the scapula, then the latter moves to perform the rest of the movement. In this case, the head of the humerus, surrounded by a joint capsule and tendinous ligament structures which are too loose, subluxates and goes beyond the edges of the glenoid cavity of the scapula.

According to the article, this is also an overall assessment according to *the clinician's experience*, an experience that is not

---

[26] Cypel D. Gleno-humeral abduction measurement in patients with Ehlers-Danlos syndrome. Orthop Traumatol Surg Res. 2019;105(2):287-290.

defined in the article. From my perspective, a doctor with personally diagnosed and followed up at least 100 to 200 patients with EDS has this experience.

I always use an inclinometer for questionable angles rather than a standard goniometer, which is imprecise and, to my sense, full of subjectivity. It is necessary to press well the inclinometer on the bone surface, on both sides of the joint. There may indeed be measurement errors if soft tissues are more important, for example, in overweight or edema. Keep in mind that this is the angle formed by the bone segments, located on both sides of the joint, which matters. So, this is not the angle formed by these two segments' skin surfaces! It is not a detail, and it is essential to differentiate.

The patient should also be carefully questioned about the history of joint dislocations and subluxations (shoulders, hips, elbows, fingers, kneecaps, temporomandibular, and more) as well as repeated sprains, which are a sign of hyperlaxity and dysproprioception.

Quite common joint crunches are considered as iterative articular subluxations: we can imagine that when a joint is in motion and that the proprioceptive messages of the joint capsules do not arrive with sufficient relevance and speed to the central nervous system, the latter does not adjust the joint positions in real-time; this misalignment causes these crackles. It should be added that the tendons and ligaments, being to loose, do not allow an adjustment that is sufficiently stable and precise.

The test of *Prayer on the back* is also very indicative of the hypermobility of the upper limbs.

The *sign of heels applied to the buttocks* in the prone position is a sign of hyperlaxity and proves that flexors are sometimes retracted, contrary to limbs' extensors. It makes us grasp the very important, and yet often neglected, notion, that hyperlaxity, linked to connective tissue modifications, can induce hypermobility, but not necessarily. It is an essential element which too often misleads physicians in the diagnostic approach of EDS.

HYPERMOBILITY IS NOT ESSENTIAL, BUT HYPERLAXITY IS!

"All truth goes through three stages:
At first she is ridiculed,
Then she is fiercely fought,
Finally, it is accepted as evidence. "
Arthur Schopenhauer
German Philosopher (1788-1860)

"What gets us into trouble
Is not what we don't know.
It is what we know for sure
That just ain't so."
Mark Twain (1835-1910)

Some Pictures (private collection)

Successively: completely bend the metacarpophalangeal joints on palm, shoulder blade detachment (scapula alata with instability shoulders), heel test on the buttocks (the extensor muscles are not retracted), 90° extension of all fingers, index finger 5-year-old girl (extension over 135°) while her fifth finger is retracted.

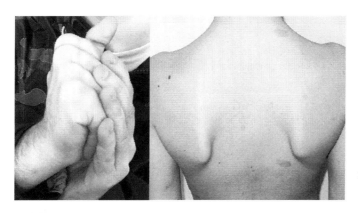

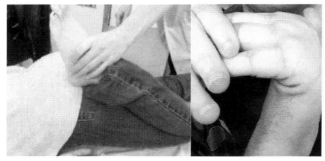

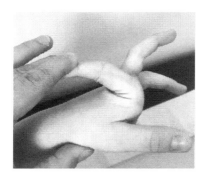

Diagnostic Criteria for EDS Hypermobile (hEDS)

Criterion I: Beighton's score

	Right	Left
Extension of the 5th finger at 90°		
Apposition of the thumb on the forearm		
Elbow recurvatum > 10°		
Recurvatum of the knee > 10°		
Palms of hands touching the ground		

Total : ☐

Joint hypermobility is approved according to the following score thresholds:

- ➤ For children and prepubescents: at least 6/9
- ➤ For 12-50-year-olds: at least 5/9
- ➤ For those over 50:   at least 4/9

If the score is one point lower in adults, the 5pHQ questionnaire must be positive, i.e. have at least 2 positive responses out of 5:

1) Can you or have you been able to put your hands flat on the floor without bending your knees?   ☐
2) Can you or have you been able to bend your thumb to touch your forearm?   ☐
3) As a child, did you entertain your friends by contorting your body in strange positions, or could do the splits?   ☐
4) Child or teenager, your shoulder or knee have they dislocated more than once?   ☐
5) You consider yourself to be disarticulated with hyperlaxity joints?   ☐

Total : ☐

If Beighton's score is one point lower, it is recommendable that other joints be considered: TMJ, shoulders, hips, flat feet, wrists, ankles, other fingers of the hand.

Is Criterion I validated?   YES   NO

Criterion II: General Clinic and History

Must be validated:

A+B or A+C or B+C or A+B+C (all 3, if autoimmune disease)

A – Clinical signs: at least 5/12

1- Unusually soft and velvety skin ☐

2- Moderate skin extensibility (between 1.5 and 2.5 centimeters on the palmar surface of the non-dominant forearm) ☐

3- Atrophic or reddish streaks, stretch marks (only man, child, and nulliparous woman) ☐

4- Piezogenic papules in both heels ☐

5- Recurrent or multiple hernias (inguinal, crural, umbilical, hiatal) ☐

6- Atrophic scar (at least 2 sites) (without hemosiderin or papyraceous - cEDS) ☐

7- Pelvic, rectal or uterine prolapse, with no major medical history (men, children, and women-only nulliparous woman) ☐

8- Irregular dentition and high or narrow palate ☐

9- Arachnodactyly (Walker's wrist sign on both sides or Steinberg's thumb sign on both sides) ☐

10- Arms span to body height ratio of > 1.05 ☐

11- Mitral prolapse ☐

12- Dilation of the aortic root with a Z score
greater than 2 ☐

Total : ☐

Is Criterion II-A validated?   YES   NO

B - Family history of hEDS in the first degree

At least one or more (father, mother, child, brother, sister)

Is Criterion II-B validated?   YES   NO

C - Musculoskeletal (at least 1 in 3)

1- Musculoskeletal Pain in at least two limbs, every day
for over three months. ☐

2- Diffuse Pain for more than three months. ☐

3- Luxations or joint instability (without trauma): at least
1 point out of 2:

° At least three dislocations of the same joint or at
least two dislocations for two different joints. ☐

° Instability of at least two sites without trauma
previously. ☐

Total : ☐

Is Criterion II-C validated?   YES   NO

Criterion III, exclusion criteria (3/3)

Tick the box if the given exclusion criterion is missing:

1- Highly extensible skin (cEDS-type). ☐

2- Other acquired or hereditary connective tissue disease, ☐
autoimmune.

3- Other genetic abnormality of connective tissue, ☐
chondrodysplasias.

Total : ☐

Is Criterion III validated?   YES   NO

Final Outcome

Choose the validated criteria

Criterion I   ☐   with a Beighton's score of: /9
Criterion II – A ☐   Criterion II – B ☐   Criterion II – C ☐
Criterion III   ☐

Diagnosis of hEDS: YES   NO

Diagnosis of HSD: YES   NO

Possible clinical observations:

Signature: Doctor's stamp:

Reviews of Part II of the New York Criteria (hEDS)
(general clinic and history)

Part II of the New York Criteria of hEDS (= csEDS, see further) is primarily concerned with the patient's clinic. It is divided into three subsections: A, B, and C.

For Part II to be completed, at least two of the three subparts must be validated (i.e., A+B, A+C, B+C, or A+B+C).

The first subpart, labeled "A," is itself divided into 12 items. At least 5 out of 12 items (see table) are required to validate this criterion IIA. It should be noted that the clinical criteria were developed WITHOUT a control group of healthy subjects (i.e., non-EDS).

The large difference in severity or clinical relevance between the 12 items is immediately noticeable:

How can piezogenic foot papules and mitral valve prolapse, or aortic artery dilatation, be put on the same level (1 point)?

Piezogenic papules are fatty hernias located at the heels and inside the foot, resulting from subcutaneous fat protrusion through gaps in the connective tissue. Histologically, there is compact hyperkeratosis, with encapsulated fat nodules protruding into the dermis. The subcutaneous adipose tissue shows a loss of compartmentalization, linked to the thinning of the connective tissue's trabeculae[27].

Before my orientation to EDS patients management I never considered that these papules would be useful for anything in my entire career as a physician. They are almost always asymptomatic (over 95% of the time). Moreover, in a standing position, 60% of the general population can be carriers of these piezogenic papules. Therefore, it is necessary to test more for their presence, patient lying on his back (dorsal decubitus), by pressing very moderately on the heel and the plantar face of the inner arch of the foot with the base of your palm. It is good

---

[27] D. Ma, S. Vano-Galvan. CMAJ 2013. doi:10,1503/cmaj.121963.

practice, but it does not seem to be specified in *Malfait et al.'s (2017)* article.

However, you will agree that mitral valve prolapse and dilatation of the aortic artery are critical clinical information and potential sources of complications. However, these criteria are only worth one point out of twelve, as are piezogenic papules.

Another example is the soft and velvety skin item. In my clinical experience, the skin on the legs is almost always dry (>90% of cases) as is the skin on the limbs' roots. On the other hand, the upper chest and neck skin can be paradoxically very soft and velvety. Therefore, validation of this item depends on whether the examiner touches the skin of the legs or chest.

I always touch the legs, the belly's skin, the skin of the chest, and the neck's skin in succession. I often tell patients, "*When you buy a bath or shower product for dry skin, it is for the whole body, not just the legs.*" That is what is unusual in EDS, and it is probably the result of leg dyshidrosis (a disorder of the autonomic nervous system) and keratosis pilaris.

Of course, patients who come to the clinic do not complain of soft, velvety skin, nor do they complain of piezogenic papules, for that matter. Suppose one is content to establish these criteria in consultation. In that case, the patient will, legitimately, not understand why the doctor is not interested in his or her main complaints (fatigue, Pain, dysautonomia, dysproprioception, dyssensoriality, and more).

As for the two marfanoid criteria (wingspan/height > 1.05, presence of Walker's or Steinberg's signs), they are, in my opinion, not relevant here. Why insert criteria from another connective tissue disease (Marfan's disease, caused by a fibrillin 1 gene mutation) that could induce diagnostic doubts? They might as well be included in the exclusion criteria. Experience has shown that marfanoid signs are not very common in EDS.

For skin stretchability, I test it in 7 different places:

➢ The dorsal side of the forefoot.

- ➢ The dorsal face of the kneecaps.
- ➢ The dorsal face of the hands (this is the Grahame's sign).
- ➢ The non-dominant forearm.
- ➢ The surface of the clavicles.
- ➢ At the neck.
- ➢ On the cheeks (the jowl sign).

If the patient is overweight or has localized lymphedema, the results will be distorted. The same applies to hypothyroidism (myxedema), for example. I, therefore, prefer a global and multi-site evaluation.

In conclusion, these items are imperfect (criterion IIA), unequal in their clinical importance and their management implications. Furthermore, frankly, it does not stick with what patients complain about.

It would have been more beneficial to replace some of these items by:

1. **Severe chronic fatigue**: this is a significant symptom for patients who feel drained of energy, powerless and exhausted. It is often confused with the Chronic Fatigue Syndrome (CFS).

2. **Proprioception disorders**: clumsiness, repeated falls, and sprains, which are not just the result of ligament and tendon hyperlaxity.

3. **Symptoms of dysautonomia**: palpitations, Raynaud's pseudo-syndrome*, chilliness, sweating upper body, unexplained fever, syncopal discomfort, headache, fatigue, concentration and memory problems, and more.

4. **The hemorrhagic diathesis**: bruising, bleeding gums when brushing, heavy periods, haematuria, a *tablecloth* digestive bleeding, and intraoperative hemorrhage.

5. **Dystonia**: muscle cramps, fasciculations, myoclonia or even chorea, choreoathetosis or hemiballism.

(*) *Raynaud's disease is idiopathic, that is to say, without an identified cause. Raynaud's syndrome is usually associated with autoimmune disease (scleroderma, lupus erythematosus, rheumatoid arthritis, and more). This coldness of the extremities, even the buttocks, of the kneecaps or the belly, often with segmental localization, is one of the consequences of dysautonomia related to EDS. Therefore, it is not part, de facto, of Raynaud's disease or Raynaud's syndrome, strictly speaking. From where the term used, in the EDS, of pseudo-Raynaud's syndrome.*

These criteria and this 2017 classification have been brought to the practitioners and published as intermediaries, for lack of better. They were to be changed at the September congress 2018, in Ghent, Belgium, but they were not.

Moreover, why a patient association (which organized the holding of this consortium) and some patients were named co-authors of a medical article that aims to establish the criteria for diagnosing a disease? It is relatively new and perhaps an interference, or even an additional bias to this classification. Several doctors, EDS specialists, consider this to be debatable. You cannot be judge and party at the same time in your cause. This admirable phrase from Latin should enlighten us: "*Aliquis non debet esse judex in propria causa, quia non potest esse judex et pars*" (No one should be a judge of his cause, because one cannot be judge and party).

Finally, another problem, and not the least, lies in the fact that doctors, who examine the most significant number of patients with EDS have been consulted very little, or listened to. We have monitored several thousand patients at GERSED Belgium and France, but we were not interviewed on this new classification, even a posteriori. I do not know all the ins and outs of this case, but expert practitioners should have been consulted.

Let us note an article published in 2019 by Canadian colleagues from Montreal. They carried out a study on the quality or precision of the New York Criteria. Indeed, they were amazed that many very symptomatic patients for hEDS did not meet the new criteria and were left without diagnostic. After a study of 231 patients, they concluded these criteria should be reviewed:

"Based on our cohort, the 2017 hEDS diagnostic criteria require refinement to improve its diagnostic accuracy".

Référence: *McGillis L, Mittal N, Santa Mina D et al. Am J Med Genet A. 2019, first published 16 December 2019.*

This article was also published in 2021 by British Colleagues about Beighton's score: *Malek S, Reinhold EJ, Pearce GS. The Beighton score as a measure of generalized joint hypermobility. Rheumatology International. doi.org/10.1007/s00296-021-04832-4.*

See also: *Aubry-Rozier B, Schwitzguebel A, Valerio F, et al. Are patients with hypermobile Ehlers-Danlos syndrome or hypermobility spectrum disorder so different? Rheumatol Int. 2021;41(10):1785-1794.*

Keratosis Pilaris

Keratosis pilaris is an inherited disease, often of unknown origin, caused by obstruction of hair follicles by keratin. It results in dry skin and lumps (somewhat reminiscent of the appearance of *goose bumps*). It is located, most often, in the buttocks and on the posterior surface of the arms and thighs, more rarely on the face. It appears as little pimples with a pinhead size, flesh-colored or red on white skin, and brown on black skin (sometimes there are white dots at the top of the lesions). It disappears, theoretically often in adults, which is not at all case in EDS patients. In my practice, over 90% of EDS patients have keratosis pilaris.

Tips: As a treatment, I recommend lotions containing urea (concentration: 10% for the body and 5% for the face), which attracts water and keeps moisture in the skin. Urea has a keratolytic effect. Use lotions without perfume or dye, as there are more allergies in EDS. Coconut oil can be used, which is very moisturizing, or a cream that contains the 3rd generation of retinoids. Treatment *per os*[28] has more side effects (especially since treatment often needs to be repeated): Neotigason® (Acitretin) has a deleterious effect on cholesterol levels, triglycerides, and the liver. It is *teratogenic*[29] (it is, therefore,

---

[28] Taken orally.
[29] May cause development abnormalities of the embryo and malformations.

contraindicated during pregnancy) and may cause cheilitis (inflammation of the lips), which can be bothersome.

Could the cause of keratosis pilaris be Ehlers-Danlos Syndrome?

No, because keratosis pilaris is not uncommon. It affects around 40% of the world's population: 50% are reached before the age of 10, and 35% are reached between 11 and 20 years. Therefore, there is an excellent sensitivity in the EDS (it is often present in EDS) but low specificity (it is often present outside of EDS). On the other hand, its persistence at an advanced age calls out and could be characteristic of EDS.

The second sub-part of Part II called "B," concerns the family history: the mother, the father, siblings, or children of one or more affected subjects also having hypermobile EDS. The goal is to affirm the patient's hereditary character, the mechanisms involved in hEDS not being known. It would be perfect if we did not have to let slip through our fingers suffering patients who have been adopted, or torn families who no longer speak to each other (see below).

Nota Bene : if there are, in the same family, several Fibromyalgia cases, it is imperative to look for an EDS in these people since Fibromyalgia is not, *a priori*, hereditary.

From Left to right, and from top to bottom:

- *Hyper-stretchable skin at the elbow.*
- *Atrophic scar on one knee.*
- *Flying bird hand sign (Professor Jaime F. Bravo).*
- *An enlarged, thinned, and hyperpigmented scar after a functional surgery shoulder in a 20-year-old man.*
- *Diffuse stretch marks in the same 20-year-old patient.*

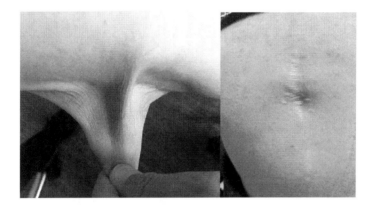

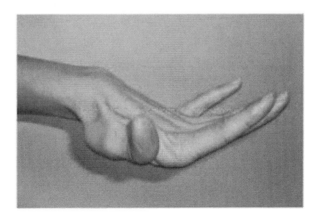

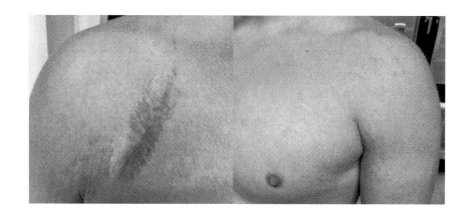

Fibromyalgia

Historically, Fibromyalgia was first given various names, such as Fibrositis, Psychogenic Rheumatism, Muscular Rheumatism, Diffuse Polyalgic Idiopathic Syndrome, or Neurasthenia. The term Fibromyalgia was first mentioned by Muhammad B. Yunus, in 1981. In an accompanying editorial, John B. Winfield, MD - Chapel Hill, NC – comments: "*Yunus is considered as the father of our modern view of fibromyalgia*".

Yunus M, Masi AT, Calabro JJ, et al. Primary fibromyalgia (fibrositis) : clinical study of 50 patients with matched normal controls. Semin Arthritis Rheum. 1981;11(1):151-71. doi: 10.1016/0049-0172(81)90096-2. PMID: 6944796.

Yunus MB, Masi AT, Calabro JJ, et al. Primary fibromyalgia. Am Fam Physician. 1982;25(5):11-21.

Yunus MB. Primary fibromyalgia syndrome: current concepts. Compr Ther. 1984;10(8):21-8.

Yunus MB. Fibromyalgia and overlapping disorders: the unifying concept of central sensitivity syndromes. Semin Arthritis Rheum. 2007;36(6):339-56. doi: 10.10.16/j.semarthrit.2006.12.009.

Then, other scientific papers have described this multifaceted affection. Among this profusion of publications, let us quote :

Treadwell BL. Fibromyalgia or the fibrositis syndrome: a new look. N Z Med J. 1981;94(698):457-9

Simons DG. Fibrositis/fibromyalgia: a form of myofascial trigger points? Am J Med. 1986;81(3A):93-8. doi: 10.1016/0002-9343(86)90885-5.

Smythe H. Tender points: evolution of concepts of the fibrositis/fibromyalgia syndrome. Am J Med. 1986;81(3A):2-6. doi: 10.1016/0002-9343(86)90865-x.

Hench PK, Mitler MM. Fibromyalgia. 1. Review of a common rheumatologic syndrome. Postgrad Med. 1986;80(7):47-56. doi: 10.180/00325481.1986.11699616.

Wolfe F. Fibrositis, fibromyalgia, and musculoskeletal disease: the current status of the fibrositis syndrome. Arch Phys Med Rehabil. 1988;69(7):527-31. PMID:3291821.

Professor Marcel-Francis Kahn (1929-) mainly described fibromyalgia in 1988 ("*Diffuse Polyalgic Idiopathic Syndrome*").

Kahn MF. Syndrome Polyalgique Idiopathique Diffus. Fibrosite. Fibromyalgie primitive. Doul. Et Analg. 1988;1:159-164.

Fibromyalgia syndrome (FMS) is often confused with EDS, even though it is not, a priori, a hereditary disease. The most widely accepted set of classification criteria for research purposes was elaborated in 1990 by the Multicenter Criteria Committee of the American College of Rheumatology (The ACR 1990 criteria). According to various papers, there is a high aggregation in FMS families, but the mode of inheritance is currently unknown, and maybe polygenic (FMS is presumably confused with EDS, I guess).

Stormorken H, Brosstad F. Fibromyalgia: family clustering and sensory urgency with early onset indicate genetic predisposition and thus a "true" disease. Scand J Rheumatol. 1992;21(4):207.

Arnold LM, Hudson JL, Hess EV, et al. Family study of fibromyalgia. Arthritis Rheum. 2004;50(3):944-52.

Professor Kahn is a rheumatologist, professor at the University and Head of the Rheumatology Department at Bichat hospital, in Paris. He supported, I dare say, unfortunately for the patients, that fibromyalgia syndrome was different from what his colleague Professor Claude Hamonet (Paris, France) had described for Ehlers-Danlos Syndrome.

For Kahn, EDS is painless...

However, in his 1988 article, Marcel-Francis Kahn wrote: "*Among the batch of patients consulting for chronic diffuse pain, a relatively homogeneous group, mostly female, has recently been isolated. Their pain is predominantly axial, without it being possible to determine the precise structure involved. Often associated with this are muscular fatigability and various non-specific disorders such as insomnia and functional coagulopathy*".../...."*we are considering either a tendinous-muscular disorder as yet unknown in its mechanism or a chronic disorder of pain perception. The treatment consists of recognizing the affection and making the patient understand that it is believed*". Further on we read: "*Although known since a 1904 description (Gowers W.R.: Lumbago. Its lessons and analogs. British Medical Journal 1904;1:117-121), the syndrome that will be discussed here, until ten years ago, at best elicited only a few lines in rheumatology treatises under the name of fibrositis.*" Alternatively, again: "*However, the pathophysiological mechanism of the disorder, as well as its etiology, and therefore its treatment, are still subject to discussion and contradictory opinions.* " .../... "*It is known that some authors have described in the SPID a Raynaud phenomenon (Dinerman H et al. Journal of rheumatology, 1986)*".../... "*For Goldenberg (JAMA, 1987), 18% of patients had signs of Goujerot-Sjögren.*"

For M.F. Kahn, in fibromyalgia, there is mainly "*a diffuse painful syndrome,*" "*a painful muscular fatigability, particularly marked in the scapular belt*" and taking up the data of Anglo-Saxon authors: "*associated functional manifestations: migraines, spasmodic coagulopathy, sexual disorders,*" "*sleep disorders with a lack of restorative sleep,*" and "*no characterized psychiatric pathology.*" However, "*anxiety*" and "*feelings of swelling and numbness*" are reported. There is a whole series of relatively constant, symmetrical, and mostly axial "*pain points*".

Surprisingly, all these symptoms are present in patients suffering from Ehlers-Danlos Syndrome, noted as co-morbidities by the New York Criteria, but described excellently by Professor Claude Hamonet in his book entitled: "*Ehlers Danlos. La Maladie oubliée par la médecine*" (Editions L'Harmattan, 2018 & 2019).

Strangely, two diseases have so many so diverse points in common.

In the long run, I would like all doctors who treat fibromyalgia syndrome (algologists, physical physicians, rheumatologists, neurologists, general practitioners) to systematically test these patients, clinically and histologically, for EDS. In my opinion, as with other practitioners, one cannot have both diseases at the same time: EDS usually explains all the signs and symptoms present in these patients. At present, I cannot say that all fibromyalgia patients suffer from EDS; it would be an intellectual drift. We will only be able to confirm that when these fibromyalgic patients have all been routinely tested for EDS.

It is necessary, even a diagnostic emergency, for EDS's hereditary implications and the potentially severe medical and surgical complications it promotes.

There is a growing body of literature on the emergence of new clinical signs and symptoms attributed to the *disease* of fibromyalgia, but more often than not, these are well-known signs and symptoms of EDS. Medical history error or not, FMS should be rethought and revised, hopefully, based on the results of future comparative studies between these two conditions, including personal and family history (the anamnesis), careful physical examination, sensitive and specific diagnostic criteria (hopefully after revision of the current EDS criteria), genetic and skin biopsy analysis.

FMS and EDS are, in fact, too clinically close to be so different etiologically. I am convinced that we have overlooked, and that we will often still miss a diagnosis of EDS, purely and simply. It is a dangerous attitude for these patients.

We continue the diagnostic wandering while it would suffice to systematically think about it in the face of hypermobility, dysproprioception, dyssensoriality, dysautonomia, hemorrhagic diathesis, and more.

Ultimately, this can only be resolved by teaching quality academics dedicated to Ehlers-Danlos Syndrome, which should be provided by customary specialists in disease and its complexity.

Maimonides' medical prayer
Moses Maimonides (1135-1204)
Philosopher, Chief Rabbi, and physician.

Attributed to Moses Maimonides, but probably written by Marcus Herz (German physician). Firstly print in 1793. Translated by Harry Friedenwald (1864-1950) in *The Bulletin of the John Hopkins Hospital*, in 1917.

"Almighty God, Thou has created the human body with infinite wisdom. Ten thousand times ten thousand organs hast Thou combined in it that act unceasingly and harmoniously to preserve the whole in all its beauty the body which is the envelope of the immortal soul. They are ever acting in perfect order, agreement and accord. Yet, when the frailty of matter or the unbridling of passions deranges this order or interrupts this accord, then forces clash and the body crumbles into the primal dust from which it came. Thou sendest to man diseases as beneficent messengers to foretell approaching danger and to urge him to avert it. Thou hast blest Thine earth, Thy rivers and Thy mountains with healing substances; they enable Thy creatures to alleviate their sufferings and to heal their illnesses.

Thou hast endowed man with the wisdom to relieve the suffering of his brother, to recognize his disorders, to extract the healing substances, to discover their powers and to prepare and to apply them to suit every ill. In Thine Eternal Providence Thou hast chosen me to watch over the life and health of Thy creatures. I am now about to apply myself to the duties of my profession. Support me, Almighty God, in these great labors that they may benefit mankind, for without Thy help not even the least thing will succeed. Inspire me with love for my art and for Thy creatures. Do not allow thirst for profit, ambition for renown and admiration, to interfere with my profession, for these are the enemies of truth and of love for mankind and they can lead astray in the great task of attending to the welfare of Thy creatures.

Preserve the strength of my body and of my soul that they ever be ready to cheerfully help and support rich and poor, good and bad, enemy as well as friend. In the sufferer let me see only the human being. Illumine my mind that it recognize what presents itself and that it may comprehend what is absent or hidden. Let it not fail to see what is visible, but do not permit it to arrogate itself the power to see what cannot be seen, for delicate and indefinite are the bounds of the great art of caring for the lives and health of Thy creatures. Let me never be absent-minded.

May no strange thoughts divert my attention at the bedside of the sick, or disturb my mind in its silent labors, for great and sacred are the thoughtful deliberations required to preserve the lives and health of Thy creatures Grant that my patients have confidence in me and my art and follow my directions and counsel. Remove from their midst all charlatans and the whole host of officious relatives and know-all nurses, cruel people who arrogantly frustrate the wisest purposes of our art and often lead Thy creatures to their death. Should those who are wiser than I wish to improve and instruct me, let my soul gratefully follow their guidance; for vast is the extent of our art.

Should conceited fools, however, censure me, then let love for my profession steel me against them, so that I remain steadfast without regard for age, for reputation, or for honor, because surrender would bring Thy creatures sickness and death. Imbue my soul with gentleness and calmness when older colleagues, proud of their age, wish to displace me or scorn me or disdainfully teach me. May even this be of advantage to me, for they know many things of which I am ignorant, but let not their arrogance give me pain. For they are old and old age is not master of the passions. I also hope to attain old age upon this earth, before Thee, Almighty God!

Let me be contented in everything except in the great science of my profession. Never allow the thought to arise in me that I have attained to sufficient knowledge, but vouchsafe to me the strength, the leisure and the ambition ever to extend my knowledge. For art is great, but the mind of man is ever expanding.

Almighty God! Thou hast chosen me in Thy mercy to watch over the life and death of Thy creatures. I now apply myself to my profession. Support me in this great task so that it may benefit mankind, for without Thy help not even the least thing will succeed."

The third part, called "C," concerns joint pain and instability.

It is divided into three points: 1, 2, and 3. One point in three is enough to validate part "C."
➤ Point One concerns joint pain of at least two members, present every day, and for more than three months.
➤ Point Two concerns diffuse pain, present for more than three months.
➤ Point Three concerns dislocations or articular instabilities (without trauma).

Point 3 is validated if at least 1 of the following two items is present:
- At least three dislocations of the same joint or at least two dislocations for two different joints.
- Instability of at least two sites without pre-existing trauma.

It is a legitimate part, on which I have no criticism.

Reviews of Part III of the New York Criteria (hEDS) (the exclusion criteria)

Part III ensures that other diseases are not present and falsely diagnosed as EDS. Alternatively, a patient may have two diseases, different EDS types, and rheumatoid arthritis or ankylosing spondylitis, for example.

This Part III is divided into three points: 1, 2, and 3. The three points must be satisfied for criterion III to be validated. For example, if there is an autoimmune disease, one cannot, according to the criteria, consider criterion IIC. It is therefore imperative that the IIA and IIB criteria are met.

The exclusion criteria are:

1. Skin fragility or stretchable skin over 3 cm, suggesting another type of EDS (such as cEDS).

Criticisms: We sometimes encounter hyperextensible skin in hEDS as well as papyraceous scars. Otherwise, and as a demonstration of the absurd, how could it be excluded that among the unknown mutations of hEDS, there is no mutation of one collagen or another substance in the extracellular matrix that could cause these characteristics punctually? It is intellectually impossible, at this time, to assert it or not.

2. The presence of other acquired or hereditary diseases of connective tissue, autoimmune such as rheumatoid arthritis, systemic lupus erythematosus, scleroderma, and more.

Criticisms: Take the case of a patient with rheumatoid arthritis, well-controlled thanks to the monthly biotherapy[30]. He or her is clinically asymptomatic, without synovitis and arthritis. His or her DAS28 score (*disease activity score-28 describes severity of rheumatoid arthritis using clinical and laboratory data, specifically erythrocyte sedimentation rate or C-reactive protein*) is less than 2.6 (indicating clinical remission), he or she has a non-inflammatory biology, and his or her bone scintigraphy[31] does not demonstrate any pathological focus. In this case, could we not consider subpart IIC as an hEDS criterion, and validate criterion II, even though one of the two sub-parts IIA or IIB, is not met?

Points IIA and IIB are not always fulfilled: either because five out of twelve items of the IIA are not present, either because the patient does not know his or her family of origin (if he or she was adopted, if he or she is the result of rape, ...) for IIB. Some families no longer speak or see each other for different relational reasons; should we penalize the patient for this and not consider him or her as hEDS?

It is also where the dermis analysis by transmission electron microscopy (TEM) is potentially useful to reinforce the diagnosis of EDS. Could we not add the results of skin biopsy as a complementary criterion or relief in some instances where the New York criteria would not be fulfilled? In Germany, for example, it is often compulsory to take this exam in order to receive certain social benefits.

---

[30] This is most often an antibody produced in the laboratory and which interferes explicitly with a molecule; these are, for example, anti-TNFα antibodies or anti-IL-6 receptor antibodies (a treatment, moreover, used in covid-19, infection during which interleukin-6 seems to have a significant role in the cytokine storm).
[31] They commonly use pyrophosphate, labeled with technetium-99m.

This is even more interesting to consider that in the article by the New York Classification (*Malfait et al., 2017*), it is written: "*In case of unavailability of genetic testing, electronic transmission microscopy (TEM) findings of collagen flowers on skin biopsy CAN SUPPORT the clinical diagnosis but cannot confirm it.*"

We often hear that this exam is useless by uninformed doctors or patients. Most people who peddle these things most often have not even read or understand the article in question (by *Malfait et al.*). It is challenging, especially in the age of social networks, to put an end to bad information that is transmitted quickly. (See below the parenthesis on received ideas and misconceptions).

3. The presence of other hereditary abnormalities of the connective tissues:

   o Stickler, Marfan, Loeys-Dietz disease, and more.
   o Neuromuscular Diseases (myopathic EDS, Bethlem myopathy, and more.)
   o Skeletal dysplasia (osteogenesis imperfecta, chondrodysplasias, and more.)

Most often, the clinical presentation and the medical history led to one of these disease diagnoses. In case of clinical suspicion, some genetic tests are available, and specific and oriented additional examinations can be carried out to specify or exclude these different conditions: ophthalmological, ENT, neurological examinations, x-rays, muscle biopsy, and more. Always keep in mind, that sporadically one of these conditions is present simultaneously with EDS. Indeed, specific mutations of other hereditary diseases can potentially be added to those of EDS.

About three years ago, I received a teenage girl, aged 17, who had Koslowski syndrome and most likely a hEDS. The clinic and the skin biopsy confirmed the diagnosis of hEDS. Here is the description of this case, extremely rare, not published to date, that I reserved for this book:

Clinical Case

By Daens Stéphane, Hermanns-Lê Trinh, Brock Isabelle,
Hougrand Olivier, Hamonet Claude, Manicourt Daniel

Regarding the clinical signs of Spondylometaphyseal Dysplasia syndrome Koslowski type (SMDK):

The clinical examination of H., 17, revealed typical symptoms of spondylometaphyseal dysplasia syndrome Koslowski type.

She was genetically diagnosed at the age of 6. She is short. It is dwarfism with a short neck, kyphoscoliosis, and a short trunk. She has a genu valgum (an angle outwards, "X" knees) and brachydactyly of the hands and feet.

The standard radiographs showed a vertebrae's platyspondyly, with anterior sliding of pedicles, and metaphyseal abnormalities in the pelvis. Radiographs of the peripheral skeleton showed enlarged joints, coxa vara-type hips (an angle inward), epi-metaphyseal deformations at femurs (prominent femoral neck, in the trochanteric region), short metaphyses, and brachydactyly of all phalanges.

The TRPV4 gene was amplified by PCR and analyzed by gene sequencing (the 12q24.1 locus, present on chromosome 12). A heterozygous variant of this gene was identified in her genotype and that of her father: the c.838G>C mutation in exon 5 of the TRVP4 gene (*Transient Receptor Potential Cation Channel Subfamily V member 4 genes*). This result confirmed the clinical diagnosis of SMDK.

Next page: X-rays

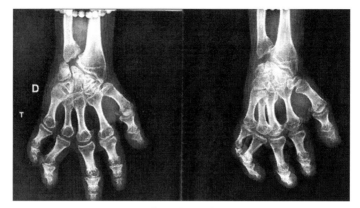

X-rays: hands and wrists

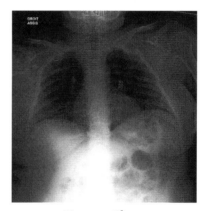

X-rays : Chest

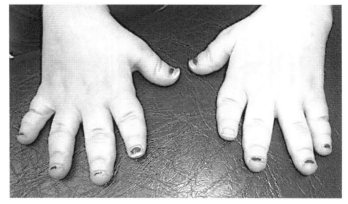

Hands and fingers

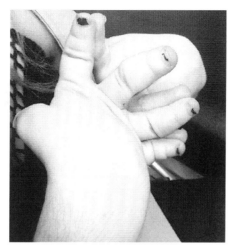
Hyperextension of the fingers (1)

Concerning the clinical signs and symptoms of hEDS:

H. suffered from chronic musculoskeletal pain, frontal headaches, severe fatigue, and sleep disturbances. She had chronic subluxations, dislocations, and sprains; she also had multiple bone fractures. The teeth are irregular, the palate is high and narrow (ogival), and the sclera is bluish. The skin is stretched over four centimeters at the neck and three centimeters at the forearm. Beighton's score was eight out of nine at the time of the clinical examination. The ankles, shoulders, and hips are also hypermobile. Stretch marks and multiple atrophic, but non-surgical, scars were also observed.

She had atopic skin, eczema, and episodes of diarrhea. The latter symptoms suggest a mast cell activation syndrome/disorder (MCAS/MCAD), which is frequently associated with hEDS. She was being treated with physiotherapy and was taking Topiramate for headaches. The latter treatment had side effects such as increased fatigue.

A skin biopsy was performed (on the upper buttock). An ultrastructural examination of the dermis revealed collagen bundles of normal size. In a few bundles, collagen fibrils of variable size and irregularly spaced were revealed. And, there were granulo-filamentous deposits between the collagen fibrils. Rare fibrils were flower-like; these fibrils were comparable in

93

diameter to typical and normal adjacent fibrils, round and regular in cross-section. It is well described in hEDS. Huge hyaluronic acid globules were also observed in the dermis.

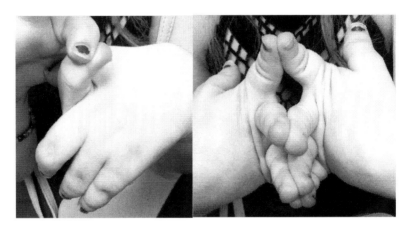

Hyperextension of the fingers (2)

Prescribed treatment:

H. began isometric physiotherapy and hydrotherapy, sequential oxygen therapy with a flow rate of 3 liters per minute, by nasal cannulas (or *glasses*), at a rate of three to four 20-minute sessions per day (for fatigue, headaches, lack of concentration and attention, and sleep disturbances). Riboflavin (vitamin B2) was introduced at 100mg/day and a combination of Levodopa 25mg + Benzaraside 6.25mg twice daily. Custom-made compression garments (vest, leggings, gloves, socks) were made to improve proprioception. Also, Levocetirizine 5mg/day for the MCAD and Melatonin 3mg in the evening to restore a correct nycthemeral rhythm and promote sleep.

After four weeks, musculoskeletal pain was drastically reduced, and sleep was improved. Headaches and fatigue had almost disappeared. MCAD symptoms were significantly less, and, most importantly, her quality of life was much improved.

Discussion:

Koslowski-type spondylo-metaphyseal dysplasia (SMDK) results from dominantly inherited TPRV4 gene mutations (one in two children is affected if only one parent carries the mutation). These mutations can induce, in 30 to 79% of cases, a limitation of joint mobility. The prevalence of SMDK does not exceed 1 over 1,000,000 people.

Unlike Koslowski dwarfism, which causes a loss of joint mobility, EDS includes patients who have, or had, joint hypermobility (in youth, for example).

Some clinical signs present in this young patient can be found in EDS's spondylodysplastic form (or spEDS). This newly described variant has mutations in β-3-Galactosyl-Transferase-6 that alter glycosaminoglycans' expression, but in spEDS, bone development in the fingers appears normal.

In this context, we tried to further differentiate our patient's clinical signs and symptoms from other diseases: spEDS due to β-4-Galactosyl-Transferase-7 deficiency or β-3-Galactosyl-Transferase-6 deficiency, but also spEDS due to SLC39A13 mutations.

Clinically, spEDS usually presents with generalized joint hyperlaxity in early childhood but stiffness and contractures in adolescence and adulthood. In hEDS, the opposite is generally observed. On the other hand, in spEDS, the fingers are typically described as slender and arachnodactyly-like (*spider legs*) or tapered with spatula-shaped or broad distal phalanges. It is different from the feet and hands of our young patient.

Her intelligence appears to be higher than average, which is essential to note because mutations in spEDS are often associated with mild mental retardation. Furthermore, the skin biopsy with the ultrastructure of the dermis, presented by *Malfait et al.* in cases of spEDS, showed different changes in the collagen bundles compared to those observed in hEDS (as in our patient). In spEDS, the collagen fibrils appear slightly packed with variable diameters, some with very irregular contours.

We compared our patient's phenotype with Spondylo-Epimetaphyseal Dysplasia descriptions with Leptodactyl Articular Laxity (SEMDJL2). Clinically, the SEMDJL2 phenotype shows differences from H. In this autosomal dominant disease, hypoplasia of the middle face, tapered fingers, macrocephaly are described. In SEMDJL2, a few mutations have been discovered, such as that of the KIFF2 gene or, more recently, homozygous missense mutations in two close genes: NIN and POLE2.

Conclusion of the H's clinical case:

We have described a case of SMDK most likely associated with an hEDS. To our knowledge, this has never been described before. This clinical case seems extremely rare when considering each of the two diseases' incidences: 1/100 for hEDS x 1/1,000,000 for SMDK = less than 1 case over 100 million people worldwide.

References:

Kozlowski K. Metapahyseal and spondylometaphyseal chondrodysplasia. Clin Orthop Relat Res. 1976;(114):83-93.

Malfait F, Francomano C, Byers P et al. 2017. The 2017 International Classification of the Ehlers-Danlos Syndromes. Am J Med Genet Part C Semin Med Genet 175C:8-26.

Hermanns-Lê T, Reginster MA, Piérart-Franchimont C, Piérard GE. (2012). Ehlers-Danlos syndrome. In: Diagnostic Electron Microscopy: A Practical Guide to Tissue Preparation and Interpretation, Ed: John Wiley and Sons, Ltd., Chichester 309-21.

Fransiska Malfait, Ariana Kariminejad, Tim Van Damme et al. 2013. Defective Initiation of Glycosaminoglycan Synthesis due to B3GALT6 Mutations Causes a Pleiotropic Ehlers-Danlos-Syndrome-like Connective Tissue Disorder. The American Journal of Human Genetics. 92;935–945.

Brady AF, Demirdas S, Fournel-Gigleux S et al. 2017. The Ehlers–Danlos syndromes, rare types. Am J Med Genet Part C Semin Med Genet 175C:70–115.

Tsirikos, A. I., Mason, D. E., Scott, C. I. and Chang, W.-N. (2003), Spondyloepimetaphyseal dysplasia with joint laxity (SEMDJL). Am J Med Genet. 2003;119A: 386–390.

Mégarbané, A., Ghanem, I. and Le Merrer, M. (2003), Spondyloepimetaphyseal dysplasia with multiple dislocations, leptodactylic type: Report of a new patient and review of the literature. Am J Med Genet, 122A: 252–256.

Grosch M, Grüner B, Spranger S et al. 2013. Identification of a Ninein (NIN) mutation in a family with spondyloepimetaphyseal dysplasia with joint laxity (leptodactylic type)-like phenotype. Matrix Biol. 2013;32(7-8):387-92.

Theoretically, there should be cases where some children have a different variant of EDS than their parent, but this would be very rare. Let us take another example, but a fictional one:

A mother is a carrier of a hypermobile EDS. She completely meets the New York criteria. Her clinical examination and the TEM examination of her skin biopsy support this diagnosis. No genetic mutation has been found in her that could give rise to another variant of EDS. Clinically, the dad is not a carrier of connective tissue disease.

The empirical view of genetics is exciting because almost anything can be considered.

In this family, let us imagine that the father is a carrier of a COL5A1 mutation that is *silenced*, and is *not expressed* in his phenotype (see below). He is, in a way, a *healthy carrier*. In this family, the father has passed this genetic mutation on to several of his children. In some of his children, the mutation has *turned on*: this mutation has activated and is expressed in the *phenotype* (see below). This COL5A1 mutation will mix with the unknown hEDS mutations inherited from the mother. These children may eventually have a genotype and phenotype of the classical variant. It is probably sporadic, but it is conceivable.

> Yes, empirically and intellectually, we can find children with a different variant than their parents.

Ultrastructural analysis of the dermis is of great help here. If this analysis shows different modifications of the collagen fibrils, elastic fibers, and fibroblasts than those of the parent with hEDS and if it is a variant for which specific genetic mutations are known (COL5A1 or A2, COL3A1, PLOD, COL1A1 or COL1A2, and more), then, a targeted blood test should be requested to look for these mutations.

On the other hand, a specific mutation (e.g., COL3A1 gene mutation) present in a parent's genotype (his or her ADN), and effectively expressed in his or her phenotype (the finished product), may very well be present but *silenced* (turned off) in his or her child's genotype. The child may then present a hEDS phenotype *(= the common systemic form, csEDS, see further)* and not the parent's phenotype (e.g., vEDS). In this case, the mutation in question has been added to the unknown mutations of hEDS *(or csEDS, see further)*, but is not expressed in the child's phenotype.

It is very important to distinguish the *genotype* from the *phenotype* (see further).

Anything is possible in human genetics and epigenetics.

Exception: a not insignificant number of patients with hEDS would have previously been diagnosed as hEDS *and* vEDS. It is what they tell us or what their testimonials on social networks tell us. It is probably wrong. Either it results from patients misunderstanding their diagnosis, or some non-traditional EDS doctors have so told them. Patients are lost in EDS's meanders, which is quite typical: it is a too complex disease and, unfortunately, unknown to the medical profession. Most often, these patients are carriers of the hypermobile variant of EDS *(or Common Systemic variant)* and have cardiovascular manifestations, such as ectasia of the aortic root, an arcuate ligament with compression of the celiac trunk, ectasia of the carotid or femoral artery, artery dissection or a family history of aneurysm, insufficiency or prolapse of a heart valve.

There may be vascular and cardiac manifestations in the common systemic form (hEDS), as well as mild to moderate scoliosis, muscle weakness or dystonia, and more. Since the mutations of the hypermobile EDS are not known, there may be some unknown mutations that lead to manifestations in the phenotype (the finished product) that can be found in other variants of EDS, but most often, they are less generalized and less marked than in the specific variants (cEDS, vEDS, ksEDS, and more).

Life is short, science is long;
opportunity is elusive,
experiment is dangerous,
judgement is difficult.

Hippocrates

Selfishness must always
be forgiven you know,
because there is no hope of a cure.

Jane Austen (1775-1817)

A Lie can travel halfway around
the world while the truth
is putting on its shoes.

Jane Austen (1775-1817)

Testimony of Florence, 46 years old

A different kind of courage.

Since I was a young girl, I have always had pain, but at first, I thought everyone was like me.

Then the pain only worsened, and I remember, stupidly, the kindergarten teacher that I was, proudly thinking that I would still make it despite everything.

Then it developed a little more and a little more... Ha! It took courage, but you should know that it took even more for me to stop.

I would say it takes courage to get up in the morning and not go to work, not have colleagues to laugh with, not have a social life, not have a life, almost ... well, I had my son.

Ha! My son! Can you imagine how much courage it took me to tell him that EDS is genetic?

Even if I had all the courage in the world, I would never accept that I passed it on to him.

I watch out for advances, especially from him...

Florence C., December 2019.

CHAPTER II

Properties of Connective Tissue in EDS or How to avoid Misdiagnosis and Inadequate Management?

By Dr. Stéphane Daens

Ehlers-Danlos Syndrome is an inherited connective tissue disease that mainly affects collagens and glycosaminoglycans, sometimes tenascin X, fibronectin, and more. In other words, the supporting tissue. This tissue is everywhere in the body: skin, tendons, ligaments, joint capsules, muscles, mesenteries, fasciae, mucous membranes of internal organs, and more. The brain and nerves are most often spared because they contain minimal collagen. On the other hand, there may be hyperexcitability and inflammation of particular brain cells, with the release of potentially toxic superoxide anions (see the chapter on central sensitization).

There is also virtually no peripheral neuropathy (there are many over-diagnoses of neuropathies of the small fibers of pain) or pure brain damage (direct damage). Small fiber neuropathies (type C) are usually related to peripheral sensitization and mast cell activation disorder (MCAD). Instead, there are more arterial vascular complications at the central nervous system level, such as aneurysms or dissections, subdural or extradural hematomas, multiple sclerosis false images, and Arnold-Chiari syndrome due to hyperlaxity of the cerebral envelopes, which are made of connective tissue (see below). However, this is rare in practice.

On the other hand, the connective tissue's particular structure may secondarily promote nerve, plexus, or truncal lesions, such as damage to the ulnar nerve in its epitrochleo-olecranial groove, located at the elbow.

In this case, repeated subluxations of the ulnar nerve, which is poorly held in place by the damaged connective tissue, would cause lesions. Pain indicating carpal tunnel syndrome is common in EDS, but it is rarely a proper compression of the nerve at the carpal tunnel, as the connective tissue of the carpal tunnel ligaments is more likely to be deformed. Dysautonomia, accompanied by swelling of the hands, is usually the cause. The topography does not usually correspond to the classic carpal tunnel syndrome: here, all fingers fall asleep or swell, whereas, in a classic carpal tunnel syndrome, only the first three fingers and the ulnar half of the fourth finger are affected. Surgical interventions to free this nerve (neurolysis) either lead to no result or fail in the medium term. It is better to treat the dysautonomia (see below) and put on compression gloves than to operate unnecessarily.

Contractures of the gluteal muscles (such as the pyramidal and gluteus medius), which are due to hypermobility of the hips and sacroiliac joints, can, for example, compress the sciatic nerve that crosses them from below and, leads to false diagnoses of sciatica of lumbar origin by disc compression (the discs are relatively soft in the EDS due to the binding properties of the intervertebral discs). There are very few true root compressions due to herniated discs, even when enlarged. Unnecessary disc surgeries are often performed. Even if they provide initial relief, probably the result of postoperative rest, the pain returns a few weeks or months after the surgery. Some local lidocaine injections into the gluteal muscles, a sacroiliac and hip belt, Bermuda shorts or compression pants with hip reinforcement, low-dose magnesium, and baclofen or levodopa, and physiotherapy/hydrotherapy sessions usually provide relief for these patients.

Scaleni muscles. Scaleni are strongly contracted muscles in the context of the instability of the craniocervical and temporomandibular joints. They are also associated with diaphragmatic weakness, which is accompanied by secondary overuse of the accessory inspiration muscles. They can cause symptoms reminiscent of a thoracic outlet syndrome, as the contracted muscles cause extrinsic compression of the adjacent vascular and nervous structures. Clinically, the upper limbs become numb, tingling, or drowsy, leading to excessive surgery in some patients.

Ortho-parasympathetic terminations, which are in the dermis and the connective tissue of the mucous membranes, among others, can also send false signals to the central nervous system and cause pseudo-Raynaud's syndrome. A true Raynaud's syndrome is usually associated with autoimmune diseases such as lupus erythematosus, rheumatoid arthritis, scleroderma, and more. Other symptoms include blood pressure and heart rhythm adjustment disorders, excessive sweating of the upper body, dry skin on the extremities, unexplained fever, chills, fatigue, concentration and memory disorders, syncopal-like complaints, orthostatic hypotension, POTS, and more. It is known as Dysautonomia.

Connective tissue receptors and sensors are remarkable diverse:

1/ Nociceptors are used for the perception of pain (of high intensity and often secondary to injury). They are often free nerve endings, which are of three types:

> Mechanoreceptors (fiber Aδ), are sensitive to mechanical deformation of the skin or intense pressure (e.g., when one hits their foot on a coffee table).
> Thermoreceptors (Aδ fiber) sensitive to extreme temperatures, above 45°C or below 10°C.
> Polymodal receptors (C fibers) sensitive to mechanical influences and temperature. These are the most common receptors.

2/ The mechanoreceptors responsible for skin sensitivity (pressure, touch, and vibration) are manifold:

> Meissner corpuscles (Aβ fibers) for a light touch in the dermis.
> Vater-Pacini corpuscles (Aβ fibers) are sensitive to pressure and deformation of the connective tissue. They provide information about the severity, beginning, and end of pressure.

> Ruffini's corpuscles (fibers Aβ), subcutaneous and articular, provide information about pressure and stretching (intensity, duration).

3/ The proprioceptors are the articular and muscular mechanoreceptors. They make it possible to perceive spatial awareness in the space of the body and its different parts. They are sensitive to posture, force, and movement.

> The neuromuscular spindles (muscle stretching) are in the muscles (fibers Aα and Aβ).
> The Golgi tendon organs (muscle tension) are in the tendons (fibers Aβ).
> The common mechanoreceptors (fibers Aβ and Aδ).

In EDS, these sensors or receptors are normal, but they are immersed in tissue with altered physical properties. They could therefore be activated either too strongly or too weakly during a stimulus. For example, when I move my elbow, the mechanoreceptors in the joint capsule inform the brain late to adjust the joint alignments and cause a subluxation, and a crackling sound can be heard when moving the joint.

If weak skin stimulation activates the nociceptors too quickly or too vigorously, the nociceptors then incorrectly inform the brain of peripheral pain. Pain is perceived where there is no real pain; and this is the same false sense of burning, numbness, or tingling in the limbs, trunk, or face.

When too much painful misinformation reaches the brain, the brain can block or unblock motor activity in one or more limbs. This can lead to pseudo-paralysis (*see below*). It is a similar mechanism to circumstantial hearing loss in hyperacusis: there is very disturbing hyperacusis, but when several people speak simultaneously, or in a common tone, they no longer understand or hear anything. The brain switches off the sensory organs' afferent fibers. Another example is the loss of consciousness or coma when pain is very severe.

Incorrect diagnoses of transient ischemic attacks, strokes, multiple sclerosis (MS), and neuropathies are therefore made too hastily in EDS patients, resulting in inadequate treatment and, in most cases, significant iatrogenic side effects. They could be avoided.

As for fibromyalgia syndrome (FMS), described, among others, by Professor M-F KAHN, it is too often evoked while an EDS differential diagnosis has not even been considered, leading to inappropriate treatment. All patients diagnosed with FMS should be thoroughly screened for EDS, as the two diagnoses are unlikely to coexist.

Often doctors maintain both diagnoses, FMS and EDS, which I think is a mistake in many patients. All signs and symptoms of EDS are usually sufficient to explain the patient's situation. There is no point in giving them a second diagnosis that does nothing, except result in ineffective treatments that can be unsuitable, or even harmful for EDS patients. This is the case with morphine, anti-inflammatory drugs, certain anti-depressants, and more.

Such an attitude is favored in internal medicine: It is better to collect signs and symptoms in one diagnosis than to misdiagnose several different diseases.

We have met patients with the misdiagnosis of multiple sclerosis (MS) despite a normal cerebrospinal fluid. Given atypical neurological symptoms and lesions of the white matter of the brain, some doctors often conclude that these patients have MS (the shortcut is quickly made), while they most often have benign leukoaraiosis (*see next page*).

Various Atypical Brain Images are Found in EDS on Magnetic Resonance Imaging (MRI)

In collaboration with Professor Daniel FREDY
Neuroradiologist, Hôpital Sainte-Anne, Paris, France

Leukoaraiosis presents a picture where the nodules are grouped in the form of a small rosary or para-sagittal splints (*white arrows*). Hyperflash nodules can be seen in the MRI at flair and spin-echo T2:

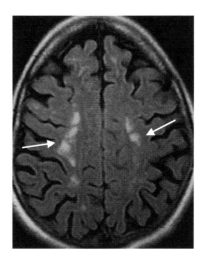

The location of these lesions often makes it possible to distinguish the diagnosis of leukoaraiosis from the diagnosis of multiple sclerosis (MS).

The lesions of leukoaraiosis are mainly found in:

➢ In the supraventricular area: in the semi-oval center. It is bilateral and is in the part of the white matter below the cerebral cortex, and above the ventricles and corpus callosum. It is located at the junction of the descending (coming from the pericortical vessels) and ascending (coming from the vessels at the base of the brain) perforating arteries. This location is not typical of multiple sclerosis lesions.

➢ In periventricular and lateral para-ventricular regions, right and left, with a T2 zone of leukoaryotic confluence covering, in front, the frontal horns, and the ventricular connections at the back.

➢ At the level of the subcortical regions.

In EDS, there are also irregular changes in the tissue of the upper part of the brainstem and the upper part of the cervical spinal cord, which take on a *leopard appearance* in a COSMIC hypo-hyper flash (white arrows):

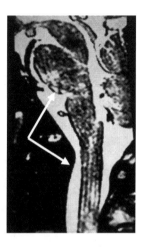

EDS can be triggered or made worse after a traumatic event such as whiplash, concussion, or road accident (see also the chapter on genetics and epigenetics).

"Shock waves can spread throughout the body, but are not damped due to the flexibility of the tissue. They arrive with all their initial force, hit the bone arch, and are distributed in the brain." Professor Claude Hamonet.

These traumatic events generate images that can be detected with refined MRI techniques such as the 3D diffusion tensor. Since 2005, Professor Claude Hamonet has been using this instrument, in collaboration with Professor Daniel Frédy, to show the after effects of a craniocerebral trauma with forensic implications.

➢ There is damage to the reticular substance. It is located at the medial and posterior pedunculopontine junction and is

107

visible axially and in the profile during irregular *Fiesta* hyper flash (black arrows).

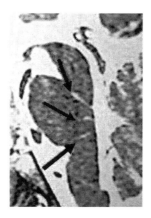

➤ There are images of remarkable cortical atrophy of the upper and middle vermis of the cerebellum (the vermis is the median region of the cerebellum flanked by the right and left hemispheres), in 2D SPGR-T1 views in profile and axially, giving it a *fern appearance*.

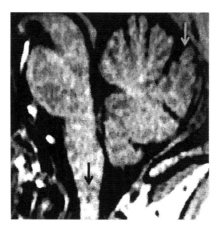

➤ There is an irregular widening of the banks of the two calcarine fissures. Each fissure contains the calcarina artery, the posterior collateral branch of the posterior cerebral artery. This damage could be part of the visuospatial disturbances. In this case, an ophthalmologist should examine the visual field, and a neuropsychological examination should be performed.

The 3D diffusion tensor (DTI) enables us to observe, in EDS, differences in the *Arcuate Fasciculus* (the Bundle of Knowledge): It is a collection of axons that connect the Broca and Wernicke areas. It is a network of interhemispheric fibers that connect the specific associative cortex, the auditory and motor cortex, and bypasses the Sylvius cleft. It is a network that enables, for example, the following chain: *I hear, I understand*, then through the bundle what has been understood is passed on to the anterior region of Broca, and *I carry out*. The fibers can be thinned or cut. The Arcuate Fasciculus is variable between the brain's two hemispheres and between individuals; it is like another personalized fingerprint.

In addition to the epigenetic postulates that would influence EDS development (see this chapter), diffusion tensor imaging (DTI) brain imaging in EDS can partially explain some post-traumatic signs and symptoms such as attention memory, visuospatial disorders, and more.

The American judicial system tolerates or, in some instances, admits the usefulness of 3D diffusion tensor imaging MRI during litigation:

➤ *Commonwealth of Massachusetts. Suffolk, SS. Superior Court Dept. Case n°08-2380, July 29, 2010.*
➤ *Florida Court upholds admissibility of DTI. Case n°08-019984. September 27, 2010.*
➤ *Colorado Court finds DTI admissible. November 19, 2010.*
➤ *Massachusetts Court finds DTI satisfies Daubert Standart. November 29, 2010.*

Note: In US federal law, the Daubert standard is a rule of evidence for expert testimony admissibility.

Hamonet C, Frédy D, Lefèvre JH, Bourgeois-Gironde S et Zeitoun JD. Brain injury unmasking Ehlers-Danlos syndromes after trauma: the fiber print. Orphanet J Rare Dis. 2016;22:11-45.

Clinical Examples of Pseudo-paralysis in EDS

♦   At the end of 2017, a 13-year-old girl came to my emergency room for consultation with her parents. Sarah presented herself with monoparesis (or even a paralysis) of her upper right extremity after a car accident in which she was a passenger. The additional neurological examinations performed were all normal: electromyography and conduction velocities of the upper limbs, somatosensory and motor evoked potentials, MRI of the brachial plexus, and MRI of the brain. Clinically she also had algoneurodystrophy of the right upper extremity (complex regional pain syndrome type 1 or CRPS-1). Beighton's score was 9/9, and the New York criteria were met. Ultrastructural analysis of the dermis by electron microscopy is compatible with hypermobile EDS. Besides, she had significant MCAD, common in both EDS and CRPS-1 (see below). As a treatment, I prescribed tailored compression garments, sequential oxygen therapy, adapted gentle physiotherapy, Alendronate 70mg 3x/week, calcium carbonate 1g/day, 25-OH-vitamin D 3000 IU/day. MCAD treatment was also started: Desloratadine 5 mg twice daily, Montelukast 10 mg/day, Ranitidine 300 mg/day, Vitamin C 1000 mg/day, and N-acetylcysteine 600 mg three times daily (as mast cell stabilizers and strong antioxidants). Low Dose Naltrexone (LDN) was started in July 2019. By the end of November 2019, Sarah had regained the function of the proximal part of her right upper extremity (shoulder and elbow). Her hand remained paralyzed, but clinically the algoneurodystrophy (CRPS-1) had decreased. She is currently still well relieved by the compression garment. This is a case of pseudo-paralysis of a limb, in an EDS context, caused by a triggering factor: a car accident.

♦   A 24-year-old woman came to my consultation with her mother. Coralie was in a wheelchair, exhausted, and had incredibly significant dystonia in all four limbs and the face, comparable to choreoathetosis. Persistent constipation with an interval of more than two weeks between each bowel movement and gastroparesis with gastroesophageal reflux were also present. The situation worsened rapidly, and when the complementary examinations all proved to be normal, she was admitted to a psychiatric clinic for hysterical conversion and treated with medication as needed. She was not able to feed herself, walk, wash, or use the amenities. She was, therefore, fully supported. Her Beighton's score was 6/9, and her Grahame's questionnaire was 4/5, meeting the New York 2017 criteria.

Treatment initiated: Oxygen concentrator with humidifier, through the fixed station, with a flow rate of 5 liters per minute, 4 to 6 sessions per day of 20 to 40 minutes each. Levocarnitine 750 mg, 3x2 tablets per day, and vitamin C 1g per day in the morning. Baclofen: 10 to 30 mg at a rate of 1 to 3 tablets per day, Nefopam hydrochloride: 30 mg, 1 to 3 tablets per day (on request). Melatonin: 4mg to 6mg/capsule in the evening. Pantoprazole or another proton pump inhibitor (PPI): 40 mg, 1 to 2/day. Prolopa® (Modopar®): 125 mg, ½ Tablet (i.e. 62.5 mg), 2x/day. Resolor®: 2mg/day, 7- to 14-day cure. Lansoÿl®: 1 soup spoon, in the evening. MetaDigest Total® 1/day with the main meal. Compression clothing made to measure: gloves, a vest with long sleeves, long pants.

Evolution: presently, she has almost no dystonia; she is autonomous and continues her studies. The intestinal transit has improved significantly. She smiles and is more fulfilled. She has significantly reduced her medication (she mainly keeps compression garments, oxygen therapy, Levodopa, and intestinal transit regulators).

This was a case of severe dystonia associated with EDS and wrongly attributed to a psychiatric origin.

◆   In mid-December 2018, anxious parents bring me their 10-year-old daughter Charlotte. For several days, even weeks, she had been suffering from sudden paraplegia of the lower limbs. The neurological examinations were all normal. Sadly, she was diagnosed with Münchhausen Syndrome by Proxy and hysterical conversion. Her Beighton's score was 9/9, and the New York criteria for 2017 were met. On the same day, I introduced compressive leggings, fixed a stationary sequential oxygen therapy (2 liters per minute, 15-20 minutes sessions per day, 3-4 times per day), and an adapted and gentle physiotherapy. After a few days, the function of her lower limbs gradually recovered. She was walking again. I saw her again in the middle of December 2019. Charlotte is smiling, intelligent, cheerful, and happy. She is doing very well. She follows a youth movement, does speleology, acrobranching, swimming, naturopathy, osteopathy, and micro kinesis on request. Her mother told me, "Charlotte is alive again!" Charlotte even made a presentation at school for her classmates and teachers in which she explained EDS with drawings. The neuropsychologist said: *"From a behavioral point of view, Charlotte was very willing and eager to do well. She shows good self-observation skills to compensate for her limitations in certain situations. She is a dynamic, smiling young girl who can interact easily. She does not hesitate to express herself at the end of a challenge."*

Conclusion

By understanding the changes in connective tissue and what the effects are, many of EDS's clinical signs and symptoms can be easily explained, avoiding misdiagnosis with potentially severe consequences for the patient.

CHAPTER III

The Interest of Skin Biopsy and Dermal Ultrastructure in EDS

In collaboration with :

Dr. Trinh HERMANNS-LÊ, PhD, Dermatologist
& Mr. Olivier HOUGRAND, Electron Microscopy - Belgium.

Skin biopsy aims to look for abnormalities in connective tissue components, including collagen, in the dermis. Since collagen is present in the tendons and in the skin, the abnormalities observed in the skin with the electron microscope reflect those present in the tendons, which is why the skin biopsy is interesting in Ehlers-Danlos syndrome, especially since it is easy to perform and minimally traumatic for the patient.

The skin biopsy is the only examination that can provide objective evidence to support the clinical diagnosis of hypermobile EDS (hEDS), as genetic mutations are currently unknown, except some genes recently described in a small number of cases which could play a role in hEDS, and other complementary examinations, such as medical imaging, are generally normal.

The biopsy is performed under local anesthesia in an area not exposed to the sun (on the buttocks, inner arm, or elbow) to avoid photo-induced changes in connective tissue that can make reading difficult.

One sample is given in formalin for histological and immuno-histochemical examination, and another in glutaraldehyde for electron microscopic examination.

Techniques for preparing skin biopsy sections:

Skin samples are fixed in 4% glutaraldehyde at 4°C, and then postfixed with osmium tetroxide at 4 °C.

By enclosing the samples, fixed in 4% glutaraldehyde, the tissue sample becomes rigid by impregnating it with a resin (Epon), which hardens when heated (oven at about 60°C) so that it can later be cut with the ultramicrotome. This inclusion process follows the fixation and precedes the embedding, which completes an Epon block's construction.

Fine cuts of 50 to 80 nanometers are then made on the ultramicrotome and placed on copper grids which are stained with heavy metals (Uranyl acetate - Lead Citrate).

The transmission electron microscope works with a flow of electrons that passes through the sections without being able to interact with the C (carbon), N (nitrogen), O (oxygen), P (phosphorus) atoms of the biological material. A contrast with the heavy metals that bind to these atoms is necessary to highlight them. The image is given in grey, black and white levels. It is, therefore, not coloring in the usual sense.

The ultra-fine sections are observed with a transmission electron microscope at various magnifications from 600x to 21,000x.

In optical histology:

Skin samples are fixed with 4% formaldehyde and coated with paraffin. For special staining and immunohistochemistry, sections of 4 to 5 micrometers are made. These samples are observed under optical microscopy at magnifications of 100 to 400x.

1) Hematoxylin-eosin: This stain is the fundamental contrast method for all conventional histological microscopic examinations.

2) Colloidal iron: This staining is used to search for acidic proteoglycan deposits, or to reveal a thickened basement membrane.

3) Orcein Light Green: This is a specific staining to Orcein - Light Green. Orcein binds with excellent selectivity and colors the elastic fibers black-brown. The Light Green provides a coloring of the collagen.

4) Sirius red: The saturated solution of Sirius red in picric acid is an elective solution for making the collagen fibers visible.

5) Investigation of factor XIII: This is the search for a decrease in the immunohistochemical expression of factor XIIIa in dendrocytes, based on an antigen-antibody reaction, revealed in the histological section and observed under the optical microscope.

A skin biopsy can be performed for two purposes:

1. For a culture of fibroblasts to look for genetic mutations. Currently, the search for genetic mutations in EDS can be done by taking blood samples, but it remains unsuccessful in hEDS. Some mutations in the collagen genes can be found in EDS and in other genetic diseases, so they are not specific to EDS.

2. For a morphological study of the connective tissue of the dermis.

Three examinations are performed on the sample:

➤ Histology (optical microscopy) sometimes shows abnormalities, such as elastopathy, which allows suspicion of a classical EDS (cEDS) or hEDS. In vascular EDS (vEDS), the thickness of the dermis and the collagen bundles' diameter are significantly reduced, which explains the transparency of the skin in vEDS.

➤ Immunohistochemistry: The anti-FXIIIa antibody marks the presence of type I dermal dendrocytes (DD-1). The number of DD-1 decreases as soon as the skin tension deviates from a specific norm. Their decrease usually indicates a form of EDS, but a normal number does not exclude EDS.

➤ Ultrastructural examination (by transmission electron microscopy) is the most crucial examination. It allows the visualization of collagen abnormalities: a variable diameter of the fibrils, irregularity of the interfibrillar spaces, and flower-like collagen fibrils. Since the number of flower-like fibrils is variable, sometimes minimal, careful examination of the sections is necessary. Other modifications can also be observed: changes in the elastic fibers, deposits of granulo-filamentous material, star-shaped globules of hyaluronic acid, etc.

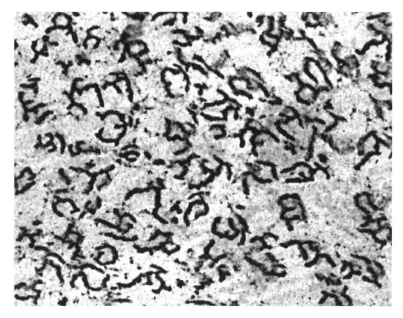

Dermatosparaxis EDS: collagen fibrils in hieroglyphs

The diagnosis of EDS, as with all pathologies, must always be based on clinic findings. Except for dermatosparaxis EDS (dEDS), cutaneous ultrastructural changes in EDS show a high sensitivity but a low specificity. Nevertheless, in the tissue sample, these modifications are reproducible in each of the different EDS types, and thus make it possible to confirm the diagnosis and classify them. Therefore, the sections must be read by an experienced examiner who is familiar with all the changes induced by the different types of EDS.

In hEDS, the diameter of the flower-like collagen fibrils is equal to that of the surrounding normal fibrils, which are rounded in cross-section.

116

Three profiles result from the ultrastructural examination of the biopsies:

➢ High variability of the diameter of collagen fibrils with few flower-like fibrils, and irregularity of the spaces between the fibrils:

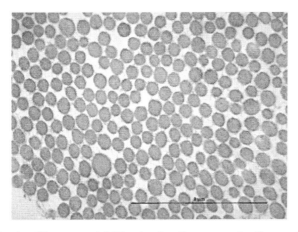

hEDS: significant variability in the diameter of collagen fibrils.

➢ Collagen fibrils of homogeneous or moderately variable diameter, with numerous flowers, and moderate to significant irregularity of the interfibrillar spaces:

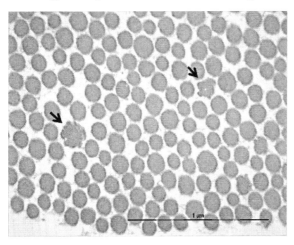

hEDS: flower-shaped fibrils (→), variable fibril diameter and irregularity of fibril spaces.

117

➤ A dense deposit of granulo-filamentous material with variable collagen anomalies:

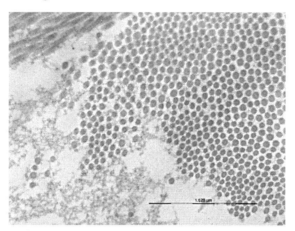

hEDS: dense granulo-filamentous deposit.

The morphological changes described in hEDS can also be observed in some unaffected family members of a patient with hEDS (healthy carrier). However, when these individuals are appropriately examined, they usually have asymptomatic joint hyperlaxity (AJH), or joint hyperlaxity associated with some signs defined by the New York criteria for hEDS, or a Beighton's score below 5/9 or 4/9, and are therefore classified as Hypermobility Spectrum Disorder (HSD). There is a continuum between AJH, HSD, and hEDS. Some patients may develop other symptoms throughout their lives, and their diagnosis may change from HSD to hEDS.

In hEDS, where genetic mutations are not known, skin biopsy for morphological examination is a valuable aid to diagnosis as it is the only way to confirm the diagnosis: other tests (Rx, MRI...) are generally all negative.

It should be noted that a healthy subject with no history of hEDS does not show these ultrastructural changes in his or her dermis.

The earlier the diagnosis is made, the earlier preventive and therapeutic measures can be taken, thus maintaining the patient's quality of life, and also limiting medical costs.

Comparative studies examining connective tissue in tendon and skin biopsies of the same EDS patient have shown that the same EDS-related changes are found at both sites. This proves the ubiquitous distribution of collagen changes. Other articles also shed light on ultrastructural changes in other connective tissues, such as human corneas.

In the new classification, the former I and II are summarized under the term classical EDS or cEDS.

In electron microscopy, the two forms look different. In addition to the variability of fibril spacing and fibrillar diameter, the presence of large flower-like fibrils is mainly reminiscent of cEDS, formerly categorized as Type II. In cEDS, which was formerly categorized as type I, the collagen bundles are disorganized.

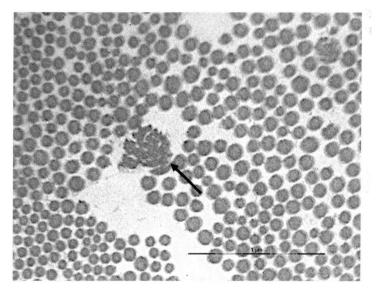

Classical EDS (formerly Type II): large collagen fibrils (→)

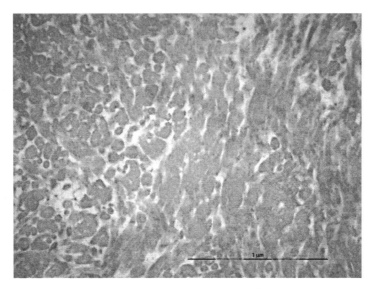

Classical EDS (old type I): Disorganization of the collagen bundles.

In vEDS, which is associated with collagen-3 mutations, on one hand, the collagen bundles are significantly reduced in size. On the other hand, the endoplasmic reticulum of the fibroblasts is expanded, and filled with granular material corresponding to the abnormal collagen that is not excreted from the cell.

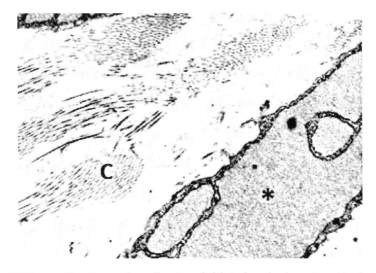

vEDS: small collagen bundles I and dilated endoplasmic reticulum filled with granular material (*).

In the publications following the International Consortium of New York in 2017, it is stated: *"In case of unavailability of genetic tests, the results of transmission electron microscopy (TEM) of collagen flowers in skin biopsies can support but not confirm the clinical diagnosis."*

To be relevant, the skin biopsy results must always be correlated with the patient's clinical examination.

Bibliography :

1. *Piérard, G.E., Piérard-Franchimont, C., Lapière, Ch.M. Histopathology aid at the diagnosis of the Ehlers-Danlos syndrome, gravis and mitis types. International Journal of Dermatology. 1983; 22: 300-4.*

2. *Piérard GE, Le T, Hermanns JF, Nusgens BV, and Lapière CM. Morphometric study of cauliflower collagen fibrils in dermatosparaxis of the calves. Coll Relat Res. 1986; 6:481-492.*

3. *Piérard GE, Le T, Piérard-Franchimont C and Lapière CM. Morphometric study of cauliflower collagen fibrils in Ehlers-Danlos syndrome type I. Coll Relat Res. 1988; 8:453-7.*

4. *Nusgens BV, Verellen-Dumoulin C, Hermanns-Lê T, De Paepe A, Nuytinck L, Piérard GE, Lapière CM. Evidence for a relationship between Ehlers-Danlos type VII C in humans and bovine dermatosparaxis. Nat Genet. 1992 Jun; 1(3):214-7.*

5. *Harvey, J.M., Anton-Lamprecht, I. (1992) Stromal aberrations, in Diagnostic ultrastructure of non-neoplastic diseases, (eds J.M. Papadimitriou, D.W. Henderson and D.V. Spagnolo), Churchill Livingstone Medical division of Longman Group, UK Limited.*

6. *Piérard GE, Hermanns-Lê T, Arrese-Estrada J, Piérard-Franchimont C and Lapière C. Structure of the dermis in type VIIC Ehlers-Danlos syndrome. Am J Dermatopathol. 1993; 15:127-32.*

7. *Hausser, I., Anton-Lamprecht, I. Differential ultrastructural aberrations of collagen fibrils in Ehlers-Danlos syndrome types I-IV as a means of diagnostic and classification. Human Genetics.1994;3: 394-407.*

8. *Hermanns-Lê T. Comment j'explore... certaines affections cutanées par examen ultrastructural de la peau. Rev Med Liège. 2000; 55:954-6.*

9. *Nuytinck L, Freund M, Lagae L, Piérard GE, Hermanns-Lê T and De Paepe A. Classical Ehlers-Danlos syndrome caused by a mutation in type I collagen. Am J Hum Genet. 2000; 66:1398-402.*

10. *Hermanns-Lê T and Piérard GE. Factor XIIIa-positive dendrocyte rarefaction in Ehlers- Danlos syndrome, classic type. Am J Dermatopathol. 2001; 23:427-30.*

11. *Hermanns-Lê T. Dendrocytes et physiopathologie de la structure du derme. Thèse de Doctorat ULg 2003*

12. *Hermanns-Lê T and Piérard GE. Collagen fibril arabesques in connective tissue disorders. Am J Clin Dermatol. 2006; 7:323-6.*

13. *Hermanns-Lê T and Piérard GE. Ultrastructural alterations of elastic fibers and other dermal components in Ehlers-Danlos syndrome of the hypermobile type. Am J Dermatopathol. 2007; 29:370-3.*

14. *Quatresooz P, Hermanns-Lê T, Piérard GE. Le syndrome d'Ehlers-Danlos. Qu'y-at-il sous la pointe de l'iceberg ? Rev Med Liège. 2008; 63 : Synthèse 2008 : 60-6564*

15. *Malfait F, Syx D, Vlummens P, Symoens S, Nampoothiri S, Hermanns-Lê T, Van Laer L, De Paepe A. Musculocontractural Ehlers-Danlos Syndrome (former EDS type VIB) and adducted thumb clubfoot syndrome (ATCS) represent a single clinical entity caused by mutations in the dermatan-4-sulfotransferase 1 encoding CHST14 gene. Hum Mutat. 2010 Nov;31(11):1233-9.*

16. *Hermanns-Lê T, Reginster MA, Piérard-Franchimont C, Delvenne P, Piérard GE and Manicourt D. Dermal ultrastructure in low Beighton score members of 17 families with hypermobile-type Ehlers-Danlos syndrome. J Biomed Biotechnol. 2012; 2012:878107.*

17. *Ronceray S, Miquel J, Lucas A, Piérard GE, Hermanns-Lê T, De Paepe A and Dupuy A. Ehlers-Danlos Syndrome Type VIII: A Rare Cause of Leg Ulcers in Young Patients. Case Rep Dermatol Med. 2013; 2013:469505.*

18. *Hermanns-Lê T, Piérard GE et Angenot P, Fibromyalgie: un syndrome d'Ehlers-Danlos syndrome de type hypermobile type qui s'ignore? Revue Médicale de Liège, vol. 68, no. 1, pp. 22–24, 2013.*

19. *Hermanns-Lê T, Reginster MA, Piérard-Franchimont C and Piérard GE . Ehlers-Danlos syndrome. In: Diagnostic Electron Microscopy: A Practical Guide to Tissue Preparation and Interpretation, Ed: John Wiley & Sons, Ltd., Chichester. 2013; 309-21.*

20. *Hermanns-Lê T, Piérard GE, Piérard-Franchimont C and Delvenne P. Gynecologic and obstetric impact of the Ehlers-Danlos syndrome: clues from scrutinizing dermal ultrastructural alterations. Gynecol. 2014; 2:1.*

21. *Symoens S, Malfait F, Vlummens P, Hermanns-Lê T, Syx D, De Paepe A. A novel splice variant in the N-propeptide of COL5A1 causes an EDS*

phenotype with severe kyphoscoliosis and eye involvement. PLoS One. 2011;6(5):e20121. Epub 2011 May 17.

22. *Hermanns-Lê T, Manicourt D, Piérard G. Familial expression of spontaneous cervical artery dissections and Ehlers-Danlos syndrome hypermobile type. J Skin Stem Cell. 2014; 1(3): e27023*

23. *Hermanns-Lê T, Piérard GE, Piérard-Franchimont C, Manicourt D. Syndrome d'Ehlers- Danlos de type hypermobile : une atteinte multi systémique. Apport de l'ultrastructure cutanée pour une prise en charge personnalisée. Rev Med Liège. 2015; 70: 325-330.*

24. *Hermanns-Lê T and Piérard GE (2015) Skin ultrastructural similarities between Fibromyalgia and Ehlers-Danlos syndrome hypermobility type. J Ost Arth 1: 104. doi:10.4172/joas.1000104*

25. *Syx D, Van Damme T, Symoens S, Maiburg MC, van de Laar I, Morton J, Suri M, Del Campo M, Hausser I, Hermanns-Lê T, De Paepe A, Malfait F. Genetic Heterogeneity and Clinical Variability in Musculocontractural Ehlers–Danlos Syndrome Caused by Impaired Dermatan Sulfate Biosynthesis. Hum Mutat. 2015, 36:535–547.*

26. *Hermanns-Lê T, Piérard GE, Manicourt D, Piérard-Franchimont C. Clinical and ultrastructural skin alterations in the Ehlers-Danlos syndrome, hypermobility type. Dermatol Open J. 2016; 1(2): 22-26. doi: 10.17140/ DRMTOJ-1-107*

27. *Low tendon stiffness and abnormal ultrastructure distinguish classic Ehlers-Danlos syndrome from benign joint hypermobility syndrome in patients Nielsen R H, Couppé C, Jensen J K, Olsen M R, Heinemeier K M, Malfait F, Symoens S, De Paepe A, Schjerling P, Magnusson S P, Remvig L, and Kjaer M, The FASEB Journal. 2014 doi: 10.1096/fj.14-249656.*

CHAPTER IV

The Paris Criteria (2017)
EDS Comorbidities and their Management
Additional Examinations

By Dr. Stéphane Daens
In collaboration with Doctor Isabelle Dubois-Brock & Professor Claude Hamonet

The Paris Criteria

The signs and symptoms of the current New York hEDS Criteria are quite limiting. Those criteria Include: Beighton's age-related score, soft and velvety skin, moderate skin stretching, atrophic striae and stretch marks, piezogenic papules on the feet, recurrent or multiple abdominal hernias, and atrophic scars. Below are some of the conditions that can be highlighted during additional examinations: pelvic prolapse without significant history, dental and palatal abnormalities, arachnodactyly, marfanoid wingspan, mitral valve prolapse, aortic root dilatation, diffuse pain, or joint instability or dislocations; and a family history of hEDS. These do not represent a complete echo of our daily clinical practice and are often subjective. In addition, these were established without a control group (healthy people, without hEDS).

The Paris hEDS criteria (*Claude Hamonet, Isabelle Brock, et al. 2017*) seem to be much more explicit and diversified (62 points). The strength of these criteria is the presence of a control group of subjects in the clinical trial, which was not the case with the New York criteria.

This study in Paris was able to highlight the most revealing and significant clinical points of hEDS:

➤ The patient suffering from hEDS is a *diffuse body of pain* with *intense fatigue*, which Professor Claude Hamonet calls *the asthenoalgic syndrome*.

➤ It could be said that in some cases, it is a hemorrhagic body, with bleeding in 83% of cases: bleeding gums, heavy menstrual bleeding, bruises, internal digestive bleeding and more.

The most important signs and symptoms of EDS examined in this study are (*C. Hamonet, I. Brock et al.*):

➤ The pain (present in 93% of cases) is articular and periarticular (98%), muscular (82%), abdominal (77%), thoracic (71%), genital (75%), headache (84%), cutaneous hyperesthesia (39%).

➤ Chronic fatigue (95%).

➤ Sleep disorders (85%).

➤ Proprioception disorders (dysproprioception): dislocations (90%), hypermobility (97% of cases, and not only based on the Beighton's score), sprains and pseudo-sprains (86%).

➤ Skin changes: excessive stretch (76%), thinness (91%), fragility (87%), stretch marks (64%), delayed healing (85%), bleeding (92%).

➤ Gastrointestinal symptoms: gastroesophageal reflux (80%), the feeling of fullness (69%), miscarriage (48%), constipation (72%).

➤ ENT symptoms: hyperacusis (89%), hearing loss (57%), tinnitus (69%), hyperosmia (69%), dizziness (80%).

➤ Ophthalmological manifestations: visual fatigue (86%), myopia (56%).

➤ Gynecological symptoms: heavy menstruation (78%), difficult delivery (78%).

➤ Dysautonomia (76%): chills (77%), profuse sweating (74%), pseudo-Raynaud's syndrome (74%), tachyarrhythmias (66%).

- Urinary disorders: pollakiuria, urgency, and leakage (59%).

- Cognitive disorders: memory, attention, concentration, orientation (68%).

- Dystonia (66%), sometimes impressive (involuntary movements, tremors, twitching, sometimes restricted to a hemibody or the extremities, contractures), pseudoparalysis or paresis of one or more limbs.

- In around 80% of cases, there is also a mast cell activation disorder, or MCAD, related to EDS. It is a non-clonal affection in which serum tryptase level is usually within the normal limits (see the chapter on mast cell disorders).

The hereditary characteristics should always be considered when informing the family about this disease's high genetic transmission rates.

With this criteria, we can often quickly detect painful family cases, whose suffering had not been considered or solved until now ("well, I was able to put a name on my suffering after so much wandering!"). In addition, we can detect and prevent individuals, asymptomatic carriers or pauci-symptomatic, from bleeding during surgery, the possible delay of healing, and potentially serious consequences such as wires reabsorbing faster than usual, and unusual healing in abdominal and thoracic surgery, for example, inducing suture release.

The presence of arterial dilatations and heart valve abnormalities should be systematically investigated: a mitral valve prolapse, micro-rupture or total rupture of cord, heart valve failure, etc.

As a result, I ask to examine all children of any parent who has been diagnosed with EDS, as soon as the child turns 15 or 16. This is the age when we see wisdom tooth extractions, a higher incidence of sports accidents, operations and the beginning of arterial dilatation. Occasionally I meet younger children who are symptomatic or whose parents are carriers of a rarer variant of the disease; if specific genetic mutations are known, we can search for them (vascular variant, kyphoscoliotic, classic, and more). In some variants of EDS, special examinations may be necessary from early childhood.

I would like to highlight a few special populations that need to be treated differently when dealing with an hEDS diagnosis and treatment plan:

> *"Health depends more on precautions than doctors."*
> *Jacques Bossuet, artist, writer, bishop (1627-1704)*

EDS Comorbidities and Their Management

Concerning Pregnancy

General information:

A pregnancy is always a sensitive time for any patient, but especially so for one with EDS. First, it is important to inform the woman that, most of the time, it is safe for hEDS patients to be pregnant and have children.

On the one hand, the patient is excited about the great news of expecting a child, sometimes after several miscarriages. On the other hand, there is the fear of complications and the fear of transmitting the disease to her child. Some patients do not want to have a child so as to not pass on the disease, the curse, that has ruined their own lives.

What we can say is: every child is different and every EDS life is unique. Sometimes they are asymptomatic or less symptomatic, and in other cases, the disease is more prominent. No one can assure the expectant mother that her child will be a healthy carrier or symptomatic.

In each case, the patient should know that they will probably be intelligent, emotional, and sensitive children. They are often creative and outgoing, beautiful people. It is the first point that we should tell her without hesitation.

As far as the pregnancy itself is concerned, as long as the patient informs their obstetrician, the risk factors can be discussed and prepared for, lessening the potential for unexpected complications.

The vascular variant of EDS:

I am personally in favor of egg donation for women, or sperm donation for men, if they have this variant and want a child. It is possible if the patient seeks our advice before conception. Adopting is also an option for this rare form, where the risk of arterial complications throughout life is significant (see the section on cardiovascular events below).

In the event of pregnancy in a patient with a vascular variant (collagen 3 A1 mutation), uterine rupture is also possible, and the gynecologist must be informed quickly.

Premature induction can be considered to avoid excessive pressure on the uterine walls. The vascular variant is scarce (less than 1% of EDS variants) and is likely to remain so, as most women have repeated miscarriages.

Here are some things that gynecologists and obstetricians should be aware of (for all variants of EDS):

> Consider pregnancies as risky to better monitor patients and be able to quickly react to possible complications (which occur in 66% of cases).

> There are more spontaneous miscarriages (26%).

> If a premature opening of the cervix is detected due to tissue loosening, one should not hesitate to cerclage the cervix around the 12th week of pregnancy (but I do not recommend this automatically).

> In case of early uterine contractions, urge rest and stop chemically the contractions.

> The risk of pre-eclampsia (with pregnancy-related high blood pressure, edema in the periphery, the presence of protein in the urine - proteinuria) does not seem to be more common in my practice. The general population's prevalence of pre-eclampsia is around 2% to 8% of

pregnancies (this varies according to country, socio-economic conditions, and risk factors such as obesity or diabetes).

➢ Premature membrane rupture may occur; the membranes belonging to the baby may be a factor in diagnosing EDS in the child. It is essential because if the father has EDS and not the pregnant mother, the baby may be a carrier, so a premature rupture of the membrane is possible.

➢ During birth, especially with the first child and sometimes with the ones after, the cervix can remain closed or open only slowly despite existing uterine contractions. Labor can then be long and painful. One should not wait unnecessarily before going into labor (chemically) or considering a caesarean section.

➢ Because the connective tissue is damaged and the skin becomes more sensitive, there is a risk of tearing during vaginal delivery. An episiotomy should therefore be considered if the skin tissue is under tension.

➢ There is a risk of bleeding during delivery, so I recommend that one or two units of blood (concentrated red blood cells) be available in the delivery room. If possible, Exacyl® 1000mg (tranexamic acid), in drinking ampoules, should be taken three times a day from the day before the birth in the morning until three to five days afterward, unless this is contraindicated. Vitamin C can be added during pregnancy at a rate of 2 to 3 grams/day (it increases collagen production, is a powerful antioxidant, reduces pre-and post-operative bleeding by increasing the adhesion of platelets to the vascular walls, and stabilizes mast cells).

➢ The risk does not seem to be more significant for vaginal delivery than for cesarean section. However, the consequences for the child's microbiota cannot be neglected. In any case, probiotics should be administered during pregnancy (see later in the chapter on the importance of the mother's microbiota for the baby).

➢ The anesthetist must always bear in mind that anesthesia in EDS can be capricious: epidurals do not always work or are only partially effective. As far as general anesthesia is concerned, early awakening or late awakening are noted. It can be the result of a variable metabolism of anesthetic substances in altered connective tissue.

➢ As much as possible, non-resorbable suture material should be used, and the quality of hemostasis checked repeatedly. External sutures should be left in place two to three times the regular duration to compensate for slower healing and avoid scaring.

In hEDS, it should be noted that there do not seem to be more cases of endometriosis, which is too often diagnosed in a context of dyspareunia (61%), dysmenorrhea (72%), and menorrhagia (76%). One can therefore speak of a quite frequent pseudo-endometriosis in EDS. The average number of children is also relatively normal for a woman with EDS (which is not the case with endometriosis).

Children and Parental Concerns

We doctors should not hesitate to see children at a young age when they complain of muscular and skeletal pain (especially in the calves, thighs, and spine). These are not growing pains, a diagnosis all too often mentioned in a hurry. Children can also experience headaches, fatigue, gastroesophageal reflux (GERD), gastroparesis, abdominal cramps, food intolerances, cyclic vomiting syndrome, diarrhea and constipation, sometimes persistent, MCAD, dysautonomia, and more.

There are more cases of dyslexia, dyspraxia, dysorthographia, dyscalculia, attention deficit disorder, hyperactivity, and high potentials.

Mostly they are intelligent, sensitive, emotional, curious, and creative children. They are often aspiring artists due to hyper-sensitivity levels: they like to draw, do handicrafts, play construction games, and more. Certainly, hypersensitivity and hypersensoriality are involved as well as dysproprioception and dysautonomia (see these chapters).

Mothers and fathers who are EDS carriers are often torn between justified concern for the future of their children (who are mostly EDS carriers) and the guilt for having passed it on to them: "It is my fault if ..."

As Professor Claude Hamonet often says, although EDS can be painful and cause situations of disability (a term described by the professor himself more than 25 years ago, and used in everyday language today), it can be also seen as *a gift*. It may be difficult to read at first, but in this world of constant stress, violence, and selfishness, EDS patients are *beautiful people*; they are good friends who listen to others well, and exercise a profession that is usually geared towards others: social work, nursing, medicine, pedagogy, psychology, personal assistance, and more. Patients can often do several things at once and manage large companies with ease.

Considering that the disease persists despite Darwinian selection, it probably brings a plus to this society and has done so for a long time. Had this not been the case, it would have been swept away by time and subsequent generations. In our societies, we not only need muscular warriors who are resistant to everything, but we also need people who communicate, who listen, who negotiate, who are artists, architects, and philosophers.

Joint hypermobility (JH) and EDS including, because it is part of the same family (which includes asymptomatic hypermobility, Hypermobility Spectrum Disorders or HSD, and hypermobile Ehlers-Danlos Syndrome), does not go back to yesterday or 1891 (cf. Chernogubow, in Russia):

Hippocrates developed a technique to reduce shoulder dislocations mainly because of young hyperlaxed archers who repeatedly dislocated their shoulders during archery.

More than 2,400 years ago, Hippocrates and Herodotus (the Father of History, 484-425 B.C.) reported on Nomads and the Scythian people's peculiarities which remind us of EDS: they had lax joints and multiple scars.

Hippocrates: On Airs, Waters, and Places, 400 B.C.
Herodotus: Histories, History of the Persian wars, 430 B.C.

As some young archers or ethnicities were suffering from joint hyperlaxity, EDS certainly already existed (since about 10% of them must have triggered an EDS during their lifetime). According to the British-American biological anthropologist John Lawrence Angel (1915-1986)[32], referring to the study of human skeletons, it is essential to know that life expectancy (mean age at death) in the 4th century B.C. in Greece (Classical Period) was around 42.6 years for men and 33.7 years for women. [33] Also, childbirth was the cause of to 10% of women's premature death. Infant mortality was also remarkably high during that era; consequently, one in two children did not reach the age of 10. They possibly suffered from Ehlers-Danlos Syndrome, but there was no reliable healthcare system to give them appropriate care and/or the necessary lifetime to develop symptoms that some authors could have reported.

The Most Common Problems in Early Childhood

Infants and toddler, carriers of the EDS, can already show unique signs and symptoms. Above all, never consider mothers as Münchhausen syndromes by proxy simply because they often go to the emergency room, genuinely concerned about their child's condition.

Some advice:

➢ Listen to and question EDS patients carefully; all systems and organs should be involved. Even if it seems strange or impossible to you, the strange and impossible is common in EDS. In my experience, patients should always be listened to and believed about their symptoms. As Professor Hamonet told me: "No EDS patient has ever lied to me!"

---

[32] J.L. Angel. The length of life in ancient Greece. Journal of Gerontology. 1947;2(1):18-24.
[33] Pearson K. On the change in expectation of life in man during a period of circa 2000 years. Biometrika. 1901;1:261-264.

Sir William Osler (born 1849 in Bone Head, Canada, and died 1918 in Oxford, Great Britain) was a Canadian doctor and one of the famous Johns Hopkins Hospital's four founders. He was considered *the father of modern Medicine*, and was often described as *One of the greatest diagnosticians ever to use a stethoscope*. He would often repeat this sentence, that no doctor should forget: *Listen to your patient, he is telling you the diagnosis.*

➢ Finally, patients should always be thoroughly examined, in underwear, on the examination table and then in a standing position. It may seem obvious, but it seems that fewer doctors are examining patients during office hours. The astonishment on the patients' faces when they are asked to undress is noticeable. It is a pity, I did not learn internal medicine this way: *Caregivers ought to listen, examine and take their time.*

➢ Do not forget the question of sexual activity, which is too little addressed by doctors, often due to prudery. We must always ask couples about their sexual habits and help them. It should be done as soon as possible before tensions arise and they separate.

➢ In EDS, there are many separations and divorces, including the actual abandonment of the marital home by some *gentlemen*, leaving behind wife and child(ren) with EDS, fleeing from their responsibilities afar as possible. Therefore, these abandoned people try to survive. In the best case, the abandoned mother has a job, often part-time or four-fifths. However, much of the time, these mothers are on disability and have low income. They often have to choose between caring for themselves or their children. The choice is often made quickly: *Once a mom, always a mom!*

This can be problematic as, with EDS, many of the treatments designed to improve the patients' condition and provide relief are available but financially inaccessible. Leaving so many patients behind, without treatment, is unacceptable in our so-called civilized societies with a high socioeconomic level.

ALWAYS BELIEVE EDS MOMS AND DADS!

In practice, unfortunately, parents of children with EDS are rarely believed when they arrive at the emergency room. However, all parents, especially those of children with special needs, always know when something is wrong with their child. In EDS, moreover, there are often strange things that are manifold, complex, and different. It is essential to avoid the abuse of mothers and fathers who only want their children's best.

Key Symptoms and Signs in Early Childhood

Some babies vomit their whole bottle or compotes, which rightly causes great concern to parents and can lead to the baby falling off the growth charts (weight and size, depending on age) or causing nutritional deficiencies (in vitamins and trace elements), metabolic alkalosis, and more. The lower esophageal sphincter (LES) between the esophagus and the stomach contains collagen and seems to be ineffective or even opens up to a greater or lesser extent over time (role of proprioception?). It is variable, which confuses some gastroenterologists, especially since examination by fibroscopy is often ordinary. The role of dysautonomia (Porges' Theory), proprioception, and mast cell activation disorder in the development of these refluxes is essential. Treatment consists of proton pump inhibitors or PPIs (be sure to choose a PPI with a lactose-free excipient, as this substance is often not tolerated), probiotics, osteopathy, physiotherapy (regularize the parasympathetic system), and more. A gastroenterologist should also look for, and treat, hiatal hernia. MCAD should be treated (see the relevant chapter) as necessary. See also the chapter concerning nutrition in EDS.

Gastroparesis and food intolerance should be excluded (see below, the chapter about nutrition). In these cases, a mix of enzymes can be administered before meals, which already cuts molecules into pieces in the stomach, facilitating gastric emptying and is also useful in food intolerance cases. A relatively large part of gastroparesis can also be related to MCAD, dysproprioception, and dysautonomia, and can be improved by specific treatment.

For information, the contents of MetaDigest Total®: ginger rhizome extract and a complete mixture of enzymes for the digestion of both lipids and carbohydrates and proteins: Protease 41,000 FCC units; Cellulase 1,750 FCC units; Amylase 1,400 FCC units; Alpha-galactosidase 300 FCC units; Maltase 16,050 FCC units; Lactase 340 FCC units; Lipase 1,050 FCC units; etc. Contents of MetaDigest Lacto® & Lactaid® : Lactase 9,000 FCC units.

Pyloric stenosis or Meckel's diverticulum (although these do not seem to be more frequent in EDS) should also be investigated in cases of significant regurgitation in an infant.

Infants may have a *mast cell activation disorder* (MCAD) associated with EDS, with ectopic skin, eczema, dermographism, food intolerance, colic, a severely distended abdomen, breathing difficulties, gastroparesis, GERD, and more. The pediatrician should be consulted immediately; he or she can administer specific MCAD treatments in pediatric doses (antihistamines, vitamin C, Cromoglycate, and more).

Constipation can be persistent. The causes may be varied and may be partly related to the particularities of the connective tissue (which is looser) that makes up the intestinal mucosa and mesentery (tissue that holds the intestine in place), but also to possible additional dysautonomia that slows down intestinal peristalsis (intestinal movements) and altered walls' proprioception.

The consequences can be an enlargement of the intestine or *megacolon*. Of course, a congenital disease called Hirschsprung's disease, the most common cause of a child's megacolon must be excluded.

Clinicians should also look out for a *dolichocolon*: a congenital total or local extension of the colon, well known in Marfan's syndrome, but also frequent in EDS.

Sometimes both conditions are present; in this case, it is a *mega-dolichocolon*. The symptoms are: constipation, feeling of fullness, partial or complete occlusion, with a severe clinical condition. This is a medical emergency and should be treated as such.

A severe complication of chronic constipation is intussusception and rectal prolapse:

Intussusception is incorporating a section of the intestine into the intestinal segment immediately downstream (above). Think of it like the folding of an extended scope or a gloved finger that turns around. It can lead to intestinal obstruction with severe pain, vomiting, paralytic ileus (the intestinal transit is stopped, with the silence of the intestinal sound at the auscultation, or *sepulchral silence*, which is a sign of a medical emergency). Intussusception can rarely lead to an intestinal rupture, with severe peritonitis: An increase in the intestine pressure leading to increased pressure on the intestinal wall, reduced blood flow, followed by hypoxia-anoxia, and the death of a part of the intestine, which is called *necrosis*. This is both a medical and surgical emergency. It is the most common cause of intestinal obstruction in infants and young children, and even more so in those with EDS. It can also occur in adults.

N.B.: Veterinarians are used to this type of problem and are generally more familiar with EDS than their human medicine counterparts.

In EDS, it is more common, on the one hand, because of the altered properties of the intestine and the mesenteries' connective tissue, and, on the other hand, the decrease in intestinal peristalsis (favored by dysautonomia).

Rectal prolapse is a prolapse of the rectum through the anus, caused by strong thrusts during bowel movements. *Fecal incontinence* is also possible.

In older children who stand on their feet, and in adults, it is essential to take abdominal standard x-rays (*blank radiological exam*) lying down and then standing up. Indeed, the laxity of the mesenteries causes the intestines, and especially the colon, to fall out due to gravity, creating a difficult path for the progress of the stool.

These children also have *anal fissures* or even *tears* in the anus during the evacuation of stools, which is very painful and aggravates constipation (they hold back to avoid pain during a bowel movement).

Recommended treatment for constipation
(except in emergency cases)

It is necessary to avoid stool softeners and instead use paraffin oils. Lansoÿl® , which has the taste of *cuberdons*, is preferred by children. Moreover, it allows the sometimes very hard stool to slide at the level of the rectum and the anus, avoiding anal tears, as the anus has fragile mucosal membrane in EDS.

Apply local heat to soften the stool: warm but lukewarm compresses or gel. Be careful not to burn the sensitive skin.

External massage of the intestine by a physiotherapist who can then teach the parents the appropriate technique.

If there is no contraindication, administer Levocarnitine orally in several doses at 50 mg/kg/day. The maximum dose is three g/day for children. Levocarnitine decreases constipation and intestinal bloating, improves fatigue, and relieves musculo-skeletal pain.

Triphala Churna powder (Ayurvedic medicine). General dosage is as follows (powder): Infants (6 – 12 Months): 500 mg – 1000 mg; Toddler (1 – 3 yo): 750 mg – 1500 mg; Preschooler (3 – 5 yo): 1000 mg – 2 grams; Grade-Schooler (5 – 12 yo):1500 mg – 3 grams; Teenager (13 – 19 yo): 2 grams – 4 grams; Adults (19 – above 60 yo):3 grams – 6 grams. Caution: Triphala extract tablets or capsules: maximum dosage is 2g per day. Generally, extract tablets of Triphala contain about 500mg to 750mg extract.

A *medial arcuate ligament* with mesenteric claudication should be excluded. The *Medial Arcuate Ligament Syndrome* (MALS), which also occurs in adults, was first described in 1963. It consists of extrinsic compression of the coeliac trunk's origin (the arterial trunk that supplies the intestine) by a ligamentum structure. Clinically, it consists of a triad: epigastric pain (upper abdomen), vomiting, and weight loss. The pain is maximal at mealtime or shortly after. Laparoscopy (small holes and insertion of a camera and instruments, without complete opening of the abdomen) is a method that I recommend, and must be performed by a digestive surgeon familiar with EDS and its possible surgical complications.

General advice: It should always be considered that the baby, born to one or both parents with EDS, is a carrier. This avoids bleeding surgical tragedies and unsightly scarring.

There are more *middle ear infections*, partly due to an excessively dilated Eustachian tube, which promotes the rise of germs to the middle ear (the part of the ear between the eardrum and the inner ear).

Thick and sticky secretions favor infections of the respiratory tract. They may be secondary to a change in the bronchial cells' ciliary activity (probably due to the connective tissue's particular characteristics on which they rest and dysproprioception) and to diaphragmatic weakness, which favors inadequate chest expansion, possible atelectasis, and stagnation of secretions. The infection should be treated, and N-acetylcysteine (NAC) tried.

NAC (Lysomucil® Junior, 2% syrup) in acute and chronic cases to prevent recurrence: 10 ml/day, divided into two or three doses in children under two years of age; 20 ml/day, divided into two or three doses in children 2 to 7 years of age; 20 to 30 ml/day, divided into two or three doses in children over seven years of age. NAC is also a potent antioxidant and mast cell stabilizer. Add vitamin C, 1g/day (anti-infective, stabilizes mast cells, antioxidant). Perform adapted respiratory physiotherapy. If there are no contraindications, try oxygen therapy coupled with percussion, performed by physiotherapists specialized in pediatric respiratory physiotherapy.

Dysproprioception of the respiratory tract and throat can also cause *wrong ways* (proprioceptive sensors misperceive the passage of water, saliva, and food) or a *pseudo asthma* (due to a poor perception of air passage). Appropriate physiotherapy and speech therapy should be offered. Singing can also improve wrong ways in EDS, probably through proprioception rehabilitation, muscle strengthening, and the improvement of the vagal brake (Porges' Theory).

IMPORTANT:

Whether children or adults, EDS patients rarely develop a fever (defined as rectal temperature > 37.5 or 38°C). Their initial temperature is often around 35.5°C (95.9°F), and when they reach 37°C (98.6°F), they are very sick as if they had 39°C (102.2°F). This dysregulation, probably associated with dysautonomia, leads to a trivialization of symptoms in hospital emergency rooms (even in case of Covid). It is, therefore, possible to overlook a potentially severe infection!

The Walking and School-age Child

A child stands, walks, and runs around. He can start walking a little later or go straight from sitting to standing without crawling. There is nothing serious about this. They should not be forced. It is advisable to look for muscular hypotonia, which can be present in EDS.

It is similar to what Professor Hamonet told me about certain native African tribes (he is also a doctor of social anthropology) where children are forbidden to crawl, because it reminds them of the migration of animals in the savannah. This makes the medical term for EDS patients of zebras funny.

Children with EDS can fall a bit more often and are often seen as clumsy due to dysproprioception. They can be hyperactive due to pain, and because of dysautonomia. They can also be distracted, leading to a possibly improper diagnosis of attention deficit disorder.
They have repeated sprains (hyperlaxity of the periarticular structures + dysproprioception), sometimes with torn bones in the ankles, but not systematically because the ligaments are so overstretched that usually they do not injure themselves.

Hypersensoriality can be very annoying and can lead to the child becoming isolated:

➢ If it manifests itself as intense photophobia (hypersensitivity to light), there are lenses, non-corrective but tinted, specially designed to attenuate this phenomenon: yellow or pink for day and night (for car headlights, the sun, too strong interior lamps) or bluish for computer work. The tint of the lenses must be adjusted from case to case. Gaming glasses might be useful.

➢ In the case of hyperacusis, some earplugs filter out specific sound frequencies. Brain habituation techniques should be tried: sound therapy, cognitive behavioral therapy. Hypoacusis is also common (see the chapter on neurology and ENT), regardless of whether the hearing loss is genuine or circumstantial (the brouhaha's sign).

➢ In case of cutaneous hypersensitivity, one should consider having custom-made compression garments (or cycling clothing sold in supermarkets, which is cheaper as custom garments are not always reimbursed).

➢ Hyperosmia (pathological increase in smell) is an unusual situation, but has been encountered. Try to put on a surgical mask, avoid unpleasant smells, and gradually get used to less aggressive smells (brain habituation). See chapters on neurology, ENT, and MCAD). Hyposmia does occur, but less frequently.

➢ Hypergeusia (heightened sense of taste) is rare. Hypogeusia (diminished sense of taste) or ageusia (loss of sense of taste) is more frequent.

As a reminder, there are five primary flavors:

♦ Sweet

♦ Salty

♦ Sour

♦ Bitter

♦ UMAMI (うま味), a taste sensation caused by the monosodium glutamate in Asian food. This is a Japanese term, derived from the terms *umai* (delicious), and *mi* (taste). This flavor was described, in 1908, by Professor Kikunae IKEDA, Imperial University of Tokyo, Japan.

Sensory isolation is not recommended for hypersensoriality, whether photophobia, hyperacusis, or hyperosmia. Sensory deprivation can aggravate these phenomena, as sensory organs no longer stimulate the brain. It will then react to stimuli even more strongly than before.

Children can later present with *nocturnal enuresis* (bed-wetting). In these cases, I recommend wearing custom-made compression pants (which restore sensations and improve proprioception). The development is often quickly favorable.

Constipation sometimes persists: see above.

Pediatric patients often express *muscle pain*, which some doctors clumsily refer to as growing pain. I often tell the parents of small EDS children: "When you see giraffes growing in the savannah, they do not cry out in pain! "

This pain is localized either in the front leg or in the lateral peroneal muscles. They are usually the result of varus on the feet. They are usually false Lelièvre hollow feet with retraction of the inner plantar arches, anterior hyper support of the feet, and heels' hyper support. These changes lead to overstimulation of these muscle groups.

Adjustment: I recommend consulting a posturologist and wearing custom insoles; the pain usually passes. For muscular-tendon-like retractions, mainly of the leg flexors, perform slight stretches (morning and evening), either at the physiotherapists or home on the bed.

They also complain about pain in the quadriceps and posterior flexor muscles (thigh muscles). In my experience this is mostly In male children.

Adjustment: consult a posturologist, have custom made posture insoles and compression shorts (after testing a Bermuda short of the cyclist type). The pain often disappears quickly, and the children begin to ask for them: *"Mum, can I put my shorts on, please? That gives me a good feeling!"* When a child is relieved by something, it spontaneously asks for it again. This is always a good sign!

At School

They are often *high potentials* or HP, which leads to attention problems because they look at everything and everywhere around them. They are often quite excited in their chair; they get up, sit down, and move all the time. They are often hyperactive. It is necessary to rule out pain in the pelvis and back and have it treated if necessary. Sometimes they simply look for sensations by moving all the time (because of dysproprioception). They are often confused with ADHD (Attention Deficit Hyperactivity Disorder). These children with ADHD usually look everywhere without fixing a precise point of the room.

Advice:

- Think about buying a memory foam cushion for school and home. It will help them move less and provide relief for pelvic and back pain. Posture will also be improved.

- Inform the teaching staff and issue certificates explaining the illness and the limits it imposes. Give copies to the class teacher, careers adviser, headteacher, and sports teacher.

- Regarding gymnastics and sports: The child or adolescent can follow the class but should not do potentially tiring or painful exercises, such as hanging from the trellis with the risk of dislocating the shoulders, jumping over structures during gymnastics (dysproprioception, clumsiness), running (risk of sprains, shortness of breath, muscular debts, fatigue). Common sense must prevail.

- We must rely on the child/youth and adapt to him/her and the expression of his/her illness day after day. Children with EDS always tell the truth about their pain because they want to be like

143

the others and do the required exercises: The way other pupils look at their disability can be devastating. They are courageous, sometimes too courageous, so they need to be moderated.

- Swimming: Avoid risky swimming movements such as back crawling (shoulder pain, the danger of bumping into the pool), butterfly, or dolphin (shoulders, spine). Crawling is advisable with caution (stress on the cervical vertebrae when breathing, pain in the shoulders, knees, hips, and ankles when moving limbs). Breaststroke swimming may be encouraged but can cause pain in the hips due to abduction movements, knees due to water pressure, and the cervical vertebrae when breathing. Swimming can be adjusted with short fins and a floating board, or a floating paddle under the armpits. One should also beware of chlorine allergies (asthma and sinusitis) and too cold water, which is often poorly tolerated by patients. There are diving suits adapted to the pool to resist the cold and improve the pool's proprioception.

- Children are more often affected by DYS, i.e., dyslexia, dysorthographia, dyspraxia, and dyscalculia. They will need to be tested quickly. Proprioception, posturology as well as speech and language therapy have their place here.

False Accusations of Child Abuse against EDS Parents

In both infants and schoolchildren, the presence of frequent bruising and almost immature fractures in EDS (for caregivers, school nurses, general practitioners, pediatric emergency physicians) falsely suggests parental abuse and *Silverman syndrome* (several radiological fractures occurring at different times and observed in abused children, especially infants and toddlers) or *Shaken Baby Syndrome*. The consequences can be devastating for parents. The social services and the public prosecutor (or the public prosecutor's office) can remove the baby or child for the wrong reasons, because they do not know EDS. Professor Claude Hamonet, also an expert at the Courts, had to defend several cases in this way. It must be proven that children have EDS and that one or both parents also have EDS. Psychiatric and psychological assessments of the child, and the parents, must be done. These procedures are very lengthy and sometimes take years, as in this case in Rennes, France, in 2019.[34]

There is radiological evidence that makes one think of EDS and should thus exonerate the parents.

Important

Typical clinical, circumstantial, and radiological characteristics of EDS children with fractures (to be presented to your lawyer and the court if necessary):

➢ Spontaneous fractures that occur without trauma, during simple movements or manipulations of the child, such as changing diapers, washing, gentle pressure on the chest to strap him/her in the pram or car.

➢ Radiologically:
  ♦ Fractures are often multiple in the same child.
  ♦ An aspect of detachment of the bony extremities (the epiphyses).
  ♦ Bony splinters (spores) on the extremities of the limbs.
    o *A splinter is a small fragment that comes off a bone after a fracture.*
  ♦ Compactions of the vertebral bodies.
  ♦ Enlargement of the cranial grooves, fontanelles, a craniotabes.

    o A *craniotabes* is a softening and deformation of the cranial bones. The cause is a decalcification or a lack of calcification, such as can occur in rickets.

Holick et al. (2017)[35] described 72 cases of children whose parents were wrongly accused of abuse and who, with a proper defense, were exonerated without trial. Their conclusion was that: "EDS,

[34] https://www.ouest-france.fr/bretagne/rennes-35000/bebe-secoue-la-mere-relaxee-demande-reparation-au-chu-de-rennes-7187887.
[35] Holick MF, Hossein-Nezhad A, Tabatabaei F et al. Multiple fractures in infants who have Ehlers-Danlos/hypermobility Syndrome and or vitamin D deficiency: A case of 72 infants whose parents were accused of child abuse and neglect. Dermatoendocrinol. 2017;9(1):e1279768, published online.

OI/EDS, and vitamin D/infantile rickets have been associated with infant fractures that can be misinterpreted as being caused by non-accidental trauma due to child abuse." [36]

The researchers suggested an alternative interpretation of the aspects of the fractures that occurred. These could be ossification disorders associated with altered maturation of the chondrocyte (the cartilage cell that produces bone) at the end of the growth plates.

These lesions occur as metaphyseal lesions, which are called *bucket handle fractures* because of the radiolucency of the bony metaphysis and epiphyseal plaques, which have an unorganized or even fragmented appearance. Identical aspects were found in osteogenesis imperfecta (OI) and rickets.

Several authors, including J.M. Leventhal[37], have examined the *Kids' Inpatient Database* to determine the percentage of children with fractures attributable to physical abuse.

In terms of age, they found a relatively low percentage attributable to abuse, estimated in 2003 at:

- 24.9% for children under 12 months;
- 7.2% for children aged 12 to 23 months;
- 2.9% for children aged between 24 and 35 months.

It should be a strong incentive for radiologists and clinicians to review the radiographs of these children carefully.

---

[36] EDS, OI/EDS and vitamin D/infantile rickets are associated with fragility fractures in infants that can be misinterpreted as caused by non-accidental trauma due to child abuse.

[37] Leventhal JM, Martin KD, Asnes AD. Incidence of fractures attributable to abuse in young hospitalized children: results from analysis of a United States database. Pediatrics. 2008;122(3):599-604.

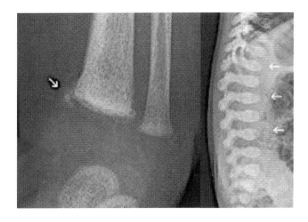

Bucket handle fracture (left)
Flattening of the vertebrae (right)

The Autism Spectrum Disorders

The term *Autism Spectrum Disorders (ASD)* is used to describe an etiologically and clinically heterogeneous group characterized by neurodevelopmental disorders that begin in early childhood. ASD are characterized by defects in communication, social interaction, and repetitive and stereotyped behaviors (*American Psychiatric Association, 1994*). The prevalence is estimated at 1% in the general population. The estimation is of 90% of ASDs occur without apparent cause (idiopathic), and 10% are secondary to a genetic disorder (known as secondary autism).

It is believed that pain, which is underestimated, is widespread in ASD. No apparent reason can causes this pain. Others pains are secondarily by self-harming, aggressive behavior, and aroused behavior (*Bursch B et al. 2004; Dubois A et al. 2017*).[38,39] Many of them have digestive and neurological disorders (e.g., seizures).

---

[38] Bursch B, Ingman K, Vitti L, et al. Chronic pain in individuals with previously undiagnosed autistic spectrum disorders. J Pain. 2004;5(5):290-5.
[39] Dubois A, Michelon C, Rattaz C, et al. Daily living pain assessment in children with autism: Exploratory study. Res Dev Disabil. 2017;62:238-246.

When reading articles on ASD, symptoms such as muscular hypotonia, joint hypermobility, apraxia, or clumsiness are mentioned. Surprisingly, these signs and symptoms are found in diseases where hypermobility is part of the clinical picture, such as hEDS. In some studies and publications, the link between EDS/HSD and ASD (or behaviors that are part of ASD) seems relatively common.[40,41]

Dysproprioception, dysautonomia, pain, fatigue, and hypersensoriality to noise (hyperacusis), light (photophobia), and touch (skin hypersensitivity, dysesthesia, paresthesia, which often lead to self-damaging behavior) lead to a tendency to develop autistic traits, in the context of the particular connective tissue of EDS that is associated with altered or distorted afferent messages.

Proprioception is also crucial for motor development, the acquisition of non-verbal communication, and social interaction. Therefore, in some cases, the autistic spectrum may become entangled with EDS, and these patients can be improved by compression garments, sequential oxygen therapy, and measures to avoid hypersensoriality.

Professor Hamonet tested this theory in Professor David Cohen's psychiatric department at the Pitié-Salpêtrière (Paris, France) with Doctor Vincent Guinchat. The results were sometimes spectacular: children and young people reopened themselves to the outside world and their families[42].

The message is: with autism, one should always look for EDS and take care of the child optimally.

---

[40] Casanova EL, Baeza-Velasco C, Buchanan CB, et al. The Relationship between Autism and Ehlers-Danlos Syndromes/Hypermobility Spectrum Disorders. J Pers Med. 2020;10(4):260.
[41] Kindgren E, Quiñones Perez A, Knez R. Prevalence of ADHD and Autism Spectrum Disorder in Children with Hypermobility Spectrum Disorders or Hypermobile Ehlers-Danlos Syndrome: A Retrospective Study. Neuropsychiatr Dis Treat. 2021;17:379-388.
[42] Baeza-Velasco C, Cohen D, Hamonet C, et al. Autism, joint hypermobility-related disorders and pain. Front Psychiatry. 2018, 9:656.

Some Data in Adults

The Announcement of the Diagnosis

The moment of diagnosis of Ehlers-Danlos syndrome is a necessary, even precious time for both the patient and the caregiver.

For the patient, it is often a time for tears, often tears of relief, and joy. "At last! After so much diagnostic wandering and abuse, you have given my suffering a name."

It can be a tetanizing news. They are so surprised while they stopped believing it. Finally, someone could put their finger on the problem that sometimes date back to childhood. They are really in shock. Tears, whether held or not, a reddening of the face, and sometimes trembling the whole body are observed.

As I often tell patients, the diagnosis's announcement leads to a real awareness and understanding of a whole life. The whole life can be explained, parading before their eyes, during this first consultation in which the Ehlers-Danlos syndrome is diagnosed. Finally, everything makes sense.

All those little symptoms that their entourage felt were normal and not so severe. All those words were spoken by the family, like: "You know, everyone in the family has that! " (since EDS is highly hereditary, most family members naturally had one or more of these signs and symptoms).

Most patients say: "Doctor, finally I understand my whole life!" It can be very moving for the caregivers, and even if they remain empathetic, the tears are hard to hold.

This emotional shock can aggravate already existing symptoms or even lead to an *asthenoalgic announcement attack*. It can be disturbing for the patient. Although a new treatment was started after this first consultation, paradoxically, the situation is getting worse and worse. Is this due to the intense emotions felt during the announcement? The decrease in chronic stress after so many years of wandering? The causes can be hormonal fluctuations, such as cortisol, adrenaline, noradrenaline, or prolactin (increasing stress). Why not let epigenetics play a role if a few days or weeks pass before this worsening?

The patient should always be warned and calmed before this possible worsening of symptoms.

After the announcement of the diagnosis, some patients go through the 5 stages of grief: Denial, Anger, Negotiation, Depression (or sadness, at the onset of the symptoms of EDS, as I tend to feel it), and finally Acceptance.

A mourning for the Self or, as I like to say, for the Old Self. Mourning about what was, what could be done before (at work, at sports, with friends) and acceptance of the illness, about what you have become and what you can still do.

It is a feeling that is difficult to describe. On the one hand, there is the satisfaction of being understood, heard, and believed by the doctor. But, on the other hand, the person will never be the same again. We regard the diagnosis as a hammer blow. Everything can finally be explained after wandering from doctor to doctor and from diagnosis to diagnosis!

Some patients first go through a phase of Denial (especially teenagers and men). "No, this cannot be it! After so many doctors have been consulted and so many tests have been done. How could a doctor make this diagnosis by merely questioning and examining me?" No, I cannot have this genetic disease!" No, I am not a carrier of this defect!"

Then the Anger rises and can burst inside, then the person might lash out at others: "This is unfair, what have I done to deserve this?"; "It is my mother's or my father's fault!" Anger can explode at home or work, with conflicts in couples and families, at work, on the street. Anger is also expressed in the following way: "How could they not diagnose me earlier after seeing all these doctors and doing all these tests? It is the doctors' fault!" Of course, no one is to blame. Relatives and family members cannot do anything about it, and most doctors hardly know anything about the disease, because it is poorly taught and rarely mentioned in general practitioners' or specialists' journals.

Then there is a Negotiation, which often takes place at the second consultation: "Do I have to undergo all these treatments? Can I not remove any of them? I can take some vitamins, but not all these potentially toxic things! Do I have to put on the compression garments, doctor? These clothes brother me. Then it is not very aesthetic!" "Are the drugs not enough? I am not ready for oxygen yet, Doctor. It makes me look sick!", and so forth.

Then comes Sadness or Depression (see next paragraph) and finally Acceptance.

In the touching book by Madame Céline Huillet (2019), "*Et si... Je devenais Pétronille*" (*What if... I became Pétronille*), we can read on page 93: "*To become the person I am today, I had to go through many important steps in the construction of 'myself' and 'mourn' certain things... The very first, the announcement of the disability, of the illness. It is the incomprehension, the hope that medicine is wrong. We must simply accept and tell ourselves that we are not responsible: "This is the law of genetics." It is a relief of being understood and well cared for, after so many years of medical wanderings, uncertainties, incomprehension, doubts in front of some doctors. You must be able to step back and ask yourself the right questions. The next phase is sadness, injustice and confusion. During this time, I had to admit that I had become different /.../ This sadness gave way to the progression of my emotions towards the path of acceptance. This last step where I accepted all my disabilities; they are a part of my life. I am different now; I have learned to love myself this way...* "

Psychological Consequences

Anxiety, depression, and eating disorders (evening cravings for sugar, anorexia bulimia) are common in EDS. They have been well studied by our friend and colleague Prof. Antonio Bulbena, a psychiatrist in Barcelona (see chapters about psychological and psychiatric aspects; and nutrition in EDS).

If the sugar craving can often be reduced by taking L-tryptophan 500mg, in the amount of two tablets in the evening (it also favors the induction of sleep), it is more complicated for anxiety and depression.

I think that patients, at the onset of their illness, are more likely to be sad than depressed, because they are no longer able to do a specific type of activities while they would like to do them. Not being able to do what one wants to do leads to sadness.

It is what they often say when they are asked what they psychologically suffer from.

If one is depressed, it does not make much difference if they are in pain, tired or not. It is usually different in EDS. If on some days the patients feel better and are less tired, they do family things or activities (even if there will be a debt of pain and fatigue for the next days), and they are not sad or depressed on those days, on the contrary. Nevertheless, they are frequently put in psychiatry for convenience, and bombarded with antidepressants, anxiolytics, or psychotropic drugs.

On the other hand, the role of the social and family environment is essential. They are not trusted; no one understands that they were in good shape one day and are *broken* the following one (the EDS's debt). Accusations, slander, "We do not understand you," "This is all in your head!" or "You are lazy!" can lead to isolation, loneliness, loss of friends, and long-term depression.

There is nothing worse than misunderstanding the people you love, and this is often their daily life. One should not hesitate or be reluctant to seek help from a psychologist or a psychiatrist before sinking deeply into depression.

Patients also have *a fear of tomorrow*, often in the evening, sometimes irrepressibly, a lump in the stomach and chest. Will I be able to get up tomorrow? Will I be able to drive my children to school and cook food for my partner? Will I be able to work tomorrow? These are the main questions they ask themselves.

In EDS, there is a big difference between *Wanting* and *Being able to*. The treatments aim, among other things, to suffer less in daily life, to be less tired, to be able to do the best they can, to extend activities with children and partners, to re-socialize with friends, and finally (in case of incapacity to work) to return to work, if possible even part-time (33%, 50% or more), by promoting teleworking, for example.

Contrary to some preconceived ideas, EDS patients have *a hard skin*, they like human contacts and work; locked up at home they are often like *lions in a cage* and sometimes lose all hope.

Also, the worry is that many patients have the feeling that their body and their brain are as if they were dissociated. They want to act; they visualize it, and their body reacts out.

For example, they see the door frame, and they know that they have to avoid it, yet they bump into it. They often think the problem is in their head, but neurological tests are normal. In most cases, it is a proprioceptive disorder.

Narcissistic Perverts and EDS Patients

In the consultation, I meet some patients who are victims of narcissistic perverts (NPs)

That is why it is crucial to tell about them, about the NPs who spot us, EDS patients, from afar. They gradually destroy us even more by exploiting our apparent fragility and weakness, our need for outside support, and our social or sentimental ties in our daily lives.

It is a species that you should run away from as soon as possible.

Many patients are involved with these narcissistic perverts, and it can take a long, long time to realize what they are.

An NP is a person with a narcissistic and perverse personality disorder (NPD). They have a self-deprecating image of themselves, but they value themselves by belittling others. Men are more often affected by narcissistic perversion than women.

This person gives himself the appearance of being superior to others, and feels an increased need to be admired. They manipulate their environment, and do not feel guilty when they hurt others. It is a severe illness. It is a white psychosis, which means that they are carriers of madness but without hallucinations.

The narcissistic pervert can be a husband, friend, colleague, or even a family member with whom the person has a close relationship. They are very bright and often apologize for their behavior, and they can be charming and adorable. Here are ten vital signs to consider when recognizing an NP, and it is not easy to recognize them as they are often just off the beaten track, in society or a couple. They are also brilliant and poisonous:

1/ The narcissistic pervert is an excellent seducer:

They know how to seduce, say what the patient likes and wants to hear. They are the ideal man in a love affair, the caring *Charming Prince*, who brings joy until the mask falls off, and they turn out to be unbearable.

2/ The double face:

The NP chooses a target, seduces it, and then gives it back its hellish life; but from the outside, nothing appears because it remains lovable with the others. People find it hard to believe the victim's statements, who is often seen as crazy, depressed, or even paranoid.

3/ Violence:

It is part of the intimidation and humiliation techniques of the narcissistic pervert towards his victim. The criticisms are permanent in public (always with finesse) or private. From verbal violence to permanent psychological violence, the manipulator sometimes crosses the barrier of physical violence when he feels that his victim is about to expose the truth.

4/ Isolate and divide in order to better reign:

To be sure that the victim always needs them, the narcissistic pervert gradually cuts off all ties that bind the victim to those close to her/him. Her/his own family might even turn against her/him. The isolation that often present in the EDS is total here.

5/ The immense attraction for money:

Narcissistic perverts are often thought to be eager for money. Because, in addition to possessing and humiliating the victim, they take a large part of the victim's income in order to gain more control over them.

6/ Beware of the honeymoon phase:

This term shows that the narcissistic pervert regularly put on their seductive mask to make the victim fall back into their nets. They do not change or ask for forgiveness. It is still a manipulative means of getting something or dulling the victim's suspicions.

7/ The narcissistic pervert lacks empathy:

To be without empathy in this perversion of personality is typical. They feel neither hot nor cold seeing their victim suffering and destroying themselves because they do not love her/him. On the contrary, they even feel an absolute joy in seeing their victim in need.

8/ Lies in everyday life:

It is pathological in narcissistic perverts. They lie all the time to make themselves look good, to be flattered, admired, and loved by their relatives. Because that is what they are looking for. They sometimes even take credit for their victims' qualities and successes, so great is their thirst for recognition.

9/ Sexual deviations:

They add a new shadow to the image of these personalities. In a couple, the pervert increasingly demands (sometimes violent) sexual demands and often opts for sadomasochism. Because he often suffered from it as a young person and lacks empathy, he can have incestuous relationships with their children or pedophilic relationships with others.

10/ Intelligent, they are often paranoid:

He is suspicious of his victim. So, if she/he wants to escape, she/he needs a lot of foresight, discretion and trust that no one will help her/him, because the narcissistic pervert will probably have spies among her/his friends and entourage. He will, by the

155

way, be ready to do anything to punish her/him for this departure.

In conclusion, NOTHING can be done for them. They will not change! They cannot be treated! They MUST be KEPT AWAY FROM OTHERS, and NEVER BE ALLOWED TO REACH OUT TO OTHERS!

To be seen:

passeportsante.net/fr/Maux/Problemes/Fiche.aspx?doc=pervers-narcissique
youtube.com/watch?v=dfGJnQGrG5w, *Clotilde Ziegler*

To read:

How to get rid of a narcissistic pervert?
Maylis Guillier
Perverted narcissists, take off your masks.
Clotilde Ziegler

INVICTUS

William Ernest Henley (1849-1903)
British writer, poet and journalist

Out of the night that covers me,

Black as the pit from pole to pole,

I thank whatever gods may be

For my unconquerable soul.

In the fell clutch of circumstance

I have not winced nor cried aloud.

Under the bludgeonings of chance

My head is bloody, but unbowed.

Beyond this place of wrath and tears

Looms but the Horror of the shade,

And yet the menace of the years

Finds and shall find me unafraid.

It matters not how strait the gate,

How charged with punishments the scroll,

I am the master of my fate:

I am the captain of my soul.

Testimony of René, 43 years old

I will be 44 years old in April 2020.

I always felt different from others until I realized that something was eating me from the inside out, making me look good on the outside, but inside was just a wreck.

From examination to examination, I went from a doctor to another, heard myself saying all the time that there was nothing, and it made me realize that everything was in my head and I should see a psychiatrist.

Eventually, I fell into a deep depression and began to believe that I was really crazy.

Ultimately, I was treated by a psychiatrist with severe antidepressant medication until I went into drug withdrawal in 2015 because nothing changed.

It was not until March 2019 that I met you and had the chance to be diagnosed with Ehlers-Danlos Syndrome with an associated MCAD.

Finally, relieved to say that I was not crazy but sick with an invisible handicap.

René R.-C., December 2019

Isolation

In EDS, there is often painful societal isolation (loss of work and relationships with colleagues) and social isolation (distance from friends who do not understand the extreme fatigue and physical suffering that varies over time and even daily). Family problems (siblings and parents who do not understand) and marital problems (misunderstandings, disputes, moral abuse, and divorce).

The patient *curls up*. Their world is *shrinking*.

It is not easily noticeable, and it starts creeping in. As I wrote above, the aim of treatment and care is also *reopening* to the outside world and resocialization.

Sleep Disorders

Typically, the sleep study (or polysomnography) shows:

> A restless legs syndrome (an almost uncontrollable urge to move the legs, usually in the evening or falling asleep).
> Nightly restlessness, dystonia, sometimes sleepwalking.
> Increased sleep latency.
> Impaired deep intermediate recovery sleep.
> Micro awakenings (superficial sleep).
> Obstructive sleep apnea (OSA).

Sleep disorders with breathing difficulties would be of multifactorial origin: changes in the cartilage development of the facial structures[43], hypotonia of the pharynx and larynx, muscle weakness of the diaphragm and accessory inspiratory muscles, disorders of pharyngeal and laryngotracheobroncheal proprioception. They should be systematically examined. Obstructive sleep apnea [44] occurs frequently and sometimes

---

[43] Guilleminault C, Primeau M, Chiu H-Y, et al. Sleep-disordered breathing in Ehlers-Danlos Syndrome : A genetic model of OSA. Chest. 2013; 114(5):1503-1511.
[44] Stöberl AS, Gaisl T, Giunta C, et al. Obstructive Sleep Apnoea in Children and Adolescents with Ehlers-Danlos Syndrome. Respiration. 2019;97(4):284-291.

requires nocturnal CPAP[45], orthodontic treatment, unique dental aligners, and myofascial rehabilitation[46].

There is also an alteration of the day/night rhythm (the nycthemeral rhythm). Melatonin is often effective in relatively high doses. Melatonin comes from the transformation of Serotonin, and therefore of tryptophan (see chapters on the gut microbiota, and nutrition). We recommend 3 to 6 mg of melatonin for adults to be taken thirty to forty minutes before bedtime. A second dose can be taken when you wake up, around two or three in the morning (but not later). In some cases, it can also be prescribed to children and teenagers in adapted doses (0.3mg to 2mg for children, and 2mg to 4 mg for teenagers; it also exists in drops or spray). Zopiclone or Cannabidiol can also be tried.

To improve the quality of average deep sleep, I prefer Trazodone in doses of 50 to 100mg at bedtime. It also improves the quality of restful sleep.

In case of MCAD, Diphenhydramine (25mg to 50 mg) or Cetirizine (antihistamines type 1, 5 to 10mg) may be useful.

For restless legs syndrome (RLS): a small dose of Levodopa (dopamine) and Benserazide (aromatic dopa decarboxylase inhibitor, it is unable to pass the blood-brain barrier) such as Prolopa® or Modopar® (31.25mg to 125mg per dose, in dispersible tablets), is preferred to Pramipexole (Sifrol®) or Clonazepam (Rivotril®) which most often do not work overtime in RLS.

As a reminder, Pramipexole is a dopamine agonist, which is similar to giving L-Dopa. Some physicians remain strangely

---

[45] Continuous Positive Airway Pressure. It is a device that maintains a continuous positive airway pressure at both times of breathing, preventing the collapse of the throat. It is used in obstructive sleep apnea.

[46] Domany KA, Hantragool S, Smith DF, et al. Sleep Disorders and Their Management in Children With Ehlers-Danlos Syndrome Referred to Sleep Clinics. J Clin Sleep Med. 2018;14(4):623-629.

reluctant to prescribe it, even though they regularly prescribe Pramipexole.

Some patients move around a lot during the night (one may notice in the morning, if the patient is in a couple, a part of the bed where the sheets are spotless and, on the side of the patient with EDS, the sheets are crumpled, the blankets are pulled in all directions). Levodopa can also be tried in these cases.

Patients also have pain when sleeping on their side, so they put pillows or intertwine the comforter between their ankles and knees, as the contact between the joints is unpleasant. They can use positioning devices, a kind of memory foam pad that looks like a nursing pillow (pillows often fall off, and the partner does not like to be without a comforter during the night, as the patient has pulled everything to him or her). Many prefer memory foam mattresses and mattress toppers, firm, neither too hard nor too soft, to properly absorb curves and joints to avoid pain and nocturnal (sub)dislocations.

Tinnitus can also interfere with sleep. Some advocate *white noise*. Devices of varying sizes generate *white noise*. They generate a continuous, composite sound of equal intensity that oscillates between 20 and 20,000 hertz, the range of audibility. It is precisely because it is supposed to include all the humanly audible frequencies that it can act on tinnitus by drowning them in the whole of the sounds perceived by the auditory cortex, which ends up getting used to them and making them pass in the background (it is the concept of auditory habituation). This would therefore be a way to reduce, but not usually eliminate, tinnitus and, consequently, improve the stress and anxiety generated, as well as sleep, by extension.

Heart palpitations, even at rest, can interfere with sleep. It is also known that there is an excess of adrenergic activity during the night in EDS, which favors lighter sleep, micro-awakenings and nightmares. The use of beta-blockers in exceptionally low doses (Bisoprolol/Nebivolol at a rate of 1.25mg or Ivabradine at a rate of 2.5 to 5 mg in the evening, for example) can reduce palpitations and improve sleep quality. Heart coherence techniques, meditation, relaxation and more, are useful (see Porges' Theory).

In the presence of asthma, Celiprolol, which is a selective beta-blocker (β-1-blocker and β-2-stimulant) may be preferred. As β-2-mimetics in puffs relieve asthma by bronchodilation, you will have understood the choice of this molecule in asthmatics. In the case of asthma, it is necessary to look for MCAD and treat it if it is the case (see below). Some studies have shown a positive effect of Celiprolol on the evolution of arterial ectasia[47]. There are also false asthmas in EDS, which can be attributed in part to proprioception disorders (a kind of secondary bronchial hyperreactivity).

Keep in mind that nighttime gastroesophageal reflux can be aggravated, causing discomfort or retrosternal pain, irritating the throat, which becomes painful upon awakening (like pharyngitis), and aggravating asthma by the passage of gastric fluid into the airways.

Many patients have bruxism (grinding their teeth) at night and clench their jaws (which are sometimes unstable and subluxate). They also wear down or break their teeth. These are most often proprioceptive disorders. A posturological and orthoptic examination and the possible use of adapted aligners should therefore be planned.

Abdominal Pain

Gallbladder:

The prevalence of lithiasis (stones) of the gallbladder appears to be higher in EDS. Some entire families have had to undergo cholecystectomy (removal of the gallbladder, with laparoscopic surgery being the most appropriate). The reasoning behind the cause is purely empirical. The gallbladder empties during meals into the digestive tract by contracting the smooth muscles present in its wall. These smooth muscles probably lean on the

---

[47] Baderkhan H, Wanhainen A, Stenborg A, et al. Celiprolol treatment in patients with vascular Ehlers-Danlos Syndrome. Eur J Vasc Endovsc Surg. 2021;61(2):326-331.

normally firm connective tissue to fully perform their role. In this case, these muscles are leaning on an altered connective tissue, and this contraction would become ineffective. This would result in incomplete emptying and stagnation of the bile (as in the bladder, for the detrusor muscle, with the consequence of repeated urinary infections). Disturbance of proprioception and dysautonomia could also be taken into account here (see also the chapter about dysautonomia and Polyvagal theory).

This stagnation could be conducive to the formation of gallstones. Moreover, the wall of the gallbladder is probably weakened, like the other tissues in EDS, so rupture is a risk to be considered. In this context, a cholecystectomy should be considered automatically in case of symptomatic macro-lithiasis (> 1cm).

Finally, it seems that gallbladder pain, usually located in the right hypochondrium with a positive Murphy's sign and irradiation of pain typically towards the right shoulder (strangely enough, it follows the gallbladder meridian in Traditional Chinese Medicine), appears in EDS as atypical: either as a subcostal bar (irradiating anteriorly and posteriorly and not towards the shoulder) or as diffuse pain in the abdomen or even in the whole body (like a diffuse hyperalgesia crisis).

It is necessary to be attentive to this specific semiology in EDS to avoid a delay in diagnosis, a potential rupture of the wall, and biliary peritonitis (bile acids are irritants for the peritoneum).

Intussusception in adults:

In case of severe colic, intussusception should also be excluded: a portion of the intestine turns over like a finger glove and enters the intestinal segment immediately downstream (just above). In 90% of cases, it affects the intersection between the ileum (the small intestine) and the colon (the large intestine). It is potentially serious and can lead to an intestinal occlusion and an interruption of the blood supply to the intestine (ischemia) with a risk of tissue necrosis (the death of part of the intestine, by the same mechanism as ischemia of the heart, for example, during a myocardial infarction), and risk of perforation of the intestine.

Complementary examinations: an ultrasound of the abdomen and, if necessary, a hydrostatic enema (injection of saline through the rectum) or a pneumatic enema (by insufflation of air), under radiological control. The latter examinations also allow the invaginated segment to be put back in place because of the pressure caused in the intestine by the examination.

Appendicitis (the vermicular appendix):

The pain may also be atypical or even almost non-existent, and, besides, they often do not have a fever. Delayed diagnosis could lead to purulent peritonitis. Therefore, it is advisable to avoid fruits with seeds (such as grapes, tomatoes, unseeded peppers), small pits, or poorly chewed peanuts (such as cherries and peanuts).

Irritable Bowel Syndrome, Food Intolerances, Deficiencies due to Malabsorption.

1/ Irritable Bowel Syndrome, or the intestinal transit pathology.

The symptoms are mainly: chronic abdominal pain, transit disorders (alternating diarrhea and constipation) with painful outbreaks (see also, further, the chapter on nutrition).

➤ *Intestinal motility disorders* are located more in the small intestine than in the colon (the term functional colopathy is obsolete). The motor disorders of the colon are mainly observed after meals (by abnormal motor response), whereas those of the small intestine is more variable during the day. This results in gas retention, with discomfort and bloating. Dysautonomia, MCAD, dysproprioception, properties of the connective tissue, and alteration of the microbiota in Ehlers-Danlos Syndrome largely explain this phenomenon. This digestive dilatation can, in turn, excite digestive sensory afferents, creating self-sustaining loops of contractions and pain.

➤ *Digestive hypersensitivity.* Dysproprioception in EDS promotes erroneous responses to food passage. The response threshold to intestinal distension appears to be lowered. These proprioceptive disorders can also be encountered at the gastroesophageal level (with dyspepsia and functional

164

pyrosis), bronchial level (with pseudo-asthmatic manifestations), bladder level (pollakiuria, incomplete emptying with infections), or skin and musculoskeletal level. At the intestine level, we can imagine a mechanical cause with a bad perception of the parietal nociceptive receptors and/or sensitization of the primary afferent neurons of the digestive wall. These primary afferent neurons may be abnormally stimulated by mediators (serotonin, cytokines) released, among others, by mast cells that are in direct contact with the sensory endings. Hypersensitivity could also be of central origin (the posterior horn of the spinal cord) or secondary to a dysfunction of the system of diffuse inhibitory controls (DIC), which modulate pain and whose role is analgesic. DICs theoretically produce a descending inhibition that reduces the activity of pain neurons (non-specific) in the dorsal horns of the spinal cord.

➤ *Mast cells* are often excited in EDS (MCAD) and could, by simple contact with poorly digested food, release a host of inflammatory and allergenic substances (histamine, interleukins, leukotriene, anti-TNF alpha, prostaglandins, etc.). These substances can cause functional colopathy symptoms and discomfort after meals (note that excessive outdoor heat, fever, intense physical exercises, and alcohol excite mast cells; e.g., the well-known case of discomfort at the family barbecue in the summer), flushing, pruritus, headaches, fatigue, orthostatic hypotension, non-specific exanthemata, etc. These substances can also sensitize the primary afferent neurons of the digestive mucosa. Tryptase levels in the mucosa may be increased.

➤ *Bacterial pieces* (or other microorganisms) that pass the epithelial barrier may encounter mucosal lymphocytes and chronically trigger an immune response with overexpression of TOLL-Like receptors (e.g., TLR-2, TLR-4). They are T lymphocytes (CD25, regulatory T lymphocytes) and not B lymphocytes (which are antibody producers). These various protagonists can recognize bacterial structures (such as pieces of their wall) with an unexplained increase in the level of CRP (C-Reactive Protein) in the blood and flu-like symptoms such as aches and pains, headaches, and inflamed lymph nodes (adenopathies).

165

➢ *The serotonin-releasing enteroendocrine cells* of the digestive tract, mainly colonic and rectal, could play a role in functional digestive disorders.

➢ *Increased digestive permeability.* Typically there are so-called Tight Junctions between cells in the intestine and colon. These junctions prevent the passage of poorly digested food or pieces of bacteria from the lumen to the mucosa of the digestive tract (more rarely, the passage of heavy metals). If they are loosened, they allow these substances to pass to the mucosa, where two crucial players are located: mast cells and lymphocytes. This can trigger a local inflammatory response with an influx of immunocompetent cells and the release of neuromediators. These can sensitize the primary afferent neurons.

Para-cellular permeability may also be promoted by bacterial proteases that activate receptors on the surface of colon cells (PAR-2-type protease receptors). Increased degradation of zonulin (which may be increased in blood and stools), occludin, and claudin by the proteasome may also play a role. It is interesting to know that stress is an enabling factor; it increases digestive permeability by involving mast cells. Finally, a high-fat diet may increase digestive permeability.

As a treatment: give foods rich in L-Glutamine (it restores the tight junctions of the small intestine) such as meat, fish, eggs, seafood, legumes, spinach, parsley, and oilseeds (walnuts, hazelnuts, almonds, etc.). There are also supplements in L-Glutamine (take about 3g per day).

➢ *Disturbances of the digestive microbiota:*
  o *It acts on digestive sensitivity and peristalsis.* The products of the activity of these bacteria, such as the fermentation of hydrogen gas H_2, methane CH_4, and short-chain fatty acids, can influence ileocolic peristalsis and interact with the epithelial cells of the digestive wall as well as with immune cells, leading to hypersensitivity (role of afferent neurons).

  o *Role of the number of bacteria and their types*: microbial overgrowth in the small intestine produces more hydrogen and methane, which can alter intestinal motility and inflame the mucosa. Bacterial stasis, in EDS, would increase this phenomenon (dysautonomia, digestive distension secondary to collagen properties, dysproprioception, etc.). It may be possible to give ten days of antibiotics such as Neomycin or Rifaximin to improve these symptoms for methano-producing patients.

o *Role of the type of bacteria, the microbiota.* Usually, 90% of the microbiota consists of Firmicutes (Eubacterium, Streptococci, Clostridium and Faecalibacterium), Bacteroidetes (Bacteroides) and Actinobacteria (Bifidobacterium). This is the dominant microbiota.

There is also a passing microbiota (food bacteria, yeasts) and a subdominant microbiota composed of Proteobacteria (Escherichia Coli, Enterobacteriacae) and Verrucomicrobia (Akkermansia sp.).

In EDS, the microbiota is often disturbed and causes excessive fermentation of carbohydrate residues (sugars).

This produces gases (H_2, CH_4). Excessive putrefactive flora and candida (mycosis) are common in EDS. The microbiota may also alter the conversion of primary bile acids (cholic and deoxycholic acid) to secondary bile acids, speeding up bowel movements.

o *Psychological disorders and stress* can alter digestive transit.

2/ Dietary deficiencies, malabsorption of nutrients.

➢ There is a possible decrease in the absorption of tryptophan and decreased serotonin levels (with a risk of depression and altered sleep).

As a treatment, we suggest an increased dietary intake of foods rich in tryptophan (banana, avocado, beet, almonds, broccoli, figs, etc.) and direct tryptophan supplements (drugstores) at a rate of 500mg around 5 and 8 pm.

➢ There is a possible deficiency of L-Tyrosine (precursor of dopamine, adrenaline, and noradrenaline; also of thyroid hormones), vitamin C, vitamin B1 - B6 - B9 - B12, vitamin A, and D, trace elements (zinc, copper, magnesium, etc.).

As a treatment: L-Tyrosine supplements can be given, for example, 500mg in the morning and around 1 pm. As a precursor of adrenaline and noradrenaline, it reduces fatigue in the late morning and afternoon. Supplements: vitamin C (1 to 3g), zinc/copper, vitamin B complex, vitamin D (3000 IU/day), magnesium.

3/ Food intolerances.

Many food intolerances are encountered in EDS. As we will see, these are generally not only type 1 food allergies. One generally sees:

➤ *Type 1 IgE allergies (so-called immediate response)*. IgE antibodies allow us to defend ourselves from parasites and intruders of all kinds. It leads, for example, to an allergy to pollens, molds, bee stings, and peanuts, but also asthma, hay fever, eczema, etc. Immediate food allergic reactions such as swelling of the lips, hives, angioedema, itching (pruritus), etc., are encountered. Rarely there is anaphylactic shock, sometimes with a life-threatening outcome. Diagnosis: specific IgE RAST assay. Treatment: Avoidance of the allergens involved.

➤ *Type 3 IgG allergies (so-called delayed response)*: an immune reaction to food proteins, with a production of specific IgG antibodies. These IgG antibodies can cause general inflammatory states. These symptoms are delayed to contact the allergen (between three hours and three days).

➤ *Lactose intolerance* (a 0% lactose diet and lactase supplementation are prescribed). Beware of frequent confusion with a true milk allergy.

➤ *Intolerance to FODMAP* (Fermentable Oligosaccharides, Disaccharides, Monosaccharides, and Polyols). In this context, one should not confuse what can happen when eating bread: an intolerance to FODMAP and gluten are different.

➤ *Pseudo-allergies - histamine intolerance.* Since mast cells are already very *excited* and release much histamine in EDS, eating a lot of it would be the last straw for your digestive system. There are lists of histamine-rich foods readily available on the web. I think it is okay to eat them, but avoid mixing several histamine-rich foods at the same meal (there is a limit to how much you can eat). One should not forget that high heat (sauna, hammam, barbecue in the middle of summer, etc.) and alcohol (wine, beer, strong liquor) aggravate the activation of mast cells (MCAD) and, therefore, the histamine levels. You can also take diamine oxidase before a meal (Daosin®), which cuts histamine into pieces, and add Riboflavin (Vitamin B2).

➢ *Fructose intolerance.* In this case, a fructose transport protein is deficient. It can appear gradually (in intestinal diseases, following antibiotic therapy, or as part of an unbalanced diet).

Symptoms: flatulence, bloating, abdominal pain, loose stools, alternating diarrhea/constipation. Acid taste in the mouth, heartburn (it promotes hyperacidity).

Treatment: avoid foods rich in fructose and fructans. Many fruits or honeys contain between 50 and 70% fructose, avoid berries, certain vegetables (often because of their inulin content) that contain fructans (artichokes, asparagus, beans, broccoli, cabbage, chicory, leeks, onions, peanuts, tomatoes, zucchini), cereal products, dried fruits, sweet wine (dessert wine, Muscadet, port wine, sherry). Fructose may also be used in some countries as a sweetener in snacks and soft drinks, for example in the form of wheat syrup. Beware of foods containing Sorbitol (E420) and Xylitol (E967), such as diet/light beverages and drinks for diabetic patients. Many diet products include fructose and fructans.

What is well tolerated: banana, Brussels sprouts, carrot, clementine, tangerine, corn, cucumber, fennel, lemon, grapefruit, potato, pumpkin, radish, currant, rhubarb, sauerkraut, spinach, sweet potato/yam.

➢ *Maltose intolerance:* there must be a hereditary, genetic deficiency in sucrase-isomaltase. Its transmission is autosomal recessive. Various mutations exist and, depending on the disease, they affect more sucrose, maltose, starch, and sometimes lactose. *The symptoms* are the same as those of fructose and lactose intolerance. They are less absorbed, and therefore they ferment in the intestine via the microbiota. Maltose intolerance also promotes intestinal hyper-permeability.

To avoid: malt sugar (consumed by sportsmen to regain strength after or during prolonged physical effort), sugar cane, beet, sorghum, powdered sugar, and powdered sugar, candy sugar, cotton candy, maple syrup, Barbados sugar, molasses, pancake syrup, gingerbread, baked beans, sometimes starch, beer, malted chocolate powders.

Possible treatment: oral enzyme replacement: sacrosidase (Sucraid®).

It is crucial to systematically think about the digestive tract in this moment of Medicine when we know that the intestine, considered the second brain, contains more than 70% of the mature immune cells of the body (lymphocytes).

It is an extraordinary fact and one that, after more than 2400 years, gives reason to Hippocrates who said, *All disease begins in the intestine*; or to Buddha: *The wise man is the one who is well from the intestine.*

Advice:

A diet that excludes FODMAPs (oligosaccharides, disaccharides, fermentable monosaccharides, and polyols) is worth trying.

I often advise a diet low in lactose (or without), fermentable sugars, unhealthy fats, ultra-processed foods, and histamine in EDS; and daily and chronic intake of probiotics and/or prebiotics. A gluten-free diet can be tried. Wheat exclusion can be successful in some of these patients. [48] Medications or supplements that contain lactose in their excipients should be excluded (e.g., maltose is preferred).

Treatment of MCAD is very important.

---

[48] Spiller R. Impact of diet on symptoms of the irritable bowel syndrome. Nutrients. 2021;13(2):575. doi: 10.3390/nu13020575

170

Tests to be done on a case-by-case basis:

- A complete blood test: blood count, liver and kidney function, ionogram, sedimentation rate (ESR), and CRP.
- If necessary, perform a blood tryptase dosage (often normal in mast cell disorders related to EDS).
- Viral, bacterial, and even parasitic serologies.
- Determination of ANF (anti-nuclear factor) with identification of subtypes, rheumatoid factor (RF, very sensitive but not very specific for rheumatoid arthritis), anti-CCP (not very sensitive but very specific for rheumatoid arthritis), anti-thyroid antibodies.
- Test for ANCA, ASCA, and calprotectin (for inflammatory diseases of the digestive tract). Search for celiac disease. Possibly perform lymphocyte typing and IgA, IgM, IgG and IgG2 testing.
- Measure specific IgE and RAST, test for lactose intolerance. Request patch tests in allergology or dermatology.
- Beware of false positives induced by polyclonal lymphocyte activation due to leaky gut: false positive Lyme serology (frequent), increased FAN and RF, etc.
- I.D.M. urine test (Intestinal Dysbiosis Mycosis): it consists of urinary determinations of specific metabolites of the activity of bacterial and/or fungal microorganisms. Their increase reflects an abnormal proliferation of certain microorganisms in the intestine (note that fecal analysis only allows us to assess 25% of the bacterial population that makes up the microbiota, so the results are variable and random).

  Urinary assays:
  - Metabolites associated with a proliferation of fermentation flora:
    - Citramalate
    - D-lactate
    - Tricarballytate
  - Metabolites associated with a proliferation of putrefactive flora:
    - Para-cresol
    - Phenol

171

- Indican
- Benzoate
- Hippurate
- Phenylacetate
- 2-OH-phenylacetate
- 4-OH-phenylacetate
- 3-OH-phenylpropionate
- Metabolites associated with fungal proliferation:
  - Arabinitol
  - Arabinose
  - Tartarate
- Zonulin assay (porous intestine, decreased intestinal tight junctions): in blood and/or stools.
- Perform a lipopolysaccharides (LPS or endotoxins) or lipopolysaccharide-binding protein (LBP) blood dosage: LPS is the major component of the outer membrane of Gram-negative bacteria. LBP is mainly produced in the liver, binds LPS, and its blood level rises with LPS.
- A lactulose test (chronic intestinal colonization).
- A test with Lactilol and Mannitol.
- Possible dosage of fecal Calprotectin (N<10mg/liter).

Treatments:

- Diet low in sugars, lactose, possibly gluten and low in histamine rich foods. Low FODMAP diet.
- Treatment of MCAD if necessary (see below): anti-H1, anti-H2, anti-leukotrienes, vitamin C, N-acetylcysteine (NAC), alpha-lipoic acid, Cromoglycate, etc.
- Decrease intestinal permeability: L-Glutamate, 3x800mg/day for the small intestine, and Butyrin 900mg (butyric acid 787mg) per day for the colon.
- Pre- and probiotics, with various flora, to restore intestinal balance.
- Special nutritional advice if there is an excess of fermentation bacteria, putrefaction bacteria and/or candida (fungus) in the I.D.M.:
  - In case of fungal overgrowth: avoid refined sugars (cookies, sweets, etc.), white flours (white bread, pasta, etc.) and alcohol.

- In case of fermentation bacteria proliferation: avoid refined sugars, white flours and alcohol. Avoid foods rich in FODMAPs.
- In case of overgrowth of putrefaction bacteria: chew properly. Decrease protein intake. Increase consumption of prebiotic foods.

Chest Discomfort

First of all, painful gastroesophageal reflux, peptic esophagitis, aneurysm or aortic dissection pain, esophageal tear, Meckel's diverticulum, pneumothorax, pleurisy or pneumonia, vertebral rotation (hypermobile structures) with secondary intercostal neuralgia, spinal tumor, or costal and vertebral metastases must be excluded. The clinic, history and anamnesis should guide further investigations.

A particular feature of EDS is weakness or blockage of the diaphragm with pseudo-paralyzing pain in the intercostal muscles and excessive and painful contractures of the accessory inspiratory muscles. Inspiration is active and expiration is passive, by relaxation of the inspiratory muscles.

The diaphragm separates the thoracic cavity from the abdomen. It is a striated muscle like the muscles of the limbs or the spine (as opposed to the smooth muscles of the intestines or the gallbladder, for example). It is shaped like a double dome. When it contracts, it lowers and flattens, increasing the vertical dimensions of the lungs and creating negative pressure in the respiratory system, allowing air to enter. The diaphragm provides 60-70% of the lung volume change during inspiration. It is composed of two muscular planes that are surrounded everywhere by altered connective tissue (in EDS).

Patients often report a feeling of blockage on inspiration (as a reminder, asthma causes expiratory difficulties, due to the increase in airway resistance). They feel like a there is a bar just under the ribs (C19, C10) and pain at the ends of the accessory ribs (C11, C12) which prevents them from breathing in fully. They feel like there is not enough air going into their lungs or that someone is pushing on their rib cage, which is also quite anxiety-provoking.

The external intercostal muscles, located between the ribs, are oriented downward and forward. They allow an increase in the antero-posterior and lateral dimensions of the thorax. They participate in 25 to 50% of the remaining inspiratory volume.

Pain in the chondro-sternal or costo-vertebral joints and their possible subluxations can lead to a limitation of the capital role of these muscles.

The accessory inspiratory muscles can intervene if necessary, or in case of weakness of the other inspiratory muscles. They are the scalene muscles, the sternocleidomastoid muscles, the trapezius muscles, and the intervertebral muscles.

Since the diaphragm and the external intercostal muscles are limited, at times the accessory inspiratory muscles contract strongly and create neck pain, torticollis (stiff neck), and vascular-nervous compressions. Patients are sometimes operated on, most often with little success, for a pseudo thoracic outlet syndrome.

These chains of events promote or accentuate tension headaches, via contractures of the occipital muscles, and trigger or aggravate Arnold's neuralgia.

Suggested treatments:

➢ Diaphragmatic re-education (through physical therapy, osteopathy, sophrology, Yoga, heart coherence, etc.) is helpful. A purely thoracic or abdominal inspiration should be avoided. A mix-type of inhalation is better: Begin by extending the belly, and in a second phase the thorax. If the lungs are chronically insufficiently unfolded, atelectasis may develop. The term atelectasis comes from the Greek: *ateles* (incomplete) and *ektasis* (extension): due to chronic or repeated diaphragmatic blockages, not all areas of the lung are adequately and/or evenly ventilated, creating areas of poor or no gas exchange: atelectasis areas. This can influence chronic fatigue and, rarely, blood oxygenation.

- ➤ Begin physical therapy sessions focusing on global postural re-education type as well as muscle chain techniques such as Sohier, Mackenzie, Struyf or GDS, Mézières, Busquet, etc. Prior posturological analysis of muscle chain asymmetries is very important.

- ➤ Gentle osteopathy of the ribs as well as of the anterior (costo-chondro-sternal) and posterior (costo-vertebral) joints. We can also decrease the activity of the orthosympathetic paravertebral chains (osteopathy, rib raising technique).

- ➤ Lidocaine injections, at concentrations ranging from 0.5 to 1%, can be given at trigger points or painful points, such as the level of the accessory inspiratory muscles, the angular muscles of the scapula, the sub-costal rim, the xiphoid appendix, the sterno-costal and the costo-vertebral joints. Results can be rapid (at the end of the needle) and lifesaving.

- ➤ A custom-made compression vest can restore the proprioception to the rib cage and spine. Both parietal and bronchial tree proprioception may play an important role in these symptoms.

- ➤ Occasional wearing of a cervical collar can relax the cervical muscles and facilitate rehabilitation as well as pain relief (maximum of 4h to 6h/day or overnight wear).

- ➤ A custom-made thoracolumbar belt with shoulder straightener or a back brace for posture correction (e.g., thoracic Medi Protect.CSB®, Elcross®) can have a stabilizing role but also a proprioceptive one at the thoracic, scapular, and glenohumeral levels.

- ➤ Sequential oxygen therapy can help and restore more appropriate proprioception of the respiratory tree. It could previously be coupled with percussion device, but this no longer seems available on the market.

Cysts and Diverticula

Cysts are significantly more common in EDS. They can be subcutaneous or articular, but they can also be present in the thyroid, breasts, ovaries, abdominal organs (liver, kidneys, pancreas), and more.

They are benign, but if the small cysts are chance discoveries, the undiscovered larger ones can cause hypothyroidism (especially if they are numerous), hemorrhages or torsions in the ovaries, possible compression of neighboring organs or even of certain blood vessels.

I consider them as structures that develop because of the particularities of the altered connective tissue, which is looser and therefore conducive to expansion, creating cystic structures. They are places of weakness. The same is true for diverticula in the colon (with a risk of diverticulitis) or rarely in the bladder, which can cause acute or recurrent urinary tract infections or even chronic infections.

Sexual Life

Many colleagues hesitate to talk to patients about their sexuality. However, this is essential in Medicine and in EDS in particular. Generally, patients will not talk about it on their own.

In some cases, a poor or absent sex life will be a destructive element for the couple, especially when pain and fatigue are already very difficult to manage on a daily basis.

The problems are many and varied, and, in most cases, there are some simple treatments.

In women:

A. Menstruation.

Menstruation can be hemorrhagic (menorrhagia), with the presence of clots, and sometimes very painful (dysmenorrhea).

For bleeding, tranexamic acid (Exacyl®) can be recommended: continuously if they are irregular or just before the period if they are regular. This does not always work, but it is worth trying. Continuous vitamin C, at a rate of 1 to 3 grams per day (in several doses), reduces the propensity to bleed of all kinds.

In the case of severe pain (which in some cases can lead to real asthenoalgic attacks at each cycle), a continuous hormonal treatment (such as Cerazette®) can be introduced. This treatment can be started at the first menstrual period in adolescents unless there are contraindications (e.g., history of venous thrombosis or pulmonary embolism).

There are also more ovarian cysts with a risk of hemorrhage or ovarian torsion. Ibuprofen 200-400mg can be used. Ibuprofen has a dose-dependent action: up to 400mg it is considered a painkiller, and above 600mg, it is more of an anti-inflammatory, which is not recommended in EDS.

B. Pain during sexual intercourse.

The first thing to ask the patient is where the discomfort or pain is felt: at the entrance to the vagina, on the vaginal wall when rubbing, at the bottom of the vagina (at the cervix) and/or as unpleasant radiations towards the lower abdomen and the ovaries. Burning sensations may be felt after the act.

The causes can be:

➢ Excessive dryness of the mucous membranes.
➢ Fragility of the walls.
➢ Hypersensoriality and dysproprioception of the genital tract.
➢ MCAD: see this chapter.
➢ Central sensitization (vestibulodynia or vulvodynia, pudendal neuralgia): see this chapter.
➢ Cystocele, rectocele, uterine retroversion.

Of course, a gynecological problem not related to EDS, such as endometriosis, must be excluded (often causing pain at the top of the vagina and in the lower abdomen). Endometriosis is a common condition in the general population (it affects up to 5 to 10% of women), but it is no more common in EDS. On the other hand, there are diagnoses of pseudo-endometriosis in the face of the triad dyspareunia-dysmenorrhea-menorrhagia, which is very frequent in EDS. Radiological and/or histological evidence is therefore always required before a diagnosis of endometriosis can be made.

Cystoceles and cysto-urethroceles occur most often when the rectovaginal and pubocervical fascia are weakened, which may, de facto, be the case in EDS. There are very few publications on this subject. These are herniations of part or all of the bladder into the vagina (most often). They are categorized in three stages: the 1st degree: there is a protrusion going to the upper part of the vagina, it is a slight descent; the 2nd degree: it is a protrusion up to the orifice of the vagina, the bladder is flush with the vulva; the 3rd degree: the protrusion is external with respect to the vaginal orifice, it goes beyond the vulva. Patients report a sensation of pelvic heaviness or organ descent. They may experience stress incontinence, urinary retention or overflow incontinence, urgency, and discomfort during intercourse.

Risk factors: intensive sports, childbirth, overweight, chronic constipation, carrying heavy loads, connective tissue diseases (including EDS).

As treatment: healthy lifestyle and correction of modifiable risk factors, perineal rehabilitation, vesicopexy. Vesicopexy is the reattachment of the bladder, but care must be taken with the techniques used because the patient's connective tissues are of poor quality; all necessary surgical precautions must therefore be taken. The use of a pessary is also possible. A pessary is a small rubber ring that is placed in the vagina; the pessary can irritate the wall, which is weakened in EDS.

Rectocele is a descent of the rectum into the vagina. It usually affects older, multiparous women, but in EDS it can affect young, nulliparous patients. Symptoms may include pain during sexual intercourse, perineal and rectal pain, rectal heaviness, constipation, rectal discharge, contraction of the anus (anism), and a feeling of incomplete evacuation of the rectum.

As treatment: introduce hygienic dietary measures, try mild laxatives, glycerin suppositories and functional rehabilitation; surgery must remain the last resort, with the usual precautions in this disease.

Uterine retroversion is common and affects 20% to 30% of women. It is a backward tilt of the uterus (the uterus is above the bladder and in front of the rectum). The complaints are mainly lumbosacral radiations, pain during sexual intercourse (mainly when the penis hits the cervix), heaviness in the lower abdomen, constipation, pain during defecation, urinary difficulties, and pollakiuria.

Treatment may include functional rehabilitation and, in some cases, a pessary; surgery is rarely required.

Some general advice:

➢ In the event of pain at the entrance, a small amount of Lidocaine gel (urethral gel type) can be applied to the vulva's edge.

➢ In the event of pain or discomfort when rubbing or at the cervix:
  - First, try a neutral lubricating gel (K-Y® gel type, used during touching by your gynecologist). Avoid scented gels or recreational gels (due to olfactory hypersensitivity or allergies).
  - If this is insufficient and/or there are unpleasant sensations outside of intimate relations, try vaginal ovules containing hyaluronic acid (5mg/ovule). Begin with one ovule in the evening for the first ten days, then one every three days thereafter. On the vaginal wall this forms a neutral film.
  - In some cases, Estriol (Aacifemin®) ovules may be prescribed at a rate of one per day in case of extreme dryness.
  - Ultimately, a small amount of Lidocaine gel (Xylocaine® urethral gel) can be placed in the vagina prior to the procedure. This raises the pain threshold to a more normal level (the woman still feels sexual stimulation). A condom should generally be used by men, as Lidocaine induces a loss of sensitivity, and therefore stimulation, of the penis. In case of multiple allergies, latex-free condoms should be used.

➢ In the event of pain or a burning sensation following a sexual encounter.
  - If genital pain exists following intercourse, (re)apply a small amount of Lidocaine gel. Lidocaine may initially aggravate symptoms of a burning sensation.

➢ In the event of mycosis and/or urinary tract infections.
- Vaginal probiotic ovules can be used to treat recurring vaginal mycosis. As a preventive measure, I recommend one per day for seven days, repeated every three months. There are a variety of creams available as well.
- To avoid urinary tract infections, take the following precautions:
o Drink in large quantities (more than 2 liters per day).
o Take 1g to 3g of vitamin C per day.
o Take juice or cranberry extract tablets (Uri-Cran® *Comfort* or *Forte*).

For Men:

1/Testicular or spermatic cord pain, or even lower abdominal pain, may occur during or after sexual intercourse. There is a slightly increased risk of testicular torsion.

2/Painful fissures in the urinary meatus or glans can potentially occur. Burning pain in the glans penis or even pain in the penis may occur due to hypersensitivity and dysproprioception. A loss of sensitivity may occur.

Treatment:

➢ Lidocaine gel (urethral), if the lubricating gel is not enough. Use a neutral gel, without dyes or odor, to avoid allergies related to MCAD.

➢ In case of cracks or dryness of the glans: try Vaseline or lip balm, neutral, natural, and without coloring.

Painful anal penetration:

This is something to think about and talk about in both LGBTQI and heterosexual men/women. There is more anal fissuring, excessive pain and/or bleeding with penetration or rubbing.

Treatment:

➢ Try lubricating gel and possibly Lidocaine gel before and/or after penetration. Keep in mind that there is also an increased risk of hemorrhoids in EDS (in the context of venous insufficiency).

Caution: if the anorectal mucosa, glans and prepuce in EDS are more fragile, the risk of contracting a sexually transmitted disease or infection (STD, STI) is probably increased. Prevention tips cannot be stressed enough.

Finally, intense fatigue and chronic pain decrease libido and this is sometimes misunderstood and/or admitted by the partner. It is important to take the time to talk about it within the couple and, if necessary, consult a therapist. Fatigue can be so intense that it can become unimaginable to consider a sexual act.

For both men and women, the problem of general musculoskeletal pain can complicate sexual life or, in any case, certain sexual positions. One should not hesitate to talk about it within the couple. It is important to insist on foreplay rather than penetration, if penetration is impossible or very painful. Look for sexual positions that are not painful: abduction of the hips, lumbosacral or sacroiliac pain, pubic pain; avoid acrobatic lifts in EDS.

For fatigue and astheno-algesic debt after the sexual act: do not hesitate to use sequential oxygen therapy, at a rate of 20 minutes per session. One session before and one session after intercourse are recommended. The flow rate that I recommend in this case is 5 liters per minute.

Anxiety should not be overlooked as it can be related to the fear of pain or of not being up to it, which can block the partner. This anxiety can lead to a lack of erection or premature ejaculation in the man, for example. There is also the fear of causing involuntary pain to the partner with EDS. Anxiety can also cause painful spasms in the vaginal or anal area. Appropriate psychological care, meditation, relaxation, sophrology, can help. Frustration, guilt, sadness and tension within couples are common.

However, when it is possible and when you overcome your kinesiophobia, the sexual act is a physical exercise that releases endorphins and well-being hormones. You feel better overall after the act, even if it doesn't always last very long. But it's already something. Then it allows to reassure oneself and to improve the perception that one has of oneself, which is often devalued: "I am not able to satisfy my partner anymore! "I have become a subhuman!", "I am not worth anything anymore!", etc. With its anthology of worries which are added to it: "He or she will go elsewhere to be satisfied", "He or she will leave me", etc.

On the next pages: Professor Claude Hamonet's model questionnaire (modified by Dr. Stéphane Daens et al.). It is easy to use in consultation, including in general medicine.

The Questionnaire and the Clinical Certificate
of Professor Claude Hamonet (Modified)

I, the undersigned, Doctor X, hereby certify that Mr/Mrs/YY born on dd/mm/yyyy is suffering from Ehlers-Danlos syndrome or HSD, a hereditary connective tissue disease, in the presence of the following manifestations, as described in the successive descriptions of Ehlers-Danlos syndrome - Villefranche/P. Beighton, Brighton/R. Grahame, Barcelona/A. Bulbena-Vilarrasa, New York/Ehlers-Danlos Society Symposium 2016, Paris/C. Hamonet & I. Dubois-Brock:

➤ Joint and periarticular pain, of multiple locations, variously distributed (neck, shoulders, elbows, wrists, fingers, back, pelvis, hips, knees, ankles, feet), of the neuropathic type, or else, brief and very violent, variable in intensity (often very strong) according to the location, usually evolving by attacks on a continuous background, and aggravated, often with a shift to the next day, by physical activity and persisting for a long time.

➤ A feeling of severe tiredness, present upon waking, with feelings of heaviness, heaviness of the body, exaggerated during unpredictable attacks, sometimes including drowsiness. Patients very often consider fatigue as the symptom responsible for the greatest number of disabling situations.

➤ Disorders in the control of voluntary movements, of proprioceptive origin, with clumsiness, collisions with obstacles, deviation of gait, and occasional falls.

➤ A joint instability responsible for pseudo sprains, osteoarticular blocks, subluxations (including joint cracks) or dislocations.

➤ Thin, pale, transparent skin, showing the subcutaneous venous network on the forearms, above the breasts and on the back, soft to the touch, not protecting against electrostatic discharge, which leads to sensations of electric discharge when touching metallic objects (car door, shopping cart, physical contact with another person).

➤ Evidence of joint hypermobility, more or less diffuse, which may be very marked in childhood (putting a foot behind the head, doing the splits) but disappear later or be masked by pain and/or muscle contractures in certain joints. Its absence does not exclude the diagnosis. Retractions (sural triceps, hamstrings) may even be encountered, especially in children.

Beighton' score = /9 ; Grahame 5pHQ = /5

➢ Gastroesophageal refluxes, which may occur early in life (bottle feeding). They cause bronchial irritation.

➢ Extensive ecchymoses, occurring after minimal trauma, often unnoticed, or purpura.

➢ Hypersensoriality such as hyperacusis with a very fine perception of sounds and intolerance to noise.

The presence of five of these 9 signs is **enough to make a preliminary diagnosis of Ehlers-Danlos Syndromes** (sensitivity: 99.6%, specificity: 98%) and start treatment. The absence of one of the signs does not eliminate the diagnosis. They vary from birth to the end of life. Some may disappear, others may appear, more or less late, sometimes on the occasion of traumatic events (e.g. road accident) or hormonal events (puberty, menstruation, pregnancy).

The following signs may coexist, forming an integral part of the clinical picture of Ehlers-Danlos syndrome, contributing to its identification and forming part of its therapeutic management: dysautonomia (vasomotor of the extremities with cold feet, wrongly evoking Raynaud's syndrome, palpitations, sweats, chilliness, unexplained fevers, low body temperature around 35,5°C), hypersensoriality (cutaneous, olfactory, light), constipation, extra-articular pains (abdomen, ribs, chest), sleep disorders, dystonia (tremors, muscle twitches, contractures), skin fragility (healing disorders, stretch marks), excessive skin stretchability, diffuse hemorrhagic tendency (gingival, genital), respiratory manifestations (blockages, breathlessness), binocular vision disorders, oral alterations, parafunctions, bruxism, vesico-sphincter disorders, sexual disorders (dyspareunia), obstetrical accidents, cognitive disorders (memory, attention, concentration, orientation, Dys- e.g. dyslexia, dyspraxia, dysorthographia, dyscalculia, and more), affectivity, behavior (anxiety, emotionality, autism spectrum disorders, emotional hypersensitivity), manifestations suggestive of MACD (superficial and deep urticaria, flush, non-specific exanthema, fatigue after a shower, pruritus, rhinorrhea or blocked nose, sinusitis, asthma, interstitial cystitis, irritable bowel syndrome, fatigue, headaches, POTS, OH, gastroparesis, musculoskeletal and joint pain, brain fog, and more).

These clinical arguments are sufficient for the diagnosis and are reinforced by observing identical family cases, which may be more or less expressive, proof of the hereditary nature of this connective tissue disease, without genetic testing in the common forms are by far the most frequent.

Doctor's name   Exam date   Doctor's stamp

Additional Examinations:
General Practical Notions

This scheme is recommendable for the examinations to do:

Before the age of 16:

➤ A transthoracic cardiac ultrasound and an electrocardiogram (ECG): An examination of the valves (bulging, insufficiency, prolapse), the valves' cords (hyperlaxity, micro ruptures, ruptures), the papillary muscles (micro tear, rupture), the root of the aorta in systole and diastole (dilation of the artery, thinning of the walls). It is advisable to look for inter-atrial (IAC) or even ventricular (IVC) communication, thinning of the myocardial walls, and signs of cardiac deconditioning (which is frequent due to kinesiophobia).

➤ A complete abdominal ultrasound, full bladder: an examination of the aorta, full organs (presence of cysts), bladder (search for diverticulum, positioning, cystocele), urinary tract, and gallbladder (vesicular stones), rectal prolapse.

➤ A posturological check-up (with the manufacture of proprioceptive posture insert), and possibly an orthoptic check-up and logopedic/speech therapy.

➤ An orthodontic assessment, temporomandibular joints (TMJ) and dental occlusion exams.

From the age of 16:

➤ A transthoracic cardiac ultrasound and an ECG. A tilt table test may be performed in case of POTS - postural tachycardia syndrome and a 72-hour holter monitoring in case of severe heart palpitations (it measures the heart rate and abnormalities of the ECG trace). The exercise stress test (using a treadmill or a bicycle, exercise ECG) does not seem to be indispensable from the outset; it should be requested on a case-by-case basis given the debt of fatigue and muscular pain that mainly patients present after this examination. This debt can last several days and generate really generalized asthenoalgic crisis. The tilt table test should be considered with caution in EDS (a few sudden death cases have been reported).

➢ An angio-MRI of the thoracoabdominal aorta and its branches: evaluate the arterial vessels and exclude vesicular stones, an abdominal arcuate ligament that may compress the celiac trunk, cysts of solid organs, colon or bladder diverticula, endometriosis, and more. Magnetic resonance imaging (MRI) is preferable to the CT[49] scan to avoid allergies or even anaphylactic shock linked to an iodinated contrast agent (allergies, MCAD).

➢ If available: carry out a skin biopsy with an optical microscopy examination (dendrocyte hypoplasia, elastopathy, and more) and an ultrastructural examination by transmission electron microscopy (evaluation of the collagen fibrils, granulofilamentous deposits, elastic fibers, and more): see chapter III.

➢ A complete ophthalmological examination in search of refractive disorders (myopia, astigmatism, hyperopia), angioid striations on the retina, lens subluxation, sicca syndrome, keratoconus, damage to the vitreous body, and more.

➢ A posturological check-up with the manufacture of posture insoles (proprioception).

➢ According to the clinical examination and the anamnesis: an orthoptic, logopedic / speech therapy, orthodontic, occlusiodontic check-up.

After the age of 40, or before if abnormalities are detected in the cardiovascular examinations, or if there is a family history:

➢ Arterial Doppler ultrasounds of the peripheral vessels (neck and cervical region, upper limbs, and lower limbs) and the lower limbs' venous.

Consider cerebral angio-MRI in case of persistent headache resistant to usual treatments, or if there is a known family history of aneurysm: exclude aneurysmal dilatation, Arnold-Chiari

---

[49] Computed Tomography

syndrome (ACS). Caution, one should not confuse lesions of leukoaraiosis with those of multiple sclerosis (see above).

Other examinations are to be considered on a case-by-case basis, in various specialties: ENT, stomatology, gastroenterology, pneumology, polysomnography (sleep study), neurology, rheumatology, and physical medicine, algology, urology, gynecology, and more.

Conclusions

Unfortunately, after its original description 130 years ago by Chernogubow, EDS is still largely unknown and often rejected by the medical world and university teaching throughout the world.

The patients suffer from a great medical wandering and from often inappropriate treatments, generating often serious, sometimes fatal, iatrogenic effects. Patients are often victims in the hands of professionals who are powerless to deal with an invisible disease, but which is a source of disabling situations.

This is further aggravated by the fact that the disease evolves according to a mode of crises of variable duration against a background of chronic pain and fatigue. The paradox of sometimes short attacks (one to several days) followed by a return to a basic situation further sows doubt in the minds of some doctors who are uninitiated to the detection of EDS and its varied clinical characteristics.

The patients are, in turn, labelled as imaginary patients, hypochondriacs or hysterics, or even as Munchhausen's syndrome. They are often diagnosed with fibromyalgia syndrome, multiple sclerosis, Lyme disease, Crohn's disease or ulcerative colitis, endometriosis, and are ultimately punished with a devastating "It's all in your head!" This is devastating and has disastrous consequences for these patients.

The delay in diagnosis since the onset of symptoms is more than 20 years, throughout the world. All this constitutes a real situation of medical abuse as Professor Rodney Grahame (University College of London, UK) points out.

To quote Professor Claude Hamonet: "A syndrome that is so frequent, so misleading and with such heavy human consequences cannot continue to be ignored. "

There are numerous, diversified and often very effective treatments to improve and relieve these patients, who must be managed and helped in all cases.

Topics for Reflection and Focus for the Future

➢ If we consider that 10 to 40% of the population worldwide is hyperlaxed (depending on the ethnicity) and that during their lifetime, more than 10% of hyperlaxed subjects will develop suggestive symptoms of EDS,

AND

➢ If it is true that the ultrastructural alterations of the dermis, observed in the so-called hypermobile EDS (or csEDS), are identical to those observed in asymptomatic hyperlaxed people, potentially all the other connective tissues of these hyperlaxed subjects can also be altered (tendons, muscles, organs, arteries, veins, etc.),

THEN,

➢ Shouldn't cardiovascular screening be performed in all hyperlaxed patients? Should we inform the hyperlaxed subjects and the medical profession of possible surgical or obstetrical complications, healing disorders, or hemorrhagic diatheses? Could this be the beginning of a much larger public health problem than Ehlers-Danlos Syndrome? Shouldn't health authorities and ministries of health around the world be informed of this problem?

This is another subject worthy of heated discussions already taking place around this Syndrome. Even if this idea might seem far-fetched to some, at first glance, it at least has the merit of raising questions.

Studies should be conducted to determine whether typical complications of EDS develop more frequently in asymptomatic hyperlaxed subjects.

Should we systematically test for collagen disease in patients with healing disorders, unsightly scars, failed functional surgeries (knee, shoulder, etc.), a bleeding diathesis, or others? Information to surgeons and anesthesiologists should be provided as quickly as possible.

These legitimate questions should not be dismissed too quickly because everything is possible in Medicine, genetics, and epigenetics.

To Remember

➢ EDS is a disease/syndrome that is not rare, and that is diagnosed seldom, leading patients to a significant medical wandering and to a major social and even societal isolation.

➢ It is a complex disease, but not so complicated when one takes the time to understand the structure of the supporting tissues. It is a disease influenced by genetics and probably by epigenetics and gut microbiota (see below).

➢ Patients present with a picture of diffuse astheno-algesic syndrome, often confused with fibromyalgia syndrome. It almost always includes the triad: Dysautonomia, Dysproprioception, and Dyssensoriality, to which cognitive disorders, mast cell activation disorder, and dysbiosis are often added.

➢ Operative precautions, drug contraindications, and the search for cardiovascular complications are essential, even vital (see below).

Bibliography:

Tinkle B, Castori M, Berglung B, et al. Hypermobile Ehlers-Danlos syndrome (a.k.a. Ehlers-Danlos type III and Ehlers-Danlos syndrome hypermobility type) : Clinical description and natural history. Am J Med Genet Part C Semin Med Genet. 2017; 175(1):48-69. doi: 10.1002/ajmg.c.31538.

Kumar B, Lenert P. Joint hypermobility syndrome: recognizing a commonly overlooked cause of chronic pain. Am J Med. 2017;130(6):640-647.

Ehlers E, Cutis laxa. Neigung zu Haemorrhagien in der Haut, Lockering mehrerer Artikulationen. Dermatologische Zeitschrift. 1901;8:173-174.
Chernogubow N. A. Über einen Fall von Cutis laxa. (Presentation at the first meeting of Moscow Dermatologic and Venerologic Society, Nov 13, 1891.) Monatshefte für praktische Dermatologie, Hamburg. 1892;14:76.

Danlos A. Un cas de cutis laxa avec tumeurs par contusion chronique des coudes et des genoux (xanthome juvénile pseudo-diabétique de MM Hallopeau et Macé de Lépinay) Bull. Soc. Fr. Dermatol. Syphilig. 1908;19:70-72.

Miget A. Le syndrome d'Ehlers-Danlos. Thèse de Médecine, Paris, 1933.

Schulman E, Lévy-Coblentz G. Hyperélasticité cutanée (cutis laxa) et laxité articulaire avec fragilité anormale de la peau et tumeurs molluscoïdes post-traumatiques (syndrome de Danlos). Bull. Soc. Fr. Dermatol. Syphiligr. 1932;39:1252-1256.

Weber, F.P. The Ehlers-Danlos syndrome. Br J Dermatol Syphil. 1936;48:609.

Beighton P, De Paepe A, Danks D, et al. International nosology of heritable disorders of connective tissue, Berlin, 1986. Am J Med Genet. 1988;29:581-594.

Beighton P, De Paepe A, Steinmann B, et al. Ehlers-Danlos syndromes: revised nosology, Villefranche, 1997. Am J Med Genet. 1998;77:31-37.

Malfait F, Francomano C, Byers P, et al. The 2017 international classification of the Ehlers-Danlos syndromes. Am J Med Genet Part C Semin Med Genet. 2017;175(1):8-26. doi: 10.1002/ajmg.c.31552.

Blackburn PR, Xu Z, Tumelty KE, et al. Bi-allelic alterations in AEBP1 lead to defective collagen assembly and connective tissue structure resulting in a variant of Ehlers-Danlos syndrome. Am J Hum Genet. 2018;102(4):696-705.

Hamonet C, Brock I, Pommeret St, et al. Syndrome d'Ehlers-Danlos (SED) type III (hypermobile): validation d'une échelle somatosensorielle (ECSS-62), à propos de 626 cas. Bull. Acad. Natle Méd. 2017;201(2) (séance du 28 février 2017).

Seneviratne SL, Maitland A, Afrin L. Mast cell disorders in Ehler-Danlos syndrome. Am J Med Genet Part C Semin Med Genet. 2017;175(1):226-236. doi: 10.1002/ajmg.c.31555.

Daens S, Grossin D, Hermanns-Le T, et al. *Severe mast cell activation syndrome in a 15-year-old patient with an hypermobile Ehlers-Danlos syndrome. Rev med Liege. 2018;73(2):61-64.*

Bulbena A, Baeza-Velasco C, Bulbena-Cabre A, et al. *Psychiatric and psychological aspects in the Ehlers-Danlos syndromes. Am J Med Genet Part C Semin Med Genet. 2017;175(1):237-245. doi: 10.1002/ajmg.c.31544.*

Guilleminault C, Primeau M, Chiu H, et al. *Sleep-disordered breathing in Ehlers-Danlos syndromes. A genetic model of OSA. Chest. 2013;144(5):1503-1511.*

Hugon-Rodin J, Lebegue G, Becourt S, et al. *Gynecologic symptoms and the influence on reproductive life in 386 women with hypermobility type Ehlers-Danlos syndrome: a cohort study. Orphanet J rare Dis. 2016;11(1):124.*

Chopra P, Tinkle B, Hamonet C, et al. *Pain management in the Ehlers-Danlos syndromes. Am J Med Genet Part C Semin Med Genet. 2017;175(1):212-219. doi: 10.1002/ajmg.c.31554.*

Daens S. *Syndrome d'Ehlers-Danlos de type hypermobile : mise au point des signes, symptômes et traitements après une histoire contrariée. A propos d'une expérience de plus de 1200 patients. Louvain Med. 2018;137(9):528-534.*

Hamonet C. *Ehlers-Danlos. La maladie oubliée par la médecine. Ed L'Harmattan. 2018, 2019*

CHAPTER V

Posturology and Proprioception

By Dr. Stéphane Daens, in collaboration with :

Mr. David LEROY,
Posturologist – Orthokinesist – Osteopath,
Tournai and Flobecq, Belgium
&
Mr. Dominique OUHAB,
Masseur-physiotherapist,
Melun, France

Posturology initially investigated postural disorders in patients. How do they maintain themselves in a standing position? What is the head, shoulder, and lap belt position, the position of the limbs? How do they walk? How are all parts of the body arranged with each other in space? Are there asymmetrical muscle contractures?

Postural Deficiency Syndrome is the name given to these disorders observed during the posturological examination.

Proprioception is often called the sixth sense. Sensors inform our brain about the body's position and the movement of connected limbs (thanks to the mechanoreceptors). The term proprioception was coined by 1932 Nobel Prize winning English neurophysiologist Charles S. Sherrington (1857-1952). Postural disorders depend not only on the proprioception of muscles, tendons, and joint capsules (the somatosensory system), but the constant interaction between various receptors that a priori come from independent systems. These sources of proprioception information interact, destabilize, or balance each other. Thus, Postural Deficiency Syndrome is too restrictive a phrase. Instead, they propose the term Proprioceptive Dysfunction Syndrome (or PDS).

Proprioception is part of a more complex system that intervenes in posture regulation, known as the Postural Control System (PCS). Proprioception is considered "the backbone or conductor of the postural system" (Dr. Patrick Quercia).

This PCS includes sensors or postural inputs:

➢ Muscles and tendons.
➢ The visual sensor and the manducator sensor (the retino-trigemal sensor).
➢ The inner ear.
➢ The podal sensor.

In my experience, EDS patients show identical disfunction. In particular:

➢ Forward curvature of the shoulders.
➢ Projection of the head forward, lateral inclination, and a rotation to the right or left.
➢ The cervicodorsal and lumbar paravertebral muscle chains are asymmetrically contracted (see Basani thumb test), as well as the muscles of the lower limbs and ankles (disorders of podal convergence). There are many scoliotic settings and lumbar hyperlordosis. The neck muscles are very tensed, which can lead to *pseudo-thoracic outlet syndrome*. Scapular and pelvic straps turn in opposite directions. There is sometimes a detachment of shoulder blades from the thorax (scapula alata), with the instability of the scapular joints (scapulohumeral joints).

The Sensors of Proprioception

1/ The sensors of the muscles (neuromuscular spindles), the tendons (Golgi tendon organs), and the joint capsules (Ruffini corpuscles) provide us, with permanent information, about the spatial position of the limbs, head, spine, and belts. These are informative sensory chains. Muscle tone, posture, and body movements are partly the result of these chains. Some muscles are more important than others in regulating posture: the paravertebral muscles, the pelvic and scapular belt muscles, the muscles that influence ankle movements, the neck muscles, and the eye muscles play an essential role.

2/ The ocular exosensor. The retina contains a proprioceptive part in addition to its nerve-sensory part (visual acuity). This system enables us to locate ourselves in space, regulate part of our balance, and allows us to go somewhere or flee.

It allows us to:

➢ Locate an object with its most central point (the fovea, located in the macula center).
➢ Perceive the verticals (we therefore continuously align our head according to this perception).
➢ Perceive differences in contrast.
➢ Perceive movements of objects on the periphery of the retina.

Example: A typical proprioceptive reflex of the retina is the body's reaction to a passing car, if it is perceived at the retina's periphery. When driving slowly, the vehicle is seen with a slow movement of the head. However, if it moves fast, even if it cannot be seen clearly, there will be a whole-body "flight" reaction (this is a proprioceptive reflex, not pure vision).

➢ Other information comes from the oculomotor muscles (especially the oblique muscles) that determine the eye's position in the eye socket (and since the body follows the gaze most often, you will understand the importance of this information). This information passes through the trigeminal nerve (V-nerve).

For example: there are often problems with eye convergence in EDS, blurred vision, especially in the morning and evening, or the transition from reading to distant vision.

3/ The manducatory apparatus. The proprioceptive information comes from the receptors located in the periodontium, in the pulpodental areas, and undoubtedly in the odontoblasts (pseudo-sensory elements), in the jaws, temporomandibular joints, lips, cheeks, and more. This information is also sent via the trigeminal nerve (a nerve connected to the eardrum tensor, which can explain tinnitus). This device is essential, from the baby's sucking reflex to actions such as tasting, swallowing, kissing, and clenching teeth.

Disorders of this apparatus can lead to incorrect positioning of the tongue in a child with dyslexia. It is often lateralized and not in the rear centered position, behind the incisors, mouth closed. There are more dyslexic children in the EDS population, and most also have generalized PCS disorders. Many patients clench their teeth (parafunctions), wear them down, or break them off. They subluxate their temporomandibular joints, even while sleeping. The pain spreads from the jaw to the ear, neck, and temples. Many patients make statements such as "the food goes down the wrong way", and more.

4/ The podal endosensor. Pressure sensors, similar to small springs, are located in the dermis. They interact with the ankles and feet muscles and tendon mechanoreceptors, and with those of the joint capsules (Ruffini's corpuscles).

5/ The proprioceptive part of the inner ear (thanks to the otoliths and semicircular channels) allows our brains to communicate our head's position. It mainly relates to the perception of acceleration and rotation and can often not be changed, or only slightly, in posturology.

All these sensors send complex afferences to the CNS, which reacts to the peripheral muscles and continuously adapts posture. This system is complicated in its interactions, and entire books on the subject are available for further study and understanding.

The most important thing to understand is that standing upright with all these elements, is a constant challenge. They are essential not only when standing upright and immobile but also when walking, running, lying down, and more.

Master Seiichi Sugano, one of my Aikido masters, and a personal student of Aïkido Founder *O'sensei Morihei Ueshiba*, used to repeat during training: "We are this unique link between Earth and Heaven."

In the eighties, he had undoubtedly understood all these aspects, which I did not understand at that time. He was aware of the enormous burden on us to Be One and Do One with the various external elements.

Imbalances in PCS usually lead to three specific Patterns

➤ The control of muscle tone, movements, and general posture is altered, resulting in asymmetric postures that cause muscle tension and pain. In the foreground is a Painful Pattern.

➤ The spatial position of the received information is changed. This localization of information allows the localization of sounds or other stimuli outside the body and the perception of a body part's position relating to others. If we cannot know the distance from an object or its characteristics relating to us (the self), a Pseudo-Vertiginous Pattern may be in the foreground. This pattern induces a permanent search for balance and leads to malicious positions. These disturbances also lead to inconveniences, as objects and distances are poorly located. One bumps, stumbles, or falls (the door sign).

➤ When multisensory perception is altered, patients experience this as a break between the body (posture, muscle contractions, overall tone) and the mind (sensory organs, altered sensory perception). Many patients tell us: "I feel like my body and mind are separated." This can lead to a Cognitive-typical Pattern. Because of the multi-sensory disturbances, we instead find ourselves in a typical picture of Dysesthesiology.

Diagram according to Dr. Patrick Quercia, Ophthalmologist, 2017

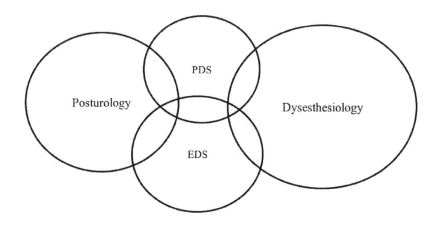

197

PDS and Dysesthesiology interconnect in the EDS

All three manifestations coincide in the same EDS patient, but one of the three patterns is usually put in the foreground.

As an acupuncturist, it is exciting to see the similarities between the pain points in PDS, the trigger points of Janet Travell, and the acupuncture points of Traditional Chinese Medicine (TCM) (see the chapter on pain). We will see later that lidocaine injection points (at trigger points) usually coincide with acupuncture points.

Different clinical tests exist to assess these different proprioceptive patterns. We will not detail them here; they are already very well explained in various books of posturology.

Here is the essential list :

For the evaluation of tone and posture:
- Rotation and extension of the head: note the asymmetries, sometimes mixed.
- The podal convergence maneuver: which evaluates posture reflexes.
- Posturo-dynamic tests: which evaluate the joint biomechanics.

For visuospatial localization:
- The pencil test.
- The eye convergence test.
- Podal perception.
- To look for vertical heterophoria (VH) in the Postural Maddox test and their reversibility after PCS correction techniques.

For disorders of sensory perception:
- After certain stimuli, whether visual, auditory, or proprioceptive, disturbances are detected in the other sensory spheres.

Example: After auditory stimuli, visual signs such as scotomas can occur in dyslexic children.

The most important thing is to process all the proprioceptive inputs disturbed and not just one of input taken in isolation. One corrected input may influence the others, but they will all need to be corrected, one after the other, to have an overall balanced effect over the long term.

Each person involved in EDS management should talk to other professionals who specialize in the field. It is a collegial work between posturologist, physiotherapist, orthotist, prosthetist, ophthalmologist, orthoptist, orthodontist, and occlusiodontist.

The work of global postural rehabilitation (Souchard's GPR), facias, and muscle chains is crucial in EDS, but it will only be positive in the long term with the implementation of other treatments:

➢ Posturological: posture insoles and other orthotic inserts.
➢ Orthoptics: re-education and placement of prisms in eyeglass lenses.
➢ Orthodontics: the placement of corrective braces, aligners, often nocturnal, or even the placement of small raider elements - the Alphs - on the labial or lingual face of the teeth in order to correct proprioceptive entries.
➢ Compression garments, which improve proprioception.

The illuminating article by *Emma Dupuis et al. (2017)* highlights that, in EDS, the combination of wearing proprioceptive (or posture) plantar orthoses and compression garments improves postural stability, especially with closed eyes, mainly in the anteroposterior axis. Proprioception is thus improved.[50]

Conclusion: All EDS patients have PDS, and it must be managed as adequately as possible. Conversely, not all patients with PDS have EDS. All caregivers can therefore use these data.

Aid in the evaluation of dysproprioception: the TINETTI test can be a valuable aid in assessing joint instability related to

---

[50] Dupuis EG, Leconte P, Vlamynck E et al. Ehlers-Danlos syndrome, hypermobility type : impact of somatosensory orthoses on postural control (a pilot study). Front Hum Neurosci. 2017;11:283. doi:10.3389/fnhum.2017.00283.

dysproprioception. Here below is the opinion of Mr. Dominique OUHAB, physiotherapist (Melun, France).

The Tinetti Test

For the record, a man standing at rest is never entirely still. He continually oscillates according to particular and complex rhythms, whose amplitude and frequency reflect the various sensorimotor systems' functioning, which places and maintains the center of gravity within the sustentation polygon. The human orthostatic equilibrium can therefore be defined as a stable, mobile equilibrium subject to constant regulation.

This equilibrium is the final result of the perception and integration of information from the three major sensorimotor systems: the vestibular system, the oculo-sensory-motor system, and the proprioceptive system (cervical proprioception, in particular, extra-cervical proprioception or exteroception, especially in the feet). The maintenance of posture (which defines balance) involves complex regulatory mechanisms involving multiple central structures (cerebral cortex, vestibular nuclei, reticular formation, and more). These central structures and the sensorimotor systems control each other, the whole constituting a model of enslaved regulation.

In the standing position, two postural reflex strategies can follow one another:

➢ As long as the body's axis varies less than 4 degrees from the vertical, postural adjustments are under continuous, automatic, and unconscious control: tonic (myotatic reflexes) and anticipated (appearing even before the start of the postural disturbance).

➢ Beyond 4 degrees, dynamic balancing reflexes appear in the form of rocking, shifting, or forward stepping reactions, more commonly known as conscious postural adjustments. It should be noted that these adjustments can be made at a greater or lesser reaction speed (calculated in millimeters per second or mm/s).

These two strategies correspond, schematically, to the two

classical forms of balance: static balance and dynamic balance.

Disorders of walking, balance, and maximal and explosive force production in EDS patients are associated with an increased risk of falls and many adverse events (subluxations, dependency, desocialization). The evaluation of walking and especially balance performance occupies, in my opinion, a central place: on the one hand, in the screening and management of these patients, and, on the other hand, in the development of targeted intervention strategies (proprioceptive re-education, support garments, orthopedic inserts).

The Tinetti test analyzes balance in different daily life situations and does not require any experience on the part of the examiner or specific equipment. It has been validated against posturography tests, and has acceptable specificity and sensitivity.

The observation is based on the analysis of static aspects with 13 tests and dynamic aspects with nine tests. A score of 0 corresponds to a normal response; when it is equal to 1, the response is adequate, and a value of 2 implies an abnormal response. These exercises present risks for EDS patients, and the evaluation of the maneuvers remains subjective. However, the parameters used to assess dynamic balance are objective and can be collected automatically.

The Tinetti test is simple and quick but does not allow for evaluating the patient in a changing environment, nor does it determine and quantify the quality of the movements used. Moreover, it does not provide information on the structures responsible for the deterioration of motor performance.

All the limitations of this clinical test make it necessary to use other approaches to understand better the risks of falling. The test also has the disadvantage of not having a threshold value that can predict the risk of falling. On the other hand, it allows materializing patients' progression during their physiotherapy rehabilitation, based on neuro-sensory-motor reprogramming.

The Tinetti Test

➤ Assessment of static balance:

- Question 1:   Sitting balance on the chair.
- Question 2:   Stand up (if possible, without the help of the arms).
- Question 3:   Attempt to stand up.
- Question 4:   Immediate standing balance (first 5 seconds).
- Question 5:   Standing balance provocation test: balance during the standing attempt with feet together.
- Question 6:   Standing balance test: push-ups (subject stands with feet together, examiner pushes lightly on sternum three times).
- Question 7:   Test of balance in standing position, eyes closed.
- Question 8:   Walking during a complete 360° turn.
- Question 9:   Balance after a complete turn.
- Question 10:   Sitting.

➤ Assessment of dynamic balance while walking:

- Question 1:   Initiation of walking (immediately after the start signal).
- Question 2:   Step length: the right foot swings.
- Question 3:   Step height: the right foot swings.
- Question 4:   Length of the step: the left foot swings.
- Question 5:   Height of the step: the left foot is swinging.
- Question 6:   Symmetry of walking.
- Question 7:   Continuity of the steps.
- Question 8:   Gap in the path (observed over 3 meters).
- Question 9:   Stability of the trunk.
- Question 10:   Width of steps.

This test does not require any specific equipment, nor does it require any specific experience. The test takes only 5 to 10 minutes.

Interpretation of the score:

- Total less than 20 points: very high risk of falling.
- Total between 20-23 points: high risk of falling.
- Total between 24-27 points: low risk of falling, look for a cause such as unequal limb length.
- Total at 28 points: average.

Testimony of Mr. David LEROY, Posturologist

Treatments Specificities for EDS Patients

As a Posturologist, Orthokinesist & Osteopath, I practice daily treatments on patients with various pathologies, especially EDS. In this testimony, I refer to patients with EDS as EDS patients and control group as non-EDS patients.

Working in close collaboration with doctors, and EDS specialists in Belgium, I have been in charge of their patients' orthokinetic treatment for several years. In this testimony, I will explain the particularities observed in the postural analysis. These notable differences facilitate detection of an EDS in a patient who is unaware of the pathology, and thus to be able to direct him/her to my medical or paramedical colleagues specialized in this field.

My consultation in postural analysis follows a well-defined structure:

➢ Anamnesis.
➢ Static postural analysis.
➢ Analysis of the foot and the sub-astragalar.
➢ Gait analysis.
➢ Posturo-dynamic analysis.
➢ Eye and jaw analysis.
➢ Palpatory analysis.
➢ Explanation to the patient and implementation of postural treatment using *Kinepod* tools.

From the anamnesis, EDS can be suspected. To the question "Where does it hurt?" The answer very often begins with "It hurts everywhere…" and often with a smile; for me, it is indicative of poor well-being; the patient does not feel well in this envelope which serves as his/her body. His/her smile says a lot, and it is rarely taken seriously. From there on, the treatment is oriented to confirm or invalidate the suspicion of EDS.

During the static and dynamic postural analysis of the gait, alterations are observable in EDS patients in 100% of cases.

In non-EDS patients, postural deficits are often related to wearing the wrong shoes, increasing inactivity in our current lifestyles, inappropriate work, and more.

In EDS patients, it is the same thing, but they also suffer from a deficit related to collagens, proteins that are very important at the structural level, found in muscles, tendons, skin, bones, and some more. It is precisely where our proprioceptive sensors are located. The purpose of these sensors is to inform the brain of our position in space. That is why EDS patients more regularly express instability disorders: "I am bumping into everything! "

It is essential to know that a postural disorder requires much energy, fatigue is quickly felt. EDS patients express instability, dizziness, fatigue, and some other symptoms. Other postural disorders are observable and accentuated in EDS patients compared to non-EDS patients: hyper pronator feet, more pronounced calcaneal valgus, disorders related to the eye. The greater the postural disorder, the stronger the compensation.

The moment dynamic proprioceptive inserts stimulate the patient, better postural tests are observable. The improvement is significant, even remarkable, in EDS patients and more marked than in non-EDS patients.

The palpatory analysis is usually the stage of my consultation that EDS patients like the least.

Why? Because EDS patients suffer from various pains, probably nociceptive, whose receptors are located in already damaged tissues, despite the characteristic hypermobility of EDS patients, this pain causes muscle retractions. There is a very significant difference between EDS and non-EDS patients.

Conclusion

As with any patient, but perhaps even more so with EDS patients, communication during a consultation is paramount. Their request is not to have an immediate solution to a specific pain. EDS patients need to understand; they are continually seeking information about their pathology, which is unfortunately still too often neglected and misunderstood. They listen and need clear and concrete explanations. On a personal level, EDS patients' consultations are incredibly enriching due to their human, social and medical particularities. Moreover, this is, in the end, what allows the therapists to blossom.

I also asked Mr. David Leroy about the architecture of the feet and ankles in EDS: "Can we talk about a false hollow foot in EDS? Can we confuse EDS patients' feet with Ledderhose disease (the equivalent of Dupuytren's disease in the hands but the feet)? "

David Leroy: "I always palpate the aponeuroses of every EDS and non-EDS patient. In most cases, the aponeuroses are painful and more intense in the EDS patients than in the non-EDS patients. When images are taken, a hollow foot is scarce in EDS. It is more of a normal or collapsed foot. In my opinion, this results from the subtalar joint eversion, which is quite pronounced in EDS patients. Therefore, if we place the subtalar joint at 0° (the arch will be more curved) and if we consider that the plantar fascia is very painful, we could talk about a false hollow foot. On the other hand, no fibrous nodule is palpated, so it is not compatible with a Ledderhose disease."

Bibliography

Alves da Silva O. Syndrome de déficience posturale : symptomatologie. 2005;121:17-20.

Gagey PM. L'examen clinique postural. Agressologie. 1980;21:125-141.

Gagey PM. L'oculomotricité comme endocapteur du système postural. Agressologie. 1987;28:899-903.

Gagey PM, Weber B. Posturologie: régularisation et dérèglements du la station debout. Edition Masson, 1995.

Gagey PM, Weber B. Entrées du système postural fin. Éditions Masson, 1995

Gagey PM, Bizzo G, Bonnier L et al. Huit leçons de Posturologie, 1995. Édité par l'Association Française de Posturologie, 4, av. de Corbéra, Paris.

Marino A, Bressan P, Villeneuve P. Bouche et Posture. Orthomagazine. 2004;54:26-27.

Martins da Cunha H. Le syndrome de dysfonction postural. Son intérêt en ophtalmologie. J Fr Ophtalmol. 1986;9:747-755.

Quercia P. Syndrome de déficience posturale : diagnostic et traitement prismatique. Réalités ophtalmologiques. 2005;121:21-30.

Quercia P. Corrections prismatiques chez l'enfant dyslexique. Les cahiers d'ophtalmologie. 2008;123-124.

Quercia P. Alteration in binocular fusion modifies audiovisual integration in children. Clin Ophtalmol. 2019;13:1137-1145.

Soulier de Morant G. L'acupuncture chinoise. Éditions Maloine, 1984.

Willem G. Le diagnostic en posturologie. Une approche globale en kinésithérapie, orthoptie, podologie et odontologie. Edition Frison-Roche, 2ème édition, 2017.

CHAPTER VI

The Autonomous Nervous System and Dysautonomia

A General Reminder of the Neuro-vegetative System

The Polyvagal Approach According To Stephen W. Porges

By Dr. Stéphane Daens, in collaboration with :

Professor Jaime F. BRAVO (Chile)

Professor Stephen W. PORGES, Dr. Katja KOVACIC,
& Dr. Jacek KOLACZ (USA)

The Autonomous Nervous System

By Dr. Stéphane Daens

The Autonomic Nervous System (ANS), also known as the sympathetic nervous system or neuro-vegetative system, is the part of the nervous system that regulates certain automatic, involuntary functions that are beyond our control. It ensures homeostasis, i.e., the internal balance of our body.

It is different from the somatic nervous system, which regulates voluntary acts such as contracting the muscles of the limbs.

In EDS, there is an alteration, or disturbance, of this ANS called Dysautonomia. It has been very well studied, especially by Professor Jaime F. Bravo (Chile and USA), Honorary President of GERSED Belgium.

Numerous publications have been made on this subject.

The ANS is divided into two parts:

➢ The sympathetic nervous system (formerly ortho-sympathetic).

➢ The parasympathetic nervous system.

    ◆ This system is of great interest and a source of many publications and books. The Polyvagal Theory, also known as the Porges' Theory, was developed by Stephen W. Porges in 1994.

In collaboration with Dr. Katja Kovacic and Dr. Jacek Kolacz (USA), Professor Stephen W. Porges (the Porges' Theory) did us the honor of writing the second part of this chapter.

Professor Jaime F. Bravo, Rheumatologist, former Professor of Medicine in Chile and the USA, and internationally recognized as one of the most outstanding specialists in dysautonomia in Ehlers-Danlos Syndrome, has kindly written the first part of this chapter.

Dysautonomia in Ehlers-Danlos Syndrome

By Professor Jaime F. BRAVO, Chile & USA

Dysautonomia is a common condition that can lead to a reduced quality of life and is a medical problem with a difficult diagnosis. Dysautonomia is often associated with hypermobile Ehlers-Danlos Syndrome (hEDS). The patients affected are often unaware they are hypermobile, and the doctors rarely look for this problem and therefore do not make the diagnosis. It is a frequent cause of fatigue, dizziness, headaches, and even syncopal episodes related to the low blood pressure frequently present in these patients.

EDS can cause various musculoskeletal complaints (joint pain, recurrent tendonitis, joint subluxations, etc.) and problems related to tissue fragilities such as dysautonomia, abdominal hernias, varicose veins, uterine descent, mitral valve prolapse, myopia, spinal disc disease, osteoarthritis, and early osteoporosis.

The autonomic nervous system (ANS) has afferent nerve roots that unconsciously regulate essential body functions and internal homeostasis. This includes control of blood pressure, electrolytes and water balance, visceral functions, and body temperature. The afferent roots are classified into two groups: the orthosympathetic adrenergic system and the parasympathetic system. A proper balance between these two systems maintains normal internal homeostasis and allows adaptation to environmental changes. Alteration of these involuntary regulatory processes leads to dysfunction of the cardiovascular system, symptoms common in chronic fatigue syndrome, fibromyalgia, and Ehlers-Danlos Syndrome.

The Physiopathology of dysautonomia is complex and not yet fully understood. For these reasons, its treatment and management remain difficult. In 1932, Lewis[1] coined the name vasovagal syncope and noticed that the cause of it was not just an increase of vagal tone (parasympathetic), but also a decrease in the orthosympathetic response. He indicated that atropine, although it increased the heart rate, did not improve either the state of consciousness or the arterial hypotension. The patient, in this case, continued to be pale due to peripheral vasoconstriction. Lewis's idea was that the parasympathetic bradycardia was particularly important in symptomatology, but it was secondary to the deep vasodilation and arterial hypotension that set in during the syncopal episode.

In some cases, rather than bradycardia, patients present with tachycardia, primarily when they suddenly rise from a bed or chair. This phenomenon is called Postural Orthostatic Tachycardia Syndrome (POTS).

Many diseases are associated with impaired autonomic nerve reflexes, such as Parkinson's disease, diabetes mellitus, amyloidosis, porphyria, and other forms of toxic, hereditary, or inflammatory neuropathies[2]. Apparently, the causes listed above are rare and, as far as I can remember in my practice as a physician, the vast majority of cases of dysautonomia are linked to Hereditary Connective Tissue Diseases (HCTD), of which Ehlers-Danlos Syndrome is one. In EDS, genetic changes in the extracellular matrix (mainly due to changes in collagens) alter the venous walls, contributing to a drop in blood pressure through venous dilatation (peripheral venous pooling). Due to an inadequate cardiovascular response to the increased splanchnic (bowel) circulation, these patients may experience postprandial (after meal) hypotension.

Because the dysautonomia arises from an alteration of the ANS, the symptoms appear unconsciously to the patient. Apart from the digestive symptoms mentioned above, other symptoms are frequent, such as alterations in body temperature regulation (e.g., unexplained fever), intolerance to cold (chilliness) or inappropriate sweating (diaphoresis). During sudden changes in position (such as getting out of bed quickly), when standing in line for a long time (at the store, post office, etc.) or sauntering in a shopping mall (or supermarket), or after eating a large meal (especially if accompanied by alcohol), the blood flow to the heart decreases, resulting in a sudden drop in blood pressure, causing hypoxia in the brain. When someone suddenly stands up, 300 to 800 milliliters of blood stagnate in the abdomen and lower limbs. In patients with dysautonomia, the body is unable to quickly compensate for this decrease in circulating volume, resulting in various symptoms: dizziness, headaches, fatigue, and syncope.

An excellent analogy to explain this phenomenon is what happens to the liquid in a half-empty bottle[2]. If we stand up a lying bottle, we can see that the liquid stagnates at the bottom of the bottle (representing the stomach and the lower limbs). When we put it back down, the liquid spills towards the neck (here the neck represents the human brain).

Experiments with rabbits show the same phenomenon. If a rabbit is held upright by its ears, it is observed that its hindquarters increase in volume, and it falls unconscious. The explanation for this phenomenon is that their veins do not contain valves that prevent blood from flowing backward. A similar phenomenon of blood accumulation in the declivities exists in patients with dysautonomia, and therefore they feel weak, dizzy and can have syncopal episodes. This is also what happens to a soldier in a parade, and he may fall unconscious after standing for a long time without moving his feet. If you lay him down, he recovers quickly because the return of blood is improved, and the blood returns from the extremities to the heart and brain.

When sitting or standing for an extended period of time, it is helpful to move the hands and feet so that the muscles can increase this blood return through their contractions; the calf muscles are thus called the second heart. In rare cases, loss of consciousness may be associated with epilepsy-like seizures (false diagnoses of epilepsy may be made).

Patients with dysautonomia are easily fatigued, drowsy and generally feel that their batteries need to be recharged in the afternoon; they have no energy. This is the cause of chronic fatigue, dizziness, and episodes of syncope.

Because of this chronic fatigue and paroxysmal feeling of generalized weakness, these patients are often misdiagnosed with depression, fibromyalgia, hypothyroidism, or hypoglycemic crises. Family and friends often view them as lazy or have antisocial behavior, simply because they lack the energy to attend meetings or do not interact with others. This happens to both women and men.

It is my feeling that fibromyalgia is part of Ehlers-Danlos Syndrome Type III (hEDS). I worked for 30 years in the USA, and I met fibromyalgia patients every day. I am now convinced that all these patients had, in fact, Ehlers-Danlos Syndrome, some with little or no joint hypermobility.

Because of the alterations of ANS and venous pooling in the lower limbs (AN: venous pooling = stagnation and accumulation of blood and therefore of blood volume in the declining parts of the body, the lower limbs for the most part), secondary to the alterations of the collagen of the vessel wall, the patients have a tendency to have chronically low blood pressure and bradycardia (AN: heart rate < 60 beats/minute), and thus they can have dysautonomia attacks when confronted with strong

211

emotions, high altitude (the mountains, visits to archaeological sites in Peru, etc.), dehydration, acute anemia, intense pain, the sight of blood for some, pregnancy, a crowded place (AN: like a church, a concert, sales, etc.).

For the past 20 years, I have been interested in studying Ehlers-Danlos Syndrome, the hypermobile type. I currently prefer the term Ehlers-Danlos type III (EDS - III), since, in a study I conducted on 2300 patients[3], I observed that 51% of them had a low Beighton's score (5/9 or less), indicating that they were not hypermobile.

Joint hypermobility is present in approximately 15% of the general population worldwide. We found that generalized joint hypermobility affected 39% of the Chilean population[4]. EDS-III is probably the most common cause of pain in rheumatology practice, but it is usually undiagnosed.

Some of these patients have very hyperlaxed joints, and are very flexible or were flexible during childhood, with recurrent sprains (e.g., the ankles) or subluxations. Other patients have low hypermobility, but they or their close relatives have fragile tissues, and, because of this, they may present with scoliosis, hip dysplasia, (false-) flat feet, lumbar problems, abdominal hernias, prolapse of certain organs, colonic diverticulosis, cracked joints, early osteoarthritis, premature osteoporosis, varicose veins in youth, etc. Frequently, they have stretchy, pale skin with visible veins, bruises due to capillary fragility (AN: and due to platelet's adhesion dysfunction). Less frequently, they have serious problems such as aneurysms, arterial ruptures, spontaneous pleural detachment (spontaneous pneumothorax), miscarriages, or a tendency to bleed. These more severe complications are mainly seen in vascular type EDS (vEDS). Both types of EDS may present with dysautonomia.

Tissue fragility is secondary to genetic alterations in collagen. Collagen is a protein that forms the extracellular matrix of all tissues, and I tell my patients that collagen is like steel in building construction. Since it is considered a dominantly inherited disease, 50% of children will inherit EDS as well. In a group of young patients under 30 years of age, we found that 84% of women and 61% of men with EDS-III had dysautonomia[3]. We agree with Rowe[5,] who reports that when a patient has fatigue and orthostatic intolerance, the diagnosis of Ehlers-Danlos or another connective tissue disease should be carefully sought.

Symptoms of Dysautonomia

The most common symptom is fatigue. Exhaustion occurs most often in the afternoon. If patients stand for too long, without moving their extremities, they begin to feel like they are at the end of their rope, their face becomes pale or grayish, they sweat and look like someone who is having a hypoglycemic attack. If they do not sit up or lie down, they may have an episode of syncope. After a while, they do not feel well; they feel weak, chronically tired, without energy, do not feel like talking to other people around them, and gradually become mute. They are more and more pale, tired, with heavy eyelids, not wanting to participate in anything anymore. At this point, because of the lack of facial expression, they may be misdiagnosed as having Parkinson's disease. These patients are mistakenly labeled as uncooperative or antisocial. It is important to recognize these early symptoms to avoid falls, fractures, or concussions. Hands and feet may feel swollen when standing, sauntering, or when the weather is too hot. The fingers may feel narrow, somewhat stiffened by the swelling, a result of poor local circulation. Clenching and unclenching the fist and moving the fingers repeatedly is essential to resolve the problem. These patients tend to have a high intolerance to cold, forcing them to expose themselves to the sun like lizards. Sometimes they have heat intolerance, so I tell them they have a bad thermostat. They get colds easily in cold weather. Some of them know they have low blood pressure, but no one has told them they have dysautonomia; that is why they have a poor quality of life (QoL). They are incredibly happy when they finally find a doctor who can explain the cause of their symptoms and give them a diagnosis: dysautonomia.

Depressed patients tend to be tired from early morning on. Hypothyroidism can also cause chronic fatigue, mainly in older people, and is also frequently under-diagnosed. Apart from fatigue and cold intolerance, these hypothyroid patients may have dry skin, a deep voice, and overweight. A lack of tendon reflex confirms the diagnosis on clinical examination, and blood tests show an increased TSH level and a lowered free T4 level.

Some patients with dysautonomia have episodes of tachycardia, mainly when they get up suddenly from a chair, for example. This orthostatic tachycardia is called POTS.

What are the phenomena that aggravate dysautonomia?

- ➢ Dehydration, due to:
    - o Excessive heat.
    - o Fever.
    - o Vomiting.
    - o Diarrhea.
    - o Taking diuretic drugs.
- ➢ High altitude, in cities such as Mexico City or when climbing mountains. It can also happen on roller coasters in amusement parks, because of the rapid succession of ascents and descents.
- ➢ Standing in a church, waiting for a long time, getting up suddenly from a bed or chair.
- ➢ Phobia of closed places (claustrophobia).
- ➢ The sight of blood, especially of a relative or close friend.
- ➢ Distressing, stressful, frightening situations.
- ➢ Intense pain or pain associated with anxiety, such as when going for an injection.
- ➢ During strong emotions or nervousness, such as when one must take an exam at school or in college.
- ➢ Acute or chronic anemia.
- ➢ Sauntering, such as in a shopping mall or supermarket.
- ➢ With certain blood pressure medications, which produce orthostatic hypotension as a side effect (such as calcium channel blockers and diuretics).
- ➢ Standing for a long time without being able to move.
- ➢ After a heavy meal or excessive alcohol consumption.
- ➢ During sexual intercourse.
- ➢ During menstruation (heavy periods).

- When coughing a lot, repeatedly, or when making efforts to defecate, in case of constipation (this causes a vasovagal stimulation).
- During pregnancy.
- During a prolonged hot bath (bathtub, shower, sauna, jacuzzi) or during Bikram yoga which is performed at 42°C.

Note. In any circumstance, the problems result from a decrease in venous return from the lower limbs, resulting in cerebral hypoxia and other symptoms of dysautonomia. Therefore, it is necessary to diagnose this situation as soon as possible, prevent it and treat it adequately, with general measures and medication.

Consequences of Dysautonomia

- A poor quality of life, because dysautonomia is not diagnosed and not treated for years.
- A tendency to fall with bruises, injuries, or fractures. EDS-III patients frequently have osteoporosis. They often feel dizzy when they jump out of bed or see little stars.
- Dizziness, headaches, and nausea at high altitudes (Machu Pichu, at 2,350 meters). They cannot stand without moving their extremities or remain standing during events, or when waiting in line, due to increasing fatigue and the tendency to syncope.
- Cold intolerance, sometimes severe, and swelling of the hands and feet due to poor circulation (acrocyanosis).
- Fatigue, drowsiness, and headaches after sexual intercourse.
- Angina pectoris in patients with coronary insufficiency, caused by a drop in blood pressure.
- Confusion with misdiagnosis: chronic fatigue syndrome, fibromyalgia, depression, hypoglycemic crisis, lack of interest in participating in events.

How is Dysautonomia Diagnosed?

It is common for a patient to be undiagnosed for years, or even never to be diagnosed, as happened to me personally. I have EDS - III, without hypermobility. As a child, I had to do all kinds of sports. I had to run every day, even at recess in school, to avoid chronic fatigue and to feel good. I was cold and had to dress

215

warmly. When I was about 35, I felt worse and started having syncope. I had difficulty with memory and concentration. Having moved to the USA, despite having had frequent syncope for 15 years, having consulted many doctors of different specialties, and having undergone multiple complementary tests, no diagnosis was made. Finally, due to age, I developed high blood pressure, and the dysautonomia disappeared. After returning to Chile 20 years ago, I made the diagnosis myself when I was interested in the study of Ehlers-Danlos Syndrome.

The diagnosis is made clinically and should be envisaged in any patient who presents with chronic fatigue, lack of energy, dizziness, headaches, with or without syncope or pre-syncopal state, especially in patients with Ehlers-Danlos Syndrome, hypermobile or not. The problem also lies in the fact that the diagnosis of EDS is rarely made, because physicians do not have this diagnosis in mind. There is ignorance about this syndrome worldwide. It is only belatedly that a major effort has been made to inform and raise awareness about EDS. The International EDS Consortium was held in 2016 in New York, and new criteria were developed.

Most cardiologists do not specialize in dysautonomia. Many think low blood pressure is normal, and some even think it is beneficial. Since pediatricians still too rarely monitor children's blood pressure, they have realized that children with attention deficit disorder (ADD) probably have low blood pressure, and these children are often hyperactive to compensate for this lowered blood pressure. I would advise them to monitor the blood pressure of these children and, if it is low, to give them salt rather than medication.

Gazit et al.[6] studied 48 EDS patients and 30 control (non-EDS) subjects. They found dysautonomia in 78% of the EDS patients and only 10% of the non-EDS (control) subjects. They concluded that dysautonomia is an extra-articular manifestation of EDS, reasoning that I fully support. As I wrote earlier, in our study of 2,300 patients, we found dysautonomia in 84% of the women and 61% of the men in a young group under 30 years of age. The frequency of dysautonomia decreases with age; older women may also have dysautonomia, but it is less frequent. With the onset of age-related hypertension, dysautonomia disappears. Usually, patients and physicians do not give importance to their dysautonomia symptoms and, thus, patients continue to feel unwell for many years with a poor quality of life.

How to Confirm the Diagnosis?

The diagnosis is clinical, and a positive response to the treatment initiated validates the diagnosis. Some cardiologists confirm the diagnosis with a TILT test. I do not recommend this test as a routine; it can cause arrhythmias, and we know of three cases of cardiac arrest. In my opinion, a doctor, who is familiar with dysautonomia, can make the diagnosis clinically without any problems.

Dysautonomia Treatment

The treatment is symptomatic, and there is no curative treatment. However, we have established recommendations, general measures, and medications that are effective.

Recommendations:

➤ It is important to avoid any factor that could aggravate the dysautonomia (see above).
➤ Avoid standing for a long time. If this cannot be avoided, various movements can help, such as crossing your legs; standing on your tiptoes and returning to the plantar sole; alternately placing one foot facing the other and changing; bending forward, as if you were going to tie your shoes; squatting and/or placing one foot on a chair with the knee extended.
➤ Avoid sauntering in shopping malls or supermarkets. Do not stay in these structures for more than one hour (less than one hour is best).
➤ When you sit in a bus or plane for a long time, it is necessary to move your knees and ankles frequently and stand up and walk. Occasionally, you can try two positions: putting your chest on your knees while bending over or putting your head between your knees.
➤ Avoid getting up suddenly from a bed or chair.

➢ After a heavy dinner or too much alcohol, try lying down for 15 minutes or more. Also, do this if you are experiencing early symptoms of dysautonomia.

- General Measures.

➢ Fluids. We recommend drinking 2 to 3 liters of fluid a day or until urine is clear as water. If the urine is concentrated and dark, the patient needs to drink more. Drinks containing electrolytes or isotonic drinks may help. Alcohol and coffee do not increase blood pressure.

➢ Compressive garments. We recommend elastic stockings, tights if possible, with a pressure measured at the ankle of at least 20 mm Hg, to increase blood return from the extremities. In Paris, Professor Hamonet[7] uses custom-made compression garments for men and women with excellent results. He also uses sequential oxygen therapy in the treatment of patients with dysautonomia, again with excellent results.

➢ Salt intake should be quantified and most often increased. Salt intake should be increased if the patient does not have hypertension or renal impairment*. This will increase venous blood return and blood pressure, making the patient feel much better. We recommend the intake of 6 grams of salt (NaCl) per day to be added to foods already cooked and salted normally. One teaspoon contains 3 grams of salt, so it will be necessary to add two teaspoons of salt per day to obtain the desired 6 grams. So it can be added to meals, but also to juices or water. Most people are afraid of salt, but they should be told that it is not bad for their health. Salt should only be avoided by people suffering from high blood pressure or kidney failure (AN: or heart failure).

➢ Increase physical activity. Moderate aerobic exercise is helpful to promote a venous return to the heart and brain through muscle contractions. The most beneficial, in my opinion, are exercises in water or exercises that involve standing for long periods. These patients need to be as active as possible. I also recommend Pilates, Yoga, Tai-Chi Chuan, swimming, or cycling three times a week.

- Medications.

➢ Fludrocortisone. This is a potent mineral-corticoid. It increases circulating blood volume and allows satisfactory venous blood to return to the heart while the patient is in the standing position. Its most significant advantage over Midodrine (Gutron® 2.5mg/tablet) is that its action lasts for more than 24 hours, unlike Midodrine's duration of action, which is only 4 to 5 hours. Its side effects are minor and include high blood pressure, peripheral edema, acne, depression, and hypokalemia. Electrolytes should be measured at the beginning of treatment and every 3 to 6 months. I most often use doses of 100 micrograms (0.1mg), once a day over a long period. The dose can be increased if necessary. It is generally well tolerated. Contraindications are glaucoma; it can be used with caution during pregnancy. When used, live attenuated vaccines, such as measles and yellow fever, are not recommended because of possible immunity problems. If the vaccine is required, then stop fludrocortisone for three weeks, administer the vaccine, and resume fludrocortisone three weeks later.

➢ Midodrine. This is an α-adrenoreceptor agonist with a peripheral action, and has no β-adrenergic effect. It increases blood pressure by increasing venous tone and peripheral vascular resistance in hypotensive patients. It is available in doses of 2.5mg and 5mg per tablet. It should be given in three doses per day (short half-life). The correct schedule is to give it at 7:00 am 12:00 pm, and 5:00 pm. It is important to tell patients that it may cause scalp pruritus and a tendency to urinary retention for the first few days.

➢ Clonidine. This is another α-adrenoreceptor agonist, partially selective. It can sometimes help some patients or be added to other medications.

➢ The β-blockers. Propranolol and Metoprolol, for example. I prefer not to use them to treat dysautonomia because their effect is to decrease cardiac contractility. If the patient also has POTS, I add it later when the dysautonomia is already sufficiently regulated (or prefer Ivabradine, see the chapter on the cardiac manifestations).

➤ Anxiolytics and antidepressants. They are useful, at least if the patient is indeed anxious or depressed.

AN: Etilefrin (Effortil® 5mg/comp). Etilefrin is a sympathomimetic amine (α-1 and β-1 adrenoreceptor agonist). It increases blood pressure and heart rate (not indicated in case of POTS or tachyarrhythmia). Usual dosage: 2 tablets tid.

In case of anemia or sleep apnea, it is necessary to correct them because they worsen the dysautonomia. A pacemaker may be indicated in some cases to prevent syncope.

Why the treatment of dysautonomia fails, while when properly administered, the treatment is remarkably effective?

➤ The fear of adding salt. It is a belief, maintained by doctors and the press, that salt is bad. This is not true because salt is good for your health. Salt, in recommended doses, does not cause any problems, but it does help to normalize blood pressure.
➤ Fear of increasing fluid intake. Unfortunately, people think that salt and fluid intake will increase leg swelling, weight gain or cellulite. This is not true.
➤ Misconceptions that treatment can lead to: weight gain, cellulite, high blood pressure or kidney damage.
➤ Refusal to wear compression stockings. This is mainly the result of their high price, and the difficulty EDS patients have in putting them on. They do not understand that this is a particularly important part of treatment.
➤ Fear of steroids. Patients think that a mineralocorticoid, such as fludrocortisone, can have the same effects as a glucocorticoid (cortisone given for inflammation). This is not true.
➤ The high cost of medication.
➤ The fear of having to take medication for life. The idea comes from treating high blood pressure, which is usually taken for life. It is important to make them aware that blood pressure tends to increase with age and that dysautonomia tends to disappear.

- Not being aware that properly administered treatment can improve memory, concentration, reduce cold intolerance, chronic fatigue, headaches, dizziness, and syncope.
- Not knowing that the treatment they stop will make them: apathetic, asocial, anxious, and depressed. With treatment, their attention deficit, quality of life and self-esteem will improve.
- Not understanding that dysautonomia can cause a decrease in brain oxygenation, which can lead to brain damage and attention deficits in adults as well.
- Because of inactivity. Because of EDS's joint and muscle pain, some people unfortunately avoid all activity (AN: kinesiophobia). However, they should be as active as possible and exercise at least three times a week. Others do not understand the importance of physical activity on the increase of blood pressure in case of dysautonomia.
- Because of the altitude, living at an altitude of 1500 meters or more aggravates dysautonomia due to lack of oxygen.
- Because of anxiety or depression. This causes a lack of compliance with treatments.
- Because of anemia. Anemia worsens the symptoms of dysautonomia by cerebral hypoxia.
- The presence of sleep apnea. Like anemia, they decrease cerebral oxygenation, which worsens the symptoms of dysautonomia.
- Because of the partial taking of the prescribed treatment, patients follow some treatments but not others or they do not take the prescribed medication (lack of compliance).
- Not regularly returning for a medical check-up. We frequently encounter patients who do not return for their follow-up visit. Some of them follow their treatment by themselves, without medical control and without regular laboratory tests (see fludrocortisone).

The Prognosis

The prognosis is generally good, but it depends on how well patients follow their treatment instructions (which are not easy to follow for everyone). If they feel they have a 30% improvement in their symptoms at the follow-up visit, it means that they are not following their treatment correctly. On the other hand, if they feel they have a 50% improvement, it means that they are following 50% of the recommendations made to them. Later, after a few months, if they say they are 80% or 90% better, they follow all the instructions given correctly. So, the effect of the proposed treatments depends exclusively on how the patients follow the prescribed treatment at the beginning.

Summary

Dysautonomia is common, but it is most often undiagnosed and leads to chronic fatigue, dizziness, syncope, and poor quality of life. It is common in Ehlers-Danlos Syndrome type III (EDS - III). Patients with dysautonomia go from doctor to doctor, undergo multiple complementary examinations, are given different medical hypotheses, but the precise diagnosis is not made. Although there is good symptomatic treatment, the results are not as good as expected because patients are worried about having to take so many salt and water supplements; they are also afraid of mineralocorticoids.

For more information : www.reumatologia-dr-bravo.cl[2]

References.

1. *Lewis T. A lecture on vasovagal syncope and the carotid sinus mechanism. BMJ 1932,1:873-876.*

2. *Dr Bravo's Rheumatology Web Page. www.rheumatologia-dr-bravo.cl*

3. *Bravo JF. Disautonomia y osteoporosis en 2300 pacientes con SED – III. Poster presentado en el Simposio Internacional de SED, Nueva York, EEUU, mayo 2016. It can be seen also in my web page.*

4. *Bravo JF, Wolf C. Clinical study of hereditary disorders of connective tissues in a Chilean population. Joint hypermobility syndrome and vascular Ehlers-Danlos syndrome. Arthritis Rheum 2006,54(2); 515-523. It can be seen also in my Web page.*

5. *Rowe PC, Barron DF, Calkins H, Maumenee R, Tong PY, Gerag MT. Orthostatic intolerance and chronic fatigue syndrome associated with Ehlers-Danlos syndrome. J Pediatr 1999, 135;494-499.*

6. *Gazit Y, Nahir AM, Grahame R, Jacob G. Dysautonomia in the hypermobility syndrome. Am J Med 2003,115;33-40.*

7. Dr Hamonet's book. Ehlers-Danlos, la maladie oubliée par la médecine, Ed. L'Harmattan 2018, 2019.

The Polyvagal Theory of Stephen W. Porges: A revolution in our understanding of the ANS.

Introduction

By Dr. Stéphane Daens

We learned in Science classes or on the benches of the School of Medicine that the autonomous nervous system (ANS or neuro-vegetative or involuntary system) was divided into two sections with opposite roles: on the one hand, the sympathetic nervous system (formerly orthosympathetic), which accelerates our functions such as heart rate, energy expenditure, stress, our reactivity, and on the other hand, the parasympathetic system (the vagus nerve) which acts as a brake as if to slow down our heart rate. However, since the American professor Stephen W. Porges's work in the 1990s, we have learned that the parasympathetic nervous system is not unique, but doubled.

We have two parasympathetic nervous systems, one ventral and one dorsal, well-differentiated by their moment of appearance during the evolution of species (phylogenesis), by the place of emergence of these in the brain stem, and by their distinct but complementary functions.

Phylogenesis is the study of relationships between living beings, and it allows us to reconstruct the evolution of living organisms.

The Polyvagal Theory

➢ The dorsal parasympathetic, the oldest system, has a global immobilizing function. It is called dorsal because the afferent and efferent nerve fibers of this system have their central point nuclei located in the posterior portion of the brain stem. It has appeared in reptiles, which can slow down their metabolism and become almost inert, possibly passing for death for very long periods. This mechanism is mediated by a neurotransmitter called acetylcholine. It is a system that is

223

very well preserved from reptiles in both mammals and humans. For example, when my cat catches a little field mouse, the mouse plays dead. The cat, disinterested in this inanimate toy, let us go of its prey, and the little mouse then starts moving again and runs.

➢ In the same way, we can be stunned by a highly stressful situation from which we cannot escape or fight, when we are trapped, without being able to find an outlet or when we are faced with a potentially fatal danger that is beyond our control. This is the case for certain situations of family abuse, rape or even when, as we experienced in 2020, an unprecedented health situation with Covid-19 (anxiety, illness, death, confinement, loss of social ties, financial problems, uncertainty for the future, etc.). In humans, this can be, unlike some animals, counterproductive. Our digestive system is out of whack; we can withdraw into ourselves, no longer feel like moving, stay cooped up at home, barricade ourselves in inaction, lack energy, desires (among others sexual), and depression can appear. During a rape, the victim can be completely overwhelmed, and instead of fighting back with all her strength, she gives in, submits, becomes a doll that her attackers can manipulate without difficulty (like a mouse in the cat's mouth, but here it is partially inappropriate, except, perhaps, to avoid suffering more violence that this act, already deeply atrocious, could induce). Immobility is the consequence of the dorsal system. It is our body's "last resort" when faced with an emergency. To get out of this state is not easy and requires adapted care and work on oneself, sometimes exceptionally long. It is like being blocked or frozen (the dorsal system has a freeze function).

Apart from these extreme situations and without any apparent way out, the dorsal system plays a regulating role for all the organs situated under the diaphragm (the viscera) but also for the heart and the lungs (inducing a vagal malaise, for example).

➢ The sympathetic system, of more recent appearance, has a Fight or Flight function: "Fight, and if you cannot, run!". It is a reaction of fight (of any kind, physical or psychic) or flight (from various situations, physical or psychic), which aims to protect us in the face of an emergency. It appears in fish during the evolution of species and is in the central part of the spinal cord in humans. The heart rate increases, bringing more blood to the brain and muscles due to the secretion of stress hormones: cortisol and adrenaline. The primary goal is to think quickly and to strengthen muscle capacity: I fight or flight. The consequences of this sympathetic activation are varied: tachycardia, high blood pressure, sleep disorders, digestive disorders, etc. But it also causes psychological disorders such as anxiety, anguish, paranoia, memory and concentration problems, rejection of the outside world, even rejection of friends and family, who are often benevolent.

➤ The ventral parasympathetic, the last to arrive in animal evolution, serves us to be safe, communicate, and engage socially to flourish. It appears, later in evolution, in mammals. The nuclei from which efferences and afferences originate and arrive are located further forward in the brain stem than those of the dorsal system. The fibers of the vagus nerve travel in two directions: upward in connection with the cranial nerves and downward to the organs. It is a vagal brake. It regulates our heart rate (it slows down our heartbeats), the bronchial tubes, the lungs (we breathe fully and calmly), the trachea, the upper part of the esophagus, the muscles of the larynx, the pharynx, the palate, and the ear (we listen, speak, show our interest by mimics, etc.) It collaborates with cranial nerves that innervate the muscles of the neck and the trapezium (through nerve XI, called accessory nerve or spinal nerve), the facial nerve (nerve VII), and the glossopharyngeal nerve (or nerve IX)[51].

All these collaborations allow us to communicate with others, talk to them, smile at them, show them mimics of displeasure or satisfaction, show them our emotions, and show interest in them by turning our heads to lend an ear and listen to them. Stephen W. Porges has shown that this ventral system is a cornerstone of what he has called the social engagement (and attachment) system. It allows for

---

[51] The term vague nerve here is quite appropriate: it comes from the Latin *vagus* which means wandering, moving, wandering, floating.

these face-to-face interactions. We are connected to others, we are hopeful and full of plans, our visceral and metabolic systems are well regulated and harmonious such as sleep, breathing, digestion, heart rate, etc. I can have fun, enjoy my life, love, build my future by being alone or with others; we feel in harmony and are in general well-being. For this ventral parasympathetic system to work, I must not be overwhelmed by the sympathetic or dorsal para-sympathetic. They must be kept on standby or activated sparingly for activities. I must feel safe; there must be no sign of permanent danger around me.

➢ In some cases, we can activate two or even three systems at the same time:

We can activate the ventral parasympathetic system and the sympathetic system, for example: when we play a board game with a friend, it is fun, we feel confident, we exchange with the other, but there is adrenaline, we compete, we can heckle each other after a while, but without aggression. Little by little, games are learned since early childhood. We can be mobilized (by the sympathetic) and be in security, in social engagement with the other at the same time (by the ventral parasympathetic). When we go beyond the limits, the other teaches us not to go beyond them anymore, to self-regulate our emotional states, without fear, without danger. In a way, it teaches us to use our vagal brake better to defuse a situation that could get out of hand and thus allow our social engagement system to play its role without having to go through the excessive activation of the sympathetic mobilization system (fight or flight).

We can also go through the three states or oscillate between the three: ventral parasympathetic social engagement, sympathetic mobilization, and dorsal parasympathetic immobilization. If there is an imbalance and the sympathetic system takes over, then on the contrary, there is conflict, fighting, insulting words etc. This is the case if the vagal brake is insufficient and/or if the ventral social engagement system is immature. The vagal brake is very quick to settle down or on the contrary to diminish, contrary to the sympathetic system and its batch of stress hormones which have a prolonged effect, and which settles down more slowly.

Making love is another example of the cohabitation between the ventral parasympathetic system of social engagement (affection, caressing, taking care of others, listening, etc.) and the dorsal parasympathetic system (one must be sufficiently immobilized in one place to be able to have a sexual act). If the sympathetic system, which produces stress hormones, takes over, there is failure, stress, fear of failing, an unconscious feeling of danger, a lower quality of erection, premature ejaculation, running away from the other person, bickering and possible conflicts.

➢ Some people are in a quasi-permanent imbalance of these different ANS systems, and they do not, or rarely, reach a state of social engagement, exchange, general well-being. They are caught between permanent danger signals (what Stephen Porges has called neuroception) and defense mechanisms (sympathetic system) and / or blockages leading to immobility, submission, depression, dissociation, or loss of consciousness (dorsal parasympathetic), if there is no possibility of fleeing for example. The lifting of the vagal brake is quickly put in place in the face of danger, but in order not to sink into these last two cases, one can then engage one's social engagement system of the ventral sympathetic and try to calm the situation (even in front of one's aggressor. For example, by talking to him and trying to defuse the situation).

➢ If the lifting of the vagal brake is insufficient or if the ventral parasympathetic system of engagement is immature (after child abuse, sexual abuse or domestic violence that did not allow for a safe relationship with the other, after a relationship with a narcissistic pervert for example), then our sympathetic system of mobilization (fight, flight) or our dorsal parasympathetic system of immobilization is triggered and takes over.

➢ Our organism must have safety cues to be able to trigger its social engagement system and prevent the defense mechanisms (sympathetic and dorsal parasympathetic).

Unfortunately, in these cases of insufficient vagal brake and immaturity of the ventral parasympathetic, the patients are often in great suffering daily. The defense mechanisms are unconscious, leading to inappropriate behaviors concerning external stimuli that are felt to be dangerous (neuroception).

➢ The Polyvagal Theory also helps to explain the different behaviors of patients with post-traumatic stress: Fight or Flight mechanism or freeze mode.

➢ Applications in Ehlers-Danlos Syndrome are potentially particularly important. Many patients have experienced a triggering factor before the onset or aggravation of their symptomatology. While we have discussed the potential role of epigenetics, it may be intertwined with inappropriate defense mechanisms of the autonomic nervous system. The role of altered connective tissue properties in afferent signal dysfunction is also of interest here.

➢ EDS patients have a great capacity for resilience and rebound. They can be in an asthenoalgic period, leading to danger messages, neuroceptive and trigger the sympathetic system (anger, aggressiveness, anxiety), then a withdrawal, kinesiophobia, and social isolation (dorsal parasympathetic of immobilization). However, when the crisis is over, they can quickly advance in phylogenetic time, from reptile to fish, then from fish to mammal. They can switch back to a ventral sympathetic mode of social engagement and exchange in a short period of time. This can be seen in one day or from one hour to the next. This can be confusing to spouses and friends. The role of the vagal theory in EDS appears to be essential and exciting. Imagine a steep road whose summit is the sympathetic ventral of social engagement. The middle of the slope is sympathetic of defense, fight, and flight. Finally the bottom of the road is the basis of phylogenesis, represented by the immobilization system of the dorsal sympathetic.

One can be at the top of the slope and feel in harmony and a ventral well-being situation. Nevertheless, in the face of danger signals (neuroception), go down the road towards the sympathetic stress level. At this level, one may be able to climb back up the slope, but one may also let oneself fall back down to the lower level of immobility and withdrawal. One can slowly descend the slope but also fall back to the very bottom. One can also firmly push with legs from the bottom of a swimming pool and get to the surface. It is this last pattern that most EDS patients seem to adopt.

➤ Professor Porges has initiated various research protocols, including "the Safe and Sound Protocol or SSP". The aim is to regain a reduction in stress to access a model of social engagement and resilience through listening to music (through headphones) that promotes a sense of security and to be able to regain a sense of the emotional meaning of language (not just listening to words) and the ability to engage. It appears that chronic pain is intertwined with the pathways of the ANS. It is noted that various pain treatments will alter the ANS, but this is not the purpose of these treatments. Consequently, we can imagine that therapies aimed at regulating the ANS pathways, which itself influences pain, will improve this suffering. Professor Porges' Listening Project Protocol or: how can music influence the vagus nerve and soothe the pain? It is, therefore, necessary to evaluate the modification of the vagus responses by examining the respiratory sinus arrhythmia (see below) on the one hand, and its repercussion in everyday life experiences on the other hand (via the Body Perception Questionnaire, see Stephen Porges' website: www.stephenporges.com).

Stephen W. Porges, Katja Kovacic, and Jacek Kolacz will tell us about their experience with Polyvagal Theory in Ehlers-Danlos Syndrome in a recent study:

Kolacz J, Kovacic K, Lewis GF, Sood MR, Aziz Q, Roath OR, Porges SW (2021). Cardiac autonomic regulation and joint hypermobility in adolescents with functional abdominal pain disorders. Neurogastroenterol Motil. Doi: 10.1111/nmo.14165

Polyvagal Theory and the Ehlers-Danlos Syndrome

By Dr. Katja KOVACIC, Dr. Jacek KOLACZ
& Prof. Stephen W. PORGES, USA

Joint hypermobility may occur along with select clinical symptoms that represent heritable connective tissue disorders known as the Ehlers-Danlos Syndromes (EDS).[1] The clinical relationship between EDS and autonomic dysregulation is well established via reports of comorbid symptoms associated with autonomic disorders and the presence of EDS. This is particularly true for the hypermobile EDS (hEDS) form, which also clusters with a number of gastrointestinal (GI) problems. The diagnosis of hEDS rests on a clinical diagnostic classification, including the Beighton joint hypermobility score, as there are no genetic or neurophysiological markers of this type of EDS.[2]

Several studies have reported a high prevalence of joint hypermobility in functional GI disorders.[3-6] There is emerging evidence for the role of the autonomic nervous system (ANS) in the pathophysiologic basis and symptoms expressed in both functional GI and hypermobility spectrum disorders (HSD).[7-9] Although the relationships between hEDS, autonomic and GI dysfunction are well documented,[10-12] a model linking or identifying the specific underlying pathophysiology of the disorder is lacking. One study documented sympathetic dysregulation and decreased sympathetic reactivity in response to postural challenge during comprehensive autonomic testing.[13] Another study documented alpha-adrenergic and beta-adrenergic hyper-responsiveness in hEDS.[7] Similarly, studies in both children and adults have demonstrated that over 50% of hEDS patients suffer from functional GI disorders.[4,9,14-16] These strong associations between ANS dysfunction, GI problems and hEDS are merely based on observational studies. There is no neurophysiological model that would lead researchers to specific metrics providing mechanistic data to explain these intriguing associations.[17] Although an abnormal autonomic response circuit may underlie the dysregulated visceral signals from the GI tract and enhanced pain perception in hEDS, the specific neural pathway that would play a causal role in this relationship is neither known nor hypothesized.

Polyvagal Theory provides a bio-evolutionary model of the ANS, which explains the dynamic bi-directional communication between brainstem structures and visceral organs that define the human brain-body connection.[18-20] The theory describes a bi-directionally integrated ANS focusing on brainstem regulatory circuits that are influenced by the central nervous system (i.e., top-down mechanisms) and afferent inputs from visceral organs (i.e., bottom-up mechanisms). This integrated model explains the role of cranial nerves (e.g., the vagus) in relaying signals controlling visceral reactivity between brainstem nuclei and specific visceral organs. A cornerstone of the research supporting the Polyvagal Theory has evolved from studying the neural regulation of the heart via vagal pathways.

AN: Top-down processes control sensory information from past experiences or knowledge. These are, therefore, high-level cognitive processes. In bottom-up processes, the information is linked to a perceived stimulus directly, for the first time.

This research has led to the development and validation of a non-invasive metric of vagal regulation of the heart by quantifying the rhythmic pattern of beat-to-beat heart rate associated with breathing known as respiratory sinus arrhythmia (RSA).[21] The RSA is a metric of the influence of vagal pathways on the dynamic regulation of the heart. It is the rhythmic fluctuation in heart rate that approximates spontaneous breathing. RSA is the primary component of high frequency heart rate variability (AN: 0.18 to 0.40 Hz, synchronous with respiration and identical to RSA), a validated index of parasympathetic tone. The amplitude of RSA provides a sensitive measure of the efferent output of the brainstem ventral vagal complex originating in nucleus ambiguus [AN: The nucleus ambiguus is a motor nucleus of the brainstem, common to the vagus nerve (nerve X), also called the pneumogastric, the glossopharyngeal (nerve IX), and the cranial portion of the spinal nerve (nerve XI): it belongs to the branchial motor column] and terminating on the sinoatrial node.[22] Due to the normal tonic inhibition of the sinoatrial node, RSA can be described as a measure of the vagal brake on the heart. The vagal brake is dynamically adjusting to deal with demands by slowing heart rate to conserve energy or enabling tachycardia to support mobilization in response to threat (i.e., fight or flight)[23] or play.

Recently, a new measure of how RSA relates to heart rate was developed.[22] This measure, termed vagal efficiency (VE), by evaluating the relationship between RSA and heart rate provides an individual, specific index of how much heart rate would change as RSA changes. Since the amplitude of RSA is a validated index of cardiac vagal tone, the new metric was labelled VE.[24] VE acknowledge that the relationship between RSA and heart rate is not a constant and is not consistent across individuals. This VE metric is extracted from the regression slopes of repeated samples of synchronous heart rate and RSA. VE therefore serves as an index of how much heart rate would change with a specific increase/decrease in the amplitude of RSA.

Our preliminary data from a cohort of 112 adolescents with functional GI symptoms indicate a link between joint hypermobility and poor VE. There is a notable decline in the VE metric with increasing Beighton scores during a supine-sitting-standing posture shift challenge. Figure 1A shows VE measured by the slope of the regression between heart rate and RSA. Note that the slope (i.e., VE) is significantly reduced in those with Beighton scores ≥4, compared to both healthy controls and children with functional GI disorders without hypermobility. The neural mechanisms involved in the dynamic changes in both RSA and heart rate induced by posture adjustments trigger shifts in heart rate, via rapid adjustments in vagal regulation, to maintain blood pressure. As seen in Figure 1B, lower VE scores relate to increased probability of joint hypermobility, based on a logistic regression. Based on these preliminary data, adolescents with a VE below about 20 had a 75% probability of having a Beighton score of 4 or higher. This suggests that hypermobile individuals have suboptimal cardio-inhibitory vagal pathways or an inefficient vagal brake of heart rate during positional changes, resulting in sympathetic excitation and postural symptoms (e.g., dizziness). This also potentially explains the neurophysiological substrate underlying states of anxiety in hypermobile individuals. These preliminary findings suggest that the subset of adolescents who present with GI complaints and have clinical and subclinical features of hEDS, have inefficient vagal regulation of heart rate during posture shifts. Further, our preliminary data indicates that VE in these adolescents is significantly lower than a pediatric healthy control population without hypermobility (Figure 2).

In conclusion, this research provides new insights into the neural mechanisms causing autonomic co-morbidities including anxiety. These findings suggest that impaired VE is reflecting a weak ANS feedback loop which contributes to gastrointestinal and autonomic symptoms in hEDS. A low VE may thus form the common substrate for the physical and psychological manifestations of these disorders.

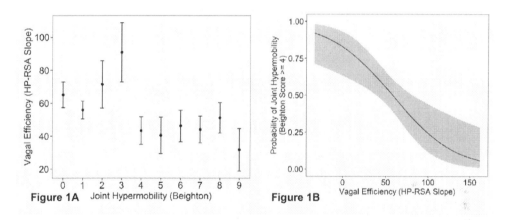

Figure 2. Model derived means and 95% confidence intervals for vagal efficiency for adolescents with functional abdominal pain disorders with joint hypermobility (FAPD + JH; n = 46) and without joint hypermobility (FAPD, No JH; n = 42) compared to healthy controls without joint hypermobility (HC, No JH; n = 19).

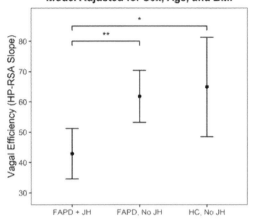

Means and 95% Confidence Intervals
Model Adjusted for Sex, Age, and BMI

References.

1. Castori M, Hakim A. Contemporary approach to joint hypermobility and related disorders. *Curr Opin Pediatr*. 2017;29(6):640-649. doi:10.1097/MOP.0000000000000541.

2. Malfait F, Francomano C, Byers P, et al. The 2017 international classification of the Ehlers-Danlos syndromes. Tinkle BT, Malfait F, Francomano CA, Byers PH, eds. *Am J Med Genet C Semin Med Genet*. 2017;175(1):8-26. doi:10.1002/ajmg.c.31552.

3. Kovacic K, Chelimsky TC, Sood MR, Simpson P, Nugent M, Chelimsky G. Joint hypermobility: a common association with complex functional gastrointestinal disorders. *J Pediatr*. 2014;165(5):973-978. doi:10.1016/j.jpeds.2014.07.021.

4. Fikree A, Aktar R, Grahame R, et al. Functional gastrointestinal disorders are associated with the joint hypermobility syndrome in secondary care: a case-control study. *Neurogastroenterology & Motility*. 2015;27(4):569-579. doi:10.1111/nmo.12535.

5. Pacey V, Adams RD, Tofts L, Munns CF, Nicholson LL. Joint hypermobility syndrome subclassification in paediatrics: a factor analytic approach. *Arch Dis Child*. 2015;100(1):8-13. doi:10.1136/archdischild-2013-305304.

6. Kishore S, Backhouse L, Rook DM, et al. Gastrointestinal manifestations of ehler-danlos syndrome type III

(hypermobility type) : A paediatric cohort. *Gastroenterology*. 2013;144(5):S610.

7. Gazit Y, Nahir AM, Grahame R, Jacob G. Dysautonomia in the joint hypermobility syndrome. *Am J Med*. 2003;115(1):33-40. doi:10.1016/s0002-9343(03)00235-3.

8. Ross AJ, Stewart JM, Medow MS, Rowe, P. C. Risk factors for postural tachycardia syndrome in adolescents and young adults. *Clinical Autonomic Research*. 2013;23(5):240.

9. Nelson AD, Mouchli MA, Valentin N, et al. Ehlers Danlos syndrome and gastrointestinal manifestations: a 20-year experience at Mayo Clinic. *Neurogastroenterology & Motility*. 2015;27(11):1657-1666. doi:10.1111/nmo.12665.

10. De Wandele I, Calders P, Peersman W, et al. Autonomic symptom burden in the hypermobility type of Ehlers-Danlos syndrome: a comparative study with two other EDS types, fibromyalgia, and healthy controls. *Semin Arthritis Rheum*. 2014;44(3):353-361. doi:10.1016/j.semarthrit.2014.05.013.

11. De Wandele I, Rombaut L, De Backer T, et al. Orthostatic intolerance and fatigue in the hypermobility type of Ehlers-Danlos Syndrome. *Rheumatology (Oxford)*. 2016;55(8):1412-1420. doi:10.1093/rheumatology/kew032.

12. Krahe AM, Adams RD, Nicholson LL. Features that exacerbate fatigue severity in joint hypermobility syndrome/Ehlers-Danlos syndrome - hypermobility type. *Disabil Rehabil*. 2018;40(17):1989-1996. doi:10.1080/09638288.2017.1323022.

13. De Wandele I, Rombaut L, Leybaert L, et al. Dysautonomia and its underlying mechanisms in the hypermobility type of Ehlers-Danlos syndrome. *Semin Arthritis Rheum*. 2014;44(1):93-100. doi:10.1016/j.semarthrit.2013.12.006.

14. Fikree A, Grahame R, Aktar R, et al. A prospective evaluation of undiagnosed joint hypermobility syndrome in patients with gastrointestinal symptoms. *Clin Gastroenterol Hepatol*. 2014;12(10):1680-87.e1682. doi:10.1016/j.cgh.2014.01.014.

15. Fikree A, Chelimsky G, Collins H, Kovacic K, Aziz Q. Gastrointestinal involvement in the Ehlers-Danlos syndromes. Tinkle BT, Malfait F, Francomano CA, Byers PH, eds. *Am J Med*

Genet C Semin Med Genet. 2017;175(1):181-187. doi:10.1002/ajmg.c.31546.

16. Beckers AB, Keszthelyi D, Fikree A, et al. Gastrointestinal disorders in joint hypermobility syndrome/Ehlers-Danlos syndrome hypermobility type: A review for the gastroenterologist. *Neurogastroenterology & Motility*. 2017;29(8):e13013. doi:10.1111/nmo.13013.

17. Hakim A, O'Callaghan C, De Wandele I, Stiles L, Pocinki A, Rowe P. Cardiovascular Autonomic Dysfunction in Ehlers-Danlos Syndrome-Hypermobile Type. Tinkle BT, Malfait F, Francomano CA, Byers PH, eds. *Am J Med Genet C Semin Med Genet*. 2017;175(1):168-174. doi:10.1002/ajmg.c.31543.

18. Porges SW. Orienting in a defensive world: mammalian modifications of our evolutionary heritage. A Polyvagal Theory. *Psychophysiology*. 1995;32(4):301-318.

19. Porges SW. The polyvagal perspective. *Biol Psychol*. 2007;74(2):116-143. doi:10.1016/j.biopsycho.2006.06.009.

20. Porges SW. The polyvagal theory: new insights into adaptive reactions of the autonomic nervous system. *Cleve Clin J Med*. 2009;76 Suppl 2(Suppl_2):S86-S90. doi:10.3949/ccjm.76.s2.17.

21. Lewis GF, Furman SA, McCool MF, Porges SW. Statistical strategies to quantify respiratory sinus arrhythmia: Are commonly used metrics equivalent? *Biol Psychol*. 2012;89(2):349-364. doi:10.1016/j.biopsycho.2011.11.009.

22. Porges SW, Davila MI, Lewis GF, et al. Autonomic regulation of preterm infants is enhanced by Family Nurture Intervention. *Dev Psychobiol*. 2019;142(Suppl. 1):565. doi:10.1002/dev.21841.

23. Berntson GG, Bigger JT, Eckberg DL, et al. Heart rate variability: origins, methods, and interpretive caveats. *Psychophysiology*. 1997;34(6):623-648.

24. Lewis GF, Furman SA, McCool MF, Porges SW. Statistical strategies to quantify respiratory sinus arrhythmia: are commonly used metrics equivalent? *Biol Psychol*. 2012;89(2):349-364. doi:10.1016/j.biopsycho.2011.11.009.

What I retain from this First Part

Second Part

Genetic and Epigenetic Postulates

CHAPTER VII

A Global Vision of EDS

Clinical Evolution and Transmission to Children

The Role of Epigenetics

By Dr. Stéphane Daens, in collaboration with :

Professor Andràs PÀLDI
Biochemist, geneticist and epigeneticist,
École Pratique des Hautes Études (EPHE),
Paris, France.
&
Professor Michel VERVOORT
Biologist and geneticist,
Université de Paris,
Institut Jacques Monod,
Paris, France.

Current EDS Classifications

This new project to classify Ehlers-Danlos Syndrome into 13 distinct subtypes is the result of a consensus reached by a group of five physicians, including four geneticists, who met in New York in May 2016 at a symposium organized by the Anglo-American patient's association, *The Ehlers-Danlos Society*. The facilitator of the symposium and working group is Lara Bloom, President of The Ehlers-Danlos Society. This paper's title on this 5th classification of Ehlers-Danlos Syndromes is: "*A Framework for the Classification of Joint Hypermobility and Related Conditions.*" The article was published in the *American Journal of Medical Genetics Part C (Seminars in Medical Genetics) 175C:148-157 (2017).*

The construction of the Ehlers Danlos Syndrome Classifications, which seeks to relate collagen mutations, or a genetic transmission pattern of specific mutations, to specific clinical pictures is ancient and has marked the history of this disease from the geneticist's point of view.

The first classification was proposed by the British surgeon A.P. Barabas in 1967, starting with 27 patients, and described three types: the Classical type, the Mild or Varicose type, and the Arterial type.[52]

The Arterial type is the same as the one described in 1932, by the German physician Georg Sack, who called it *Status Dysvascularis*.[53] The Sack-Barabas Syndrome became the Ehlers-Danlos Syndrome type IV in the Villefranche's classification. It is characterized by the detection of various COL3A1 mutations. Johnson and Falls provide proof of the dominant hereditary character of the syndrome based on a family tree of 123 people, over six generations. No mutations were found at that time. It was purely deductive, as with subsequent classifications, until the New York classification in 2016-2017.

The second classification dated from 1969 and was made by Peter Beighton, based on an observation of 100 patients.[54] He proposed five distinct, clinically detectable forms: the gravis type (or type I), the mitis type (or type II), the benign hypermobile type (or type III), the ecchymotic type (or type IV, which corresponds to Barabas' arterial type) and the *X-linked syndrome* (or type V, an X-linked syndrome).

---

[52] Barabas A.P. Heterogeneity of the Ehlers-Danlos Syndrome: Clinical types and a hypothesis to explain the basis defect(s). Brit Med J. 1967,2;612-613.
[53] Sack G. Status dysvascularis, ein Fall von besonderer Zeereislichkeit der Blutgefässe. Deutsches Archiv für klinische Medicin (Leipzig). 1935-1936, 178;663-669.
[54] Beighton P., Price A., Lord J., Dickson E. Variants of the Ehlers-Danlos Syndrome: clinical, biochemical, haematological, and chromosomal features of 100 patients. Ann Rheum Dis. 1969,28(3);228-245.

The 3rd classification was the Berlin classification in 1988.[55] It included 11 forms, which were then reduced, at the time of its revision, to form the 4th classification (known as the Villefranche classification, 1997), to six distinct forms: the classical form, the hypermobile form, the vascular form, the kyphoscoliotic form, the arthrochalasic (aEDS) form, and the dermatosparaxic form (dEDS).[56]

The latest classification of Ehlers-Danlos Syndromes (see table below) was established at the 2016 International Consortium, in New York, USA. The articles were published in March 2017 in the *American Journal of Medical Genetics part C*. The Ehlers-Danlos Syndrome classification was thus reviewed for the first time in 20 years. Some mutations have been identified over time (i.e., genotypes), and some of them have been correlated with different specific clinical pictures (i.e., phenotypes).

Because geneticists have identified specific mutations associated with particular phenotypes, they have fragmented EDS into different subtypes. They believe that one particular mutation could induce one particular phenotype and, in turn, all the clinical manifestations expressed in that phenotype.

Thirteen subtypes have been categorized. The most common subtype, that affects more than 90% of patients seen in consultation, has been called Hypermobile Ehlers-Danlos Syndrome (or hEDS, formerly known as type III EDS). For hypermobile EDS, which is extremely common compared to other EDS subtypes, no conclusive mutation could be found.

In my opinion, and that of other scientists, the mistake, and we are several scientists to think this, is that some geneticists wanted to establish a classification of EDS based on a few mutations found in a few rare subtypes. On the other hand, these subtypes' complete phenotype is not explained by the rare mutation(s) found. At best, specific rare mutations explain an alteration in

---

[55] Beighton P., De Paepe A., Danks D. (1988) – International nosology of heritable disorders of connective tissue, Berlin. Am J Med Genet. 1986,29:581-594.
[56] Beighton P., De Paepe A., Steimann B. Ehlers Danlos Syndrome: revised nosology, Villefranche, 1997. Am J Med Genet. 1998,77:31-37.

certain collagens or glycosaminoglycans. These particular mutations would induce an alteration in certain specific tissues but within a florilegium of symptoms that are not explained by these point mutations alone.

This 2017 classification is based exclusively on molecular genetics; the mode of transmission has been described as Mendelian, autosomal, dominant or recessive, without further nuances. The mode of transmission would vary according to the subtypes described in these articles. hEDS is considered to be an autosomal dominant trait with variable expressivity (this still has to be proven; see further discussion and demonstration on this subject).

Castori M, Tinkle B, Levy H, Grahame R, Malfait F, Hakim A. 2017. A framework for the classification of joint hypermobility and related conditions. Am J Med Genet Part C Semin Med Genet 9999C:1-10.

Tinkle B, Castori M, Berglund B et al. 2017. Hypermobile Ehlers-Danlos syndrome (a.k.a. Ehlers-Danlos syndrome type III and Ehlers-Danlos syndrome hypermobility type) : Clinical description and natural history. Am J Med Genet Part C Semin Med Genet 175C:48-69.

Surprisingly, the International Criteria of the 13 EDSs have been established without a control group, which in Medicine and research is, a priori, inconceivable.

Indeed, as in any scientific study, the proposed criteria for EDS subjects must be compared with a group of so-called healthy people, i.e., people who do not carry EDS, such as subjects from preventive and/or occupational medicine, for example.

Only then, can it be established whether these criteria are sensitive and specific (the most frequent and relevant for a given disease) to diagnose a specific subtype of EDS. These criteria could then be validated and applied with relative certainty that healthy people are not classified as EDS, and EDS patients are not classified as healthy (or non-EDS). Some may think this seems obvious (or even Evidence-Based Medicine, as we say in the scientific community). But here, it has not been done. The question of why has it not been done is then legitimately raised.

To further complicate matters, subgroups have been created in the same clinical spectrum:

➢ Asymptomatic Joint Hypermobility (AJH)
➢ Hypermobility Spectrum Disorder (HSD)
➢ The real hEDS (which these authors say that it is rare)

The aim of these actors was, it seems, to isolate a homogeneous group of patients in order to carry out genetic studies to discover the gene(s) involved in hEDS.

In the article, the following points should be noted:

➢ In this classification, HSD patients do not meet all the hEDS criteria (criteria I + II + III), but they still have specific characteristics of hEDS.
➢ Besides, HSD patients may be clinically much or even more symptomatic than patients labeled hEDS.
➢ Patients may move from one subgroup to the other throughout their lives. For example, they may move from the HSD subgroup to the hEDS subgroup or vice versa. They might be reclassified into the Asymptomatic JH (AJH) subgroup (localized, peripheral or generalized JH).

Furthermore, since that was not complicated enough, HSD was divided into four forms:

➢ A Localized form (L-HSD): when it only affects, for example, joints such as the elbow, hip, knee, or shoulder;
➢ A Peripheral shape (P-HSD): when it touches only the extremities such as the fingers of the hands of the toes;
➢ A Generalized shape (G-HSD): in this case, Beighton's score is high and touches the extremities as well as the proximal joints;
➢ A Historical form (H-HSD) : when the patient is no longer hyperlaxed at all at the time of diagnosis, but has a high score on the historical Grahame questionnaire (5pHQ); he was therefore hypermobile in his youth.

In order to plunge patients and doctors even further into vagueness, the mutual health insurances were not warned of these name changes, nor of the fact that patients should enjoy the same rights and benefits, whether they are diagnosed as HSD or hEDS, as is the case for the FPS Public Health and the AVIQ/PHARE/VAPH (i.e., agencies dedicated to people with disabilities, in Belgium). The situation is identical in France, and in many other countries.

According to the New York Classification: AJH – HSD - hEDS

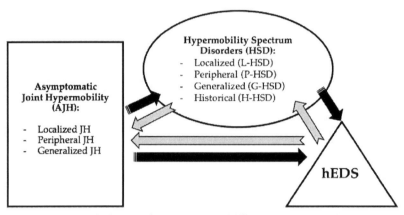

According to: *Castori M, Tinkle B, Levy H, Grahame R, Malfait F, Hakim A. 2017. A framework for the classification of joint hypermobility and related conditions. Am J Med Genet Part C Semin Med Genet 9999C:1-10.*

© Stéphane Daens

In 2021, *Aubry-Rozier et al.* wrote at the end of their article: "hEDS and HDS patients showed similar disease severity score except for pain, motricity problems and bleeding, and similar spectrum of extra-articular manifestations. Long-term improvement was observed in > 50% of patients in both groups. These results add weight to a clinical pragmatic proposition to consider hEDS/HSD as a single entity that requires the same treatments."[57]

Currently, if a diagnose of HSD is made in a medical report, in good faith and following the rules established in New York, most of the time, patients do not receive the status of severe pathology (e.g., *type E pathology*, in Belgium). Nor do they receive

---

[57] Aubry-Rozier B, Schwitzguebel A, Valerio F, et al. Are patients with hypermobile Ehlers-Danlos syndrome or hypermobility spectrum disorder so different? Rheumatol Int. 2021;41(10):1785-1794.

the status of chronic disease to the mutual insurance companies, nor the status of invalidity to the FPS Public Health (in Belgium). In France, the situation is identical with most often a refusal of ALD (Long Term Disability) and recognition by the Departmental House for the Disabled (MDPH).

Where is justice for these patients?

There is not adequate dedicated training on EDS in Medical Schools. It is most often taught in 5 to 10 minutes. Students are taught that it is a sporadic condition, that all patients are very hypermobile, and all have incredibly elastic skin. Students are told EDS patients are fairground animals, and they never feel pain, and there is no treatment for them. The student has to be in the class at that time, which, from experience, is not always the case.

Since doctors are already not trained on EDS itself, they will, of course, not understand these new complex classifications, which moreover do not bring anything new to the patients; and it will still be the patients who pay the bill in terms of wandering and medical abuse.

Demonstration by the absurd of a classification without clearly identified genes

Since the mutations and genes involved are not identified in hEDS, the most common form, how can it be said that these same unknown mutations are not present in the other EDS subtypes, defined in the 2017 classification? How can we prove that something unknown (in this case, the mutations in question) does not exist in the other EDS subtypes? It is, in the current state of knowledge, simply impossible. It is intellectually limiting and circular.

According to our clinical experience, with more than 10,000 to 15,000 patients followed by doctors familiar with EDS (trained by obtaining a university degree in France or by clinical training with competent doctors), the transmission does not seem to be autosomal at all, nor Mendelian for that matter. On the one hand, it was observed that more than 90% of children are carriers of signs and symptoms suggestive of hEDS, while only one of the two parents is affected. This impression is confirmed by the study of the dermis under electron microscopy: almost 100% of children of EDS patients have an altered connective tissue. On the other hand, patients with other subtypes of EDS, although they have some identified mutations (i.e., in their genotype) and sometimes singular clinics (i.e., in their phenotypes), have in common signs and symptoms of the hypermobile form, such as fatigue, pain, dysautonomia, dysproprioception, dys-sensoriality, MCAD, and more.

Finally, never mentioned in these classifications is the probability that a known mutation remains unexpressed in the phenotype. We are all carriers of various known mutations that are not clinically expressed, which is not a new thing in genetics.

We can thus be carriers, in our genome, of a known mutation of collagen 3A1, which could give a vascular form, without this being expressed in the phenotype. It can lead to false diagnoses of vascular shape and cause anxiety for some patients, who imagine having a Sword of Damocles over their head for the rest of their lives, and, even more traumatically, on the heads of their children. On the other hand, not all the mutations of collagen 3 (alpha one or A1 chain), which could give vascular (vEDS, old type IV) forms (phenotypes), are currently known.

As a reminder, collagen 3 is an essential constituent of hollow organs, such as arterial blood vessels, the uterus, the bladder, and the intestine; this explains the complications of tissue rupture reported in the vascular variants of EDS. Type 3 collagen is also involved in platelet plug formation, and healing.[58]

So, can we really confirm to a patient, who does not have a known mutation of collagen 3A1, that he does not have a so-called vascular form?

This would be to say to certain patients: "We have not found any known mutation of COL3A1 that could lead to a vascular form",

---

[58] Kuivaniemi H, Tromp G. Type III collagen (COL3A1) : gene and protein structure, tissue distribution, and associated diseases. Gene. 2019;707:151-171.

with the corollary: "You are not at risk of anything serious!". This is false and extremely dangerous.

In our practice, we see patients with a hypermobile form who have ectasias of the aorta or its branches. We regularly see hEDS patients who have undergone surgical disasters or organ ruptures (e.g., such as during colon or tracheal exploration).

This is a serious matter because, in these cases, patients are over-reassured. It would be wrong to say: "You do not have a vascular form, so you are not at risk! There is no need to screen for arterial complications."

The best thing to say, in my opinion, is: "You have a hypermobile type of EDS. Do not worry, I will order additional tests to rule out arterial or visceral complications. I will also give you a Care and Emergency Card, to alert the medical professionals to your situation's potential risks and complications. Besides, many drug, vitamin, and orthotic treatments are available, and we are going to make sure you get better. "

The best thing for the patient is always to know.

At this point, doctors will take precautions. They will be cautious about surgeries and invasive procedures such as colonoscopy, laryngoscopy, bronchoscopy, oeso-gastro-duodenoscopy, etc. Thus everything goes well, most of the time.

The danger in EDS is not to know that one is a carrier, and not to say so. In these circumstances, the iatrogenic risk (the risk inherent in medical care) is considerable.

It is a real headache, isn't it? But a puzzle with significant repercussions!

At least one hour should be devoted to an initial consultation, as the disease is extremely complex and multifaceted, not 15 or 20 minutes, as in some hospital departments in which efficiency is, unfortunately, increasingly taking precedence over the excellent Medicine that every patient is entitled to receive.

In Medicine, the clinic should always take precedence over theories that do not fit the reality of patients' lives and what they endure daily.

Of course, this matter of phenotype variations between individuals is well known for some genetic diseases, as Professor Vervoort[59] rightly pointed out to me. This is true for mutations with variable expressivity and incomplete penetrance.

According to what is called genetic backgrounds, the same mutation can give specific phenotypes (a variable expressivity). Genetic backgrounds are innumerable factors in the genome, often very subtle, that differ between each individual and affect the function of our genes. Not everything is understood in this case, but it is exciting.[60]

He reminded me of the case of polydactyly: in this case, the same mutation can lead to supernumerary fingers on all limbs or three, two, or even one limb, without it being known precisely why. By analyzing family trees, one can conclude, in some cases, that the mutation may well not give the phenotype in some individuals (incomplete penetrance), again without knowing why.

This may be the case in EDS, but I would argue that in EDS, the phenotype is so complex and so polymorphic that one mutation, detected in a rare subtype (kEDS, for example), never explains the whole phenotype encountered in the patient.

Secondly, the genetic background does not take away our questions and our reflections regarding epigenetics and the exposome[61], which we will describe later. Indeed, even if the phenotypes are different between the children of the same sibling because of the genetic background, the latter does not a

---

[59] Biologist and geneticist, Professor of genetics, Université de Paris, Institut Jacques Monod, Paris, France. Developmental Genetics, Comparative Genomics, and Neurogenesis, Phylogeny, and Stem Cells.
[60] Fournier T, Schacherer J. Genetic backgrounds and hidden trait complexity in natural populations. Curr Opin Genet Dev. 2017;47:48-53.
doi: 10.1016/j.gde.2017.08.009
[61] That is to say: all the factors which are external to DNA, but which could influence its expression, its "reading".

priori explain, in each patient, the variations of phenotypes during his or her life, according to his or her experience. Epigenetics can absolutely come into play at this level, and it is essential to understand what we encounter daily in Ehlers-Danlos Syndrome.

Some clinically-based postulates need to be brought up sooner rather than later. Unfortunately, it may be late or even too late, I fear, We fear. Many preconceived notions are propagated in the medical world and on social networks, which EDS patients often run.

Preconceived ideas

Some preconceived ideas are dangerous and confuse people. Some people propagate the idea that EDS is rare or is an orphan disease, that we should not consider other possibilities for the classification of EDS variants, for its transmission between generations, or for its clinical evolution during the course of life.

I can already hear some of these comments about the Global Vision of EDS and Epigenetic Postulates of EDS:

- *"There is nothing new; we know about epigenetic diseases!"*
- *"It has no evidence! These are just ideas put forward to stir up trouble! "*
- *"Only the criteria established in New York are the right ones!"*
- *"He is against genetics!"*

Etc.

At the risk of disappointing those with a thirst for blood instead of a thirst for knowledge, I will never write that epigenetics is something new or a scoop, but, on the other hand, its influence was never mentioned in the articles published in 2017, following the New York Consortium.

A scientist has to think and innovate.

To quote the Hungarian biochemist Albert Szent-Györgyi of Nagyrápolt (1893-1986, Nobel Prize in Physiology and Medicine in 1937):

251

"Research is seeing what everyone else sees and thinking what no one else has thought of."

Preconceived ideas are dangerous:

➢ For each disease, there is proven scientific knowledge and postulates. The postulates are based on science and knowledge, and also on personal or collective experience. They are intuitively true. When we read them, doubts must creep into our minds, even though they have not been scientifically proven in each situation, in this case Ehlers-Danlos Syndrome.

➢ One must, as a good father or a good scientist, always make a distinction between what one knows for sure (Mendel's laws, natural selection, ontogeny, phylogeny, etc.) and postulates when writing a scientific article or book. These precautions are not only oratorical (or scriptural), but they are also fundamental to a good understanding and a favorable reception by the scientific world. If not, they would be, at best, false truths and, at worst, real lies.

Some examples of preconceived ideas to illustrate my point

➢ Real lies breed misconceptions. The controversy over vaccination speaks for itself. According to the WHO, we are all familiar with the example of the eradication of smallpox, a virus that has the potential to continue to cause two to three million deaths each year worldwide. Routine vaccination of the world's populations made it possible to eradicate it. Although vaccination of populations has made it possible to eliminate certain deadly diseases from the face of the earth, an anti-vaccination movement is increasingly present around us, in the media, and on social networks. It is absurd, of course, yet this is a common misconception about vaccination with potentially severe consequences. A British doctor, surgeon and researcher, Andrew Wakefield (b. 1957), has intentionally confused this significant advance in vaccination. This unscrupulous individual wrote an article in 1998 on the risks of the Measles-Mumps-Rubella (MMR) vaccine to cause autistic spectra (*autistic enterocolitis*, a term he coined).[62,63]

Wakefield intentionally manipulated his data to arrive at this disastrous conclusion.

Vaxxed: From Cover-up to Catastrophe, is a 2016 American conspirational film directed by Wakefield, arguing that the Center for Disease Control (CDC) covered the existence of link between MMR vaccine and autism.[64]

Despite press releases, scientific articles invalidating his writings[65,66,67], and having banned Wakefield from practicing Medicine in the UK (*General Medical Council*, UK, 2010), the damage was done, and it was spreading. Famous, sensationalist talk shows added fuel to the fire, and the fire spread rapidly. More and more families refused to have their children vaccinated, and we watched helplessly as the number of polio cases, measles, diphtheria, and more increased dramatically. It is a fine example of a scientific article that should never have been believed and disseminated; critical thinking, verification of experience, and methodology are essential to Science.

> False truths lead to misconceptions. These are ideas that are peddled, word-of-mouth, unscientific, and sometimes born of the collective imagination. The well-known example of the blue-blooded nobles is a false truth that has been jabbered

---

[62] Wakefield AJ. MMR vaccination and autism. Lancet, 1999,12;353(9169):2026-2029.

[63] Wakefield AJ et al. Autism, viral infection and measles-mumps-rubella vaccination. Isr Med Assoc J. 1999;1(3):176-177.

[64] Duchsherer A, Jason M, Platt CA, et al. Immunized against science: Narrative community building among vaccine refusing/hesitant parents. Public Underst Sci. 2020;29(4):419-435. doi: 10.1177/0963662520921537.

[65] Hviid A, Hansen JV, Frisch M, et al. Measles, Mumps, Rubella vaccination and Autism: A Nationwide Cohort Study. Ann Intern Med. 2019;170(8):513-520.

[66] Dyer C. Wakefield was dishonest and irresponsible over MMR research, says GMC. BMJ. 2010;29:340:c59.3.

[67] Flaherty DK. The vaccine-autism connection: a public health crisis caused by unethical medical practices and fraudulent science. Ann Pharmacoth. 2011;45(10):1302-1304.

about as early as the 17th century. It was thought to be accurate by merely observing the blood's color through the nobles' skin compared to that of the peasants (blood is always red, bright in arterial when oxygenated, and darker in venous when it returns to the heart, deoxygenated). Explanation: the nobles took less sun than the peasants, sheltered in their castles, which gave them pale skin. Moreover, the skin is a color filter, and the color blue dominates the spectrum. Thus, the blue of the veins stood out more than that of the peasants who had sun-tanned skin.

➤ Unconscious transpositions give preconceived ideas. Dinosaurs ruled our Earth for 185 million years (from the Triassic period, 250 million years ago, to the end of the Cretaceous period, 65 million years ago). Their presumed and generalized appearance of large lizards, heralded by many Hollywood movies (including *Jurassic Park*), made them scaly in the collective unconscious, before modern scientific studies on the subject. This idea is widely held in the general population, while current research supports that a particular subgroup of dinosaurs were covered with feathers. Yes, some of these terrifying dinosaurs probably looked, to caricature, like huge pollards. Of course, the majority of dinosaurs did not have feathers, but the generalization is dangerous too. Only birds [68] are the descendants of dinosaurs, the other subgroups of dinosaurs having disappeared.

All these preconceptions prevent Science from being updated in the minds of real-time, and it can take decades for discoveries to enter the public world and even, strangely enough, in doctors' minds. These delays lead to errors in diagnosis and treatment, as in the case of Ehlers-Danlos Syndrome. In today's age of social networking, hearsay about EDS has catastrophic consequences in properly managing many suffering patients.

All these preconceived ideas lead to dark ideas in many patients: "There is no treatment," "I will never get better," "It is a rare

---

[68] Brusatte SL, O'Connor JK, Jarvis ED. The origin and diversification of birds. Curr Biol. 2015;25(19):R888-98.

disease with no treatment," "It is a genetic disease that affects one child in two or one child in four," and more.

So, we need to have clear ideas:

➢ No, EDS is not a rare disease. According to the European regulatory definition, a rare disease affected less than one individual in 2000.[69] There are estimated to be between 5000 and 8000 rare diseases. 80% of rare diseases are genetic diseases. Many articles deny these figures for EDS and instead put forward prevalence figures of 0.5 to 4% of the general population, depending on ethnicity. There is probably an interest in keeping EDS in rare diseases, but I do not see it personally. The more a disease remains in the rare disease category, the fewer young researchers there will be interested in it, the less money there will be for research, the less it will be taught at the university in the Faculty of Medicine, and the less information about it will be available in the general population. Diabetes, for example, will affect 5% of the French population in 2016 and rheumatoid arthritis 0.5%; for these two conditions, medications are reimbursed, doctors are very knowledgeable, and the social benefits are significant. Many patients believe that the more frequent an illness is, the less it will be covered by social security. That is not true! So, there is no benefit, either social or financial, in keeping the name rare disease for EDS.

➢ No, EDS is not an orphan disease. An orphan disease is a disease for which there is no effective treatment. When we talk about effective treatments, we are not talking about curative treatments that would eradicate the disease, but about treatments that improve quality of life and maintain a normal life expectancy. Otherwise, the majority of diseases would be so-called orphan diseases. When a patient is treated for diabetes, hypertension, HIV, and even alcoholism, their disease does not disappear, the symptoms are relieved, and it is made more livable. When treatment for these conditions is stopped (including psychotherapy and talk and support groups such as Alcoholics Anonymous), symptoms and

---

[69] Rath A, Bailly S. La prévalence des maladies rares évaluée. Pour la science. 2019;506:7

complications return. Except for some infectious diseases, other illnesses are only relieved by current medicine. Many medications, often natural or orthotic, are available in EDS. Not all doctors are familiar with them, and it is different! They then wrongly tell their patients that there is no treatment for EDS. It is due to a lack of training and information for doctors, but not an intrinsic property of the disease.

➢ No, the so-called New York Criteria should not to be taken for granted. They have been described as intermediate, however they were not reviewed in 2018 in Ghent, as they were supposed to be. We all have the right to think about improving these criteria, penalizing many patients as they stand. We cannot leave so many people undiagnosed and untreated, in suffering and distress. It is unfair and unjustified mistreatment of patients who are already suffering multiple punishments (a *sevenfold punishment*, as Dr. Daniel Grossin states in his public interventions).

➢ No, immobility should not be the law. We must listen, think and reflect together to inform and develop new management strategies for these vulnerable patients. It must be done without further delay!

➢ Speaking of postulates is neither a weakness nor an oratory precaution, but a contained strength to move forward.

My First Postulate:
The Global Vision of EDS

➢ How to explain this transmission, a priori, non-Mendelian, encountered in our daily practice? How can we explain that almost 100% of children are carriers of EDS when only one parent has it?

➢ How can we explain that some patients are more symptomatic than others when, a priori, according to some, the genetic cause is the same?

➢ How can we explain the worsening of symptoms after specific traumas or hormonal variations, when genetics are unchanged and stable (except for *de novo*, spontaneous, mutations)?

➤ How can it be explained that women are more symptomatic than men? Is it only related to hormonal factors?

➤ How can it be explained that some children of EDS patients, who are themselves affected, are more or less strongly symptomatic when, a priori, the same mutations are found in all of them (i.e. transmission of mutations in an autosomal mode)?

The New York Classification does not provide the answers, nor were the questions asked. This is a simple observation of things, and I would like to open other avenues of reflection. I think that there is only one basic form of EDS (more or less equivalent to the hypermobile form, whose mutations are unknown) that could be called the COMMON SYSTEMIC FORM or, in short: csEDS. Other mutations, which are eventually known, can then be added to this basic form, and induce specific phenotypes (such as a mutation of collagen 5A1 and A2 leading to a so-called classical variant, or a mutation of collagen 3A1 for vascular variants). This is an approach that I have called: The Global Vision of EDS.

This is not a simplification whose aim would be to denigrate the work of eminent doctors who are incredibly involved in research on EDS. It is not a question of pointing the finger at these colleagues who, after long reflections, repeated meetings, and exhausting corrections, participated in elaborating the 2017 Criteria.

Important Warning

I certainly would not want my words to be taken as denigrating or as if I were against someone or against the current Classifications. I bring here my vision of things, a stone in the building, a drop in the ocean of understanding of EDS's complex disease. This casuistic vision is based on the current knowledge of EDS and my clinical experience, with more than 3,000 patients followed during my consultations. These are postulates and lines of thought. It is crucial to take it as such. Furthermore, if it can move things forward, that would be good; if it can open up avenues of research, that would be perfect.

EDS appears to us as a complex genetic disease with epigenetic marks. Complex genetic diseases have an evident genetic determinism but whose transmission does not correspond to any classical Mendelian modes or to a mitochondrial-type transmission mode.

Indeed, the monogenic genetic disease can be summed up in a simple model (as opposed to complex genetic diseases): alteration at the level of one gene is necessary and sufficient to be accompanied by the appearance of the genetic disease (except for mutations with incomplete penetrance).

In complex genetic diseases (such as EDS, probably), it is most often a polygenic genetic determinism: many alterations exist at the level of many different genes, which are the multiple determinants of the disease. This is also known as a multifactorial disease. We will study the genetic and epigenetic mechanisms in greater depth later.

In this Global Vision of EDS, the other subtypes described by the New York Classification could result from unknown alterations to csEDS to which other mutations have been added. These mutations are known in some cases, such as COL3A1 or COL5A1 & A2. These results would then lead to the other 12 identifiable phenotypes (Table 2).

Examples:

In the so-called classical form (cEDS), one could say that there is the basis of the Common Systemic form. One mutation of collagen five on its alpha one or alpha two chains (COL5A1, or COL5A2) would have been added to these unknown mutations of the csEDS. That additional mutation would influence the phenotype so that the skin would be more stretchy. So, the scars are even less easy to form (large, pay rate and often hyper-pigmented), and the hyper-elasticity of all the other conjunctive is more marked (leading to ptosis of the organs, diverticula in the colon or bladder, eye damage with a detachment of the vitreous body, and more). However, in this variant, the basis of the csEDS form is well present with its share of fatigue, dyssensoriality, dysproprioception, dysautonomia, and diffuse pain. In consultation, a priori, one does not meet patients with classical EDS who would only come to complain that their skin is too elastic or that they heal poorly. They come especially for everything else, i.e., the typical picture of csEDS form.

The same is true for the vascular form (vEDS), in which specific mutations of collagen 3 are known that weaken the arterial vessels (they contain more than other tissues). Patients can consult us for personal or family aneurysms, but they also complain of symptoms and clinical signs encountered in the csEDS form. Nevertheless, these mutations in collagen 3 bring the vascular phenotype to the forefront.

I also encountered a few cases of the Kyphoscoliotic form (kEDS). These are confirmed by the ultrastructural study of the skin and by the detection of specific mutations in the PLOD1 gene or the FKBP14 gene. They often consult for something other than their child's severe scoliosis, possible eye or hearing damage. The demonstration is the same.

On the other hand, it is wrong to think that in the so-called hypermobile form, there is never any arterial dilatation or increased risk of organ rupture or perforation. I regularly see patients with a clinic and dermal ultrastructure typical of the hypermobile form. They do not carry a known COL3A1 mutation. However, some of them do have arterial ectasias, often discrete, but they are there. It is important to note that these arterial dilatations are mainly located at the root of the thoracic aorta or at the arteries that originate in the abdominal aorta and feed various structures as kidneys, liver, spleen, intestines, and others. These are atypical localizations in vascular surgery, and they generally begin before the age of 40. The age distribution curve peak for the onset of arterial dilatation is at about 25 years of age. Nevertheless, the curve's extremities are at about 15-16 years of age, to the left of the Gauss curve, and before 40 years of age, to the Gauss curve's right. After the age of 40, arterial vessel dilatation mainly affects the central body of the aorta (the large trunk rather than the branches) and more in patients with cardiovascular risk factors such as smoking, high blood pressure, high cholesterol (its role is controversial for some cardiologists), diabetes mellitus, being male and sedentary (lack of regular exercise).

The brain can also be affected at the vascular level. The subclavian arteries (under the collarbone), carotid arteries (at the neck), femoral arteries (in the groin), and sometimes the tibial arteries (in the legs) too. Cerebral artery damage mainly affects the ophthalmic arteries, cavernous sinus, communicating arteries, and some more.

Therefore, it is always necessary to be on the lookout, watch, listen, examine, and be careful. One examination too many, out of caution, is better than a ruptured aneurysm, with potentially catastrophic consequences!

After 40, and regardless of the variants, even in the common systemic form, one must always keep in mind the risk of potential arterial wall tears, called dissections. They are usually extremely painful and localized mainly in the abdominal area.

It should be noted that there may exist, and more frequently in EDS, an abdominal arcuate ligament that could compress the artery that feeds the intestines (most often the celiac trunk). It can give intense abdominal pain while eating or just after eating (this is called mesenteric claudication). When we eat, we need more blood flow to the intestine to absorb nutrients and oxygen. If this is not the case, the digestive tract suffers and causes significant abdominal pain, predominantly cramps. I, therefore, ask that the arcuate ligament be systematically sought on thoracoabdominal MRI. A minor laparoscopic procedure (small holes in the abdomen to introduce instruments and a camera) is sufficient to cut this ligament and free the artery from its compression.

Note: One should always be wary of gallbladder stones in abdominal pain; they can be atypical in a presentation in EDS. Cysts (fluid surrounded by a membrane) are also much more common. Cysts in the thyroid, breasts, ovaries (which can become twisted or bleed), kidneys, liver, pancreas, joint or skin cysts and even cysts in the epiphysis (pineal gland). Most often they are benign (i.e., non-cancerous) and pose little health concern. Pituitary cysts can cause hormonal disturbances or compression of the optic chiasm (the place where the right and left optic nerves cross in an X shape), resulting in vision problems.

I would like to take this opportunity to emphasize that EDS does not always explain everything in a patient! We must remain general practitioner or internist doctors.

Several independent diseases can coexist with EDS in the same patient, such as osteoarthritis, rheumatoid arthritis, inflammatory spondylo-arthropathies, inflammatory connective tissue disease, cancer, Parkinson's disease, Alzheimer's disease, etc. These must always be excluded in the presence of new specific complaints. At the slightest doubt, a complete blood test should be performed, including viral or bacterial serologies and autoimmune factors, focused radiological examinations, specialized scans, PET-CT scans, and if necessary, the patient should be referred to a colleague specialized in another branch of Medicine. A good doctor must always know his limits.

> This Global (or Holistic) Vision of EDS is more in line with our daily clinical practice and constitutes my 1st Postulate.

In order to understand these complex notions of genetics and epigenetics, we need to recall:

- The basics of molecular genetics (i.e., DNA, histones and non-histone proteins, nucleosomes, chromatin, chromosomes, RNA, proteins, etc.).

- The different modes of transmission of this genetic information to children, as well as the mechanisms that sustain the phenotype's differences and modifications throughout their own lives and/or between siblings (i.e., meiosis, autosomal recessive and dominant transmission, the non-protein coding DNA and RNAs, the epigenetic profile of genes, X-linked transmission, Y-linked transmission, the double exposure' phenomenon, the histone code, the bistable states of chromatin, the X-chromosome inactivation (XCI) and XCI bias, the notion of parental genomic imprinting, and more).

Why Use the Term Postulate?

Of course, as has been pointed out to me, I might have preferred the more familiar term hypothesis; this is probably true. But I am a complex and sometimes narrow-minded person, probably because of my EDS... A postulate can be used in Mathematics, Science, or Philosophy. The term postulate comes from the Latin, *postulatum*, which means *to ask*.

In Science, a postulate is an unproven principle that is accepted and formulated as the basis of research or theory. In philosophy, it is a proposition which is not self-evident, but which one is led to conceive because one sees no other principle to which one can attach, either a truth which cannot be questioned, or an operation or an act whose legitimacy is not contested. (LAL 1968).

Diagrams of the Global Vision of EDS

The following two diagrams show, on the one hand, the current fragmented view of the classification of Ehlers-Danlos Syndromes according to the International Consortium of New York and, on the other hand, my Global Vision of Ehlers-Danlos Syndrome. A Common Systemic form arise from this global view, from which different variants emerge due to additional genetic mutations.

In the current New York view, there are 13 subtypes of EDS that are independent of each other, with autosomal recessive or autosomal dominant transmission to offspring.

In the Global Vision of EDS, there is a central type of EDS, the Common Systemic form (csEDS), and twelve variants of the same csEDS.

The mode of transmission appears to be complex, polygenic. It includes the basics of classical molecular genetics and epigenetics (i.e., everything that is not transmitted by the protein-coding DNA).

Figure 1. The New York Classification (2017): 13 Subtypes of EDS

Name of EDS Subtype	IP*	Genetic Basis	Protein Involved
Classical EDS (cEDS)	AD	Major: COL5A1, COL5A2	Type V collagen
		Rare: COL1A1 c.934C>T, p.(Arg312Cys)	Type I collagen
Classical-like EDS (clEDS)	AR	TNXB	Tenascin XB
Cardiac-valvular EDS (cvEDS)	AR	COL1A2 (biallelic mutations that lead to COL1A2 NMD and absence of pro α2(I) collagen chains)	Type I collagen
Vascular EDS (vEDS)	AD	Major: COL3A1	Type III collagen
		Rare: COL1A1 c.934C>T, p.(Arg312Cys) c.1720C>T, p.(Arg574Cys) c.3227C>T, p.(Arg1093Cys)	Type I collagen
Hypermobile EDS (hEDS)	AD	Unknown	Unknown
Arthrochalasia EDS (aEDS)	AD	COL1A1, COL1A2	Type I collagen
Dermatosparaxis EDS (dEDS)	AR	ADAMTS2	ADAMTS-2
Kyphoscoliotic EDS (kEDS)	AR	PLOD1	LH1
		FKBP14	FKBP22
Brittle cornea syndrome (BCS)	AR	ZNF469	ZNF469
		PRDM5	PRDM5
Spondylodysplastic EDS (spEDS)	AR	B4GALT7	β4GalT7
		B3GALT6	β3GalT6
		SLC39A13	ZIP13
Musculocontractural EDS (mcEDS)	AR	CHST14	D4ST1
		DSE	DSE
Myopathic EDS (mEDS)	AD or AR	COL12A1	Type XII collagen
Periodontal EDS (pEDS)	AD	C1R	C1r

Figure 2. First Postulate:
The Common Systemic EDS and Its Variants

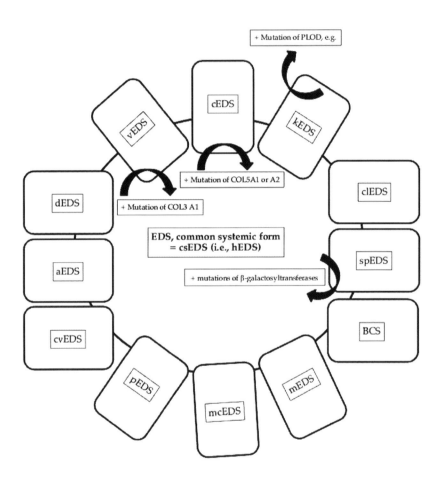

Abbreviations : *h = hypermobile; c = classical; cl = classic-like; v = vascular; d = dermatosparaxis; a = arthrochalasia; cv = cardio-valvular; p = periodontal; mc = musculocontractural; m = myopathic; BCS = brittle cornea syndrome; sp = spondylodysplastic; k = kyphoscoliotic.*

The Classical View of Molecular Genetics:
The Central Dogma

➢ Gregor Mendel (1822-1884): this monk, a Czech botanist, and biologist (Moravia, Austrian Empire at the time), made crosses of various lines of peas according to two characteristics: smooth or wrinkled. He observed how the characteristics (the term gene was only proposed in 1909 by Wilhelm Johannsen) were expressed (the phenotype) in successive generations. These were the premises of what would later be called the modes of gene transmission (the recessive mode and the dominant mode).[70]

➢ Charles Darwin (1809-1882): The theory of evolution by natural selection (1859).[71] Evolution is based on the selection of hereditary traits (genes), which vary randomly. The most suitable traits persist from generation to generation because they give others an advantage; other traits are destined to be eliminated. From this comes the evolution of the plant, animal, and even human species. EDS has withstood the test of time. Why has it withstood the test of time? See an attempt at an explanation, discussed later in the chapter.

➢ It was a deterministic vision of things: everything is written in the great book of DNA (genes, mutations). Most geneticists today, fortunately, no longer think that everything is written in DNA.

➢ One could compare this deterministic vision to a dish that one would eat, made from a cooking recipes' book (DNA) and that would always taste the same, or compare it to a sheet of music that would always give the same melody, regardless of who plays it, the symphony orchestra that plays it, or even the person listening to it.

➢ It is called the Central Dogma of molecular biology, i.e., the cascade: DNA, RNA, proteins.

---

[70] Gregor Mendel. Versuche über Plflanzenhybriden. Verhandlungen des naturforschenden Vereines Brünn, Bd. IV für das Jahr 1865,Abhandlungen, 3-47.
[71] Charles Darwin. On the Origin of Species by Means of Natural Selection, or the Preservation of Favoured Races in the Struggle for Life (November 24, 1859).

Do you already sense a clash in this orthodox view of genetics?

Is there a problem in this way of conceiving food or music?

You're right!

Even if DNA is like a cook book or a musical score, the recipes that will be made or the music that will be listened to will not, in fact, always be of the same quality or flavor. Even if they come from the same instruction manual, the taste and sensations generated by a dish or a piece of music could be very different from one individual to another, and even from one moment to another in the same individual.

Likewise, each patient with EDS is different, even slightly from another. All patients have common characteristics, but some of them standing out and coming to the forefront.

The zebra emblem for EDS patients makes sense:

➢ When you hear hoof sounds behind you, it is probably a horse. That is, a sign or symptom should evoke the most common diagnosis. For example: if one has a burning sensation behind the sternum, palpitations, and goes to the bathroom 30 times a day. He or she has to go to the doctor and do further tests. Doctor may diagnose a hiatus hernia, extrasystoles, and a descending bladder. The conclusion could be that it is gastroesophageal reflux because of a hiatal hernia. He or she might have palpitations because of the extrasystoles and have frequent urinary needs (pollakiuria) because his or her bladder has descended. Result: there are three different diseases for three different symptoms. The diagnosis of EDS could explain all three symptoms simultaneously, but they do not generally think about it. So, in EDS, the story is reversed: when you hear the hoof sounds behind you, think of something other than a horse, a zebra, for example.

➢ From afar, zebras look the same: zebras! However, closer, they are all slightly different in their stripes, and that is how they recognize one another. In EDS, it is the same thing. Overall, the patients are quite similar in their experience of

266

the disease, their symptoms, and clinical signs. Nevertheless, on closer inspection, they are all slightly different. The group of EDS patients is not so homogeneous when viewed under a magnifying glass.

We will see why, although the genetic information remains the same (the DNA), the manifestation of the disease is not ever the same according to patients, and the events they have experienced in their lives (what is currently called the Exposome), and maybe even according to the events their parents and grandparents have experienced. This is the notion of acquired characteristics. We are glimpsing epigenetics! The Environment and the Life of each person interact with the expression of our genes, and, as you will see, this is only the tip of the iceberg. Epigenetics is an upheaval and even a revolution when applied to Man, Nature, animals, plants, and of course to EDS. But this vision is still not orthodox for many geneticists (see below).

Before doing so, we need to remind ourselves of the basic notions of genetics, which can be put in the form of our previous metaphors: a cookbook or a musical score.

The Basics of Molecular Genetics

DNA is, therefore like a cookbook or a musical score. The letters or musical notes are here composed by the succession of four different nitrogenous bases (nitrogen-containing base or nucleotide base; they are molecules): A, T, G, and C (for Adenine, Thymine, Guanine, and Cytosine). The successive, specific combination of the four nucleotides forms DNA (deoxyribonucleic acid). Nucleotides are assembled by an enzyme called ADN polymerase.

A nucleotide (nt) is composed of:

- One nucleobase (or nucleotide base): adenine (A), thymine (T), cytosine (C), or guanine (G). A and G are purines, C and T are pyrimidines.
- A sugar molecule, comprising five carbon atoms (or pentose) : β-D-2'-desoxyribose (for DNA).

- A phosphate group, attached to the 5′ carbon atom of deoxyribose.

A nucleoside is an association of a nucleotide base and a pentose (a deoxyribose for DNA, and a ribose for RNA). Therefore, there are four different nucleotides found in DNA: deoxyadenosine monophosphate (dAMP), deoxyguanosine monophosphate (dGMP), deoxycytidine monophosphate (dCMP), (deoxy)thymidine monophosphate (dTMP or TMP).

DNA is organized in a double helix (*Crick and Watson, 1953*) and is in the nucleus of cells. The nucleotide bases of the two DNA strands are complementary (an A sticks to a T, and a C to a G).

These two DNA strands of the double helix are strongly linked to each other by hydrogen bonds (A to T, by 2 hydrogen bonds; and G to C, by 3 hydrogen bonds), but less strongly than the links between the different nucleotides (phosphodiester's bonds).

These two strands of DNA are condensed around small coils (like sewing thread coils): the histones (which are formed by 4 x 2 pairs of proteins).

The assembly formed by this DNA, wrapped around each histone, is called a nucleosome. These histones make it possible to compact about two meters of DNA. The succession of nucleosomes results in a structure reminiscent of a pearl necklace, the chromatin. The pearls representing the nucleosomes, and the small piece of thread visible between the pearls is unwound DNA.

The increasing compaction of the chromatin results in the formation of the 23 pairs (total of 46) of chromosomes in humans. 23 chromosomes are inherited from mom, and 23 are inherited from dad. Of these, 22 chromosomes are homologous and called autosomes, numbered from 1 to 22. The last pair of chromosomes is sexual, and these sex chromosomes are only partially homologous. There is a sex chromosome called X and a sex chromosome called Y. The XX pair results in a generally female phenotype, and the XY pair generally results in a male phenotype. The X chromosome is longer than the Y chromosome, so there are fewer genes on the Y chromosome than on the X chromosome.

It is crucial to conceptualize that chromosomes formed by two chromatids (with the appearance of a cross) are present ONLY during the metaphase of cell division (mitotic chromosomes). The DNA is less condensed outside this stage, and the different chromosomes are not identifiable (these are the non-mitotic chromosomes). The chromatin (which is the whole DNA + histones + non-histone proteins) appears as a ball of wool with a fibrous aspect. Each non-mitotic chromosome is composed of a single chromatid with a centromere.

During interphase, each chromosome is formed by duplication (or replication) of two identical chromatids, linked at their centromere. The chromatids are copied identically during mitosis to give each of the two daughter cells several chromosomes with identical DNA structures. The centromere is important to assemble the kinetochore, which links the chromosomes to the microtubules. The microtubules will allow each chromatid to be drawn to one side of the cell or the other before division (thus creating two daughter cells with 23 pairs of identical chromosomes each).

Each chromosome has two small protective caps that terminate them, the telomeres. It is interesting to note that telomeres shorten with each cell division (via the enzyme called DNA polymerase). A sort of programmed death is underway from the start because the shorter the telomeres, the shorter the life expectancy. However, there is an enzymatic complex (called telomerase) that can stabilize or even lengthen telomeres.

Centromeres and telomeres are non-protein coding parts of DNA, i.e., they do not code for proteins.

Except in certain mitosis and meiosis phases, DNA and chromosomes are located in the nucleus to not be denatured or damaged by being outside this latter. The nucleus is thus a kind of protection, a shield.

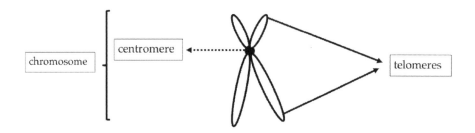

As it coils, some parts of the DNA are partially decondensed and therefore more exposed than others. Thus, the genes found are more easily read into proteins: this is euchromatin; other parts are more hidden, more condensed inside the coil: this is heterochromatin.

The 22,500 known genes[72] from our DNA book are transcribed into pre-messenger RNAs (ribonucleic acids) thanks to a complex set of proteins which includes enzymes known as RNA polymerase. These pre-messenger RNAs are then processed (splicing) to remove some of their parts (introns) and reassemble the kept parts (exons)[73] to form a messenger RNA (mRNA). Splicing is achieved by the activity of a complex molecular machinery, the spliceosome, which includes enzymes that cut the pre-messenger RNAs into pieces and that ligate exons to each other's.

These mRNAs are then translated into proteins, outside the cell nucleus, at the ribosomes' level (they are small translators-interpreters) with the help of transfer RNAs (tRNAs). Proteins are composed of amino acids (mostly of 20 different types) that are added one by one according to the succession of nucleotide bases present in the mRNAs. Proteins display a large variety of three-dimensional structures and functions: they can be enzymes, hormones, structural proteins, collagens, glycosaminoglycans, in short, everything that makes up our body and makes us who we are.

---

[72] These days, the span of estimates has shrunk, with most now between 19,000 and 22,000 protein-coding genes, and between 15,000 and 20,000 non-coding genes. Willyard C. New human gene tally reignites debate. Nature. 2018;558(7710):354-355.
[73] Mnemonic reminder: **E**xons = **E**xpressed; **I**ntrons = **I**ntruder.

Of course, most Human genes can code for more than one protein and, in many cases, the activity of the encoded proteins influences positively or negatively the expression of many other genes.

Only 1-2%[74] of the DNA is used to directly code proteins but this does not mean that the rest of the genome is functionless as we will see later in the chapter.

"It was done!"
"We had been talking about it for many years!"
"We finally knew the 22,500 genes of the human genome!"
"We finally knew everything, we thought."

The (first draft of the) human genome was finalized in 2003, they said...

Every cell in our body contains these same 22,500 genes, whether they are liver or brain cells, bone or intestine, white blood cells, or skin.

We were there, and we had read the whole book, the ecstasy!

I remember hearing this great news when I was already a 3-year rheumatologist. We were already predicting all the diseases to be cured by knowing the genes involved. Gene therapy, manipulating the genome at will, creating replacement organs from the patient's genome, even considering cloning at will!

In fact, it was not. [75,76,77]

---

[74] FYI : https://medlineplus.gov/genetics/understanding/basics/noncodingdna/

[75] Nurk S, Koren S, Rhie A, et al. The complete sequence of a human genome. doi:10.1101/2021.05.26.445798.

[76] Miga KH, Koren S, Rhie A, et al. Telomere-to-telomere assembly of a complete human X chromosome. Nature. 2020;585(7823):79-84

[77] "But actually, the human genome was still not complete. Even the revised draft was missing about 8 percent of the genome. These were the hardest-to-sequence regions, full of repeating letters that were simply impossible to read with the technology at the time." (Zhang S, The Atlantic, 2021)

It should be stressed that the Human Genome Project, however, only dealt with euchromatin (the partially decondensed, and therefore more exposed part of the DNA) and not with heterochromatin (the more condensed part whose genes are less, or not exposed, to transcription).

Parenthesis

Speaking of cloning, we all remember the cloning of the sheep named Dolly in 1997, which had already raised a great deal of concern in public opinion (from Doctors Frankenstein), but we should also welcome this significant advance in understanding the Living. As for the machismo of the scientific world, here is another example: Dolly was inspired by the singer Dolly Parton, born in 1946 in Sevierville (Tennessee), in the USA. Since the ewe came from the cloning of an adult mammary gland cell, the researchers, mostly men, quite naturally thought of the singer's breasts to give her first name. Dolly Parton is a multi-instrumentalist musician, singer-songwriter, actress, scriptwriter, and producer. In a second, and this emanating from brilliant brains of male scientists (there were far fewer women researchers than men), the undisputed queen of country music was reduced to her breasts! Still, in many scientific studies, there are fewer women, especially in the reproductive age group, i.e. in the immense range of 12 to 50 years, than men who have been enlisted and studied since the stilbene - phocomelia affair. It often leads to statistical bias in scientific studies and possible dosing errors in drugs by gender (see below). As a result, most drugs have been designed for men, without regard to the different metabolism they might have in women (see below).

Machismo is decidedly everywhere, including in Science and, for what we are interested in here, in EDS: it is mainly women who consult (80%), and women are, for many doctors, all hysterical, so they have nothing, so it is in their head.

We often hear from colleagues that EDS is the new fashionable disease! It does not hurt (*since it is in their head*), or some colleagues say to patients: "I do not believe in EDS!". They are not asked to believe. Beliefs are based on other levels of values: religions, animist ancestral rites, or others. This has nothing to do with it. EDS is a disease. People suffer, people are in disabling situations, and sometimes, by negligence or because some do not believe, they could die.

Uh, if these disbelievers could spend a day, or even an hour, in our EDS body, they would beg to be taken out!

This reminds me of a story of a patient who was telling me about the epic of her pregnancy. She was not yet diagnosed with EDS at the time. She was complaining of repeated palpitations and malaise. Doctors blamed her symptoms on stress, hormones, or whatever. She was systematically sent home with various ineffective treatments. Complaining more and more, having to insist, even beg, after several months of pregnancy, that more thorough examinations be done, they granted her anyway, out of spite and to reassure this hypochondriac woman, a standard chest X-ray. The result was that the diaphragm had been torn, and the uterus and the fetus had been pushed up into the chest. This is what caused the symptoms that this woman, who was supposedly hysterical, was experiencing. Had this condition lasted longer, both woman and baby could have died.

After the sequencing of the human genome in 2003[78], there existed the prospect of scientists becoming Masters of the Living, of being able to predict the future of individuals. They were like the Pythia of Delphi, describing to kings and army leaders the course of their lives, or of this or that epic battle, and even being able to influence their outcome. It was certainly an intoxicating idea, at least among the general population. It would even come close to the power of God (to put it mildly), or even the possibility of removing that God from the equation. But, if we want to get too close to the sun, like Icarus, we burn our wings. When we think we have finally reached our goal, when we cross a wall that we thought was impassable, then we realize that behind it rises another wall, even bigger, and that upsets everything we thought we knew. This is the story of all our lives.

One surprising finding of the analysis of the Human genome is that only 1-2 % of our DNA is used to encode proteins. The rest,

---

[78] We now know that this was the first draft of this discovery!

from 98 to 99% of the DNA, uncovers a large variety of different types of sequences, including introns of protein-coding genes, sequences required for the control of transcription (gene regulatory regions), and genes that can give non-coding RNAs (ncRNAs), i.e., RNAs that do not give rise to the production of proteins, but which nevertheless have specific functions.

Among these latter, there are microRNAs (miRNA, 21-23 nt), small interfering RNA (siRNA, 20-25 nt) and Long non-coding RNAs (lncRNAs, >200 nt) which can interact with the expression of the genetic information (e.g., the degradation of specific protein-coding RNA) (see below).

Finally, an important part of our genome (roughly 50%) is made of Transposable elements, or TEs (e.g., LINEs and SINEs) or Endogenous retroviruses (ERVs). [79],[80],[81] Together with the remains of mutated genes that have lost their functions, TE are thought to form what has been called junk DNA, the part of our genome with no clear roles in our cells and body.

Please note: many ncRNAs have been discovered but some of them will not be detailed here, such as: rRNA (ribosomal RNA), tRNA (transfer RNA), snRNA (small nuclear RNA), snoRNA (small nucleolar RNA), TERC (telomerase RNA), tRF (tRNA-derived fragments), tiRNA (tRNA halves), piRNA (piwi-interacting RNA), eRNA (enhancer RNA), circRNA (circular RNA) or Y RNA.[82]

One Gene, Many Alleles, Many Functions

On each chromosome, there are nucleotide sequences (DNA) that correspond to genes. These genes are then transcribed into

[79] Wells JN, Feschotte C. A field guide to eukaryotic transposable elements. Annu Rev Genet. 2020;54:539-561.

[80] Saliminejad K, Khorram Khorshid HR, Soleymani Fard S, et al. An oberview of microRNAs: Biology, functions, therapeutics, and analysis methods. J Cell Physiol. 2019;234(5):5451-5465.

[81] Kazimierczyk M, Wrzesinski J/ Lon non-coding RNA Epigenetics. Int J Mol Sci. 2021;22,6166. doi: 10.3390/ijms22116166.

[82] Zhang P, Wu W, Chen Q, et al. Non-coding RNAs and their integrated networks. J Integr Bioinform. 2019;16(3):20190027.doi: 10.1515/jib-2019-0027.

mRNA and translated into proteins. The proteins then have various functions (structure, enzymes, hormones, transcription factors, and some more), including regulating the gene expression that produced them (this is the notion of *feedback*). The genotype is all the genetic information of an individual.

The nucleotide sequences (A, T, C, and G) of a gene can be different on each of the two homologous chromosomes, and this is called the alleles of a gene. For example, one allele is present on chromosome 2, inherited from the father, and the other allele is present on the homologous locus of chromosome 2, inherited from the mother. The locus is the place in the DNA where the gene is located. Usually, there are two alleles for each gene, but some genes have more than a dozen different alleles.

A phenotype is a character that we observe. For example, peas have a smooth or wrinkled phenotype, in Mendel's experiment.

The influence of this or that allele of a gene on the individual's phenotype (the finished product, the individual himself, what is observable) is most often of variable intensity.

If the allele is dominant, a single copy of the allele is sufficient to give the phenotype. Whether there is only one copy (therefore in the heterozygous state) or two copies of the allele in question (in the homozygous state), the phenotype is expressed. Remember that a gene gives proteins in variable quantities. If a recessive allele is poorly or not transcribed, only the dominant allele proteins will be apparent in the phenotype.

On the other hand, if it is recessive, both alleles (each carried by one of the two homologous chromosomes) must be present (i.e., in the homozygous state) to give a particular character in the phenotype. If it is present in only one copy (in the heterozygous state), the characteristic is not expressed.

There may also be alleles of identical strength; this kind of transmission is called codominance. When there are two codominant alleles of a gene, each of the two alleles can independently give a particular phenotype. It is the case with *Wyandotte* hens' plumage: one of the alleles gives a black color, the other allele gives white color. If the two alleles present are identical (homozygous), the hen will be either white or black, depending on the alleles present. When the two different and codominant alleles are present together (heterozygous), the plumage's color will be variegated, mixed white and black. For codominant alleles, the two alleles are expressed in the same way (50/50 ratio of proteins produced).

These *Wyandotte* hens' plumage could have been grey if the dominance was incomplete, which exists in Nature. For example, one of the two alleles is not expressed at all, but the other is expressed incompletely: this is called partial dominance when the observed phenotype is an intermediate between the phenotypes that would have been obtained for each of the two alleles taken separately.

In X-linked transmission, the mutations are located on the sex chromosomes (X, Y). Most often on the X chromosome. A recessive mutation on one of the X chromosomes does not usually result in an altered phenotype in women with two X chromosomes. Since men have only one version of the X chromosome, even a recessive gene is enough to influence the phenotype because he does not have an *alter ego* on the Y chromosome. There are also dominant mutation. Nevertheless, these diseases are mostly expressed in men, which is absolutely not the case in EDS. We find this kind of mode of transmission in color blindness, for example. There used to be a form of EDS called X-linked (formerly type V), but it has been removed from the New York classification.

There is also a transmission linked to Y chromosome, but these mutations often lead to fertility disorders (impaired spermatogenesis). The transgenerational heredity thus stops quickly.

In the ovaries and testes, meiosis is the diploid cell's division mechanism (which contains 46 chromosomes). It results in the formation of four haploid cells: oocytes or spermatozoa (to be correct, this gives one oocyte, the other three being atrophied, or four spermatozoa). A haploid cell contains only 22 chromosomes and one sex chromosome (or gonosome), X or Y.

During conception, an egg comes into contact with a sperm cell and creates, again, a diploid cell, a mixed form whose genetic information has been inherited half from the mother and half from the father. It is what patients remember most of all: we are half daddy's and half mummy's genotype.

It could be so simple if it did not exist, during the phases of meiosis, an important mixing of alleles.

Meiosis takes place in two parts:

➢ During the first part of meiosis, the homologous chromosome pairs, each composed of two chromatids formed by replication, are paired in bivalent or tetrad. During this phase, pieces of homologous chromosomes are exchanged, which is called a crossing-over or intra-chromosomal mixing. Then, the homologous chromosomes, with two chromatids, separate and migrate independently, randomly, towards the two poles of the cell, which results in a genetic inter-chromosomal mixing. The cell will divide the first time into two haploid daughter cells, each containing 23 chromosomes with two chromatids. This first phase is called reductional division.

➢ During the second division of meiosis, or equational division, the chromatids separate and result in the formation of two haploid daughter cells composed of 23 chromosomes with one chromatid.

At the level of spermatozoa and oocytes, the genetic mixing is so important during meiosis that it is impossible, contrary to what one could believe, at first sight, to have two identical children, from a genomic point of view, resulting from two different fecundation events. Indeed, with crossovers and the random distribution of homologous chromosomes, it is possible to produce 2^{23} different gametes in both men and women. The probability of having two genetically identical children is therefore $1/2^{23} \times 1/2^{23} = 1/2^{46}$!

Another thorny issue in the transmission of EDS is the lack of knowledge of which traits to look for mutations. It is easy to study the transmission of innate traits if they are known, simple and if they are dominant or recessive. To have a smooth or wrinkled pea, it is easy to distinguish. It would be less easy if it were a partial dominance with more or less smooth or wrinkled peas. The subjectivity of the observer would take over. It would be even more complex in the case of polygenic disease. Even more so when we talk about epigenetics.

EDS has many diverse and varied manifestations, with phenotypes as particular as the patients affected. It is currently almost impossible to know which genes to look for and in whom. Who is normal and who is not normal? Who is severe, and who is mild or intermediate? There are so many affected EDS systems, the symptomatology is so rich, and the affected organs so varied, that it is very difficult to categorize people with the required precision. The phenotype changes between generations, but it changes over time in the same individual and changes within siblings.

Please note. In a pilot study of 105 Italian hEDS/HSD patients, the authors proposed to separate the patients into two severity classes: a *complex/severe cluster*, and a *simplex/milder cluster*.[83] "Patients completed a set of questionnaires exploring pain, fatigue, dysautonomic symptoms, coordination and attention/concentration deficits, and quality of life in general. Severity class distinction (complex vs simplex) may reflect different management programs in hypermobile Ehlers-Danlos syndrome/hypermobility spectrum disorders."

In the present state of knowledge, it is impossible to say whether the transmission of Ehlers-Danlos Syndrome is autosomal dominant or recessive.

Conrad Hal Waddington (see below) had already understood this kind of picture or *Landscape* of phenotype versus genotype. He called the process by which the genotype produces the phenotype: the *Epigenetic process*. The genotype does not entirely determine this or that phenotype; there is a certain amount of

---

[83] Copetti M, Morlino S, Colombi M, et al. Severity classes in adults with hypermobile Ehlers-Danlos syndrome/hypermobile spectrum disorders: a pilot study of 105 italian patients. Rheumatology. 2019;58:1722-1730.

chance that a particular phenotype will emerge from the same genotype.

Theodosius Dobzhansky (1900-1975) was an eminent Ukrainian-born biologist, geneticist, and evolutionary theorist. He proposed that the genome is capable of determining a set of possible phenotypes (this is called the *Reaction Norm*). The influence of factors, possibly external, favors the emergence of one phenotype over another. It is, for example, seen in monozygotic twins growing up in different environments. Their morphology, psychology, and the ailments they suffer from, change, even though all their genes are, by definition, identical. While the genes do not change, the phenotype is still different.

Epigenetics is the Science that will try to understand all those elements not part of the protein-coding DNA, but that influence the phenotype of an individual. In any case, EDS does not fit with the Mendelian transmission of a particular mutation, monosomal, for a variety of reasons.

Let us look at the theoretical autosomal dominant mode of transmission and apply it to Ehlers-Danlos Syndrome

IF:

F is the set of chromosomes passed down from the father;
M is the set of chromosomes inherited from the mother;

Fw is noted to indicate that the paternal chromosomes are free of the mutation being studied; Mw is noted to indicate that the maternal chromosomes are free of the mutation being studied;

Fd is noted to indicate that the paternal chromosomes carry a dominant EDS mutation; Md is noted to indicate that the maternal chromosomes carry a dominant mutation of the EDS;

W indicates that the gene under study's allele is in the baseline or wild-type state.

Since humans get half of their chromosomes from their father and a half from their mother. If one of the parents is a heterozygous carrier.

THEN:

If the mother is MwMd (EDS patient) and the father is FwFw (non-EDS carrier), there are four possible phenotypes in children: MwFw, MwFw, MdFw, and MdFw.

We will therefore have, on the one hand, a girl and a boy who does not carry the mutation, and, on the other hand, a boy and a girl who are heterozygous carriers of the dominant mutation, thus expressing the mutated phenotype. There will therefore be 50% non-EDS children and 50% EDS children, according to this mode of transmission (this is the first generation).

Then, however, the children will meet life partners and have children. The mutated character will then be diluted little by little over the generations:

MwMw x FwFw will give children: MwFw, MwFw, MwFw and MwFw: 100% non-EDS individuals (50% girls and 50% boys).

MwMw x FwFw will give children: MwFw, MwFw, MwFw, and MwFw: 100% non-EDS individuals (50% girls and 50% boys).

MdMw x FwFw will give children: MdFw, MdFw, MwFw and MwFw: 50% EDS and 50% healthy. One girl and one boy EDS, one girl and one boy healthy.

MdMw x FwFw will give children: MdFw, MdFw, MwFw, and MwFw: 50% EDS and 50% non-EDS subjects. One girl and one boy EDS; 1 healthy girl and one healthy boy.

In this case, out of 16 grandchildren, only four would be EDS carriers, and 12 would be non-EDS carriers (i.e., 25% EDS/75% healthy).

Following this logic, out of 64 great-grandchildren, eight would be EDS carriers or only 12.5%. 48 would be healthy.

In the fourth generation, out of 256 children, 16 would be EDS carriers (or 6.25% of children), and 240 would be healthy (or 93.75% of children).

There would thus be what I call a *transgenerational dilution* of the dominant EDS allele.

By proclaiming loud and clear that, on the one hand, the hypermobile EDS is autosomal dominant (and monogenic) Mendelian-transmitted and that, on the other hand, EDS is rare (and therefore, the probability of encountering another EDS carrier in the general population to procreate is low): they have, so to speak, shot themselves in the foot. If EDS represents only 1 case in 2000 people, the probability that an EDS patient, heterozygous for a dominant monogenic mutation, will meet a partner with the same characteristic is $1/2000 \times 1/2000 = 1/4,000,000$ (one chance in four million). It is, therefore, improbable that two partners, each carrying EDS, will meet.

Based on the prevalence of EDS that they estimate in the general population, and the transgenerational dilution of EDS mutation: EDS, which has probably been mentioned at least since the time of Hippocrates and Herodotus, should have been less and less frequent, which is, de facto, absolutely not the case. Of course, a certain number of *de novo* mutations could have appeared over time.

Does the Modeling of the Mendelian transmission of EDS clinically hold up ?

In our daily practice, we do not see this kind of transmission with a dilution of character over generations.

On the contrary, we often notice that the parents and grandparents of patients who spontaneously come to us for a diagnosis of EDS are or were less symptomatic than the patients in question, or even are or were asymptomatic (healthy carriers).

On the other hand, when EDS is clearly expressed in the phenotype of the patients who spontaneously consult us, the children and grandchildren of these patients are, in turn, almost all symptomatic, even slightly.

It is, therefore, an inverse logic to autosomal dominant transmission (see above).

It is as if, once the EDS phenotype is established, it would tend to become self-reinforcing and to persist by not following Mendel's laws. Epigenetics appears here as a possible outlet.

EDS, a disease that upsets Genetics: The role of Epigenetics?

It was Aristotle (384 - 322 B.C.), the Greek philosopher, who was already asking the question: Which came the first, the chicken or the egg? He, therefore, observed hen embryos developing, dissected them, and followed their evolution. He introduced the term *epigenesis* to describe this state of affairs (it was thought before, like Hippocrates, that the child or young of an animal existed as it was, but in miniature in the egg or germ and therefore in the testicles of a macho, patriarchal society).

However, from Aristotle, let us move forward in time to the British developmental biologist and geneticist Conrad Hal Waddington (1905-1975). In 1942, he named *epigenetics* (formed by the contraction of the terms epigenesis and genetics) everything that was outside of DNA but that interacts with its expression, i.e., the interaction of genes with their environment.

Epigenetics has developed mainly in the last 20 years or so. That was yesterday! Some say that it is one of the most significant advances in genetics since discovering the double helix of DNA in 1953.

Note: the conformation of DNA is said to have been discovered by the English biophysicist Francis H.C. Crick (1916-2004) and the American geneticist James D. Watson (born in 1928).[84] This discovery earned them the Nobel Prize for Medicine and

---

[84] Watson JD, Crick FH. Molecular structure of nucleic acids for deoxyribose nucleic acid. Nature. 1953;171(4356):737-8.

Physiology in 1962. Looking more closely at this discovery, we realize that it had already been mentioned (1951) before by the British physicochemical Rosalind Elsie Franklin (1920-1958), who worked at King's College London. Rosalind seems to have been plagiarized by Crick and Watson, who never mentioned her primary role in discovering DNA's structure. In tribute to this great scientist, the Royal Society created a Rosalind-Franklin Prize in 2003, and the future Martian automobile (ESA ExoMars) bears her name.

The three other postulates proposed later on about EDS, and its transmission to children and its evolution over time, will be based mainly on epigenetics. It is, therefore, necessary to understand and identify this significant advance.

Let us take a few examples from animal biology to introduce this reflection:

In reptiles, turtles, eggs are initially neither male nor female but become one or the other depending on the outside temperature. The temperature (the environment) influences the DNA expression towards one or the other sex. Therefore, the temperature does not influence the written book, the DNA itself, which does not change, but it does influence its expression, it is reading.[85,86]

In bees[87], it is the social role, morphology, life expectancy, and reproduction possibilities that change according to the food. Let us take bee larvae that are identical from the genetic code's point of view, the book, the DNA; they are randomly separated into two groups. The first group is fed only with royal jelly, and the second group of larvae with pollen and nectar. The larvae fed with royal jelly will all become queens, which are larger, lay eggs, and live longer. The other larvae, fed with pollen and

[85] Weber C, Zhou Y, Lee JG, et al. Temperature-dependent sex determination is mediated by sSTAT3 repression of Kdm6b. Science. 2020;368(6488):303-306.
[86] Ge C, Ye J, Weber C, et al. The histone demethylase KDM6B regulates temperature-dependent sex determination in a turtle species. Science. 2018;360(6389):645-648.
[87] Lyko F, Foret S, Kucharski R, et al. The honey bee epigenomes: differential methylation of brain DNA in queens and workers. PLoS Biol. 2010;8(11):e1000606.

nectar, will become workers, smaller, do not lay eggs, and live shorter lives. Feeding alone changes the phenotype.[88,89]

In humans, as a reminder, epigenetics can already be approached when studying the morphological and even psychological changes in identical twins (so-called monozygotic twins, having, by definition, the same genetic information) that were separated at birth. Raised in different families, they have been immersed in a social and economic world that is sometimes very different: with variables such as diet, stress, socioeconomic, occupation, life-course, tobacco, alcohol, drug use, and more, all of which are essential factors in the development of a healthy lifestyle. Comparing the pictures of these twins as adults, one would sometimes think they are not even brothers. The genetic information has not changed, but the reading of it has.[90]

Another example is the differentiation of the cells in our body according to the tissue they make up or their body functions. Nothing is more different between them than a liver cell, a brain cell (neurons, glial cells), and a white blood cell, for example. However, all the cells in our body start as a single cell divided repeatedly to form an embryo, a fetus, a child, and then an adult. The DNA is, therefore, the same in all the cells of our body. Depending on the tissues, roles, and functions, some of their 22,500 genes are better expressed; on the contrary, others are relatively extinct. Epigenetics would also have its role here.[91,92]

If it was not the DNA that changed, i.e., there were no mutations in the DNA gene sequences that would have in turn induced these changes, then what happened?

[88] Rasmussen EM, Amdam GV. Cytosine modifications in the honey bee (Apis mellifera) worker genome. Front Genet. 2015;6:8.

[89] Yagound B, Remnant EJ, Buchmann G, et al. Intergenerational transfer of DNA methylation marks in the honey bee. Proc Natl Acad Sci USA. 2020;117(51):32519-31527.

[90] Bell JT, Spector TD. A Twin approach to unraveling epigenetics. Trends Genet. 2011;27(3):116-125.

[91] Tammen SA, Friso S, Choi SW, et al. Epigenetics: the link between nature and nurture. Mol Aspects Med. 2013;34(4):753-764.

[92] Pàldi A (2020). Random walk across the epigenetic landscape (chapter 3). In: Phenotypic switching: implications in Biology and Medicine. doi.org/10.1016/C2018-0-02645-6. ISBN 978-0-12-817996-3

The Non-Coding RNAs and the DNA Methylation

1/ Non-coding DNA is not so useless, and codes, in part, for non-protein coding RNAs, such as: miRNAs[93] (micro-RNAs), siRNAs (small interfering RNAs), and lncRNAs (long non-coding RNAs). They could prevent messenger RNAs from fulfilling their role as carriers of information to the ribosomes (and then the production of particular proteins). They can act by neutralizing or destroying those protein-coding mRNAs (thanks to a sophisticated mechanism involving DICER and RISC enzymes). In recent years, many other mechanisms have been discovered that could turn on or turn off some of our genes.

In a recent article written by an Italian team, the roles of miRNAs in HSD and hEDS were brilliantly discussed. Analysis of the transcriptome (the set of RNAs derived from the genome transcription) allowed them to highlight differences between different subtypes of EDS (cEDS, vEDS, hEDS/HSD). In hEDS/HSD, some connective tissue alterations may be due to the excessive production of extracellular matrix degradation enzymes and the acquisition by fibroblasts of a particular myofibroblast phenotype. The latter cells have increased contractility and other structural changes. These particularities could explain specific manifestations in EDS (gastrointestinal dysfunction, increased susceptibility to osteoarthritis, chronic musculoskeletal pain, soft tissue inflammatory lesions, neurological disorders, and more.).[94]

2/ DNA methylation. DNMTs (DNA methyltransferases) are a family of enzymes that catalyze the reaction of addition of the methyl group to cytosine residues of specific genes, within CpG dinucleotides using S-adenosylmethionine as a methyl donor. The more methylated a gene is, the less it is expressed. Of course, genes can, in turn, promote or repress other genes in cascade, and some more. Many mechanisms act on the histones

---

[93] miRNAs are small molecules of non-protein coding RNA, composed of about 20 to 25 nucleotides (nt).

[94] Chiarelli N, Ritelli M, Zoppi N, et al.. Cellular and molecular mechanisms in the pathogenesis of classical, vascular, and in hypermobile Ehlers-Danlos syndromes. Genes. 2019;10:609. doi :10.3390/genes10080609.

themselves, allowing the chromatin to unwind and expose genes to be encoded or, on the contrary, to wind up further, causing the opposite effect. These mechanisms are methylation, but also acetylation, phosphorylation, ubiquitylation, sumoylation, and more. In other words, histone acetylation generally results in the unwinding of the DNA, making other parts of the DNA more exposed to transcription into RNA.

On the other hand, histone methylation has the opposite effect. It hides specific genes. No need to go into details for all these mechanisms; the important thing is to know that there are a variety of mechanisms. These phenomena can be influenced by the environment, our lifestyles and life events, and sometimes by those of our parents and grandparents.

A few years ago, it was thought that these phenomena were non-reversible and not transmissible to children via male or female gametes. At that time, we were convinced that there was a reset of epigenetic markers in the gametes before conception, that these were purely and simply erased. We now know that it is much more complicated than that, that some epigenetic marks may persist and can be transmitted, at least partially, to children during procreation.

Prof. Andràs Pàldi[95] adds:

It was a revolution in the conception of genetics and heredity, that called in question the role of DNA as the only carrier of heredity. The idea that acquired characters can be transmitted to the next generation was generally accepted during the 19th century. It is erroneously attributed to Jean-Baptiste Lamarck, a French naturalist and usually believed to be opposed to Charles Darwin's views on biological evolution. The truth is that both Lamarck and Darwin strongly believed in the possibility of transmission of acquired characters. It was August Weismann, a German scientist at the end of the 19th century who put forward the idea that characters acquired by the soma during the life leave unaffected the germ plasma. The concepts of *soma* and *germ plasma* were also coined by him to differentiate the parts of the

---

[95] Biochemist, Geneticist and Epigeneticist, Paris, France.

body executing normal functions and the germ line that carries hereditary information. The impossibility of transmission of acquired characters became at the beginning of the 20th century one of the basic tenets of the emerging science of genetics. Research on epigenetics over the last 20 years has demonstrated that the situation is more complicated. Environmental perturbations during the gestation have been shown in animal models to interfere with the epigenetic reprogramming and induce epigenetic changes in the fetal germ line. These environmentally induced phenotypes can persist during the postnatal life and transmitted to the subsequent generations. Fetal development appears particularly sensitive to nutritional stress that may generate transgenerational phenotypic effects though epigenetic mechanisms such as chromatin modifications or microRNAs.

Although there are more and more known and well documented examples, the mechanisms are not yet fully understood. This makes the issue of transgenerational inheritance of acquired phenotypes a matter of controversy between *orthodox geneticists* and epigeneticists. It is clear that the exact place of epigenetic transgenerational inheritance is still to be determined. More specifically, in human examples of non-Mendelian inheritance it is currently difficult to estimate the relative weight of epigenetic mechanisms as compared to genetic or non-biological (maternal effect, cultural etc.) transmission. Nevertheless, in the light of the available evidence it is not only impossible to deny the existence of transgenerational transmission, but it should be considered as a serious candidate every time when non-Mendelian patterns of transmission are observed in the human population.[96,97,98,99]

---

[96] Radford et al. In utero undernourishment perturbs the adult sperm methylome and intergenerational metabolism. Science. 2014;345:1255903. doi.org/10.1126/science.1255903.

[97] Tuscher et al. Multigenerational epigenetic inheritance: One step forward, two generations back. Neurobiology of Disease. 2019;132. doi.org/10.1016/j.nbd.2019.104591.

[98] Kazachenka et al. Identification, Characterization, and Heritability of Murine Metastable Epialleles: Implications for Nongenetic Inheritance. Cell. 2018;175:1259-1271.

[99] Huypens et al. Epigenetic germline inheritance of diet-induced obesity and insulin resistance. Nature Genetics. 2016;48:497-500.

In summary, epigenetic marks could therefore not only be acquired and stable over time, but could also be reversible depending on life events and the environment. Furthermore, extraordinarily, they could, at least in part, be passed on to children (they are hereditary).

It was a revolution in the conception of genetics and heredity, which were thought to be immutable in time (and therefore in human life), apart from spontaneous mutations in DNA (*de novo mutations*).

As time goes by and Science evolves, things change, and we must adapt ourselves to these rapid changes in the understanding of the Living in Medicine.

EDS, a Genetic and Epigenetic disease?

Some may ask, "how could you have this crazy idea of transposing epigenetics to Ehlers-Danlos Syndrome?"

At a GERSED France board meeting in Paris in 2017, to which Prof. C. Hamonet and Prof. M. Vervoort were also invited, I asked Prof. Vervoort whether what we were encountering in our daily clinical practice, i.e., transmission to almost 100% of children when only one of the two parents was suffering from the syndrome, could be found in nature, in animal biology, or otherwise? Prof. Vervoort answered in the affirmative. He said first of all, that as a biologist and geneticist, "If you tell me that you encounter this in your daily clinic, I believe you".

What we encounter in our clinic must be believed, nice first message.

Then, He confirmed that in animal biology, we could meet individuals who, as carriers of a particular biological particularity (thus, the phenotype), irreparably transmit it to the young (even if there are 100 of them), and even if the other parent is not a carrier of this particularity.

It immediately reassured our EDS vision and our practices as physicians.

Time passed, and since then, I came across a few articles talking about epigenetics applied to animals and humans. After reading a few books, and talking with some geneticist and epigeneticists, I quickly realized the incredible potential of this Science of understanding the Living.

After studying EDS with Professor Claude Hamonet in Paris and listening to his experience and vision of EDS, after meeting, listening to, and examining more than 3,000 patients: epigenetics appeared as a piece of evidence in this disease. EDS had to be, in addition to a genetic disease, an epigenetic disease!

Among the various studies that concern epigenetics, here are some that made me think:

Post-traumatic stress disorder (PTSD). A few dozen pregnant women were directly exposed to the trauma of the September 11, 2001 attacks in New York. They were in or near one of the twin towers, at the time. Some of them experienced significant PTSD. Women with PTSD reported more depression ($P = 0.002$) than women without PTSD, but did not differ in self-reported postpartum depression. Examination of PTSD effects in each trimester separately revealed a significant effect of maternal PTSD in infants born to mothers pregnant in the third trimester ($P = 0.012$), but not in infants born to mothers in the first or second trimesters.[100] After a year, researchers found that these PTSD women had low levels of cortisol in their saliva. More surprisingly, their children, who were one year old at the time, also had decreased levels of this stress hormone. However, as far as they were concerned, they had not suffered any direct trauma during the attack since they were in their mothers' wombs. The most likely origin of these hormonal disorders (cortisol level) was epigenetic marks transmitted to children by the mother during pregnancy. The low levels of this hormone were, a priori, secondary to an induced change in the expression of one or more genes that regulate this hormone's levels. The correlation between maternal PTSD and cortisol levels in infants was

---

[100] Yehuda R, Mulherin Engel S, Brand SR, et al. Transgenerational effects of posttraumatic stress disorder in babies of mothers exposed to the World Trade Center attacks during pregnancy. J Clin Endocrinol Metab. 2005;90(7):4115-4118.

remarkably similar to that reported between parental PTSD and urinary cortisol levels in adult offspring of Holocaust survivor.[101,102]

Stress is an environmental factor that can induce, for example, DNA or histone methylations or acetylations, or even miRNA-mediated actions.[103]

Other studies were published concerning the same traumatic event.[104,105]

Another study looked at the case of pregnant women at the time of the genocide in Rwanda, which sadly took place from 7 April 1994 to 17 July 1994, and which decimated an estimated 800,000 to over one million people.[106] Scientists looked for methylations of a gene, which influences chronic stress and sensitivity to external stresses, in women who were pregnant at that time and who had directly witnessed unspeakable and horrific massacres. At the same time, they analyzed DNA sequences from other women, of the same ethnicity as the previous ones, but who had not directly witnessed these events. The results were incredible! Mothers exposed to the genocide as well as their children had lower cortisol and GR (glucocorticoid receptor) levels and higher MR (mineralocorticoid receptor) levels than non-exposed mothers and their children. Moreover, exposed mothers and

---

[101] Yehuda R, Teicher MH, Seckl JR, et al. Parental posttraumatic stress disorder as a vulnerability factor for low cortisol trait in offspring of holocaust survivors. Arch Gen Psychiatry. 2007;64(9):1040-8.

[102] Yehuda R, Halligan SL, Bierer LM. Cortisol levels in adult offspring of Holocaust survivors: relation to PTSD symptom severity in the parent and child. Psychoneuroendocrinology. 2002;27:171-180.

[103] Pfeiffer JR, Mutesa L, Uddin M. Traumatic stress epigenetics. Curr Behav Neurosci Rep. 2018;5(1):81-93.

[104] Kuan PF, Waszczuk MA, Kotov R, et al. An epigenome-wide DNA methylation study of PTSD and depression in World Trade Center responders. Transl Psychiatry. 2017;7(6):e1158.

[105] Brand SR, Engel SM, Canfield RL, Yehuda R. The effect of maternal PTSD following in utero trauma exposure on behavior and temperament in 9-month-old infant. Ann NY Acad Sci. 2006;1071:454-458.

[106] Vukojevic V, Kolassa IT, Fastenrath M, et al. Epigenetic modification of the glucocorticoid receptor gene is linked to traumatic memory and post-traumatic stress disorder risk in genocide survivors. J Neurosci. 2014;34(31):10274-84.

their children had higher methylation of the *NR3C1* exon 1_F (promotor regions) than non-exposed groups (*Perroud N et al., 2014*).[107] Not only were the genes of the women who had directly witnessed these horrors more methylated than those of other women, but so were their children! The transmission of these acquired epigenetic marks was therefore hereditary (i.e. biological alterations of the hypothalamic-pituitary-adrenal axis – HPA axis). Moreover, the children who did not experience these atrocities were much more sensitive to stress than those whose mothers had not witnessed these dramas.[108,109]

It is naturally more challenging to study transgenerational transmission in humans, where each generation is about 20 years apart than in mice, which reproduce much faster. It has also been observed that the intensity of gene methylation may decrease over time, after x generations. It is therefore also encouraging to know that the induced phenomenon can potentially diminish.

The environment and pesticides. [110 , 111] Studies show that exposure to pesticides induces DNA methylation in mice and that these methylations can be transmitted to the young over several generations. Even more impressive, even dramatic, was the observation of decreased fertility in these mice. Imagine, with all that we breathe, what will become of our epigenome and that of our children![112] It is high time to act. The good news is that

---

[107] Perroud N, Rutembesa E, Paoloni-Giacobino A, et al. The Tutsi and transgenerational transmission of maternal stress: epigenetics and biology of the HPA axis. The World Journal of Biological Psychiatry. 2014;15(4):334-345.

[108] Vukojevic v, Coynel D, Ghaffari NR, et al. NTRK2 methylation is related to reduced PTSD risk in two African cohorts of trauma survivors. Proc Natl Acad Sci USA. 2020;117(35):21667-21672.

[109] Perroud N, Rutembesa E, Paoloni-Giacobino A, et al. The Tutsi genocide and transgenerational transmission of maternal stress: epigenetics and biology of the HPA axis. World J Biol Psychiatry. 2014;15(4):334-345.

[110] Rajender S, Avery K, Agarwal A, et al. Epigenetics, spermatogenesis and male fertility. Mutat Res. 2011;727(3):62-71.

[111] Menezo Y, Dale B, Elder K. The negative impact of the environment on methylation/epigenetic marking in gametes and embryos: A plea for action to protect the fertility of future generations. Mol Reprod Dev. 2019;86(10):1273-1282.

[112] Carlsen E, Giwercman A, Keiding N, et al. Evidence for decreasing quality of semen during past 50 years. BMJ. 1992;305(6854):609-13.

these marks can be gradually erased over time if we do everything we can to prevent them from being left behind.

Childhood maltreatment[113] (such as sexual abuse, physical or emotional abuse, emotional neglect). Studies have been conducted on the methylation levels of the NR3C1 gene (a gene that codes for a nuclear cortisol receptor) in childhood maltreatment (such as sexual abuse, physical or emotional abuse, emotional neglect).[114] Theoretically, when we are under great stress, we secrete special hormones to react quickly and promptly to the situation (cortisol, adrenaline, etc.). Once the stress has passed, we must return to normal levels of cortisol to avoid being in a state of chronic stress (*see also the Polyvagal Theory of Stephen W. Porges*).

This is when the NR3C1 gene becomes active and causes the cortisol level in the blood to drop. In children who were abused as children, this gene is more methylated. This chronic stress has probably increased the activity of specific enzymes (methyltransferases). These methylations inactivate the gene and the cortisol level remains chronically too high. This leads to borderline personalities in adulthood with significant emotional instability. The more the abuse was important, the more the gene seemed to be methylated; the more the gene was methylated, the more the pathologies generated in adulthood were marked.[115]

The positive point is that psychotherapy could reduce the methylations of this gene (NR3C1) and antidepressants (pharmacogenomics studies how drugs act on the genome).[116]

---

[113] McGowan PO, Sasaki A, D'Alessio AC, et al. Epigenetic regulation of the glucocorticoid receptor in human brain associates with childhood abuse. Nat Neurosci. 2009;12(3):342-8.

[114] Stenz L, Schetchter DS, Serpa SR, Paoloni-Giacobino A. Intergenerational transmission of DNA methylation signatures associated with early life stress. Curr Genomics. 2018;19(8):665-675.

[115] Perroud N, Paoloni-Giacobino A, Prada P, et al. Increased methylation of glucocorticoid receptor gene (NR3C1) in adults with a history of childhood maltreatment: a link with the severity and type of trauma. Transl Psychiatry. 2011;1(12):e59.

[116] Xulu KR, Womersley JS, Sommer J, et al. DNA methylation and psychotherapy response in trauma-exposed men with appetitive aggression. Psychiatry Res. 2021;295:113608.

The same is true for studies on the effects of alcohol consumption or smoking during pregnancy[117]: these are, at least partially (*see teratogenic effects*), epigenetic phenomena.

It reminded me that smoking increases the probability of developing rheumatoid arthritis. So, it could, a priori, be due to epigenetics. I did not know this at the time when I was consulting at the University Hospital.

There are also studies about epigenetics' effects of endocrine disruptors (e.g., phthalate and dioxin).[118,119,120,121]

Mass traumas, massacres, and wars imprint in people methylations of genes that are transmitted from generation to generation, causing, for example, an increased susceptibility to stress. We are all the epigenetic result of what our parents and grandparents experienced[122], during the Second World War, for example, and, who knows, during earlier wars.

An estimated 89.7% of adults have been exposed to at least one traumatic event in their lifetime[123], with the norm being multiple trauma exposures.

---

[117] Stouder C, Somm E, Paoloni-Giacobino A. Prenatal exposure to ethanol: a specific effect on the H19 gene in sperm. Reprod Toxicol. 2011;31(4):507-12.

[118] Dutta S, Haggerty DK, Rappolee DA, Ruden DM. Phthalate exposure and long-term epigenomic consequences: a review. Front Genet. 2020;11:405. doi: 10.3389/fgene.2020.00405.

[119] Prados J, Stenz L, Stouder C, Dayer A, Paoloni-Giacobino A. Prenatal exposure to DEHP affects spermatogenesis and sperm DNA methylation in a strain-dependent manner. PLoS One. 2015;10(7):e0132136.

[120] Somm E, Stouder C, Paoloni-Giacobino A. Effect of developmental dioxin exposure on methylation and expression of specific imprinted genes in mice. Reprod Toxicol. 2013;35:150-155.

[121] Anway MD, Cupp AS, Uzumcu M, et al. Epigenetic transgenerational actions of endocrine disruptors and male fertility. Science. 2005;308(5727):1466-9.

[122] Kaati G, Bygren LO, Pembrey M, et al. Transgenerational response to nutrition, early life circumstances and longevity. Eur J Hum Genet. 2007;15(7):784-90.

[123] Kilpatrick DG, Resnick HS, Milanak ME, et al. National estimates of exposure to traumatic events and PTSD prevalence using DSM-IV and DSM-5 criteria. Journal of traumatic stress. 2013;26(5):537-547.

Dietary deficiencies during wars can also induce methylation of genes, which will lead to an eating disorder, such as bulimia, in the offspring, even though there was no deficiency at the time. It is as if the lack of food from parents or grandparents had induced a mark involving an exaggerated search for food.[124]

The examples are to be multiplied *ad infinitum* when one applies these searches to the Living and Man, and it almost makes one dizzy!

I must mention here that the transmission of epigenetic marks and the heredity of acquired traits remains a controversial subject among researchers. Many geneticists do not accept the existence of epigenetic heredity. There is a grey area where it is difficult, if not impossible, to distinguish between epigenetic transmission and culture-like transmission, including that related to variations in the microbiota (see below).

These findings are controversial and are mostly valid for human studies. Animal studies are more convincing.[125]

In EDS, however, there are many arguments for epigenetic influence, in practice. There are specific repetitions in the disease history of patients which are almost constant:

- The frequent presence of a disease trigger: trauma, rape, abuse, road accident, concussion, post-traumatic stress disorder, burn-out, divorce, bereavement, sudden hormonal changes, and more.

- If the disease was of classic genetic transmission, why do people who are carriers of EDS, but not symptomatic, trigger the disease at variable times in their lives? Why is it that sometimes the disease is triggered in childhood and other times only around the age of 20, 40, or 60? It does not seem to

[124] Heijmans BT, Tobi EW, Stein AD, et al. Persistent epigenetic differences associated with prenatal exposure to famine in humans. Proc Nat Acad Sci USA. 2008;105(44):17046-9.

[125] Deichmann U. The social construction of the social epigenome and the larger biological context. Epigenetics & Chromatin. 2020;13(1):37. doi: 10.1186/s13072-020-00360-w.

make sense. If one has a genetic disease, it usually manifests itself from birth or childhood (as with cystic fibrosis, for example) and not suddenly after a life event.

- The variation of symptoms and their intensities over time: there are moments of crises, with possibly difficult situations of disability, which are sometimes surprisingly temporary. These crises are often favored by a trigger and most often occur a few days, weeks, or months after the event. Could this be the time it takes for epigenetic factors to take place?

Since EDS patients' life courses are very different, the evolution is exceptionally variable over time, variable between individuals, and often variable between family members.

The transmission of the disease, or specific disease features, occurs to virtually all children and not just to one child in two or one children in four, as expected in Mendelian genetics. It is not a myth or a fabulation of a few enlightened doctors. It is a general feeling among clinical physicians who see patients with EDS daily. The transmission is more than Mendelian, more important than if it were based only on orthodox or classical molecular genetics.

The variable and diverse expression of the disease in children and the presence of healthy or non-symptomatic carriers are striking. If mutations are transmitted to children, then why are they not all affected in the same way? Why are some only healthy carriers (but sometimes transmit the disease to their children who may, in turn, become more symptomatic than their healthy carrier parents) and others are somewhat, mildly or very symptomatic? It is because there are other factors to consider, such as epigenetic factors.

In Mendelian genetics, innate traits tend to dilute over generations (see EDS transmission modeling above). Children and grandchildren have an increasingly lower probability of carrying the mutation(s) due to a variety of mechanisms: firstly, they link up with healthy individuals who do not carry the mutation(s) in question; secondly, due to the meiosis inducing intra- and inter-chromosomal mixing, and thirdly, due to the chance of chromosomal transmission by gametes over successive generations.

On the one hand, in EDS, in practice, we note that the parents and grandparents of patients who consult us are or were, more often than not, less symptomatic than them. On the other hand, once the EDS phenotype appears in a family, it seems to be maintained over generations.

We will see later what the notion of bistable states is and what it can bring us to understand this phenomenon.

My Second Postulate:

Exposome Influences the Evolution of EDS during the Life of the Patient

Some patients, as we observe daily, present aggravation of their symptomatology after a life event and/or life accident, as I call them: the first menstrual period, menopause, childbirth, a road accident, an assault, a rape, child or adult abuse, a concussion, a bereavement, or separation, a burn-out, etc. It seems obvious to us that this aggravation of the symptoms of EDS, and even of various clinical signs, most often occurs a few days, weeks, or months after this event. It is as if it took some time for the epigenetic marks to set up, then increase and/or decrease the expression of certain genes and, ultimately, influence the production of certain specific proteins.

It is also very surprising that it not only affects pain, but also muscle fatigability, the autonomic nervous system, sense organs, proprioception, and even the appearance of bruises (via an influence of epigenetics on platelet function, for example?) or other clinical phenomena.

At other times, their lifestyle habits, stress management and other factors (see below: "How can epigenetics be positively influenced?") seem to improve their clinical condition over time. Epigenetics, as we have seen, is potentially reversible. The Environment permanently influences patients' clinics.

I have imagined a fictional story, that of Zebrin. This story could schematize the evolution of an EDS patient's life according to innate traits (genetic and epigenetic) and acquired traits (epigenetic and, rarely, a *de novo* genetic mutation).

Here it is:

Zebrin is born!

This beautiful baby, whom her parents named Zebrin in memory of their honeymoon in Cameroon in 1997, is in good health. Her mother, Ida, was diagnosed with EDS a short time ago by Dr R.G., a rheumatologist in Brussels.

This little baby, then this little girl, whom her friends will later mischievously nickname Z, is hyperlaxed but has no other clinical signs or symptoms. She is a good student, highly intelligent and lively, full of energy, and a little ballet dancer.

At 19, she meets a nice guy, Guy, a 21-year-old architecture student. They move in together, and Z is pregnant when she turns 20.

Everything went smoothly during her pregnancy, the doctors having been warned that her mother had Ehlers-Danlos Syndrome and that Z was hypermobile, therefore probably a potential healthy-carrier of EDS and at risk of obstetrical complications. Her gynecologist followed her sympathetically, and she delivered her baby without any problems. However, it was necessary to induce labor because the baby did not want to show up, Z's cervix was not dilated despite uterine contractions, and she had been in labor for over 10 hours. But in the end, she gave birth vaginally without any major problems, except for an episiotomy.

She gives birth to Alex, on her 21st birthday. Alex is a beautiful and healthy baby, 3kg700g and 51cm. What a joy!

Two to three months after giving birth, Z felt very tired and drained when she got up in the morning, and felt as if she had been under a steamroller all night. She had more and more frequent headaches, almost daily.

A few weeks later, palpitations and night sweats (especially on the upper body, between the breasts and on the head) started. This surprised her GP because Z's family life was great, and she was not under any stress. She is on maternity leave; Guy has a good final year internship position with a well-known architect in the Kingdom's capital, and is already earning a small salary.

Z cannot take it anymore and returns to her general practitioner again, but he finds nothing special in her blood tests or her cardiological examination. He still sends her to her mother's rheumatologist to rule out manifestations of Ehlers-Danlos Syndrome since her mother has it.

Dr. R.G. questions and examines Z from every angle, writes down tons of things, fills out all kinds of papers, puts crosses in boxes and announces his diagnosis with a frank but reassuring tone: "Zebrin, like your mom, you have developed a common systemic form of Ehlers-Danlos Syndrome, or hypermobile as they say, you meet all the criteria of the New York International Consortium. Do not worry, we will do some additional tests and start a treatment to relieve you. This is probably due to the sudden fluctuations in your hormones during pregnancy and especially during childbirth. They must have influenced and triggered the disease; it happens often." (This is the consequence of the first event on the diagram below). Z then carefully follows Dr. R.G.'s recommendations and treatments, and feels better. She returns to work in her restaurant after her maternity leave. She manages her pains and headaches as best she can, but this is not obvious with the restaurant's heavy loads and the omnipresent noise in the room.

Time goes by, Alex is growing up; he is 11 years old. He is an intelligent young teenager, a bit turbulent, diagnosed dyslexic and dyscalculic, but the follow-up in speech therapy improves his little worries. He is clumsy, a little awkward as his grandmother Ida says, "he was like me when I was young," she often says. Alex started practicing aikido under the guidance of Master Seiichi, a Japanese expert, eighth dan from the Tokyo World Center. He is evolving well, thriving, and has good company, which is not easy in these troubled times. He even dries classes on Thursdays to go and demonstrate for the climate.

While Guy finally returns from his trip a week later, Z is in her eighth month. Z is sad, isolated, and cowering in her corner. Guy does his best, but nothing helps. They often quarrel, their complicity slowly fades away. They tear each other apart just before giving birth, and they hardly speak to each other anymore. In this chilly half of April, she gives birth two weeks later at the Eddy Cavelle Clinic. Her delivery is fast, but she lost much blood during the cesarean section; she even has to be transfused with two units of concentrated red blood cells.

One year later, several events jostle in Zebrin's life, significant events, blow after blow, follow one another.

First, her father, brought in on the night of September 11th, died suddenly in the emergency department of St. Paul's Hospital in Brussels. We had not seen anything coming. Z is collapsed. Almost at the same time, Z learns that she is expecting a second child with Guy. The grief brought on by the death of her father will follow her throughout her pregnancy. Her work at the restaurant is difficult and stressful. In the fifth month of her pregnancy, she ends up developing a burn-out and stays at home, alone and without friends, while Guy is on a business trip to Qatar. She receives her dismissal, clearly abusive, from her boss. She is devastated.

Z is physically and morally exhausted. She is 33 years old. Fortunately, little France is doing well and displays 3Kgs 900g for 50cm. She raises her little girl alone, Guy having decided to move.

Suddenly, one day of July of the same year, her legs do not answer any more, Z is paralyzed. After various tests, all normal, she was diagnosed with "conversion hysteria" and put on antidepressants and antipsychotics. She knows that she is not crazy and consults Dr. R.G.; She is very worried.

After careful examination, he is sure that it is pseudoparalysis related to EDS; all neurological tests have come back negative.

This is the consequence of all the upheavals she has undergone, grouped under event 2.

Dr. R.G. prescribes compression garments, sequential home oxygen therapy, physiotherapy, and hydrotherapy.

Things improve in the following weeks; Z walks a little, but she cannot get off her crutches or wheelchair when she has to go out, for limited shopping or a short walk. She gradually gets back on her feet, but she does not regain her full independence. To keep herself busy, she swallows book after book, looking after her two children as best she can, with the help of Ida.

Zebrin's Life

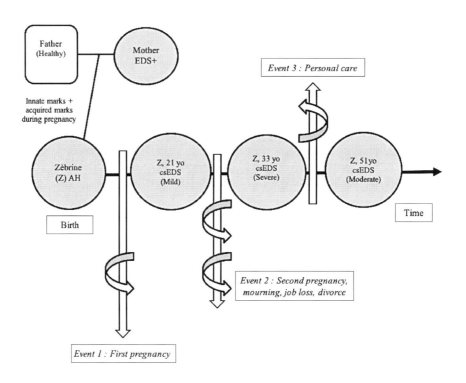

Legend : AH = asymptomatic hyperlaxity; csSED = common systemic EDS.

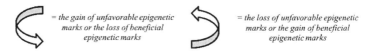

= the gain of unfavorable epigenetic marks or the loss of beneficial epigenetic marks   = the loss of unfavorable epigenetic marks or the gain of beneficial epigenetic marks

One day she came across a book about epigenetics, which advocates some simple principles to improve gene expression. Z decides to get her life back on track, gets back to regular exercise and heart coherence, eats

healthier, and begins to write, with satisfaction, a novel telling the story of a zebra in perdition but who, in the end, regains his honor and becomes the leader of his group. Z is satisfied with her writing. She goes out again, sees long-lost friends, and registers for a yoga class (this is 'event 3' in the diagram).

A few months later, she no longer uses her wheelchair, her Ferrari, as she called it; she walks with only one crutch and feels much better.

At 51, Zebrin is a happy mother and grandmother. She has found a life companion who fills her with joy.

An empirical explanation of Zebrin's evolution according to the events of her life.

Zebrin was born with half of her parents' genetic code, which includes mutations in collagen, GAG, and more, but she also received part of their epigenetic markers (from each of the two parents).

During her mother's pregnancy, depending on whether the environment was calm, serene, or unfortunately agitated (mistreatment, malnutrition, mother's fall, and stress, mourning in the family, separation of the couple), she also acquired beneficial or unfavorable epigenetic marks. It is the same during Z's pregnancies.

Throughout her life, Z has accumulated or lost epigenetic marks (e.g., cytosine methylation). It may have worsened or improved her disease's clinical significance, her phenotype.

It is crucial to note the dynamics and temporality of the events.

The case of Zebrin, exemplary and purely fictitious, clearly shows that the worsening of symptoms and clinical signs take a particular time to set in: days, weeks, or months. Moreover, their improvements are no exception to the rule. It is a reflection of what we encounter every day.

In the history and experience of patients, we follow, there is almost always one or more successive triggers that favor the appearance of Ehlers-Danlos Syndrome. The same is true for the transition from an asymptomatic hyperlaxity (JHS) to a common systemic EDS form (csEDS), often wrongly categorized as hypermobile (hEDS), and/or the worsening of pre-existing EDS symptoms.

The same is true for clinical improvements when specific treatments are adequately implemented, and when the patient's lifestyle changes, whether positive or negative.

Life accidents such as abuse, psycho-emotional damage, hormonal variations, and trauma can influence our epigenetics and therefore the expression of our genes and, by extension, the production of proteins (enzymes, structural proteins, hormones).

The notion of Bistable Chromatin States, and the Histone Code

The crucial point, the cornerstone of the production or not of proteins (structural proteins, enzymes, transcription factors, hormones), is the state in which chromatin is found. This state makes it accessible or not to RNA transcription. As a reminder, chromatin is composed of the DNA sequence and proteins called histones (composed of 4x2 subunits). The DNA wraps firmly, around these histone molecules, which condenses it, and forms nucleosomes. When chromatin is very condensed, it is called heterochromatin, and when it is partially decondensed and therefore more accessible to transcription factors, it is called euchromatin.

In this structure, one thing is remarkable: the conservation, through time and species, of the structure of these histone molecules. Natural selection has carefully preserved them. They are, therefore, essential and have a crucial role for the Living.

For DNA to be transcribed, it must be accessible to this enzymatic machinery thanks to transcription factors (TFs). Histone acetylation makes the nucleosomes less stable, which allows the histone molecules to temporarily detach from the

DNA. This allows the two complementary strands of DNA to separate at this point and then be accessible to TFs.[126]

Euchromatin is characterized by an increased amount of histone acetylation and cytosine acetylation on regulatory regions of the DNA sequence, for example, on transcription factor binding sites (promotors, enhancers). Simultaneously, specific enzymes are noted to remove methyl groups from histones and various DNA sequences; methylation decreases DNA gene expression, and further stabilizes nucleosomes.

These activities are thus complementary and could give a partially deterministic character to these epigenetic mechanisms. It would indeed be very unlikely that such complementary epigenetic machinery would be set up by simple chance.

Would there then be a pre-ordained code or pattern of epigenetics?

This is becoming more and more intriguing, and it upsets the established thinking of classical (or orthodox) molecular genetics.

Some epigenetic memory is, therefore, imprinted in the DNA. Once these epigenetic marks are put on histones and DNA, they can be passed on during mitosis and meiosis for future generations.

In contrast, transcription factors, which are protein structures floating between the DNA structures in the cell nucleus, are not inherited during meiosis. These protein structures are not inherited, but their instructions for use are inherited.

It is possible that the epigenetic marks are set up from the start on the two homologous chromosomes and therefore transmitted to the children, regardless of which of the two homologous chromosomes is inherited by the haploid cells during meiosis.

---

[126] Mukhopadhyay S, Sengupta AM. The role of multiple marks in epigenetic silencing and the emergence of a stable bivalent chromatin state. PLoS Comput Biol. 2013;9(7):e1003121.

Let us insist on the fact that the phenotype will change because of the epigenetic marks, but not the genotype (which is the sequence of the nucleotides of the DNA). This is how we can obtain several phenotypes from the same genotype in addition to the genetic backgrounds (see above). This is a real revolution in the thinking of the All Genetic and the Central Dogma of classical molecular biology. Although it should be remembered, most geneticists have outgrown this way of thinking.

Epigenetics was only possible when the resources of classical genetics were almost exhausted. That is to say, when it was realized that, although we had deciphered the human genome (or at least euchromatin) as a whole, we still faced seemingly impassable walls in certain diseases. Diseases that clinical presentations in patients differ, while the genetic damage involved is the same. It is the case for many diseases, including EDS.

Therefore, the state of activity of the genes can be, in some cases, transmitted to the descendants; this discovery, which seems banal at first sight, is extraordinary. It is essential for understanding the transmission of EDS and its phenotypic modifications over time in a patient or even across generations.

Transmission of various combinations of histone modifications (acetylations, methylations, and more) that influence the state of gene expression, could explain variations in phenotypes (i.e. the reading of the book) without any change in the genotype (i.e. the writing of the book).

There would be a histone code, i.e., specific combinations of histone modifications that would have specific outcomes in terms of gene expression. One way to view this histone code is to consider that it would be deterministic as is the genetic code.

In this view, it is as if the genetic information (DNA, the book) provided the blueprint for the layout of a train, its switches, and the various possible routes to be taken. In this scheme, indeed, the train is well built and its multitude of possible tracks. If the histone code determines the track that this train will systematically have to use (the phenotype) to the detriment of other tracks, the result will be the same, with or without epigenetics, in any case in the stability of the long-term transmission of information. It does not suit us intellectually to explain the variations in the train's paths in different individuals or the same individual throughout his or her life (as in EDS).

Prof. Andràs Pàldi adds:

"The state of gene activity correlates with the combination of epigenetic modifications of the chromatin of the gene's regulatory region. It has been proposed that the epigenetic profile can be seen as an extension of the genetic code. The so called histone code would contain the information required to the correct regulation of the gene. However, this idea is now almost completely abandoned. Indeed, contrary to the genetic code, the epigenetic modifications are either stable or reversible depending on the circumstances. The epigenetic profile of a gene usually remains stable in a cell, unless biological stimuli or large environmental perturbations come to modify it. The induced modifications remain stable until the perturbation. The capacity to resist to small fluctuations but change under the pressure of physiological induction or large perturbations confers to epigenetic mechanisms the capacity to keep the record of the past changes. This is a kind of molecular memory underlies the capacity of the cells in a tissue to maintain their normal or pathological phenotype even in the absence of the original trigger that induced it. The mapping of the epigenetic profiles of the genome in normal and pathological tissues is an important step toward a better understanding of the physiological or pathophysiological process."

The dynamic heredity theory with bistable chromatin states proposes an interactive system, in which the likelihood of the train taking one track, rather than another, will be influenced by epigenetic marks, which are, by definition, stable but reversible over time. Like stationmasters, epigenetic markers will direct DNA genes to a greater or lesser probability of being expressed and producing one phenotype over another. It is only a probability, more or less intense, but not an obligation.

In one part of the genome, epigenetic marks can accumulate, little by little, increasing the likelihood of switching from heterochromatin to euchromatin. This phenomenon is established and then reinforced over time and from generation to generation at the cell level.

It should be understood that enzymatic reactions, such as acetylation (via enzymes called acetyltransferases) or methylation (via methyltransferases), are dynamic and act together on the genome and histones, promoting stability in a given state. They act in the opposite direction, maintaining equilibrium in one of the two chromatin states. It is like a ball continuously oscillating around its equilibrium point, pushed on both sides by opposing but equal forces.

A system can be called cooperative between the different enzyme systems, influenced by epigenetic events: when certain enzymes promote histone acetylation, other enzymes act synergistically by increasing the demethylation (demethylases) of various other sites in the genome located near the former. Similarly, deacetylases act synergistically with methyl-transferases.

It is all lively, fast, and fleeting!

The stability of chromatin in one of the two states (euchromatin or heterochromatin) is constantly dependent on these antagonistic interactions (methylation, demethylation, acetylation, deacetylation, and more). Euchromatin and heterochromatin are two stable states of chromatin.

Switching from one to the other requires breaking this stability. To do this, epigenetic marks must be repeated and/or strong enough to switch the chromatin from one state to another and make certain genes express or not.

There is a point of no return (a *turning point*) that must be reached. Once reached, the epigenetic mechanisms are self-reinforcing to maintain this new stability. As it becomes more and more stable with time, it becomes more difficult to change its state. One can think of water that is brought to a boil. The

Brownian agitation of the atoms is more vigorous until a point of no return where the water is vaporized: it has passed from one stable state to another.[127,128]

This is, I think, one of the most interesting theory to understand the evolution of Ehlers-Danlos syndrome throughout a lifetime. It could partially explain the different phenotypes that are possible over a lifetime from the same genotype.

Thus, when an individual goes from the stable state asymptomatic hyperlaxity (A-JHS) to another stable state, low symptomatic EDS, or even high symptomatic EDS, the genome has not changed. On the other hand, sufficiently repeated epigenetic marks in a short period of time, or fewer but powerful epigenetic marks may have shifted the patient from one stable state to another.

The consequences could be important for the diagnosis and management of EDS patients: one could say that the sooner patients are diagnosed and managed correctly, the easier (or less difficult) it will be to switch them from one stable chromatin state to another. This is quite an attractive vision, but it needs to be studied further.

These studies are currently impossible due to the lack of doctors who diagnose and treat EDS, or even those who do not over-psychiatrize these patients who are in great pain. I remind you that the delay between the onset of symptoms and the diagnosis of EDS in our countries is more than 20 years on average. The delay in getting a consultation with an EDS specialist is usually more than one year. Epigenetics has plenty of time to strengthen and take hold during this time, and it will be increasingly difficult to act on the state of the chromatin.

This is an additional punishment to the sevenfold punishment evoked by Dr Grossin: not only do patients suffer, but they are also not listened to, they are psychiatrized (it's in your head),

---

[127] Sood A, Zhang B. Quantifying the stability of coupled genetic and epigenetic switches with variational methods. Front Genet. 2021;11:636724.
[128] Taherian Fard A, Ragan MA. Quantitative modelling of the Waddington Epigenetic Landscape. Methods Mol Biol. 2019;1975:157-171.

they are misdiagnosed and mistreated, and then, finally diagnosed with EDS, doctors do not believe them, refute the diagnosis of EDS, and put them back into a state of total wandering.

> In the light of these epigenetic postulates: by delaying the diagnosis of EDS patients, on the one hand, we could aggravate their disease, and, on the other hand, we could reduce their chances of returning to a stable state with fewer symptoms.

It is a real Stephen King nightmare!

It would be probably wrong to say that epigenetic mechanisms are all related to DNA, histones, and chromatin. Epigenetic marks are all events not related to DNA information's, and nothing more. There are probably epigenetic markers whose mode of action, or whose very existence, remains totally unknown to this day.

We still have a long way to go, even though we thought we knew everything, until very recently, with the decoding of the human genome. It was only the first draft in 2003.

This takes some time to set up. It is not directly after the accident of life that things change. It is sometimes difficult to link a whiplash accident with a worsening of symptoms that occurs weeks after the accident.

When it is commonly said that a tragedy changed someone, it is meant literally and figuratively in EDS and many other conditions.

You can see the medico-legal implications of this epigenetic setting up. How could lawyers and medical advisors believe this when abuse and "I do not believe it" are their daily lives?

Diagram of bistable states

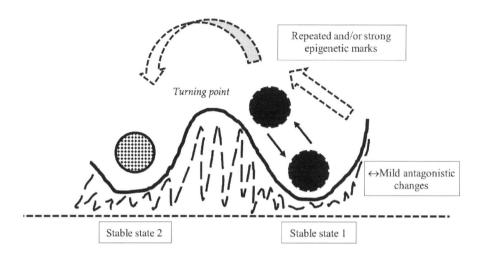

And human suffering, who cares?

Some doctors and scientists remain anchored in their knowledge of Medicine, sometimes outdated, and they are satisfied with this: no self-criticism, no questioning, no desire to learn and improve.

A doctor must be curious about everything and remain humble before patients and the "Symphony of the Living" (*Joël de Rosnay, LLL, 2018*), which still holds many unknowns. I had to update, like other EDS practitioners, a good part of my knowledge, my a priori about a disease that I thought it was rare, and that should only concern circus artists with extreme hypermobility and hyper-stretchable skin, to the point of wrapping it around their necks (the case of Danlos). In short, they are like fairground animals. It happened to me, and I did not believe it, I did not know that it could happen to me too!

I had to update my knowledge and go to Paris to train with Professor Hamonet and his team.

In my career as a rheumatologist, I had to accept that I had certainly missed certain diagnoses of EDS or that I had diagnosed them as fibromyalgic, without paying more attention to them, or even as psychiatric.

You must dare to question yourself, learn and forgive yourself. Then you must go further and further in your knowledge of Medicine.

Testimony of Sylvie, 39 years old

I thought I was just a girl, a woman, an unlucky mother...

An intestinal resection ended in internal bleeding with a stay in intensive care and additional surgery to repair the damage.

A few years later, a pregnancy brought me to the emergency room because the base of the ugly scar on my belly was leaking a strange fluid. After blood work and an ultrasound, a wire remained "stuck" in my abdominal wall. The surgeon saw no other option but to operate as soon as possible to avoid infections and worries for my baby. At 31 years old, my son was born by cesarean section and stayed in the neonatal unit for just under two months. When my son was five months old, I had to undergo a re-operation for a ventricular cure, as a large abdominal hernia was found!

Despite this experience and being eager to have a large family, I became pregnant again, but it was soon disillusioned. I had a miscarriage at 12 weeks of gestation. The second attempt was the right one, my pregnancy went perfectly until one morning, I was seized with horrible abdominal pains. I went directly to the emergency room, I was at 35 weeks of gestation, my gynecologist was in the Alps, but my file was nevertheless transmitted to the right person. This did not prevent me from being insulted as a "mythomaniac" when I described my pains: an impression of tearing in me. It turned out to be real at one point: "I passed out". They tried to get the baby's heartbeat, and there was no heartbeat for my future daughter. At that moment, an alarm sounded, people arrived in my room, and I left immediately for the operating room. Diagnosis: uterine rupture and placental abruption. The baby was passing right through my abdominal wall. My daughter was resuscitated, intubated, and spent a little less than two months in the NICU.

We tried for a third, but after a dozen miscarriages and a D&C, we decided to stop our family expansion!

Three years ago, in 2016, my primary care physician asked me to go see Dr. D., who specializes in an improbably named disease. Finally, my misfortunes have a name, my misfortunes are, in fact, linked to one and only one disease.

I have four autoimmune diseases and EDS. It is not easy every day, but now I know that "I'm not crazy", that I have real pain, and that some doctors finally understand me.

Unfortunately, I am often confronted with people who tell me that my pain is "because I am too fat", that "I have to lose weight," that "I have to eat healthily", etc. I know all this, but 20 years ago, I was told that I was not in pain. I know all this, but 20 years on cortisone leaves its mark! Being called a liar and an imaginary patient also leaves psychological scars and compulsive problems with food.

So dear Doctors, who only see me as a fatty, learn to treat your patients with kindness, as my GP, my gynecologist, and especially Dr. D. did.

I could not stop writing this text, and it did me good to "empty" myself. I am in tears as I close it.

Sylvie D, December 2019.

A historical aside

Not so long ago, Louis Pasteur (1822-1895), a French chemist and microbiologist, fought against the theories of spontaneous generation, adopted by everyone at the time, scientists or not. It was previously thought that vermin or rats, fleas, and moths could be born spontaneously from a bag of dirty laundry, therefore without a progenitor.

In the 18th century, it was thought that the air itself made microscopic living beings appear. Not from pre-existing life, transported by the air, but by the reproductive power of the air itself from Nothing. This conception was called heterogeny or spontaneous generation.

Yes, we believed this in my great-grandmother's time, it is not that far away, is it?

Fortunately, Louis Pasteur was rigorous, and his demonstration was without appeal. He created, among other things, what is still called pasteurization. He heated wine to 57° to kill germs and improve its transportation and conservation. He is in a way the founder of oenology.

In 1881, he isolated the anthrax bacterium and attenuated it with potassium dichromate (an antiseptic). In Pouilly-Le-Fort, close to Melun in France, he injected it into sheep.[129,130] It can be said that he vaccinated them this way two weeks apart. Then, the sheep had made, a priori, what was later called antibodies, he inoculated them with the unattenuated anthrax bacillus, and they survived. He had proved that it was possible to protect animals (by extension, later humans) against certain diseases by injecting them with less virulent microbes beforehand. However, he also proved that the disease was caused by microbes that could be seen and isolated.

These beliefs persisted mainly for religious reasons (how else can we explain Adam and Eve in Genesis? No, Adam was not born from the clay made by God who would have breathed life into his nostrils so that he could take life). It is a good thing, and the Catholic Church has long allowed the reader to interpret Genesis. Here, it is that religion influenced Science and its advances, while elsewhere it is beliefs, superstitions, or merely the received ideas of Science.

Another telling example is the life of Galileo de Vincenzo Bonaiuti de' Galilei (better known as Galileo). He was a mathematician, astronomer, physicist, and surveyor, born in Pisa in 1564 and died near Florence in 1642.

This brave man had tried to reaffirm what had already been proposed in 1539 by Nikolaus Kopernikus (Copernicus, 1473-1543), 32 years before the birth of Galileo: Yes, the Earth does

---

[129] Pasteur L, Chamberland, Roux. Summary report of the experiments conducted at Pouilly-le-Fort, near Melun, on the anthrax vaccination, 1881. Yale J Biol Med. 2002 Jan-Feb;75(1):59-62.
[130] Pasteur L. Remarks on Anthracic Vaccination as a Prophylactic of Splenic Fever. Br Med J. 1882 Apr 8;1(1110):489.

revolve around the Sun (heliocentrism, Copernican) and not the opposite (Aristotelian or Ptolemaic geocentrism).

Interestingly, and this takes us back to my previous statement; the jealous academics and proud scientists were the ones who brought Galileo before the Holy Inquisition's tribunal. Contrary to popular belief, clerics were Galileo's staunchest defenders.

In short, after virulent accusations and twists and turns, the Church condemned Galileo, despite a clear and partly correct vision (he was wrong about the revolution of the Earth and did not admit its elliptical movement around the sun), of what was then inconceivable. Galileo also had a strong character to provoke Pope Urban VIII, which did not help him. Fortunately, Galileo recanted, he always affirmed his Faith (so he was not burned alive), and since he was old and docile at the time of his trial, he ended his days relatively quiet, at home, in a beautiful Florentine villa.

One may ask, what can we learn from these ancient stories?

1/ If some agree with the current consensus, they will not be remembered as scientists (thank you, Galileo). That is pretty reassuring!

2/ The second lesson, Science evolves, and false ideas fall (thank you, Louis Pasteur).

On the one hand, to assert theories, they should have experimental proof. It is a lesson to be given to specific criteria established without a control group and, to be honest, with my postulates even though they hold up pretty well. That is also why I chose the term Postulate; it protects me from some spiteful tongues.

Secondly, since this book does not have a suicide mission, aiming at emitting a dogma to be believed without proof and which would be immediately condemned by my peers (or by the Academic Inquisition), I strongly appeal to You, researchers, to make scientific studies on EDS and Epigenetics.

313

At best, they will keep what they have learned; at worst, we will confirm what we are sensing daily, thus moving forward together!

Unfortunately, it is more comfortable to believe without checking, I think; this is true for everyone, especially if the theories have been sitting for a long time and taught, as such, in Universities and in some international articles that are well established.

It would be nothing if it were not for the patients who had to foot the bill daily; some are deaf, blind and dumb, like the three monkeys, to the changes, or rather to the restoration of truth, and the correction of decades of medical history errors that Ehlers-Danlos Syndrome has undergone.

Wouldn't the truth be sufficient enough? Moreover, if not for the truth, let them grant reasonable doubt to this case.

To quote Andràs Pàldi: "Finally, epigenetics allows us to progress in our understanding of hereditary diseases. Even in the case of so-called monogenic diseases, whose heredity obeys Mendel's laws, a diversity of symptoms can be observed and evolution over time that genetics alone cannot explain. Epigenetics may provide a better understanding. In the same way, thanks to epigenetics, we can hope to understand better complex diseases where the role of heredity has been suspected for a long time, but for which genetic analyses have been unsuccessful." (AN: as for hEDS/csEDS)

My dear readers, as in the Myth of Pandora's box, once everything was out, there was still one priceless thing left at the bottom of it: Hope!

My Third Postulate:

Phenotypic Differences Between Children Could Be Explained, in Part, by Epigenetics?

Unquestionably, patients with Ehlers-Danlos Syndrome all have the same disease; they are roughly clinically remarkably similar. However, each one has its differences, its particularities, and this or that symptom is often brought to the forefront. For some, it will be sprains and dysproprioception; for others, dysautonomia, MCAD, POTS, highly hyper-stretchable skin, aneurysms, or dystonia.

Why these inter-patient phenotypic differences? Different genetic mutations? Maybe... But not only!

Parents and children are sometimes, not to say often, clinically different, less or more affected, even between siblings. Yet, theoretically, although this is certainly not the case, they inherit the same EDS mutations. The genetic reassembly can vary depending on whether one inherits one or the other of the two homologous chromosomes from each of the two parents, but also because of chromosomal shuffling. This is relatively simple and well known.

But there is something more, and this something is huge, unpredictable, and destabilizing: their epigenetics is certainly different! These epigenetic markers are acquired, either via their parents' gametes, or in the womb, or later, throughout their lives.

Our lives are so different. Our successes, failures, and accidents of life are so multiple and varied that they influence the expression of our genome.

"Repetition is the strongest of all rhetorical figures."
Napoleon Bonaparte (1769-1821)

315

Consequences:

Let us take the example of a mom, let us call her Constance, and a dad, let us call him Theophilus. This couple gives birth to three children during their lives: Stéphane, Patricia, and Dominique. The children were naturally conceived at different times. I know it is normal, but it is important. For example, they were conceived respectively at the age of 21, 25, and 34 for Constance and 25, 29 and 38 for Theophilus.

Depending on whether Constance and Theophilus carried epigenetic marks (DNA methylations, for example) at a given time in their lives, they could transmit, via their gametes, different epigenetic baggage to each of their children.

This is a legitimate statement, and even a Postulate, which would have exciting consequences in clinical practice if it turns out to be true.

This could explain, in part, the differences in phenotypes (by the expression of more or less genes, modulated by epigenetics) and therefore the different severity of EDS between children from the same parents but conceived at different times!

This becomes even more complex if positive or negative events occur during Constance's pregnancy, such as relaxation, musicology, hydrotherapy, meditation, yoga, or, in contrast, an emotional shock, abuse, stress, alcohol consumption, or smoking. As the embryo or fetus may lose or acquire epigenetic marks, they may influence the presentation of the (eventual) EDS of their future child. Of course, since each child has different life accidents and different environmental or psychological contributions, the evolution of the disease will also be different between the children and then between the adults, they will become.

Finally, if Constance and/or Theophilus are affected by a form of csEDS, but at the same time they also carry one or more silenced mutations (by epigenetics) in genes coding for specific collagens, GAGs, TNXB, PLOD, β-3-Gal-t-3 or β-6, for example, they will not present a more particular clinical variant of EDS (such as classical, classic-like, myopathic, kyphoscoliosis, spondylo-dysplastic, etc.). But, if these mutations turn on in children, then the phenotype of this or that child may be different from that of the parents. This is an interesting notion because it is usually thought that children (except for spontaneous mutation of a gene) have the same variant of EDS as their parents. With this demonstration, once again, we show that in modern genetics, everything is possible!

The phenomenon of double exposure:

For example, if the mother suffered certain accidents in her life or had a certain deleterious lifestyle during her pregnancy, then epigenetic marks could have been imprinted in the fetus but in a silenced way. If later in life, as a child or adult, the child is exposed to the same type of behavior or the same type of life accident, he or she may then develop the disease, or strongly aggravate the pre-existing symptoms. This second exposure will then be a trigger factor. Therefore, the history should also focus on the lifestyle of the patient's mother during pregnancy (alcohol and tobacco consumption, malnutrition, etc.) and question her about any life accidents she may have suffered (abuse, domestic violence, traffic accidents, etc.). This could lead us to use a preventive discourse for EDS patients who wish to have a child. We could recommend a healthy lifestyle, stress management, etc. This could positively influence the future of their children[131]. There can therefore be preventive medicine in EDS pregnant women.

*"Imagination is used to invent the impossible.
Then one day, the impossible becomes possible."
Alain Sauvé, guitarist and musician
Montreal, Canada, 1947*

---

[131] Messer LC, Boone-Heinonen J, Mponwane L, et al. Developmental Programming: Priming disease susceptibility for subsequent generations. Curr Epidemiol Rep. 2015;3(1):37-51. doi: 10.1007/s40471-014-0033-1.

Illustrative Diagram of the Third Postulate

Epigenetic events in the life of the parents; three children conceived at different times.

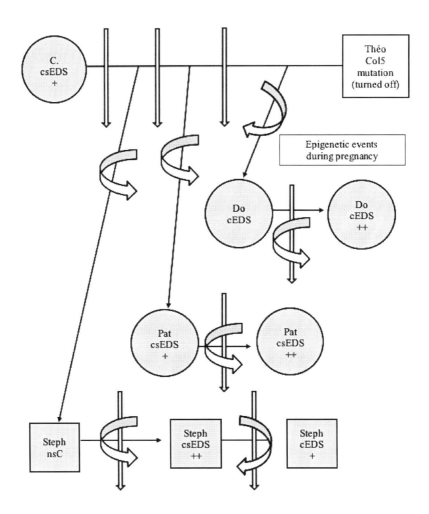

Legend:

cEDS: Classical EDS
csEDS: Common Systemic EDS
nsC: Non-Systemic Carrier.

Explanations of the exemplary scheme
of the 3rd Postulate

Constance (C) carries a common systemic form (or hypermobile) of EDS of moderate-intensity (csEDS+). Throughout her life, she acquires or loses epigenetic marks. It is, therefore, more or less symptomatic throughout its life.

Theophilus (Theo) does not have EDS, at least clinically. However, he does carry a COL5A1 mutation, but this is silenced, and is not expressed in his phenotype. It acquires or loses epigenetic markers, like everyone else, throughout its life.

Constance and Theo have three children (Steph, Pat, and Do) during their married life. Depending on when Steph, Pat, and Do were conceived, they receive more or less epigenetic marks from their parents (methylations, acetylations, and more).

During the gestation of each child, as an embryo or fetus, epigenetic marks can be added or even lost, depending on the environment (the exposome) and Constance's life accidents. At birth and in childhood, Stephane is a non-symptomatic (or non-systemic) carrier of EDS (noted nsC), and Patricia is a common systemic EDS with moderate presentation (noted csEDS+). Dominique has a mild form of EDS but also a classical variant (cEDS): she has received Theophilus COL5A1 mutation in addition to the unknown mutations of the csEDS (by Constance and Theophilus). In her, the COL5A1 mutation has turned on, and is therefore expressed in her phenotype.

Stephane becomes highly symptomatic EDS (rated csEDS++) after difficult life events, then, thanks to appropriate medical and personal care, he becomes moderate EDS (csEDS+). Theophilus did not transmit to Stephane the COL5A1 mutation.

Patricia, following difficult life events, becomes highly symptomatic EDS (csEDS++) and so on. She is poorly or not taken care of medically; she becomes more isolated and remains significantly affected throughout her life. The COL5A1 mutation was transmitted by Theophilus but remains silenced.

On the other hand, Dominique becomes very symptomatic, with a classical variant phenotype (noted cEDS++), and remains so throughout her life.

That is an example of a family with different phenotypes, gain or loss of epigenetic marks, and the expression or not of a COL5A1 mutation (which is either *turned off or turned on*).

Epigenetics has changed our view of what is innate and what is acquired. Genes are continually interacting with our exposome: what we eat, what we drink, what we breathe (pesticides, smoking, harmful particles in the air), the day/night cycle (nychthemeral), the microbiota, regular physical exercise, physical or psychological stress, and more.

"Contrary to the definition of genetic mutations, epimutations are defined as potentially (but not necessarily) reversible changes in gene activity not involving DNA mutations, but rather, gain or loss of DNA methyl groups conserved in cells through mitosis" (*Fiorito G et al., 2019*).[132]

My Fourth Postulate:
EDS could be a Complex Gendered Genetic Disease

> « *Let us strive for the impossible. The great achievements throughout history have been the conquest of what seemed the impossible* »
> *Charlie Chaplin (1889-1977)*
> *Actor, artist-filmmaker, scriptwriter*

Often, at the end of the first appointment, I ask the diagnosed patients if they think that the disease would come from their father's or their mother's side. If it is their mom, they usually spontaneously say, "Yes, mom has always had pain everywhere, she is clumsy and flexible, etc. ". If it is the father who has passed it on, then these patients say, for example: "I do not know, mom

---

[132] Fiorito G, McCrory C, Robinson O, et al.; BIOS Consortium; Lifepath consortium. Socioeconomic position, lifestyle habits and biomarkers of epigenetic aging: a multi-cohort analysis. Aging (Albany NY). 2019;11(7):2045-2070. doi: 10.18632/aging.101900

is in great shape and dad complains about few things, he has pain in his back and hands, but it is probably osteoarthritis. Very often, when the father is the carrier, he is less or not symptomatic. Sometimes the patients go back to their paternal grandmother, and they say: "I remember that dad's mother always complained of having pain everywhere, but at the time, you know doctor, we didn't pay attention to it".

Some food for thought:

1/ The parental imprint in Genetics (genomic imprinting).[133]

In this transmission mode, specific genes are expressed in the children's phenotype only if their inheritance is maternal or paternal. Some genes would carry a kind of mark or imprint that would allow the embryo to differentiate between copies of the genes (alleles) inherited from the mother and those inherited from the father. The copy of the most activated allele (depending on whether it comes from the mother or the father) produces more protein than the other copy that is relatively inactivated. These proteins are, as always, architectural proteins, enzymes, or hormones. The genomic imprinting is a form of epigenetic gene regulation that results in expression from a single allele in a parent-of-origin-dependent manner.[134,135,136]

"Genomic imprinting is an epigenetic regulatory mechanism consisting of the monoallelic expression in the function of the parental origin of a subset of genes, located in specific regions, called differentially methylated regions (DMRs). These differential methylation sites located on the maternal and paternal alleles are protected from the wave of global demethylation that occurs immediately after fertilization, giving rise to a specific epigenetic signature of the parent of origin. The

[133] Barlow DP, Bartolomei MS. Genomic imprinting in mammals. Cold Spring Harb Perspect Biol. 2014;6(2):a018382. doi: 10.1101/cshperspect.a018382.

[134] Idereebdullah FY, Vigneau S, Bartolomei MS. Genomic imprinting mechanisms in mammals. Mutat Res, 2008;647(1-2):77-85. doi: 10.1016/j.mrfmmm.2008.08.008.

[135] Noordermeer D, Feil R. Differential 3D chromatin organization and gene activity in genomic imprinting. Curr Opin Genet Dev. 2020;61:17-24. doi: 10.1016/j.gde.2020.03.004.

[136] Hirasawa R, Feil R. Genomic imprinting and human disease. Essays Biochem. 2010;48(1):187-200. doi: 10.1042/bse0480187.

imprinting of these loci, that is the regulation of their gene expression, plays an essential role in the normal growth and development of placental mammals.../... Many of these imprinted regions contain lncRNAs, which function as silencers of complementary sequences"[137]

In this case, if a gene, whether mutated or not, is with maternal imprint, it will be expressed in the children's phenotype if the mother passes it on; but if a mother' son has children, the gene passed on is turned off (silenced) and is not, or possibly hardly, expressed. The situation is reversed if it is with paternal imprint. The gene maybe could be turned on again in one of the following generations if one of the son's daughters has children. The disease then reappears in this family branch, where it had previously seemed to be unaffected.

Example below (maternal imprinting): It is interesting to note, in these healthy male (noted *) subject's family, that his father does not suffer from the disease, but his paternal grandmother has this last. This phenomenon of genes being on or off is also due to epigenetics (e.g., via lncRNA), which acts like an on-off switch.

If so, then the son and the daughter of a female EDS patients might be more affected. The daughters of this female EDS patient could then later transmit the disease to their children (via the maternal imprint). But, in this case, the daughters and the sons of the EDS male patient could not express a marked EDS.

> This is not what we encounter in our daily consultations: this not explain the phenotype's expression difference between siblings of different sex, because the most important in the parental imprint transmission is the sex of the parent, and not that of the child.

[137] Migliore L, Nicolì V, Stoccoro A. Gender Specific Differences in Disease Susceptibility: The Role of Epigenetics. Biomedicines. 2021;9(6):652. doi: 10.3390/biomedicines9060652.

Maternal imprinting transmission scheme

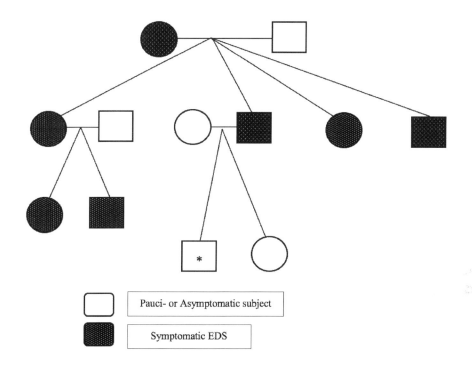

Pauci- or Asymptomatic subject

Symptomatic EDS

2/ Epigenetics acts as a dimmer switch? These epigenetic influences are multiple (dozens or even more) and can reach only 10%, 20%, 50% or 99% of an organ or tissue cells. This is highly complex, but here again, it could play a role in the clinical expression of EDS: if 10%, 20%, 50% or 99% of the connective tissue of an organ (intestine, skin, artery walls, etc.) or of a supporting tissue is affected, the impact on the severity of the disease will vary. Not only will the severity change between generations, but also between siblings. Epigenetics can be an on-off switch, but not only that: it can also be a dimmer switch.[138,139]

---

[138] Liang R, Bates DJ, Wang E. Epigenetic Control of MicroRNA Expression and Aging. Curr Genomics. 2009 May;10(3):184-93.
[139] Nehila T, Ferguson JW, Atit RP. Polycomb Repressive Complex 2: a Dimmer Switch of Gene Regulation in Calvarial Bone Development. Curr Osteoporos Rep. 2020;18(4):378-387.

EDS could maybe have a mode of transmission of varying intensity This could also fit with what we encounter in our daily consultations.

In EDS, it is known that women are generally more symptomatic than men. Could this intensity switch be one of the explanations for these findings? Is this sex-linked, and why?

3/ The X-Chromosome Inactivation (XCI) in females. Skewed (biased) XCI and diseases.

Let us cite the explanations of an enlightening article on this subject which could give us some leads for thoughts to the usually stronger phenotypic EDS' expression in women than in men (*Migliore L et al., 2021*)[140]:

"In female mammalian cells, one of the two X chromosomes is randomly inactivated early during embryogenesis in all cells, to balance the expression dosage between females and males, the latter having only one X chromosome. This X chromosome inactivation (XCI) represents a well-known epigenetic mechanism of gene regulation. Thus, females are mosaics for two cell populations: cells with the paternal X active and cells with the maternal X active. Since it is assumed that the choice of the X chromosome to inactivate is random, the result is that on average 50% of the cells express the paternal genes and the remaining 50% express the maternal genes. However, there are two phenomena in this regard that can interfere with what is expected: (1) in many cases, an unbalanced X inactivation has been recorded; (2) not all genes on the inactivated chromosome are silenced " (= escape genes).

.../... An asymmetric selection of the X chromosome to inactivate often occurs: it is known as skewed XCI (or non-random XCI). This is observed when more than 75–80% of the cells within a tissue inactivate the same X chromosome, while the extreme skewing of the XCI involves 90% of cell populations. Thus, skewed XCI could be detected in a tissue-specific manner

[140] Migliore L, Nicolì V, Stoccoro A. Gender Specific Differences in Disease Susceptibility: The Role of Epigenetics. Biomedicines. 2021;9(6):652. doi: 10.3390/biomedicines9060652.

or could affect the whole organism, depending on the gene-specific function and activity.

.../... A recent study, based on over 5500 transcriptomes from 449 individuals spanning 29 human tissues, provided an exhaustive survey of sex-biased gene expression in humans and demonstrated that expression of escape genes outside PARs (pseudo-autosomal regions) is usually female-biased. At least, 15–20% of X-linked genes outside of PARs escape silencing and show a gene-specific bias. Moreover, most escape genes have shown a substantial heterogeneity across cell types, tissues, individuals, and experimental settings. Tukiainen and co-workers showed that incomplete XCI affects at least 23% of X-chromosomal genes, and they identified seven genes that escape XCI. They suggested that escape from XCI results in sex differences in gene expression, thus, establishing incomplete XCI as a mechanism that is likely to introduce phenotypic diversity (*Tukiainen T et al., 2017*).[141]

.../... skewed X chromosome inactivation has been extensively investigated as a potential mechanism that contributes to the strong female preponderance observed in certain diseases.

.../... As described above, XCI is the strategy adopted by females to balance the gene dosage between sexes. However, the mechanism of silencing is incomplete, resulting in 12% of genes that escape inactivation and another 15% of genes varying in their X chromosome inactivation status across individuals, tissues or cells: the expression levels of these genes are attributed to sex-dependent phenotypic variability. Moreover, the sex chromosome complement was observed to influence the expression of autosomal genes, suggesting an additional global effect.

.../... Many complex traits have a deviation of the gender ratio in humans. We have seen that epigenetic mechanisms are often involved in processes responsible of differential expression sex-related. We have also mentioned that, in the literature, there are

---

[141] Tukiainen T, Villani AC, Yen A, et al. Landscape of X chromosome inactivation across human tissues. Nature. 2017;550:244–248.

several hypotheses to explain the deviation of the relationship between the sexes, mainly the hormonal and the genetic/chromosomal ones. Indeed, both can be interpreted in the light of epigenetic processes.

.../... A sex bias in DNA methylation levels, usually associated with sex-biased gene expression, was found in many animal and human studies. In addition to gender effects for methylation loci on the X chromosome due to the X-inactivation dosage compensation mechanism in females, hundreds of autosomal CpG loci showed strong differences in the methylation between males and female.

.../... A significant proportion of human imprinted genes are realistically involved, as well as altered expression of critical regions, due for instance to a skewed inactivation of the X-chromosome in females, or to the presence of genes that escape to X-inactivation or to a deregulation of miRNAs located on the X chromosome. Moreover, the expression of specific genes can be modified epigenetically by many intracellular (hormones) or extracellular environmental factors. Likely, all these players act in the most vulnerable stages of our life, such as pregnancy, by interfering with fetal programming and making individuals more susceptible to developing diseases later in life."

Can we do something about his epigenetics? Are we the actors of our lives, and can we improve it?

For some authors, key factors could influence and improve our epigenome (removing, for example, DNA methylations):

➤ Food: Nutrigenomic[142] is a new science that aims to influence favorably, through nutrition, the expression of our genes. The main foods of interest would be folates, turmeric, resveratrol (present in wine), green tea, broccoli, tomatoes, all colored fruits and vegetables, pomegranate juice, apples (pectin),

---

[142] Aruoma OI, Hausman-Cohen S, Pizano J, et al. Personalized Nutrition: Translating the Science of NutriGenomics Into Practice: Proceedings From the 2018 American College of Nutrition Meeting. J Am Coll Nutr. 2019;38(4):287-301. doi:10.1080/07315724.2019.1582980. PMID: 31099726.

dark chocolate (it contains flavonoids). They could also act synergistically if consumed regularly.
- ➤ Regular physical exercise.[143]
- ➤ Stress management, meditation, yoga, psychotherapy, heart coherence, and more.[144]
- ➤ Having fun, doing daily activities (self-satisfaction).
- ➤ The social network (friends, family, and more).

Note: these factors could also play a role in the profile of the gut microbiota.

Most researchers disagree with these assertions: as mentioned above, this view is still controversial, essentially because of the lack of detailed mechanistic description and the need for appropriate methodology allowing the clear differentiation between phenomena conveyed by epigenetic mechanisms or resulted from direct environmental effects.

In practice, however, the beneficial influence of these factors on EDS development in an individual can be seen. It is clear that when the patient is well surrounded, has a right circle of friends, has a fulfilling job, exercises regularly, and is not too stressed, he or she is often less symptomatic than other patients with unfavorable epigenetic factors. Stress, junk food, lack of meaningful work, and sedentary lifestyle are increasingly present in our Western societies and affect mainly, but not exclusively, people from low socio-economic backgrounds.[145,146]

---

[143] Di Liegro I. Genetic and Epigenetic Modulation of Cell Functions by Physical Exercise. Genes (Basel). 2019;10(12):1043. doi:10.3390/genes10121043. PMID: 31888150; PMCID: PMC6947840.

[144] Jiménez JP, Botto A, Herrera L, et al. Psychotherapy and Genetic Neuroscience: An Emerging Dialog. Front Genet. 2018;9:257. doi:10.3389/fgene.2018.00257. PMID: 30065751; PMCID: PMC6056612.

[145] Fiorito G, McCrory C, Robinson O, et al. BIOS Consortium; Lifepath consortium. Socioeconomic position, lifestyle habits and biomarkers of epigenetic aging: a multi-cohort analysis. Aging (Albany NY). 2019;11(7):2045-2070. doi:10.18632/aging.101900. PMID: 31009935; PMCID: PMC6503871.

[146] Notterman DA, Mitchell C. Epigenetics and Understanding the Impact of Social Determinants of Health. Pediatr Clin North Am. 2015;62(5):1227-40. doi:10.1016/j.pcl.2015.05.012. PMID: 26318949; PMCID: PMC4555996.

Epidemiological studies should be carried out to highlight the influence of the socio-economic environment (and of the microbiota) on Ehlers-Danlos Syndrome's symptomatology. It is an exciting avenue, which could provide additional clues as to the critical role of epigenetics in EDS.

The Microbiome and Metagenome

There are up to 39 trillion (39×10^{12}) microorganisms that live in our bodies (mainly in the gastrointestinal tracts, and in the skin, saliva, oral mucosa, and conjunctiva). The total number of cells that make up our body is estimated at 30 trillion (30×10^{12}).[147] The bacterial to human cells ratio = 1.3, with an uncertainty of 25% and a variation of 53% over the population of standard 70 kg males.[148]

The genes of bacteria are called the microbiome[149] (by analogy to the human genome). The microbiome consists of several million genes, i.e., more than a hundred times the total number of genes in the human body (i.e. about 22,500 genes).

These microorganisms are commensals and are useful to us: they protect us against other microbes, they produce vitamins, hormones, and increase our immunity, communicating with our brain by producing neuroactive substances. We are continually interacting with this microbiome. By analogy, we talk about virome for viruses and mycobiome for fungi.

The metagenome analyzes the genomes of all microorganisms in an ecological niche such as the intestine. The MetaHit study (*Metagenomics of Human Intestinal Tract*, started in 2008 and coordinated by INRA - the French National Institute for Agricultural Research) was able to identify 3.3 million different

---

[147] The standard person used in the literature is defined as a "reference man being between 20 to 30 years of age, weighing 70 Kg, is 170 cm in height" (Snyder et al., 1975).
[148] Sender R, Fuchs S, Milo R. Are we really vastly outnumbered? Revisiting the ratio of bacterial to human cells in humans. Cell. 2016;164(3):337-340.
[149] Lloyd-Price J, Abu-Ali G, Huttenhower C. The healthy human microbiome. Genome Med. 2016;8(1):51.

genes in the intestinal metagenome comprising more than 1,000 different microorganisms species. It is estimated that each individual carries an average of 540,000 microbial genes from 160 species, divided into seven family groups (or phyla).[150]

We can influence this metagenome by what we eat, probiotic and prebiotic supplements, and more.

The microbiome can communicate with our brain, and vice versa, via interactions with the central nervous system, the autonomic nervous system, the neuroimmune and neuroendocrine systems. Thus, our intestine is a second brain, an enteric brain, indispensable to our life. Without a microbiome, it would be a disaster!

Over the last few decades, numerous studies have been conducted to discover the complex interactions between microbes in the intestine and patients' phenotypes, with various pathologies. The analysis of these microbes' different genetic sequences occupies many scientific minds (*Human Microbiome Project, Human Gastrointestinal Bacteria Genome Collection*). However, despite significant efforts, many unknowns persist.

The term dysbiosis refers to situations in which there is a disturbance in the microbiota's composition, leading to adverse effects on the patient. Variations in the composition of the gut microbiota have been associated with various digestive and non-digestive conditions: inflammatory bowel diseases (IBD), irritable bowel syndrome (IBS), functional colopathies, colorectal or thyroid cancer (via its role in carcinogenesis), food allergies, obesity, hypertension, type 2 diabetes mellitus, asthma, nonalcoholic steatohepatitis (NASH), cardiovascular diseases, neuropsychiatric diseases (such as bipolar patients, autism, epilepsy, Alzheimer's disease), muscle mass, chronic kidney disease, certain immune disorders, longevity, etc.

On the other hand, factors specific to individuals influence, in the opposite direction, the composition of the microbiota.

---

[150] Qin J, Li R, Raes J, et al. A human gut microbial gene catalogue established by metagenomic sequencing. Nature. 2010;464(7285):59-65.

Studies have compared the microbiota of monozygotic and dizygotic twins, showing that the former had a closer microbiota than the latter.

These individual-specific factors are very well explained in Chang and Kao's *(2019)* article[151]:

> *Innate immune sensors.* Enterocytes express receptors (Pattern Recognition Receptors or PRRs) on their surface, capable of recognizing various microbiota-specific molecules (microbe-associated molecular pattern or MAMPs).
> *Antimicrobial peptides.* The secretion of specific peptides by the individual influences the importance of a particular microbiota population.
> *The mucus barrier produced by enterocytes.* Intestinal cells produce transmembrane mucin, a large protein highly loaded with sugars that acts as a barrier, maintaining the intestinal epithelium's integrity and limiting the passage of various molecules. Mucins also act as a communication system between gut immunity and the microbiota.
> *Secretory IgA.* They are produced by plasma cells in the mucosa and are transported through the enterocytes (intestinal cells) to the digestive lumen (the interior of the tube where the bacteria of the microbiota and the food are located). They, therefore, have an obvious role in the compositions of the microbiota.
> *The intestinal microvilli.* They create an electrostatic barrier, negatively charged, which influences the adherence of some microbes rather than others to the cell surface.
> *Tight junctions.* They create a physical barrier to the intercellular passage, whether with poorly digested or poorly digested food or intestinal microbiota. Certain bacteria can secrete substances capable of degrading these junctions and promoting an increase in intestinal permeability. The immune cells of the mucosa are thus stimulated by antigens, which pass the barrier and participate, in return, in the regulation of the bacterial populations of the intestinal lumen.

---

[151] Chang CS, Kao CY. Current understanding of the gut microbiota shaping mechanisms. J Biomed Sci. 2019;26:59.

➤ *Intestinal metabolism*. The human being ingests nutrients that are useful to him, but which are also used by the different kinds of bacteria for their survival. There is a kind of competition between the individual and his microbiota to use the ingested substances, substances that are essential for their development and maintenance. The way an individual absorbs and metabolizes, less or more, certain substances, will influence the type of populations found in the intestine.

➤ *Lionel Rigottier-Gois proposed the oxygen hypothesis* in IBD.[152] In this case, lesions of the epithelium favor the passage of oxygen from the intestinal wall to the lumen and influence the development of bacteria that develop in facultative anaerobia (they can develop with or without oxygen) and obligate aerobic bacteria (Salmonella, for example). It does not necessarily take intestinal damage to encounter this type of situation. In general, the cells of the small intestine function by using glucose and glutamine (in anaerobic glycolysis), which increases the concentration of oxygen on the surface of the cells (and thus favors the proliferation of facultative anaerobic bacteria - Enterobacteriaceae, Enterococcus, Streptococcus - and obligate aerobic bacteria). On the other hand, colon cells generally prefer to use butyrate (a short-chain fatty acid) by oxidation. They consume oxygen, so the epithelial surface of the colon becomes hypoxic, which favors the growth of obligate anaerobic bacteria (Bifidobacterium, Clostridium, Veillonella, Bacteroides, Eubacterium, Ruminococcus). Therefore, it is sufficient for the epithelial cells to change their mode of energy production, from anaerobic to aerobic or vice versa, for the bacterial populations residing in the intestinal lumen to change.

➤ *MicroRNAs*. These are sequences of 18 to 23 nucleotides that do not code for proteins (see the chapter on genetics and epigenetics). They can be found in the stool. Some of them are used as markers for colitis or dysbiosis. It seems that they also participate in the composition of the intestinal microbiota. It is interesting to note that animal or plant microRNAs (e.g., ginger) can also affect the microbiota.

---

[152] Rigottier-Gois L. Dysbiosis in inflammatory bowel diseases: the oxygen hypothesis. ISME J. 2013;7(7):1256-1261.

The microbiota plays an essential role in the mechanisms of chronic pain, both in the periphery and in the central nervous system. There are different mechanisms involved in the so-called [microbiota - gut - brain] axis:

➢ *An increase in intestinal permeability* that leads to the passage of certain endotoxins into the bloodstream, such as lipopolysaccharides or LPS. LPS are inflammatory molecules contained in the walls of gram-negative bacteria. They potentially increase central sensitization (by acting as TLR4 agonists, for example). High LPS' blood levels may indicate gut dysbiosis and intestinal barrier dysfunction (Leaky gut).[153]

➢ *Modulation of local and peripheral inflammation.* The microbiota influences the development of lymphoid structures and the differentiation of immune cells. These phenomena have been implicated in developing psychiatric disorders (in psychotic disorders and autism spectrum[154,155] disorders) and chronic fatigue.[156]

➢ *Dysbiosis causes a decrease in the absorption of nutrients* that are useful or even essential: amino acids such as tryptophan (the precursor of serotonin), and phenylalanine (the precursor of tyrosine, dopamine, epinephrine and norepinephrine), but also vitamins or polyunsaturated fatty acids). Dysbiosis also increases toxic substances such as ammonia, phenols, indoles, sulfides, etc.

➢ *The important role of the microbiota in the activation or inhibition of the autonomic nervous system* (ortho-parasympathetic) which interacts with the CNS (nucleus of the solitary tract). This nucleus in turn, influences centers involved in anxiety and stress (amygdala, cholinergic system, cerebral cortex).

---

[153] Ghosh SS, Wang J, Yannie PJ, Ghosh S. Intestinal barrier dysfunction, LPS translocation, and disease development. J Endocrin Soc. 2020;4(2):bvz039. doi:10.1210/jendso/bvz039.

[154] Fattorusso A, Di Genova L, Dell'Isola GB, et al. Autism Spectrum Disorders and the Gut microbiota. Nutrients. 2019;11:521. doi: 10.3390/nu11030521

[155] Srikantha P, Mohajeri MH. The possible role of the microbiota-gut-brain-axis in autism spectrum disorder. Int J Mol Sci. 2019;20:2115. doi:10.3390/ijms20092115.

[156] Safadi JM, Quinton AMG, Lennox BR, et al. Gut dysbiosis in severe mental illness and chronic fatigue: a novel trans-diagnostic construct? A systematic review and meta-analysis. Molecular Psychiatry 2021. doi:10.1038/s41380-021-01032-1.

> *The microbiota* also interacts directly with the digestive tract, bypassing the [gut-brain] axis. It sends signals to the enteric nervous system, a network of neurons located in the digestive wall, and can thus directly influence intestinal secretions and peristaltic movements.
> See also *the Polyvagal Theory* of Stephen W. Porges (The Porges' Theory).

It is easy to understand that the interaction between the individual and the microbiota is a two-way process: from the individual to the microbiota and from the microbiota to the individual.

> The microbiota is often altered in EDS patients. The study of the influences of the microbiome in EDS and its phenotypic expression would therefore be an exciting avenue of exploration.

Many EDS patients present with a chronic inflammatory state of unexplained origin, sometimes with temperature peaks or a sub-febrile state, a feeling of flu-like syndrome all year round, digestive disorders, food intolerances, etc. The cause is most often intestinal dysbiosis and/or a porous intestine (Leaky Gut).

I recently read some remarkably interesting articles about microbiota variations:

The authors evaluated the microbiota of children born by vaginal delivery or cesarean section, as well as the influence of the mother's microbiota during pregnancy on the allergic outcome of the children:

The microbiota present in the mother's digestive tract and her breast milk, on her skin and in her vagina, contribute to developing the child's microbiota. Although this influence acts during childbirth (via the mother's skin, vagina, and stools), it seems that this maternal microbiota may already play a role during pregnancy (in utero). Although it is accepted that the uterine environment is sterile, this is not the case for the placenta! This placental microbiota can act on the neonatal immunity of the baby.

Not only can the exposome (stress, life events, nutrigenomics, pharmacogenomics, toxins, emotional shocks, abuse, smoking, alcohol, etc.) modify, as we have seen previously, the expression of genes during pregnancy, but so can the microbiota.

The mother's gut microbiota also influences the innate immunity of babies on the 14th day postpartum. It is understandable that taking antibiotics during pregnancy, for example, can significantly influence the maternal microbiota and, therefore the baby's innate immunity (which is received at birth).[157]

This can lead to a predisposition in the child to develop various illnesses or diseases.

So, be careful when administering antibiotics during pregnancy; think about prebiotics and probiotics! Or even suggest giving them routinely.

There is also mother-to-child transmission via breast milk (*Martin et al.*). Intestinal bacteria, from the pre-delivery and post-delivery microbiota, are found in the mother's mammary glands and her milk; this is the entero-mammary route. These bacteria also influence the baby's immune system.

The vagina contains more than 170 species of bacteria, whose composition is very stable during pregnancy. Various studies have also compared the microbiota of children born by vaginal delivery or by cesarean section. The fact that the baby is in contact or not with the vaginal flora during delivery will influence, later in life, its allergic state.

It is well known, for example, that pregnant women exposed to animals and livestock in rural areas will have less allergic and asthmatic children than those living in urban areas.

AAgard K, Riehle K, Ma JA. A metagenomic approach to characterization of the vaginal microbiome signature in pregnancy. PloS ONE. 2012;7:e36466.

---

[157] Nyangahu DD, Lennard KS, Brown PP et al. Disruption of maternal gut microbiota during gestation alters offspring microbiota and immunity. Microbiome. 2018;6:1-10.

Fall T, Lundholm C, Örtqvist AK et al. Early exposure to dogs and farm animals and the risk of childhood asthma. JAMA Pediatr. 2015;169:e153219.

Jhun I, Phipatanakul W. Early exposure to dogs and farm animals reduces the risk of childhood asthma. Evid Based med. 2016;21:2015-201.

Yu J, Liu X, Li Y ret al. Maternal exposure to farming environment protects offspring against allergic diseases by modulating the neonate TLR-Tregs-Th axis. Clin Trans Allergy. 2018;8:1-13.

Therefore, prebiotics and probiotics to mothers during and after pregnancy are essential to prevent allergies and eczema in the baby. Postnatal administration only is probably not enough.

Not only does the maternal microbiota play a vital role in these allergic conditions, but it also plays an essential role in the risk of developing inflammatory bowel disease (IBD), type 1 diabetes mellitus, and more.

Hu Y, Peng J, Tai N et al. Maternel antibiotic treatment protects offspring from diabetes development in nonobese diabetic mice by generation of tolerogenic APCs. J Immunol. 2015;195:4176-484.

Örtqvist AK, Lundholm C, Halfvarson J et al. Fetal and early life antibiotics exposure and very early onset inflammatory bowel disease: a population-based study. Gut. 2018,68:218-225.

The microbiota and the metabolites generated by these bacteria (butyrate, propionate, acetate, and more.) probably pass to the baby during pregnancy via the placenta and the ingestion of amniotic fluid, on the one hand, and via the mammary glands and milk in the post-natal period, on the other hand. Metabolites directly influence the baby's immunity, but more than that, they also influence it, again via Epigenetics (see this chapter).

Holmes E, Li JV, Marchesi JR et al. Gut microbiota composition and activity in relation to host metabolic phenotype and disease risk. Cell Metab. 2012;16:559-564.

Kato K, Uetake C, Kato T et al. Commensal microbe-derived butyrate induces the differenciation of colonic regulatory cells. Nature. 2013;504:446-450.

Thorburn AN, McKenzie CL, Shen S et al. Evidence that asthma is a developmental origin disease influenced by maternal diet and bacterial metabolites. Nat Commun. 2015;6;7320.

Michel S, Busato F, Genuneit J et al. Farm exposure and time trends in early childhood may influence DNA methylation in genes related to asthma and allergy. Eur J Clin Immunol. 2013;68:355-364.

Cesarean section births (the upper route) can potentially lead to more immune disturbances in the child than if they were born by the lower route (no passage through the vagina during cesarean section, and therefore no exposure to the vaginal microbiota). However, a positive intestinal flora during pregnancy and breastfeeding can, in practice, improve this risk.

To Remember

Chronic treatment with probiotics of various bacterial strains, and prebiotics, should be taken from the outset in EDS, including during pregnancy. Symptoms are generally significantly improved in patients who ingest them; these substances also promote a favorable development of the unborn child's immunity. L-Glutamine can also be added at a dose of 3 to 4 times 800mg/day in patients to improve the porous intestine (*Leaky gut*).

Probiotics: WHO (World Health Organization) and FAO (Food and Agriculture Organization of the United Nations) definition from 2001: "Probiotics are living microorganisms which, when ingested (or administered) in sufficient quantities, exert positive health effects beyond the traditional nutritional effects."

Prebiotics: These are food substances, mainly composed of bound sugars, known as short-chain oligosaccharides and polysaccharides, which are believed to selectively promote the growth of certain probiotic-type bacteria or the activity of the microbiota and provide a health benefit.[158]

---

[158] Reid G, Verbeke K, Cani PD, Swanson KS. Expert consensus document : The international scientific association for probiotics and prebiotics (ISAPP) consensus statement on the definition and scope of prebiotics. Nature Reviews Gastroenterology & Hepatology 2017,14(8):491-502.

Relevant articles:

Almeida A, Mitchell AL, Boland M et al. A new genomic blueprint of the human gut microbiota. Nature. 2019;568(7753):499-504.

Guo R, Chen LH, Xing C. Pain regulation by gut microbiota: molecular mechanisms and therapeutic potential. Br J Anaesth. 2019;123(5):637-654.

Chang CS, Kao CY. Current understanding of the gut microbiota shaping mechanisms. J Biomed Sci. 2019;26:59.

Roy Sarkar S, Banerjee S. Gut microbiota in neurodegenerative disorders. J Neuroimmunol. 2019;328:98-104

Fattarusso A, Di Genova L, Battista Dell'Isola G et al. Autism spectrum disorders and the gut microbiota. Nutrients. 2019;11(3). Doi: 10.3390/nu11030521.

Molina-Torres G, Rodrigues-Arrastia M, Roman P et al. Stress and the gut microbiota-brain axis. Behav Pharmacol. 2019;30(2&3):187-200.

Bejaj JS. Alcohol, liver disease and the gut microbiota. Nat Rev Gatsroenterol Hepatol. 2019;16(4):235-246.

Aresti Sanz J, El Aidy S. Microbiota and gut neuropeptides : a dual action of antimicrobial activity and neuroimmune response. Psychopharmacology (Berl). 2019;236(5):1597-1609.

Zhao W, Ho HE, Bunyavanich S. The gut in food allergy. Ann Allergy Asthma Immunol. 2019;122(3):276-282.

Noce A, Marrone G, Di Daniele F et al. Impact of gut microbiota on onset and progression of chronic non-communicable diseases. Nutrients. 2019;11(5):1073

Nutrigenomics

Nutrigenomics is an emerging science. Geneticist Claudine Junien defines it as follows: "Nutrigenomics also called nutritional genomics, establishes interactions between genes and food. It is interesting, among other things, in the genes involved in the absorption, transport, fate, and elimination of nutrients and their mechanisms of action. Nutrigenomics is concerned with how foods, nutrients, and certain dietary practices can affect gene expression through epigenetic modifications during development and throughout life." [159,160]

Pharmacogenomics and Pharmacoepigenomics

I will only mention what is called pharmacogenomics and pharmacoepigenomics, or how medications affect the expression of our genes. This is also Epigenetics.[161]

A Gendered Medicine

Some studies would indicate that medications work differently, depending on whether the patient is male or female.[162] In 2013, the American FDA (*Food and Drug Administration*) announced that Zopiclone doses (Zolpidem®10mg) used without distinguishing the sex of the patient was a mistake.[163] The dose for women should be half that of men! Women would also be more sensitive to the toxicity of Paracetamol on the liver than men, so the doses should be lower.[164] Various studies show that women are 50 to 70% more likely than men to have undesirable effects from medication! The desired effects of medication also vary according to the patient's sex. Physiology, fat distribution, metabolism, hormones, for example, are naturally different according to gender. Absorption, metabolism, excretion by the

---

[159] Claudine Junien, « Qu'est-ce que la nutrigénomique ? » (What is nutrigenomics?), https://www.dailymotion.com/video/x7qtw2_claudine-junien-qu-est-ce-que-la-nu_lifestyle

[160] Paoloni-Giacobino A, Grimble R, Pichard C. Genetics and nutrition. Clin Nutr. 2003;22(5):429-435.

[161] Kalinin AA, Higgins GA, Reamaroon N, et al. Deep learning in pharmacogenomics: from gene regulation to patient stratification. Pharmacogenomics. 2018;19(7):629-650. doi:10.2217/pgs-2018-0008.

[162] Zopf Y, Rabe C, Neubert A, et al. Women encounter ADRs more often than do men. Eur J Clin Pharmacol. 2008;64(10):999-1004. doi:10.1007/s00228-008-0494-6.

[163] Kesselheim AS, Donneyong M, Dal Pan GJ, et al. Changes in prescribing and healthcare resource utilization after FDA Drug Safety Communications involving zolpidem-containing medications. Pharmacoepidemiol Drug Saf. 2017;26(6):712-721. doi: 10.1002/pds.4215.

[164] Liu Y, Chen Y, Xie X, et al. Gender Difference on the Effect of Omega-3 Polyunsaturated Fatty Acids on Acetaminophen-Induced Acute Liver Failure. Oxid Med Cell Longev. 2020;2020:8096847. doi: 10.1155/2020/8096847.

liver or kidney may vary and lead to different effects at the same doses or side effects that could be avoided.

"The different efficacy of drugs in women and men is due to biological differences that may be caused by sex-specific gene expression, which is likely triggered by sex- specific epigenetic modifications. Furthermore, gender plays a role in drug efficacy as a sociocultural dimension that can lead to differences between women and men. The same considerations can also be valid for vaccines. Many studies clearly demonstrate that the development of vaccines against infections should carefully consider the effect of differential immune response in males and females. Moreover, also an accurate analysis of outcomes as well as of adverse effects should be performed (*Migliore L, et al., 2021*)"[165]

More women (all age groups) are now included in clinical studies to optimize the medicine of tomorrow, a gendered, preventive, and curative medicine.

In EDS, this is even more important: more than 80% of the patients who consult us are women, and it is precisely for this population that studies are lacking.

Jeremias G, Gonçalves FJM, Pereira JL, Asselman J. Prospects for incorporation of epigenetic biomarkers in human health and environmental risk assessment of chemicals. Biol Rev Camb Philos Soc. 2020. Doi: 10.1111/brv.12589.

Thiagalingam S. Epigenetic memory in development and disease: untraveling the mechanism. Biochim Biophys Acta Rev Cancer. 2020;1873(2):188349.

Duempelmann L, Skribbe M, Bühler M. Small RNAs in the transgenerational inheritance of epigenetic information. Trends Genet. 2020;36(3):203-214.

Tikhodeyev ON. Heredity determined by the environment: Lamarckian ideas in modern molecular biology. Sci Total Environ. 2020;710:135521.

---

[165] Migliore L, Nicolì V, Stoccoro A. Gender Specific Differences in Disease Susceptibility: The Role of Epigenetics. Biomedicines. 2021;9(6):652. doi: 10.3390/biomedicines9060652

David I, Canario L, Combes S, Demars J. Intergenerational transmission of characters through genetics, epigenetics, microbiota, and learning in Livestock. Front Genet. 2019;10:1058.

Liberman N, Wang SY, Greer EL. Transgenerational epigenetic inheritance: from phenomena to molecular mechanisms. Curr Opin Neurobiol. 2019;59:189-206.

Schlissel G, Rine J. The nucleosome core particle remembers its position through DNA replication and DNA transcription. Proc Natl Acad Sci USA. 2019;116(41):20605-20611.

Morgan HL, Watkins AJ. Transgenerational impact of environmental change. Adv Exp Med Biol. 2019;1200:71-89.

Sciamanna I, Serafino A, Shapiro JA, Spadafora C. The active role of spermatozoa in transgenerational inheritance. Proc Bio Sci. 2019;286(1909):20191263.

Lempradl A. Germ cell-mediated mechanisms of epigenetic inheritance. Semin Cell Dev Biol. 2020;97:116-122.

Cavalli G, Heard E. Advances in epigenetics link genetics to environment and disease. Nature. 2019;571(7766):489-499.

Bianco Rodriguez J, Camprubi Sànchez C. Epigenetic transgenerational inheritance. Adv Exp Med Biol. 2019;1166:57-74.

Sarkies P. Molecular mechanisms of epigenetic inheritance: possible evolutionary implications. Semin Cell Dev Biol. 2020;97:106-115.

Perez ME, Lehner B. Intergenerational and transgenerational epigenetic inheritance in animals. Nat cell Biol. 2019;21(2):143-151.

Stewart KR, Veselovska L, Kelsey G. Establishment and functions of DNA methylation in the germline. Epigenomics. 2016;8(10):1399-1413.

Clarke HJ, Vieux KF. Epigenetic inheritance through the female germ-line: the known, the unknown, and the possible. Semin Cell Dev Biol. 2015;43:106-116.

Paldi A. Effects of the in vitro manipulation of stem cell: epigenetic mechanisms as mediators of induced metabolic fluctuations. Epigenomics. 2013;5(4):429-437.

What I retain from this Second Part

Part Three

Mechanisms of Pain

Special Treatments of EDS

Emergencies in EDS

CHAPTER VIII

Mast Cell Activation Disorders in EDS

By Professor Anne Maitland, MD, PhD
& Doctor Stéphane Daens, MD, DATC

1.   Physiopathology, Clinical Signs and Symptoms

By Professor Anne Maitland, MD, PhD

They are the most reviled cells in the body.

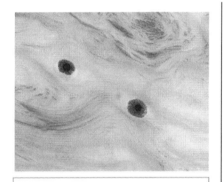

Two mast cells with granules, situated in unstained connective tissue

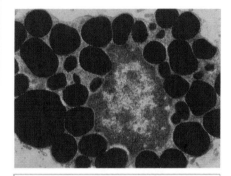

Mast cell with cytoplasm filled with granules (dense, black structures) containing histamine, proteases, cytokines, growth factors

Their meddling makes our skin itch, our eyes swell, and our noses stream; the cells even provoke suffocating asthma attacks that kill thousands of people every year. In fact, these villains, known as mast cells, are responsible for so much suffering that some researcher have proposed eradicating them. That could be a big mistake. *(Leslie, 2007)*

Before the rise of mast cell activation disease:

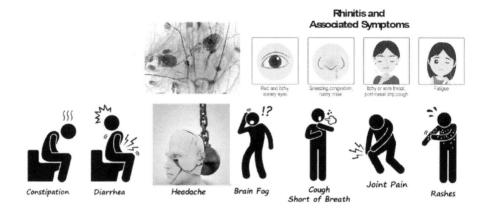

Before:

- Rhinitis became more than a nuisance of condition, contributing to other illnesses, such as headache and sleep disorders as well as respiratory infections and asthma;
- Asthma became a common chronic condition, leading to millions of urgent care visits as well as hospitalizations, and nearly ten neighbors dying, on daily basis, before their time;
- Food intolerances led to a growing number of children and adults avoiding eating unfamiliar restaurants as well as near friends or home of family members, to minimize risk of gastrointestinal distress or worse; and
- One out of every fifty Americans have been treated for anaphylaxis and many more instructed to carry rescue adrenalin auto-injectors;

.... A sore throat ended the lives of the young and old.

According to early medical journals, public health enemy #1 were infections (*Godlee, 2007*):

	Dysentery
Abscess	Fever
Burns	Worms
Croup	Syphilis
Colic	Whooping Cough

Diarrhea	Consumption
Tooth Decay	(Tuberculosis)
	Sore throats

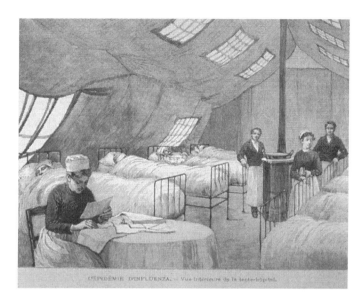

From www.shutterstock.com. Asian Flu epidemic of 1889-90. In Paris, a supplemental tent hospital. A nurse attends to patients during winter of 1889-90. Wood engraving from L'ILLUSTRATION, Jan 4, 1890.

But in the mid 1800s, several medical advances started to usher ways to ensure safety of the food and water supplies, raised our understanding of the role of infections as well as the immune system in health and disease, implemented sanitation and anti-septic techniques to reduce the spread of infectious agents, in public and during surgery; and, incorporated routine vaccinations, of the young and old, as well as the use of antibiotic agents, which prevent and treat a range of infections, respectively. *(Jones, et al., 2012) (Godlee, 2007)*

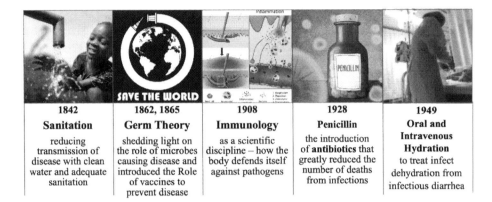

1842	1862, 1865	1908	1928	1949
Sanitation	**Germ Theory**	**Immunology**	**Penicillin**	**Oral and Intravenous Hydration**
reducing transmission of disease with clean water and adequate sanitation	shedding light on the role of microbes causing disease and introduced the Role of vaccines to prevent disease	as a scientific discipline – how the body defends itself against pathogens	the introduction of **antibiotics** that greatly reduced the number of deaths from infections	to treat infect dehydration from infectious diarrhea

Public sanitation, which reduces the spread of disease, with use of clean water and protection of our food sources; the germ theory, that diseases arose from the breach of our bodies' borders, by invasive microbes; the use of vaccines, starting with smallpox (variolation) vaccine, boosted immune responses to prevent several infectious diseases; the emergence of Immunology as a scientific discipline, providing insight of the body's defenses against infectious and toxic challenges; and the development of germ killers -antibiotics.

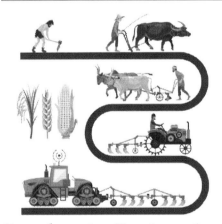

By the end of the 20th century, our habits and habitats had dramatically changed, and so did "the burden of disease". In less than two centuries, there was a dramatic decline in killer infections, such as tuberculosis, measles, whooping cough, hepatitis and polio. However, as medical miracles and scientific advances saved millions of lives, those dwelling in modernized environs started to acquire chronic disorders, such diabetes, neuropathies, inflammatory bowel diseases and chronic respiratory disorders, including asthma.

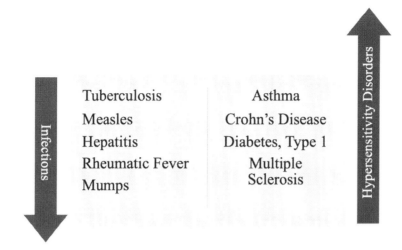

Tuberculosis   Asthma

Measles   Crohn's Disease

Hepatitis   Diabetes, Type 1

Rheumatic Fever   Multiple

Mumps   Sclerosis

From 1950 to 2000, as prototypical infectious diseases were on the decline, the incidence of immune mediated, hypersensitivity disorders started to rise. Adapted from Bach, 2002

The Human race has come to dominate its environment so completely that any analysis of the increase or appearance of a disease has to take changes in our lifestyle into account. In the case of [mast cell activation] disease changes in our environment, diet, water quality, and personal behavior over the last 150 years have played a dominant role in the specificity of these diseases, as well as in prevalence and severity. *(Platts-Mills, 2015)*

NHAPS (National Human Activity Pattern Survey) [166] respondents reported spending an average of 87% of their time in enclosed buildings and about 6% of their time in enclosed vehicles. *(Klepeis, et al., 2001)*

Nowadays, we are now living longer. However, nearly 1 out of 2 us has a chronic disorder and more than likely, the ailments are associated with recurrent tissue injury and persistent inflammation. Children and then adults started developing immediate and delayed hypersensitivity disorders:

---

[166] The National Human Activity Pattern Survey (NHAPS): A resource for assessing exposure to environmental polluants. Klepeis NE, Nelson WC, Ott WR, et al. Journal of Exposure Analysis and Environmental Epidemiology. 2001;11(3):231-252. doi: 10.1038/sj.jea.7500165. PMID: 11477521.

- Food sensitivities,
- Rhinitis and asthma,
- Itchy skin disorders,
- Drug intolerances,
- Anaphylaxis.

Vitamin D is crucial for immune health –

make sure you're getting enough

The surprising role it plays for your body's immune system and how it can ward off respiratory infections. (cnet, 2021)

In less than a century, the systems of the human body that evolved over millennia, to detect and battle a sea of pathogens and naturally occurring toxins, now must learn to navigate and negotiate a dramatically new set of exposures, both infectious, physical and chemical challenges (National Geographic, 2021):

- Labile outdoor climates, more storms = crop failures, higher humidity for insect borne diseases, such as Lyme, and more exposure to indoor pollution;
- Indoor pollution, both naturally occurring substances, such as mold, as well as manufactured, such as cleaning agents, and gasses from indoor electronics to engineered building materials;
- Food sources, no longer locally raised, with additives, and stored in plastic, not paper (cardboard), tin, or glass.

It is the epithelium, the tissue-based mast cells and nerves interact with this "new" outside world, detect and then respond to these challenges. Moreover, this triad of body systems contribute to around-the-clock barrier function and homeostasis.

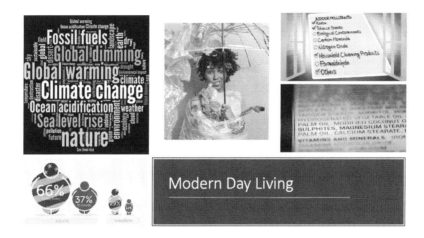

Along with change in our activities, more screen time than outdoor exercise, e.g., there is now an obesity epidemic and a rise of micronutrient deficiencies, such as vitamin D. These medical conditions have been shown to alter the bodies' responses to extrinsic challenges- infectious agents, chemicals- naturally occurring or manufactured, and climate. These insults, in turn, have been linked to chronic tissue injury and inflammation.

Interconnected relationships and mast cell activation orders:

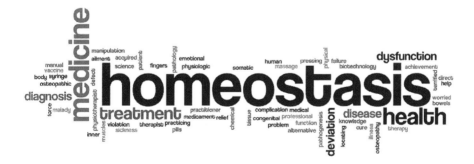

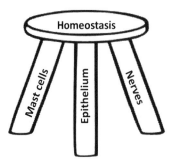

Homeostasis is the body's efforts to maintain internal harmony against the backdrop of constant challenge from external threats and the expected wear-and-tear of its internal structures. The key to surveillance of damage, coordination of the body's responses to various dangers and the repair efforts to damaged tissue, is the immune system; and, the immune cell population, which is recruited and trained to meet the needs of its assigned micro-environment, is the mast cell.

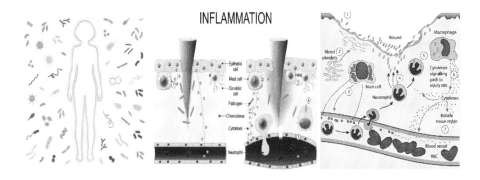

Our) immune systems ... (are) embodied expectations of injury and the corresponding programs of protection and repair."
-Peter Sloterdijk

This is evident in children and adults with connective tissue disorders, who exhibit a constellation of symptoms of the musculoskeletal system and beyond, highlighting the dysfunction of these innate, tissue-based immune cells. Although the mast cell was originally described in the mid 1800s, it is only now that efforts are being re-focused to better understand the role of mast cells, not only in allergic inflammation, but in the overall health and disease of our connective tissue. In the adult, of average stature, there is nearly 3 yards of epithelium - the skin and the linings of the gastrointestinal, the respiratory and urogenital tract - which separates our bodies' inner workings from the external world. Closely associated with these epithelial borders are the resident mast cells and nerve endings.

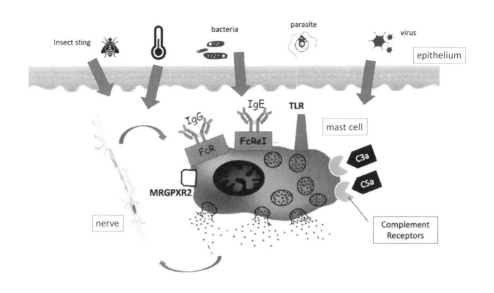

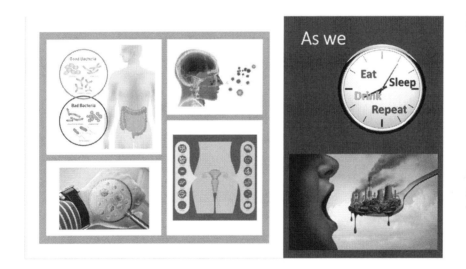

So, as we ingest, breathe, eliminate waste products, wear clothing or apply substances to our skin, it is the epithelium and this resident immune cell population that vets all encounters, including organisms- "good vs bad" bacteria, e.g: biological matter and chemical substances; as well as physical changes, such as water content, acid-base balance, pressure and temperature. The triad, of [connective tissue - mast cell - nerves],

353

detects and coordinates responses to impending dangers and tissue injury, including:

- An infectious agent, such a virus, parasite or bacteria.
- A toxic chemical, either natural occurring substance, such as the venom from an insect (spider, mosquito), snake bite or sea creature (jellyfish, sea urchins) or manufactured chemicals, such as lye, bleach, formaldehyde;
- A physical insult, such as penetrating trauma, barometric pressure, etc.

Mast cells have been detected in all types of species, sea life, fowl and mammals;

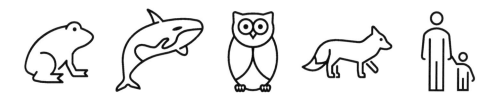

and, in humans, not a single child has been born without mast cells, indicating that this resident immune cell population has been preserved across species and time, playing a central role in tissue defense and repair.

After being recruited from the bone marrow, its "birthplace," progenitor or "rookie" mast cells undergoes further instruction, called differentiation, from signals derived from the surrounding environment. This results in a diverse population of mast cells operating throughout the human body, due to the varied signals of each micro-environment in every organ system. That is, the tissue, which surrounds the solitary mast cell, dictates which surface receptors are expressed as well as the contents of the granules, which give the mast cell its distinctive appearance amidst the connective tissue of each organ in the body.

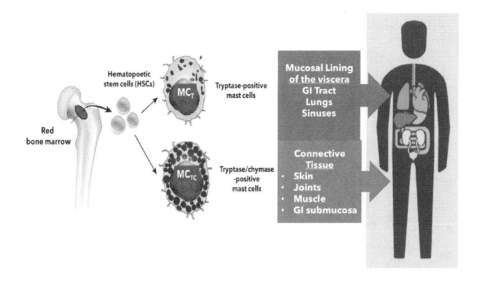

Describing these cells, which contained numerous sacs or granules, as well-fed or well-nourished cells, the German pathologist Paul Ehrlich ostensibly likened mast cells, 'mastzellen,' to the patrons of the arts and sciences, the German nobility, who were living well off their landholdings. Yet a different picture emerges, regarding the dynamics of the mast cell and the surrounding structures and cells. There is a growing body of evidence that indicates a role in our homeostasis, beyond allergic inflammation.

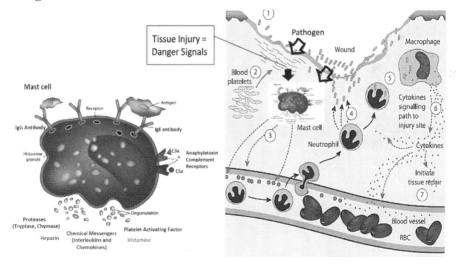

With their numerous surface receptors, which allow surveillance of the surrounding tissue, and the action of the numerous chemical mediators, which can impact the functions of every organ system, both nearby and distant, mast cells appear to be a central regulatory cell population. A multifunctional cell, mast cells apparently are regulated by the actions of the micro-environment. Local signals shaped the last stages of mast cells' development into tissue sentinels, and likely regulate the ability of mast cells to unload its payload of potent chemicals, in the presence of detected encounters, via its surface receptors *(Akin, 2017) (Galli & Tsai, 2010) (Sandig, et al., 2013) (Theoharides & Kandere, 2002)*

By recognizing and responding to dangers, inside and out of our borders, mast cells play a key role in our homeostasis. Think of mast cells as command central for border defense and tissue repair. With numerous surface receptors, mast cells can detect tissue injury or ongoing inflammation and then "usual suspects," such as dangerous bacteria, viruses, as well as chemicals (from poisonous plants or venomous insects and snakes) that pose a threat to our internal balance, homeostasis.

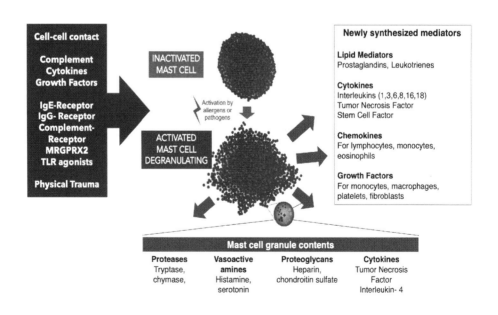

Mast cells can be triggered into a different set of actions, from their vigilant, resting state into danger detected, spring-into-action response. They are equipped with receptors that can detect substances derived from harmful microbes and injured tissue, and as part of the body's first line of defense, mast cells are the first responders to foreign invaders in our bodies.

Upon detection of tissue injury, mast cells have an armamentarium of chemical mediators and hardwired actions, tailored to different types of dangers. Moreover, a growing body evidence points to the mast cell compartment as one of the key regulators of the innate and adaptive immune system, given:

- their strategic location, underneath the epithelial lining that interfaces with the external world as well as clustering near nerves, blood vessels and lymphatics, and
- their multifunctionality, with the capacity to recruit and activate other immune effector cell populations, regulate angiogenesis, tissue remodeling, wound healing, and tumor repression growth.

The power of the mast cell derived chemical mediators and actions is evident, if one looks how a honey badger can recover from the venomous bite of a deadly snake *(Galli & Tsai, 2010)*. Moreover, a good way to describe the role of mast cells is as "border defense and tissue repair," recognizing and responding to pathogens, addressing tissue injury, and participating in tissue homeostasis.

However, if mast cells are activated improperly, these "false alarms" can lead to the release of tissue-cutting enzymes, such as tryptase, as well as distress signals. Depending on the offending agent, these chemical mediators can call in a flood of cell-lysing, complement proteins, or a cavalry of eosinophils or neutrophils. In every instance, the body's first responder, the mast cell, will sacrifice healthy tissue and inflict collateral damage, in order to contain a pathogen or life-threatening injury. Therefore, mast cell activation must be tightly regulated, to "prevent the pathology associated with unnecessary immune activation". *(Sandig, et al., 2013) (Rossi & Pitidis, 2018) (Platts-Mills, 2015)*. However, given the rise of hypersensitivity disorders, the inter-connectedness of [the connective tissue - mast cells and nerves] has been disrupted by the industrial revolution of our daily habits and living environments. That is, before the COVID-19 pandemic, one out of two us have been coping with a different epidemic, that of immediate and delayed hypersensitivity disorders *(Weiler, et al., 2091) (Mathis & Benoist, 2002).*

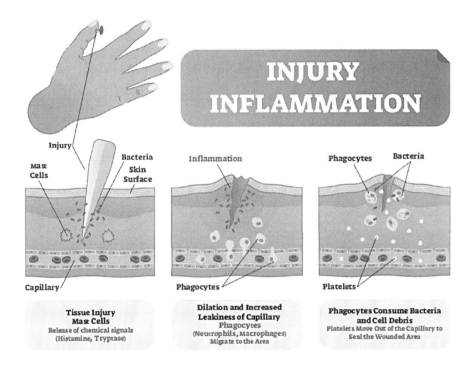

Loss of tolerance in the mast cell compartment can lead to excessive, unnecessary inflammation and aberrant tissue remodeling. In the past 30 years, dysregulation of the mast cell compartment has been on the rise, in the form of immediate and delayed hypersensitivity disorders.

In addition to classic mast cell activation disorders, such as rhinitis, asthma, urticaria, food allergies, and anaphylaxis, a growing body of evidence points emerge to the role of mast cell dysfunction in autoimmune disorders, such as rheumatoid arthritis, Sjogren's syndrome, and immune mediated neuropathies, including multiple sclerosis. *(Theoharides, et al.,*

2015) (Theoharides & Kandere, 2002) (Benoist & Mathis, 2002) (Lee & Mueller, 2017)

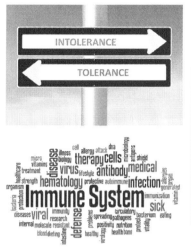

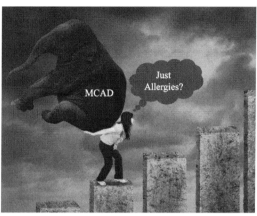

Beyond allergies, an epidemic of mast cell activation disease:

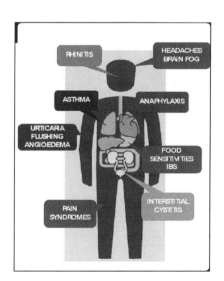

Sneezing? Congested? Runny Nose? Mucus in the throat?

- ▸ 4 out of 10 children
- ▸ Up to 30% of the adult population

Coughing? Wheezing? Breathless?

- ▸ 8 – 9 Million children with asthma
- ▸ Nearly 18-20 Million Adults

Itchy, red rashes of eczema or atopic or contact dermatitis

- ▸ 2% US population affected

Food Allergies? Itchy mouth with fresh fruit?

- ▸ 4-8 % US population have food allergies

Urticaria / Angioedema

- ▸ 1 out 5 individuals will experience hives/swelling

Anaphylaxis

- ▸ 1 in 50 have been treated for this severe allergic reaction

When a child or adult has nasal congestion, recurrent hives, asthma attacks or reaction at a medication, triggering anaphylaxis, most healthcare professionals focus on the most well-known mast cell activation inflammatory pathway, "allergies," also known as allergen bound to allergen-specific Immunoglobulin E (IgE) triggered mast cell activation (MCA).

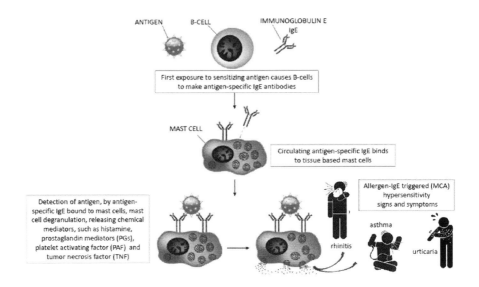

Scientists Find How Allergic Reaction Works

New York Times Jan. 12, 1989 (Schmeck Jr., 1989)

Unlike white blood cells readily detected in circulation, little was known about mast cells in health and disease, besides the rare clonal mast cell disorder, systemic Mastocytosis. Then, in 1989, scientists described the relationship of Immunoglobulin E and mast cells, in the growing burden of allergic disorders. Ever since this cardinal observation, linking allergen specific Immunoglobulin E (IgE) antibodies and mast cells to atopic or allergic reactions, it is difficult for most health care professionals to think of mast cells in other contexts, other than allergic inflammation *(Galli & Tsai, 2010)*. But remember that there are numerous receptors detected on the surface of mast cells besides the Immunoglobulin E (IgE) receptor, called FcRe. This is reflected by all the allergic (allergen specific IgE) and nonallergic triggers of a very common, itchy skin condition called urticaria (hives).

360

Smear of peripheral blood

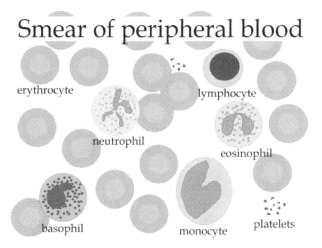

erythrocyte

lymphocyte

neutrophil

eosinophil

basophil

monocyte

platelets

Immunologic Triggers		Non-immunologic Triggers
Allergen-Specific IGE (foods, medications, supplements, airborne)	Allergy skin testing	Physical triggers (pressure, solar, cold, vibration, heat, exercise
Autoimmune urticaria (thyroid autoantibodies		Hormones (thyroid disease, estrogen, progesterone)
Complement		Medications (opoids, anesthethic agents, antibiotics- Vancomycin)
Cytokine/ Chemokines		
Immuno-deficiencies		Neoplasms
Infections		

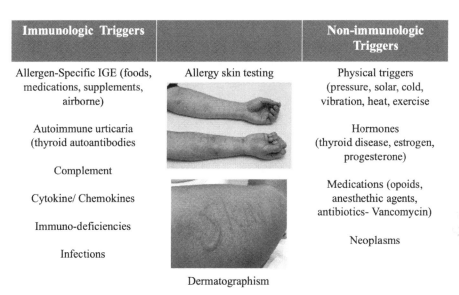

Dermatographism

If one can see the different ways mast cells can be activated in the skin, then there will be a greater appreciation of the numerous triggers causing mast cell activation throughout the body, given that mast cells are situated in every organ system. As seen above, chronic, recurrent mast cell activation of the skin, called chronic spontaneous urticaria, individuals can react to physical, nonimmune-mediated triggers, such as sudden changes of body temperature, either cold or heat, vibration, pressure, more intense waves of sunlight when changing geography, penetrating trauma, as well as chemicals derived from naturally occurring substances or manufactured.

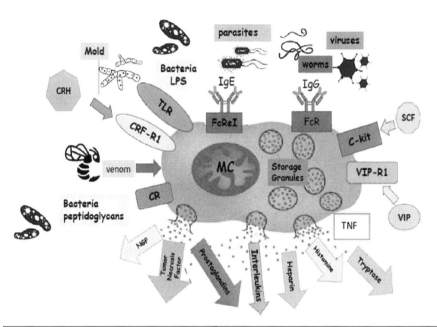

Alarming Receptors	Pathogen Receptors
Heat Shock Protein (HSP)	Toll Like Receptors (TLRs)
Interleukin-33 (IL33)	Complement (C) Receptors
Complement (C3A, C5A)	Immunoglobulin (Ig) Receptors

	Direct Pathogen Receptors	Indirect Pathogen Receptors	
	TLRs	C-Receptors	Ig Receptors
Chemical Mediators Released	**Only Secretion of:** Leukotrienes (LTC4) Interleukins (IL-1, IL-6) Tumor Necrosis Factor (TNF) Chemokines, Cytokines	**Degranulation:** Proteases (Tryptase, Chymase), Histamine	
		Secretion: LTC4, IL-1, IL-6, TNF Chemokines, Cytokines	

All of these can stimulate mast cell activation, via different receptors found on the surface of mast cells. In addition, upon engagement via different surface receptors/triggering events, mast cells can release a variety of different types of mediators – all of which can cause different combinations of the classic hallmarks of inflammation: dolor (pain), rubor (redness), calor (heat), and tumor (swelling).

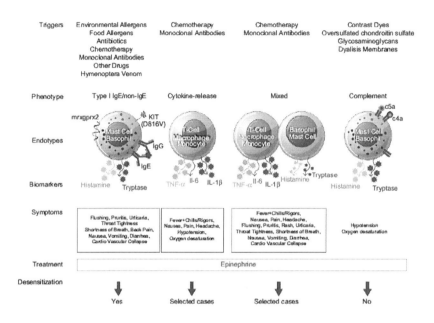

Figure. Since mast cells bear an array of receptors, it is important to remember that there are a number of triggers that activate mast cells, a variety of different mediators that they secrete (which can serve as biomarkers of mast cell activity), and a range of programmed responses to those challenges detected, including the cardinal signs of inflammation. Figure adapted from Dr. Castells (Wilfox , et al., 2018).

Given their location and expression of receptors that look out for dangers and monitor the normal wear and tear of our bodies' organs, mast cells and mast cell activation play a key role in homeostasis: surveillance, initiation of innate and adaptive immune system responses to numerous insults, and coordination of tissue repair, after harm has been cleared. Wellness depends on the integrity of the innate immune cell compartment, and, if mast cells go awry, illness is sure to follow.

MCs can tailor their responses, depending on the stimulus encountered and the tissue in which they are stimulated. MCs differentially process various stimuli into distinct degranulation programs. (Karhausen & Abraham, 2016)

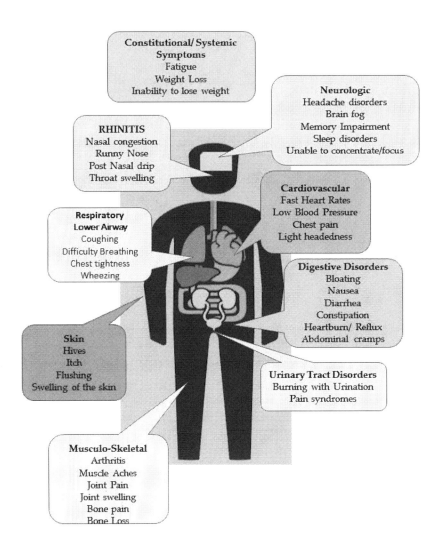

Most practitioners are familiar with allergen-IgE driven mast cell activation as well as an uncommon mast cell disorder, Mastocytosis. The latter occurs as an individual mast cell acquires a mutation in the c-kit surface receptor, or the associated downstream signaling pathway. However, by 2010, there was a growing appreciation that children and adults were experiencing immediate hypersensitivity reactions/aberrant release of chemicals, without having Mastocytosis or identified allergen-specific IgE. Therefore, according to the Mast Cell Disorders Working Group of the World Health Organization (WHO), mast cell dysregulation put forth criteria for patients exhibiting symptoms worrisome for dysregulation of the mast cell compartment - mast cell activation syndrome (MCAS).

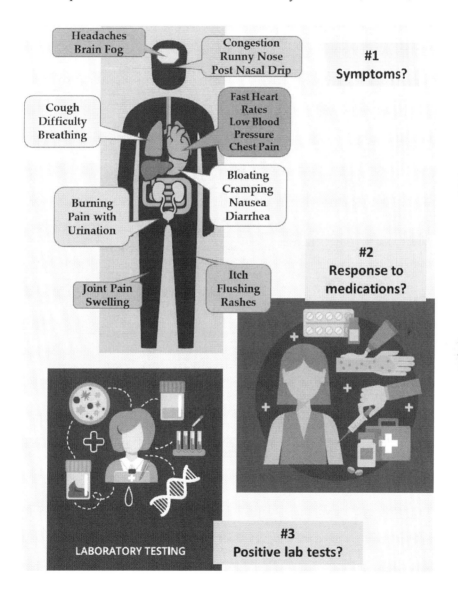

Criteria for Mast Cell Activation Syndrome:

Mast cell activation disorders are common, a severe form of mast cell activation disease (MCAD) is mast cell activation syndrome (MCAS), which identifies children and adults at risk for recurrent or severe hypersensitivity reactions. MCAS is characterized by the combination of the following three criteria:

1) Typical symptoms,
2) Laboratory abnormalities and
3) Response to treatment.

Proposed Criteria for MCA Syndrome Diagnosis	
Symptoms present in two or more organ systems:	**Skin:** urticaria, angioedema, flushing **Gastrointestinal:** nausea, vomiting, diarrhea, abdominal cramping/pain. **Cardiovascular:** hypotensive syncope or near syncope, tachycardia. **Neuropsychiatric**: brain fog, anxiety, depression. **Respiratory**: wheezing. **Naso-ocular:** conjunctival injection, pruritus, nasal. **Genito-urinary**: pain with urination, urinary frequency females- pain with intimate relations; heavy-painful menses.
An elevated biomarker for mast cell activation syndrome, which can include serum tryptase or urinary mediators, such as prostaglandin and histamine metabolites (prostaglandin D2, 11-Beta-prostaglandin F2 Alpha, or methylhistamine.	
A decrease in the frequency, severity, or resolution of symptoms with histamine receptor antagonists or other mast-cell targeted medications, such as ketotifen, omalizumab, cromones or tricyclic agents.	

MCAS is assigned to patients who have the combination of hypersensitivity symptoms, response to medications that uniquely damper mast cell activation, and test results indicating aberrant mast cell activation.

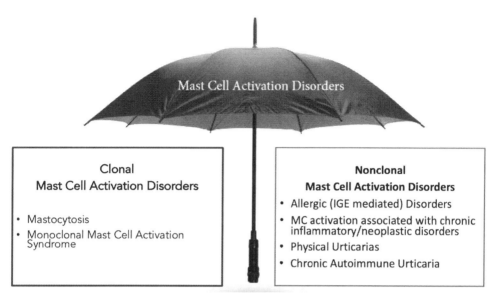

Mast Cell Activation Disorders

Clonal Mast Cell Activation Disorders	Nonclonal Mast Cell Activation Disorders
• Mastocytosis • Monoclonal Mast Cell Activation Syndrome	• Allergic (IGE mediated) Disorders • MC activation associated with chronic inflammatory/neoplastic disorders • Physical Urticarias • Chronic Autoimmune Urticaria

Hypertryptasemia – Mast Cells that have increased copies of the tryptase gene, patients exhibit MCAS signs and Symptoms
Idiopathic – Idiopathic anaphylaxis, Idiopathic Urticaria

Once the 3 criteria have been fulfilled, the next step focuses on the known causes of mast cell dysfunction:

• **Primary MCAS** = clonal or identified intrinsic defects, such as mutations in the c-kit gene or downstream signaling molecules, such as systemic Mastocytosis;
• **Secondary** = nonclonal, or extrinsic factors, causing the nearby upstanding mast cells to "break bad", such as detected allergen-specific IgE (food, airborne substances or medications), physical urticarias (solar, cold, cholinergic, and pressure); and autoimmune disorders, such as Sjogren's disease, Hashimoto's thyroiditis and autoimmune urticaria); and,
• After much scientific pursuit with available tools and no current answers for mast cell activation (MCA) events, patients receive the diagnosis of **Idiopathic MCAS** - " to be determined".

Note that at least two organ systems must be involved to be considered for a MCAS diagnosis.

The first diagnostic challenge of mast cell dysfunction is that both patients and medical providers tend to focus on a single sign or symptom, rather than the constellation of symptoms that readily involve different organ systems. Or the patient has a constitutional symptom, for which one organ system may be involved, such as fatigue, headache, or abdominal pain. With few healthcare systems integrated or lacking specialists, such as an allergy/immunology specialist, the opportunity to see the connections between or the overlap of symptoms often is lost.

The next diagnostic challenge is the detection of biomarkers that indicate increases in tryptase level, and even a small increase in serum total tryptase over baseline levels is considered proof of systemic MCA. Additionally, it might take a while to identify the biomarkers. However, it is nearly impossible to get emergency department personnel to assess a serum tryptase level within hours of a suspected MCAS flare. A baseline serum tryptase level should be measured at the initial visit, and then the patient should be provided with a script to check a serum tryptase with 4-6 hours of a suspected mast cell activation event, and then at least 24 hours after complete resolution of all signs and symptoms. If the patient shows an elevated baseline level of tryptase, this suggests systemic Mastocytosis, which warrants an evaluation for this clonal mast cell activation disease. Systemic Mastocytosis should be suspected in patients with flushing, abdominal pain, diarrhea, unexplained syncope, anaphylaxis to stinging insects, and classic urticaria pigmentosa lesions. *(Akin, 2017) (Theoharides, et al., 2015) (Hamilton, 2018) (Golden & Carter, 2019).*

Other mast cell-derived mediators are suggestive of MCAS, but take note that other cells, including basophils and neutrophils, can produce histamine or prostaglandin D2 metabolites. Also, two markers that have been utilized by some providers, but has little primary data supporting a MCAS diagnosis, are serum histamine, chromogranin A and heparin. Utilization of these unvalidated markers can lead to delayed diagnosis and under-utilization of corresponding treatments of "an unrelated, overlooked disease" *(Fuerst, 2014) (Akin, 2017) (Valent & Akin, 2019).*

Unlike most immune cells, which can be readily detected with blood tests, mast cells live in the tissue. Therefore, checking for atypical mast cells, in the tissue of affected organ systems, such as the gastrointestinal tract, bone marrow and skin, can also fulfill the lab requirement for the MCAS diagnosis. Often, patients that have already undergone repeat endoscopies and colonoscopies, but the pathologists were not made aware to use the correct stains to detect mast cells. All is not lost; if there are fresh tissue blocks frozen and stored, then a request can be sent to run stains that detect mast cells: CD117 and Tryptase, for example. A classic clonal mast cell activation disorder, such as systemic Mastocytosis can be detected with biopsy of an affected organ, including bone marrow, gastro-intestinal tract *(Akin, 2017) (The Mastocytosis Society, 2017) (Theoharides, et al., 2015) (Valent & Akin, 2019).*

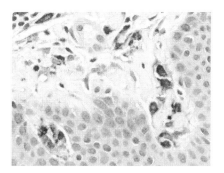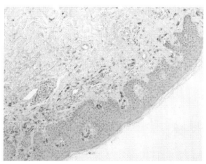

Figure. Systemic Mastocytosis (SM) Typical anti-tryptase immunohistochemistry in skin biopsies: Diagnostic criteria include the detection of multifocal dense infiltrates of mast cells (≥15 mast cells in aggregates) or >25% of all mast cells are atypical cells, or in bone marrow biopsies and/or in sections of other extracutaneous organ(s), such as the skin or gastro-intestinal tract.

> *On a good day, my shoulders, knees, and hips will dislocate two to five times apiece. The slightest bump into a table or door will bloom new bruises on my arms and legs or tear a gash in the thin skin on my hands. My blood pressure will plummet each time I stand, making me feel woozy, nauseated, and weak. I'll have trouble focusing and remembering words. I'll run my errands from underneath an umbrella to prevent an allergic reaction to the Sun. I have Ehlers-Danlos Syndrome (EDS), Postural Orthostatic Tachycardia Syndrome (POTS), and Mast Cell Activation Syndrome (MCAS) – a trifecta of weird diseases. POTS, EDS, and MCAS are so obscure that many doctors have never even heard of them. – Kate Horowitz, 2016*

369

Another genetic disorder associated with mast cell activation disease is hyper-alpha-tryptasemia (HαT). Associated with either a modest elevation or a normal serum tryptase, this autosomal dominant, inherited disorder has been associated with dysregulation of the three cell populations that underprop our bodies' homeostasis. HαT is associated with multisystem complaints including (1) cutaneous flushing and pruritus; (2) dysautonomia, functional gastrointestinal symptoms, chronic pain; and (3) connective tissue abnormalities, including joint hypermobility.

In addition to detection of duplications, triplications and quadruplications of the TPSAB1 gene encoding α-tryptase, a recent report noted subtle, but significant, changes in the appearance of mast cells in HαT patients. Compared to normal controls and patients with other forms of non-clonal MCAS, HαT patients exhibited an increased number of these normally solitary immune sentinels form a greater number of small clusters. Moreover, these observations shows promise in pointing to a potential connection between variations in mast cell endotypes and some of these multi-systemic complaints in individuals with hypermobility disorder, where tryptase may possibly be playing a role in modifying the connective tissue.

Please note that you and your health care professional need to look for MCAS, like emergency departments and cardiologists do so for heart attacks. When investigating whether a heart attack has occurred, there are electrocardiograms, stress tests, blood tests to detect for leaked cardiac specific proteins, enzymes, and MRI/MRA exams. For mast cell dysfunction, one also needs to look at different angles at different times to understand whether the mast cell compartment has gone awry. Do not give up on a single blood test, such as urine methylhistamine or tryptase.

The third criterion, for the MCAS diagnosis, focuses on the improvement of symptoms with medications that either directly target the mast cell compartment or that attenuate the action of mast cell derived mediators. As seen in other disorders associated with recurrent mast cell activation, such as asthma and chronic spontaneous urticaria, patients with suspected mast cell activation disease who note an improvement of their symptoms with the following agents, fulfills the last proposed criterion for MCAS diagnosis:

Mast Cell Targeted Therapies				
Histamine Receptor-1	Histamine Receptor-2	Tricyclic Agents	Leukotriene Antagonists	Mast cell Stabilizers
Chlorpheniramine	Famotidine	Amitriptyline	Montelukast	Ketotifen
Diphenhydramine	Cimetidine	Doxepin	Zafirlukast	Cromones
Hydroxyzine		Imipramine	Zilueton	
Cetirizine		Nortriptyline		
Desloratadine				
Loratadine				
Levocetirizine				
fexofenadine				

Reflecting the need for practitioners to team up in the diagnosis and management of mast cell activation disorders, one of the first reports describing non-clonal MCAS (not Mastocytosis) was a joint effort between the Allergy/Immunology and Gastroenterology specialists at Brigham & Women's Hospital. Stepping outside their area of clinical expertise, the gastroenterologists decided to ask patients, who had been followed in this clinic for Irritable Bowel Syndrome, for years, whether they have or ever had symptoms of rhinitis, neurocognitive challenges, asthma, urticaria, or anaphylaxis. In this prospective study, eighteen patients, who had been in the IBS clinic on average for 5 years, met the first criterion of symptoms: beyond the gastro-intestinal tract, each individual reported at least one organ system, whether it was rhinitis, mood disorder, or itchy skin, such as the physical urticaria, dermographism. Subsequent testing, which had not been performed before, revealed that these patients had elevated mast cell derived mediators (serum tryptase or urinary mediators,

371

such as prostaglandin D2, 11-Beta-Prostaglandin F2 Alpha, or methylhistamine). Interestingly, most of these patients with the newly diagnosed MCAS refused to give up the medications that targeted MCs, after changing the medical regimen away from conventional IBS medications. The effectiveness of histamine receptor-1 (cetirizine, loratadine, diphenhydramine) and histamine receptor-2 blockade (famotidine, cimetidine, ranitidine) in the reduction of symptoms in this former group of just "IBS" patients fulfilled the 3rd criterion for MCAS diagnosis.

What if I only meet two of three MCAS criteria? Be prepared for MCAS masqueraders.

> The [MCAS] diagnosis is sometimes applied to patients with vague yet suggestive symptoms. These patients may suffer from an unrelated, overlooked disease. Applying solid diagnostic criteria when considering the [MCAS] diagnosis helps avoid wasting time and money. Certain cardiovascular disorders, endocrine disorders, neoplasms, GI diseases, primary skin diseases, infectious diseases, and neurologic or psychiatric disorders are among the numerous conditions sometimes confused with [MCAS]. (Fuerst, 2014)

Of the 3 criteria, obtaining data supporting aberrant mast cell action is the most challenging. Gratefully, while efforts are being coordinated to investigate the role of mast cells in your constellation of symptoms, medications used to target mast cells have a benign side effect profile compared to agents that treat cancer, for example. Nonetheless, you must be also prepared to consider that MCAS may not be the driving force. That is, symptoms such headache syndromes, abdominal pain, neurocognitive disorders, and fatigue can be caused by illnesses other than MCAS.

Conditions that can mimic MCAS	
Cardiovascular	Coronary hypersensitivity (the Kounis syndrome), Postural orthostatic tachycardia syndrome.

Endocrine	Fibromyalgia Parathyroid tumor Pheochromocytoma Carcinoid syndrome.
Digestive	Adverse reaction to food, Eosinophilic esophagitis, Eosinophilic gastroenteritis, Gastroesophageal reflux disease, Gluten enteropathy, Irritable bowel syndrome, Vasoactive intestinal peptide–secreting tumor (VIP).
Immunologic	Auto-inflammatory disorders such as deficiency of inter-leukin-1–receptor antagonist, Familial hyper-IgE syndrome, Vasculitis.
Neurologic/psychiatric	Anxiety, Chronic fatigue syndrome, Depression, Headaches; Mixed organic brain syndrome, Somatization disorder; Autonomic dysfunction, Multiple sclerosis.
Skin	Angioedema, Atopic dermatitis, Chronic urticaria, Scleroderma.

Disorders that can mimic MCAS, or that have symptoms that overlap with MCAS, include dysautonomia/postural orthostatic tachycardia syndrome (POTS), neuropsychiatric conditions, certain ailments involving the cardiovascular and endocrine systems, infectious disorders, gastrointestinal illnesses, some cancers, as well as primary skin disorders. So, it is important to be diligent in applying the MCAS diagnostic criteria when undergoing an evaluation of your symptoms. This will prevent delays to securing the best working diagnosis and tailored, more effective treatments.

Mast Cell Activation Disorders

Sneezing? Congested? Runny Nose? Mucus in the throat? Rhinitis affects nearly one in three of us, which predisposes to headache syndromes.

Can take a deep breath? Notice chest tightness that comes and goes? Coughing? Wheezing? Breathless? Because general practitioners do not screen for asthma, the actual prevalence of those affected by this common lung disorder is a 'guess – estimate': approximately 1 of 10 have been treated for asthma exacerbation, and nearly 10 people die from an asthma exacerbation daily.

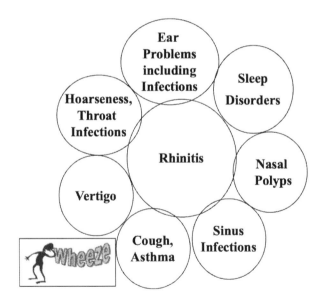

Itchy, red rashes? Scratching from eczema or atopic or contact dermatitis? There is 1 out 5 individuals will experience urticaria (hives)/angioedema (swelling) and 2% US population affected sleep disturbing eczema;

Itchy mouth with fresh fruit? Feel lightheaded or difficulty breathing or increased gastro-intestinal distress after eating a meal that you did not prepare? 4-5 % US population have food allergies, and more have food intolerances, not explained by classic food allergy testing.

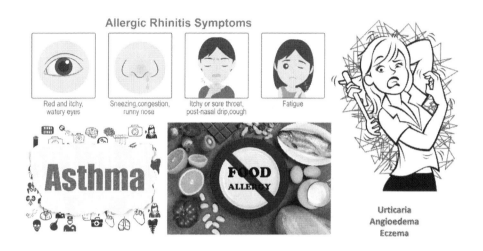

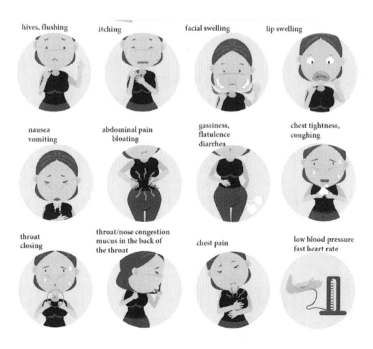

Anaphylaxis

By 2015, nearly 2 out of 100 of Americans had been treated for anaphylaxis, and more are carrying emergency medications, such as oral histamine blockers and epinephrine, in case of a serious hypersensitivity reaction to insect sting, foodstuff, medication, airborne chemical, and, for some, physical changes.

MCAS Treatment / Management Recommendations:

> Translational research and precision medicine are based on a profound knowledge of cellular and molecular mechanisms contributing to various physiologic processes and pathologic reactions in diverse organs. Whereas specific molecular interactions and mechanisms have been identified during the past 5 decades, the underlying principles were defined much earlier and originate from to the seminal observations made by outstanding researchers between 1850 and 1915. One of the most outstanding exponents of these scientists is Paul Ehrlich. His work resulted not only in the foundation and birth of modern hematology and immunology, but also led to the development of chemotherapy and specific targeted treatment concepts. (Valent, et al., 2016)

In addition to describing the presence of mast cells throughout the human body, Paul Ehrlich is also considered to be one of the pioneers of translational, if not personalized medicine, which focuses on the development of treatments based on the identified dysregulated pathways, contributing to disease.

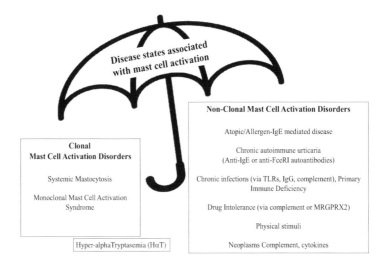

Given that mast cell activation disease comprises a heterogenous group of "mast cell mediator disorders" *(Theoharides, et al., 2019)*, treatment must be tailored to counter the triggers of aberrant mast cell activation and key mediators released by the distinct MC degranulation and secretion events. For example, mast cell activation events triggered by Toll like receptors (TLRs) leads to increased secretion of de novo produced pro-inflammatory cytokines, such as tumor necrosis factor, TNF alpha (TNF), and Interluekin-6 (IL-6), but not the release of histamine and tryptase. In contrast, Immunoglobin or Complement receptor engagement leads to degranulation events, including release of cytokines, histamine and proteases, such as tryptase. Consequently, using histamine blockers to reduce inflammation triggered by an infection in the nose recognized by TLR, will not block several components of this MC activation event. While allergen-specific IGE triggered MC degranulation, likely respond to therapies that block mast cell degranulation and the release of histamine, for example. Moreover, different MC activation disorders can overlap, as described in a recent case report of a patient has systemic Mastocytosis, venom specific serum IgE, hyper-alpha-tryptasemia, and alpha gal syndrome *(Golden & Carter, 2019)*; patients with immunodeficiency syndromes can present with non-clonal mast cell activation disorders *(Arkwright & Gennery, 2014)*; and several reports have described an increased prevalence of **MCAD in Ehlers Danlos Syndrome and autonomic dysfunction disorders**. *(Cheung & Vadas, 2012) (Louisias, et al., 2013) (Chan & Jongco, 2015) (Lee & Mueller, 2017)*

MCAD is a chronic hypersensitivity disorder, with distinct phenotypes, based on range of triggers, route of exposure, pattern of chemical mediators released, organ involvement, severity, and co-morbid disorders (Wilfox , et al., 2018) (Sala-Cunil, et al., 2018). Consequently, therapeutic recommendations should be based on organ system involvement, severity, co-morbid disorders, and identified inflammatory phenotypes – allergy? Nonatopic, including physical triggers? Autoimmune disorders? Primary immunodeficiencies? Current treatment recommendations should be tailored to address the identified phenotypes/endotypes, with implementation and appropriate follow-up to assess efficacy and identify potential adverse reactions to the recommended therapies.

In addition to medications known to attenuate the action of mast cells or mast cell-derived mediators, such as the use of H1 – and H2 – histamine receptor blockers, anti-leukotriene medications, mast cell stabilizers, and the monoclonal antibody omalizumab, treatment recommendations should be designed to target the identified co-morbid illnesses that are driving mast cells to "misbehave".

Mast Cell Phenotype	Possible Treatment Options
Allergen-IgE (Atopic) Nonatopic (Irritant, Vasomotor, e.g.)	Avoidance measures (Diet, Environment) Histamine blockade Leukotriene blockade Tricyclic agents Ketotifen Cromolyn Corticosteroids Desensitization/Immunotherapy Omalizumab Dupilumab
Infections	Targeted anti-microbial therapy
Primary Immune Deficiency	Prophylactic Antibiotics Immune Globulin Anti-inflammatory Agents
Autoimmune Disorders	Anti-inflammatory Agents Immune Globulin
Autonomic Dysfunction	Physical / Occupational Therapy Oxygen Therapy Acupuncture

Figure. Treatments listed above are for informational purposes only and not intended to be a substitute for professional medical advice, diagnosis, or treatment. Always seek the advice of your physician or other qualified health providers with any questions you may have regarding a medical condition.

Moreover, partnering with a heath care practitioner who is willing to learn about your disorders, select appropriate testing, coordinate referrals to other specialists, and review potential therapies is key to restoring homeostasis, with reformed mast cells.

Key Points:

• Mast cell disorders can be detected with the use of multiple diagnostic approaches, starting with a thorough review of systems and personal history taking. Repeat testing, over time, may be needed to capture that elevated mast cell-derived marker, the type of mast cell dysregulation, and to measure mediator release following a triggering event.

• Medications targeting mast cells not only help secure the diagnosis of MCAS, but hopefully provide temporary relief to one's symptoms. Then, these can be used to calm down inflammation, so that mast cells are not called into action.

• Mast cells have a myriad of surface receptors that allow interaction with surrounding structures and cells. As a result, dysregulation of the mast cell compartment can result in a host of symptoms and likely contributes co-morbid illnesses.

• The MCAS diagnosis is assigned to patients with at least two organ systems with mast cell-driven signs and symptoms.

Therefore, a multi-disciplinary team, with team effort across specialists, and with you and your primary care physician as copilots, is needed to start feeling better. Remember, mast cells have a job to do: tissue surveillance, defense, and repair. Therefore, mast cells are in constant bi-directional communication with the surrounding connective tissue and nearby cells. So, it should not be surprising that disorders arising in connective tissue or impacting nerve function may mimic mast cell activation syndrome. Efforts are now focused on understanding the miscommunication between the mast cell compartment, connective tissue and the nervous system.

2. Complements and Practical Aspects

By Doctor Stéphane Daens, MD, DATC

Mast cell activation disorders (MCADs) are condition in which mast cells have an excessive propensity to degranulate, i.e., to release various substances previously concentrated in intracellular granules. They can mass degranulate from mild, unusual or inappropriate stimuli, the origin of which may or may not be known. The mast cell count is within normal limits, thus eliminating a diagnosis of Mastocytosis. Its diagnosis is usually based on the patient's clinic. The blood tryptase level (tryptasemia) is usually normal in MCADs related to EDS, in contrast to other conditions such as Mastocytosis or MCAS (mast cell activation syndrome); the same for idiopathic anaphylaxis, hereditary tryptasemia syndrome, or certain hematologic malignancies (elevated blood tryptase level).

➢ In Mastocytosis, there is a local or generalized proliferation of mast cells; thus, it is a neoplasia secondary to a genetic mutation that results in clonal proliferation (a cell begins to divide wildly). The tryptase level is elevated (see below).

➢ In hereditary α-tryptasemia syndrome (HαT)[167], the patient has inherited several copies of the TPSAB1 gene. This syndrome was only discovered in 2016 by researchers at the *National Institute of Allergy and Infectious Diseases*. It is an autosomal dominant genetic disorder. The TPSAB1 gene is located on chromosome 16 (locus 16p13.3) and codes for either β1-tryptase or α1-tryptase (these are the two alleles of the gene). In almost 90% of cases, patients with hereditary α-tryptasemia have duplicated the TPSAB1 gene on chromosome 16 (they have two copies rather than one). In less than 10% of cases, patients have a triplication (they have three copies of the TPSAB1 gene on one of the two homologous chromosomes). In rare cases, there are more additional α-extra-copies. The more copies of this gene in the

---

[167] Sprinzl B, Greiner G, Uyanik G, et al. Genetic Regulation of Tryptase Production and Clinical Impact: Hereditary Alpha Tryptasemia, Mastocytosis and Beyond. Int J Mol Sci. 2021;22(5):2458. doi: 10.3390/ijms22052458.

patient, the higher the tryptasemia level and the more marked the symptoms. Note that 4-6% of the general population would have elevated baseline tryptasemia (>11.4 µg/L), without apparent cause. The majority of these may have hereditary α-tryptasemia syndrome.

➤ A variety of other hematological conditions may also present with elevated tryptasemia, such as chronic eosinophilic leukemia, myelodysplastic syndrome (MDS), acute myeloid leukemia (AML), or chronic myeloid leukemia (CML), etc.

The mast cell was discovered by Paul Ehrlich (Prussia 1854 - German Empire 1915), a physician considered the Father of chemotherapy. He was awarded the Nobel Prize in Physiology and Medicine in 1908 for his work on immunity in collaboration with Ilya Ilitch Metchnikov (Russian Empire 1845 – France 1916).

The mast cell comes from a pluripotent stem cell of the bone marrow and belongs to the innate branch of the immune system. Although it is known to be of hematopoietic origin, its precise origin remains uncertain: does it derive from a common precursor with the myeloid lineage in general (CD34+/CD117+ progenitor) or, more specifically with that of the basophil polynuclear cell? In any case, they emerge relatively *adolescent* from the bone marrow, finishing their maturation and becoming adult in particular tissues, in interface with the environment: the skin, the digestive mucosa, the respiratory mucosa in the broad sense (nose, sinuses, respiratory mucosa including bronchi but also laryngeal or pharyngeal regions), the urogenital mucosa; but also in the dura mater (spinal cord), the cerebral meninges, the muscles and joints. Mast cells have a sentinel role, one could say.

I often picture, for patients, the mast cells of MCADs to the Taz in Warner Bross cartoons, a furious and touchy little Tasmanian devil, versus Tex Avery's Droopy, a calm and phlegmatic little dog, in people without MCADs. This is an easy metaphor to remember.

Mast cells and basophils have in common that they are the only ones to express on their surface the complete tetrameric form (αβγ2) of a receptor with a high affinity for IgE: the RFcεI. The chain αβγ2 allows to increase their signaling capacity very strongly. This allows a very rapid release (within minutes) of the substances stored in their granules (degranulation). Degranulation, of course, occurs because of the [allergen-IgE-receptor] interaction, but not only. This rapid release of granules can also occur in response to other stimuli such as neuropeptides, microbial substances, cytokines, lysosomal enzymes, venoms or anaphylatoxins, NO synthetase, endothelin, kinins. The release of granules to the outside of the mast cell is massive, complete, and rapid. These granules contain various substances: histamine, serotonin, enzymes such as proteases (tryptase, chymase, carboxypeptidase A), cytokines, and chemokines (TNFα, IL-8, MCP-1), proteoglycans (e.g., heparin).

- Their effects: vasodilation, increased vascular permeability, increased white blood cell adhesion, bronchoconstriction (which can induce asthma).

In a slightly later or semi-delayed phase, between 15 and 30 minutes after the stimulus, lipid mediators, formed from phospholipids located in the cell membrane, are released: prostaglandins, leukotrienes, PAF (platelet aggregation factor).

- Their effects: they prolong the effect of the first rapid phase and prepare the ground for the delayed phase.

Finally, after several hours (this is the delayed-release or delayed phase), de novo synthesized substances are released, such as cytokines, chemokines, and growth factors (IL-3, IL-4, IL-5, IL-6, IL-8, IL-10, IL-13, TNFα, etc.).

- Their effects: they maintain inflammation, increase the recruitment and the activation and survival of white blood cells, influence the response of lymphocytes, etc.

These three successive steps allow an excellent adaptation of mast cell action. In contact with nerve endings and blood vessels, mast cells have a role in nociception and central sensitization (see this chapter). The interactions between immune cells and the central nervous system, the so-called neuroimmune interface, in the genesis and maintenance of peripheral and central sensitization phenomena have been the focus of many studies in recent years.[168]

In MCADs, the diagnosis is essentially clinical and can be made without difficulty. The blood levels of tryptase are usually within the normal range, the release of substances by mast cells being intermittent and less important than in Mastocytosis or MCAS.

The American Academy of Allergy Asthma and Immunology (AAAAI), recently described the diagnosis and management of MCAS: *Weiler CR, Austen KF, Akin C et al. AAAAI Mast Cell Disorders Committee Work Group report : Mast cell activation syndrome (MCAS) diagnosis and management. J Allergy Clin Immunol. 2019;144:883-896.*

"This classification includes three types of 'MCA Syndromes' (MCASs), namely primary MCAS, secondary MCAS and idiopathic MCAS. MCA is now defined by robust and generally applicable criteria, including (1) typical clinical symptoms, (2) a substantial transient increase in serum total tryptase level or an increase in other MC-derived mediators, such as histamine or prostaglandin D_2, or their urinary metabolites, and (3) a response of clinical symptoms to agents that attenuate the production or activities of MC mediators. These criteria should assist in the identification and diagnosis of patients with MCAS, and in avoiding misdiagnoses or overinterpretation of clinical symptoms in daily practice. " [169]

These attacks must be accompanied by an increase in certain mediators' blood or urine levels released by the activated mast cells. This increase in levels must be found on two or more occasions to establish a definite diagnosis.

---

[168] Aich A, Afrin LB, Gupta K. Mast Cell-Mediated Mechanisms of Nociception. Int J Mol Sci. 2015;16(12):29069-92. doi: 10.3390/ijms161226151.

[169] Valent P, Akin C, Arock M, et al. Definitions, criteria and global classification of mast cell disorders with special reference to mast cell activation syndromes: a consensus proposal. Int Arch Allergy Immunol. 2012;157(3):215-25. doi: 10.1159/000328760

Mediators:

Urinary:
  ➤ N-Methyl-Histamine (NMH)
  ➤ 11β-$PGF_{2\alpha}$ (platelet growth factor)
  ➤ LTD_4 / LTE_4

At the blood level:
  ➤ Tryptase

Histamine (2-[4-imidazolyl]-ethylamine) is produced from a semi-essential amino acid, L-Histidine. It is produced by mast cells and eosinophilic cells, and other cells such as lymphocytes, neutrophils, monocytes, macrophages, and keratinocytes. Bacteria can also release histamine (from mucous membranes or a contaminated meal). It is rapidly metabolized and results in the production of N-Methyl-Histamine (NMH). The determination of urinary NMH is of little interest in the diagnosis of MCAD, but it can help in combination with other markers.

The serum tryptase level (tryptasemia) can be useful if the baseline level is compared with the level in the MCAD crisis. Blood should be drawn between 30 minutes and 2 hours after the onset of clinical symptoms, but significantly elevated levels may be found up to 4-6 hours after the onset of symptomatology. This acute tryptase level (sAT) should be compared with the baseline tryptase level or the level in a blood sample taken at least 24 hours after signs and symptoms have resolved (sBT). A formula has been established to determine whether the level is significantly pathological or not:

$$[sAT > (1.2 \times sBT) + 2]$$

The specificity is high (>90%), but the sensitivity depends on the time of sampling, the severity of clinical signs and symptoms, and the trigger.

Prostaglandin (PG) is produced from arachidonic acid. This is first converted by the action of COX-1 or COX-2 (cyclooxygenases) to PGH_2. PGH_2 is in turn transformed into PGD_2 via PGD synthetase. PGD_2 is metabolized to 11β-$PGF_{2\alpha}$, which can be assayed in blood or 24-hour urine (11β-PGF2$_\alpha$/creatinine) according to the European Competence Network on Mastocytosis Consensus Conference (2012). The currently available test is a urine test. If the level is high in EDS, treatment with Aspirin is preferred to non-steroidal anti-inflammatory drugs (NSAIDs).

Leukotrienes are produced from arachidonic acid. Under the action of 5-lipoxygenase, LTA$_4$ is obtained. Then, thanks to a particular synthetase, LTA$_4$ is transformed into LTC$_4$ (cysteinyl leukotriene), which can be measured in the urine. One of its metabolites, LTE$_4$, which is more stable, can also be measured. In patients with high levels, Montelukast is the drug of choice.

It is inappropriate to measure heparin, chromogranin A, or plasma histamine.

Conclusions regarding biomarkers:
- An increase in one or more markers indicates mast cell disease in the broadest sense.
- Baseline levels should always be compared with acute levels (anaphylaxis, Quincke's syndrome), especially for blood tryptase, but certainly also for urinary NMH.

In Mastocytosis, the serum tryptase level is generally higher than 20 µg/liter (in 75% of cases), and a mutation of the c-kit gene (CD117, receptor for the stem cell factor, the main growth factor of mast cells) should be sought. The D816V mutation is the most common and is detected in more than 70% of patients with indolent systemic Mastocytosis (look for it in blood, skin, bone marrow, or other extracutaneous organs).

Note that significant external heat (weather temperatures, hot shower, or bath, etc.), intense physical activity, variation in atmospheric pressure, stress, and alcohol intake increase mast cell degranulation. A typical example is barbecuing in summer.

Tissue hypoxia causes mast cells to release interleukin 6. Interleukin-6 increases the survival and degranulation of mast cells and thus the release of their cytokines. This is a self-perpetuating loop. In EDS, disorders of respiratory proprioception, muscle fatigability, blockages and weakness of the diaphragm and accessory inspiratory muscles may also promote or aggravate hypoxia in certain pulmonary zones attacked by the infection. This could, in turn, exacerbate mast cell activation and locoregional inflammation. Treatments aimed at blocking interleukin-6 receptors would therefore be useful in certain infections such as covid-19. Such substances (Tocilizumab or RoActemra, a monoclonal antibody directed against the interleukin-6 receptor) are used to treat rheumatoid arthritis that is refractory to conventional treatments such as DMARDs (immunosuppressive drugs). In the case of covid-19, there is what is called a cytokine storm (cytokine release syndrome), with an increase in IL-6 concentrations.[170]

Regarding oxygen therapy: Sequential oxygen therapy in EDS patients could therefore also calm mast cells, and thus reduce the signs and symptoms of MCAD.

Until recently, it was considered that about 66% of EDS patients were MCA carriers, but now the trend is towards 80%! The cause of this high prevalence of MCA in EDS is not fully understood. Perhaps it is a consequence of the maturation of mast cells in connective tissue altered by EDS. The interactions and relationships between the central nervous system, the peripheral nervous system, the ANS, the gut microbiota, and mast cells (and their role in central sensitization) are avenues to investigate in EDS.

My opinion

In practice, it is illusory to measure serum tryptase in EDS patients with MCA. Indeed, these patients do not go from one angioedema or anaphylactic shock to another! They usually have an MCA every day of the year.

---

[170] Zhang Z, Wu Z, Li J-W et al. The cytokine release syndrome (CRS) of severe COVID-19 and interleukine-6 receptor (IL-6R) antagonist tocilizumab may be the key to reduce the mortality. Int J Antimicrob Agents. 2020. Doi:10.1016/j.ijantimicag.2020.105954.

So when should tryptase be measured? How do you compare the baseline level with the acute level? This is almost impossible in practice. On the other hand, bone marrow biopsy is not recommended in EDS, at least not routinely. The risk of bleeding is present and makes these procedures dangerous. Therefore, it is more appropriate to base oneself on the clinic and try a trial treatment, than to carry out useless or even dangerous examinations. All this, keeping in mind that potentially 80% of EDS patients have signs and symptoms of MCA.

This attitude is, to me, pure conjecture and completely counterproductive. It reminds me of the classification of hEDS and HSD, which is confusing for both caregivers and patients. Whether it is hEDS/HSD or MCADs/MCAS, it does not matter which box you are in; the care and treatment should be the same. This is an intellectual complication, not a simplification to treat the most patients efficiently. We need to stop creating mazes from which it will be more complicated than for Icarus to get out. And once again, who will pay the bill? The patients...

The treatments of MCAD can therefore complement those of EDS if necessary:

➢ Anti-H1 antihistamines combined with anti-H2 antihistamines used in the first line to block mast cell histamine receptors. Anti-H2 drugs help the action of anti-H1 drugs, especially in the case of cardiovascular events.

   o Example : Desloratadine, Rupatadine, Ketotifen, Levocetirizine, etc.

➢ Montelukast may have value as a leukotriene receptor antagonist; it is also a mast cell membrane enhancer. It works well in case of respiratory symptoms (bronchospasm) and/or digestive disorders related to MCAD. Cautions have been brought to the attention of physicians by drug monitoring agencies regarding the risk of psychological disorders when taking this molecule. [171] Therefore, it is not a first-line

---

[171] Clarridge K, Chin S, Eworuke E, et al. A Boxed Warning for Montelukast: The FDA Perspective. J Allergy Clin Immunol Pract. 202;9(7):2638-2641. doi: 10.1016/j.jaip.2021.02.057

treatment, except in the case of initial treatment that proves insufficient to control MCAD.

➤ Oral sodium Cromoglycate is interesting as a mast cell membrane enhancer, especially in case of digestive food intolerance.

➤ Simple medications such as vitamin C, N-acetylcysteine, alpha-lipoic acid, and even cannabinoids or flavonoid analogs can be added.

➤ Aspirin (or acetylsalicylic acid) is interesting at doses of at least 625mg, twice a day. It is highly active in case of signs and symptoms related to prostaglandins (flush, hypotension). Use with caution in EDS due to increased risk of bleeding.

➤ Corticosteroids are not encouraged, except in cases of acute airway involvement or incredibly significant skin involvement (anaphylaxis, Quincke's syndrome).

PRACTICE SHEET: What to do?

Examinations to be done in the emergency room:

➤ Complete clinical and anamnestic examination.

➤ Determination of serum tryptase (normal baseline values up to 13.5µg/liter, to be determined during and 24 hours after the attack); exclusion of Mastocytosis (tryptase >20µg/liter).

➤ Measure NMH, PGD_2 and LT_4/LTE_4, if available routinely.

➤ Rx thorax (front and side).

➤ Rx abdomen blank lying and standing.

➤ Microscopic and chemical examination of urine.

➤ Electrocardiogram (ECG) + continuous heart rate monitoring and repeated blood pressure measurements.

➤ Oxygen saturation (finger oximeter).

> Advice from a dermatologist and/or hematologist and/or internist familiar with MCAD. Seek advice from an allergist, if necessary.

Treatments to start in the emergency room (personal regimen):

> Type 1 antihistamines: for example, combine Desloratadine 5mg (or another molecule) morning and evening + Rupatadine 20mg at lunchtime (i.e., three or sometimes four doses of anti-H1 per day). Ketotifen (Zaditen®) can also be used (evening).

> Type 2 antihistamines: Ranitidine 300mg, Famotidine 40mg or Cimetidine (if available). Preferably taken in the evening (to also decrease acid reflux during the night).

> Anti-Leukotrienes: Montelukast 10 mg in the morning (in the evening, it often gives nightmares and sleep disorders in EDS). Beware of psychological precautions.

> Vitamin C, 3 x 1 gram/day. Vitamin C increases degradation of histamine and decreases histamine formation by inhibition of histidine decarboxylase.

> N-Acetylcysteine 600mg, twice a day. It can also be given intravenously (300mg/3ml ampoules, slow IV or infusion).

> Aspirin (acetylsalicylic acid): 625mg, twice daily.

> Gastrointestinal protection (e.g., pantoprazole 40mg).

> Trendelenburg position (lumbosacral position): the patient lies on his back; his legs are placed higher than his head: useful in hypotension.

If necessary:

> Sequential oxygen therapy (with humidifier), 5 liters per minute (nasal canula, oxygen mask), with or without breathing difficulties (asthma, bronchial hyperreactivity, asthmatic bronchitis).

- ➤ Bronchodilators (in aerosols, if necessary): in case of asthma, bronchial hyperreactivity. Beware of secondary tachyarrhythmias.

- ➤ In case of extreme necessity: methylprednisolone 125mg bolus IV. Then 40mg, 2 to 3x/day in the acute phase.

- ➤ Aprepitant is a neurokinin 1, NK1 receptor agonist (tachykinin receptor); it is antagonistic to substance P (SP). SP is known to be involved in the development of pain, nausea, vomiting, and pruritus (skin itching). It is also used as an antiemetic (against vomiting) during certain cancer chemotherapies. Various studies show its interest in managing specific manifestations of MCAD, such as intense refractory pruritus, by acting on skin cells called keratinocytes. There are 80mg and 125mg tablets. A dose of 125mg can be used on the first day and then 80mg/day (variable duration from a few days to a few weeks or months).

Bibliography:

He A, Alhariri JM, Sweren RJ et al. Aprepitant for the treatment of chronic refractory pruritus. BioMed Research International 2017. Doi.org/10.1155/2017/4790810.

Li W, Guo T, Liang D et al. Substance P signaling controls mast cell activation, degranulation, and nociceptive sensitization in a rat fracture model of complex regional pain syndrome. Anesthesiology. 2012; 116 (4):882-895.

Kwatra SG, Boozalis E, Huang AH et al. Proteomic and phoshoproteomic analysis reveals that neurokinine-1 receptor (NK1R) blockade with Aprepitant in human keratinocytes activates a distinct subdomain of EGFR signaling: implications for the anti-pruritic activity of NK1R antagonists. Medicines. 2019;6(114). Doi:10.3390/medicines6040114.

Blank U, Vitte J. Les médiateurs des mastocytes. Revue française d'allergologie. 2014

Aich A, Afrin LB, Gupta K. Mast Cell-mediated mechanisms of nociception. Int J Mol Sci. 2015;16:29069-29092; doi:10.3390/ijms161226151.

Gullikson M, Carvalho RFS, Ulleras E et al. Mast cell and mediator secretion in response to hypoxia. PLoS one. 2010;5(8):e12360.

Yang J, Wang J, Zhang X et al. Mast cell degranulation impairs pneumococcus clearance in mice via IL-6 dependent and TNF-α independent mechanisms. World Allergy Organization Journal. 2019;12:e100028. Doi.101016/j.waojou.2019.100028.

Seneviratne L Maitland A, Afrin L. Mast cell disorders in Ehlers-Danlos syndrome. Am J Med Genet C Semin Med Genet. 2017;175(1):226-236.

Lyons JJ. Hereditary alpha tryptasemia: genotyping and associated clinical features. Immunol Allergy Clin North Am. 2018;38(3):483-495.

Gao Y, Li T, Han M et al. Diagnostic utility of clinical laboratory data determinations for patients with the severe COVID-19. J Med Virol. 2020;10.1002/jmv.25770. doi:10.1002/jmv.25770.

CHAPTER IX

Central Sensitization and Chronic Pain Algoneurodystrophy and Causalgia

By Dr. Stéphane Daens, in collaboration with:

Dr. Pradeep CHOPRA,
Pain Management Center of RI and
Assistant Professor at Brown Medical School, RI, USA

Central Sensitization and Chronic Pain

By Dr. Pradeep Chopra

Pain can be classified as two types – acute pain and chronic pain. Acute pain is provoked by a specific disease or injury and is self-limited. Chronic pain may be considered a disease state. It is pain that lasts the normal time of healing. Chronic pain serves no biologic purpose, and has no recognizable end point. The management of acute pain and chronic pain are very different. Management of acute pain depends on treating the underlying cause and interrupting the pain signals. The management of chronic pain is far more challenging because it may persist even after the underlying cause has healed. One of the phenomena about chronic pain is that it persists and even increases. This can be explained by Central Sensitization. Central Sensitization is a key concept in understanding the development and maintenance of chronic pain.

Central Sensitization is the increased responsiveness of nociceptive neurons in the central nervous system to their normal or subthreshold afferent input. There is an increase in membrane excitability, synaptic efficacy or reduced inhibition as a result of increase in the functional status of neurons in the nociceptive pathways.

Under normal circumstances, the spinal cord sends modulatory signals to suppress pain signals. When a constant barrage of pain signals reaches the spinal cord, it causes a shift in the dorsal horn cells to a sensitized mode. The constant barrage of pain signals cause sensitization of the dorsal horn cells resulting in the central nervous system switching from one that suppresses signals to one that enhances its response to a stimulus.

Studies in clinical cohorts of chronic pain states in fibromyalgia, osteoarthritis, musculoskeletal disorders with generalized pain hypersensitivity, headache, temporomandibular joint disorders, dental pain, neuropathic pain, visceral pain hypersensitivity disorders, and postsurgical pain reveal changes in pain sensitivity. These changes have been interpreted as a result of Central Sensitization. Ehlers Danlos Syndromes is one such cohort that presents with all the above clinical pain conditions.

Patients present with heightened sensitivity to pain. This heightened sensitivity can extend to other senses such as sounds, light and smells. Ambient sounds and light can either sound louder or even increase pain in the affected area, a phenomena commonly seen in acute migraine. Some of the other effects are cognitive issues such as poor concentration, insomnia, anxiety, and mental fog. Clinically, in some chronic pain conditions, pain is no longer a protective mechanism. These patients present with spontaneous pain. They may have an exaggerated response to a noxious stimulus, which is called hyperalgesia. They present with allodynia (pain with an innocuous stimuli). These are features of Central Sensitization.

The best way to explain Central Sensitization is by changes to the neuronal NMDA (N-methyl D-Aspartate) receptors in the dorsal horn of the spinal cord. In Central Sensitization, the dorsal horn neurons in the spinal cord develop an increase in spontaneous activity, increased response to suprathreshold stimulation, enlargement of the receptive field and a reduction in the threshold for activation by peripheral stimuli. The nociceptive neurons now behave as wide dynamic range neurons that respond to noxious and non-noxious stimuli (AN : this is the basis of the *wind-up,* or amplification, mechanism. There are two types of neurons in the spinal cord's posterior horn: neurons specific to nociception and non-specific neurons called *wide dynamic range* which react to painful and non-painful stimuli). This progressively leads to an increased response to non-painful stimuli (e.g., mechanical) that lasts much longer than the initial trigger.

Glutamate binds to the AMPA, NMDA (N-methyl D-Aspartate) and KA (Kainate) receptors. When the NMDA receptor is activated it initiates and maintains Central Sensitization. Normally, the NMDA receptor is blocked by magnesium. A continuous barrage of nociceptive pain signals releases glutamate, Substance P and CGRP (Calcitonin Related Gene Peptide). As a result, there is sufficient membrane depolarization to force magnesium to the unblock the NMDA receptor. Once the NMDA receptor is unblocked this allows glutamate to bind to the NMDA receptor, thus generating an inward current. As the voltage dependent block is removed, it boosts the synaptic efficacy and allows calcium to enter the neurons. This helps maintain Central Sensitization. Thus activation of the NMDA receptors is critical in increasing excitability of the neurons.

Substance P is also released with glutamate is important in maintenance of Central Sensitization. It is released by unmyelinated peptidergic nociceptors. Substance P causes long lasting membrane depolarization by binding to the NK1 (Neurokinin-1) receptor.

The effect of substance P is enhanced by CGRP (Calcitonin gene-related Peptide). CGRP is produced by small diameter sensory neurons and increases Central Sensitization by acting on the post-synaptic CGRP1 receptors.

Brain-derived neurotrophic factor (BDNF) is also a synaptic modulator synthesized by nociceptor neurons. It is released into the Central Nervous system in an activity dependent manner. BDNF also plays role in Central Sensitization. The release of BDNF is enhanced by CGRP from Trigeminal nociceptors, thus contributing to the development of migraine.

Painful stimuli activate sensory neurons leading to the release of chemical inflammatory mediators such as Substance P and

Excitatory Amino Acids, which activate pain projection neurons in the CNS. When there is a constant barrage of painful stimuli, spinal cord neurons are persistently depolarized by Substance P and glutamate is released. Magnesium dissociates from the NMDA receptors, thus allowing Calcium influx into the cell and facilitating signal transmission. This also causes the release of nitric oxide and prostaglandins (PGE2) by cyclooxygenase enzymes. The release of nitric oxide and prostaglandins increases the excitability of the neurons in the spinal cord and cause an exaggerated release of neurotransmitters from sensory neuron presynaptic terminals to the spinal cord. Thus, NMDA activation results in amplification of pain signals being relayed to the higher brain centers.

The constant barrage of signals from the periphery results in activation of the low threshold T-type calcium channel levels, NMDA and NK1 receptors in the lamina I of the dorsal horn. Increased input from the nociceptors causes activation of glutamate NMDA receptors, brain-derived neurotrophic factors (BDNF), Tropomyosin receptor kinase B (trkB) receptors and SP neurokinin 1 (NK1) receptors. As the glial cells in the central nervous system are activated, there is an up-regulation of the pro-inflammatory cytokines IL-6, IL-12 and IL-18. Presynaptic release of neurotransmitters and increased post- synaptic excitability, facilitate pain signal processing.

Subtle brain dysplasia based on structural tissue characteristics, known as microdysgenesis, may accompany EDS. It is unknown whether this disorder of neuronal cytoarchitecture and connectivity could cause Central Sensitization by creating a chronic state of hyperexcitability.

The key feature of Central Sensitization is that it is induced with a very short latency period of a few seconds that results in intense, repeated and sustained nociceptor inputs that can last from many minutes to hours, even without any further nociceptor input. This happens as a result of NMDA receptor activation which then contributes to maintenance of pain as result of Central Sensitization. There are multiple other triggers that can contribute to the maintenance of Central Sensitization, such as Substance P, CGRP, BDNF and the effect of glutamate on

NMDA receptor and AMPA receptor. Thus, there are many parallel inputs to the dorsal horn neurons that can collectively initialize Central Sensitization. There is no single mechanism for Central Sensitization but a collection of initiating and maintaining factors that produce a change in somatosensory processing. In Central Sensitization when there is a nociceptor input several different processes take place in the dorsal horn: facilitated synaptic strength, increased membrane excitability and decreased inhibition.

The above-described processes also known as *inflammatory soup* are identified at the first order synapses. Recent developments have shown that neuronal activity does not provide a complete understanding of Central Sensitization.

Glial cell activation has been shown to be the common underlying mechanism. Glial cells are made up of astrocytes, oligodendrocytes, resident microglia, perivascular microglia. Glial cells have been shown to play a role in pain facilitation by modulating neuronal synaptic function and neuronal excitability by several mechanisms. Anatomically, glia out number neuronal cells. Astrocytes, resident microglia and perivascular glia have a modulating function in pain processing. Astrocytes completely encapsulate synapses and are in close contact with neurons. This close contact between the astrocytes and neurons allows for astrocyte activation by neurotransmission. Perivascular microglia alter the blood brain barrier and have an anti-inflammatory response. Resident microglia rapidly proliferate on activation and have an inflammatory and anti-inflammatory effect. Activated microglia produce and release other chemicals that activate astrocytes in close proximity.

Astrocytes and microglia express Toll Like Receptors (TLR). There are 13 TLR's that have been identified. When TLR's are activated they release pro-inflammatory cytokines. Microglia express TLR2 and TLR4 which then release TNF-alpha, IL-1beta and IL-6. Activation of TLR in the CNS creates an excitatory positive feedback loop in the pain pathway.

Activated glia release pro-inflammatory cytokines which then result in a neuroinflammatory response in the neurons.

Astrocytes release TNF-alpha and IL-1beta which increase neuronal excitability by increasing the conductivity of NMDA and AMPA receptors. They also increase the density of these receptors on the neurons. IL-1beta increases calcium conductance of NMDA receptors in the pain carrying neurons of the spinal cord. TNF-alpha, IL-1beta and IL-6 cause sensitization of the DRG and sensitization of the dorsal horn resulting in an exaggerated response. Glia do not relay pain information. They release neuro-inflammatory cytokines which amplify neuronal pain signaling and excitation.

Algoneurodystrophy and Causalgia

By Dr. Stéphane Daens

Algoneurodystrophy, recently renamed Reflex Sympathetic Dystrophy (or RSD), and Causalgia have been grouped under the term Complex Pain Syndromes. This recent classification was established because of the inconsistent and non-permanent nature of the sympathetic system's action on Pain. The dystrophy is also not systematic.

They have therefore been separated into two distinct entities:

➢ RSD is Complex Regional Pain Syndrome Type 1, or CRPS-1.
➢ Causalgia is Complex Regional Pain Syndrome Type 2, or CRPS-2.

The precise mechanisms of CRPS-1 are multiple and partially unknown:

➢ A disturbance in the autonomous nervous system (ANS).
➢ A dysfunction of the central nervous system (CNS), by abnormal integration of Pain. The notion of central sensitization (see above).[172]
➢ Neuropeptides, including Substance P, would play a role in vasomotor phenomena.

---

[172] Ji RR, Nackley A, Huh Y, et al. Neuroinflammation and central sensitization in chronic and widespread pain. Anesthesiology. 2018;129(2):343-366.

> The inflammatory hypothesis: after a trauma, lymphocytes and mast cells (MCAD) release pro-inflammatory substances such as cytokines.

Ambroise Paré (1510-1590), a French barber surgeon (one of the Fathers of Surgery), made the first clinical description of what was to become algoneurodystrophy (CRPS-1) in 1557, and its mechanism is still imperfectly understood after 465 years!

The pain of CRPS-1 is characterized as continuous, constant, extremely intense, even at rest, and disproportionate to the triggering trauma. It has intermittent exacerbations.

CRPS-1 is currently considered one of the most intense forms of chronic pain, according to the McGill Pain Index.

> The McGill Pain Index[173] is a scale that determines the level of intensity of pain. Two researchers at McGill University originally developed it: Ronald Melzack (Quebec psychologist, also the author of the *Gate Control theory*, 1929-2019) and Warren S. Torgerson (American psychologist, 1924-1999), in 1971. It is divided into four categories (and has 20 items in total): sensory, affective, evaluative, and indeterminate (or varied).

    The top 10 most severe pains are: CRPS, sting of a bullet ant or Paraponera ant, childbirth, finger amputation (index finger), Crohn's disease, rheumatoid arthritis, fibromyalgia (EDS?), renal colic, migraine with aura, trigeminal neuralgia (this ranking changes periodically).

It does not follow a radicular or even metameric pathway, and occurs rapidly after the trigger. It is most often described as a burning beginning at, or around, a joint and then spreading distally (from the hip to the knee, for example) or proximally (from the hand to the shoulder, with a *shoulder-hand syndrome*). It can even start from the spine, abdomen, or pelvis.

---

[173] Melzack R. The McGill pain questionnaire. In : Pain measurement and assessment, edited by R. Melzack. New York: Raven Press, pages 41-47.

The pain is continuous, with *hyperalgesia* (an exaggerated sensitivity to a painful stimulus) and/or *allodynia* (a painful sensation to a non-painful stimulus, such as touch, sounds and vibrations, as well as wind and outside temperature). Loud or even moderate sounds and light exacerbate the pain. There is also edema, dyshidrosis (a sweating disorder), skin discoloration, faster nail growth with nail deformities; hair growth is faster, darker and may fall out early. There are also inflammatory signs, spastic vascular and muscular damage (dystonia), as well as insomnia, fatigue, and emotional disturbances (including changes in the limbic system such as short-term memory problems, concentration problems and irritability).

The diagnosis of CRPS-1 is purely clinical. Additional examinations, such as bone scans with early time studies and bone x-rays (with *speckled osteoporosis* images), should only be performed if there is a doubt about another, potentially more serious pathology (e.g., neoplasia).

CRPS-1 occurs in more than 50% of cases after trauma (sprain, fracture, musculotendinous strain, etc.), limb surgery and/or cast immobilization.

Non-traumatic causes include inflammatory rheumatism, carpal tunnel or tarsal tunnel syndrome, stroke, myocardial infarction, multiple sclerosis, certain cancers (paraneoplastic CRPS-1), deep vein thrombosis (DVT), infections such as panaritium or shingles, metabolic disorders such as diabetes or dysthyroidism.

It also develops following the use of certain medications (such as phenobarbital, a barbiturate) or during pregnancy (CRPS-1 can be found in the hip, for example).

Recovery is often long with possible functional sequelae.

The concept of Central Sensitization (summary)

By Dr. Stéphane Daens

This is an increase in the excitability of the neurons of the central nervous system (CNS). The consequences: normal nerve impulses can produce abnormal responses in the CNS.

There is an activation and proliferation of receptors called NMDA. These are glutamate receptors that a pharmacological agonist, N-Methyl-D-Aspartate, activates. These receptors are essential to memory and synapses' plasticity (the communication junctions between neurons). They are more numerous and activated, leading to an exaggerated response of the CNS to pain, and a decrease in sensitivity to opiates.

There is an activation of the glial cells (microglia), which constitute more than 70% of the cells of the CNS. Normally, these cells remain dormant, they have functions of nutrition and synthesis of myelin sheaths. They also have an immune function within the CNS. When glial cells are activated, they release substances that inflame and damage the nerves such as cytokines, nitric oxide, and superoxide anions. The nerves in turn release substances that keep the microglia activated, creating a self-perpetuating cycle.

The link between the CNS (glial cells, neurons) and the immune system is still not fully understood. IgG (immunoglobulin type G) antibodies directed against the autonomic and peripheral nervous systems have been identified. Thus, glial cells' cytokines may modulate pain by affecting the CNS and the immune system. [174] MCAD and central sensitization are intimately related.[175]

In CRPS-1, pain can be maintained by the ortho-parasympathetic nervous system (sympathetically maintained pain or SMP), but,

---

[174] Lacagnina MJ, Heijnen CJ, Watkins LR, et al. Autoimmune regulation of chronic pain. Pain Rep. 2021;6(1):e905. doi: 10.1097/PR9.0000000000000905.
[175] Hendriksen E, van Bergeijk D, Oosting RS, Redegeld FA. Mast cells in neuroinflammation and brain disorders. Neurosci Biobehav Rev. 2017;79:119-133.

there is also pain independent of the ortho-parasympathetic nervous system (sympathetically independent pain or SIP).

Among the differential diagnoses of CRPS-1, we can mention, in a non-exhaustive way: CRPS-2 (causalgia), traumatic vasospasm, Raynaud's syndrome, arterial or venous thrombosis, etc.

In EDS, in addition to musculotendinous, para-articular, capsular, and cutaneous-mucosal disorders, there are also motor proprioceptive disorders (87%), neuro-vegetative disorders (76%) and hypersensoriality (69%). Also found are cognitive disorders (68%), dystonia (66%) as well as fatigue (95%) and multiple intractable pain (93%) (*Hamonet et al. 2017*).

It should be noted that many of these impairments may be mixed and confused with some of the signs and symptoms included above in CRPS-1; they are also well known in MCAD.

CRPS-1 is largely related to vasomotor disorders (dysautonomia). Previous research found that 70 to 80 percent of CRPS-1 patients were female. This is the same prevalence we saw in EDS patients during our consultations: 75-80 percent of women and 20-25 percent of men. Moreover, in more than 80% of cases, patients with EDS seem to have symptoms suggestive of MCAD.

The term EDS/MCA is suggested: Mast cell activation associated with Ehlers-Danlos Syndrome.

In EDS/MCA, mast cells are more prone to release (degranulation) substances such as: histamine, tryptase, heparin, interleukins, prostaglandins, Tumor Necrosis Factor alpha (TNFα). There are also neuro-inflammatory mechanisms, which underlie the pain associated with CRPS-1 and which are intimately linked to the substances released by mast cells.

"Thus, CRPS is a neuroinflammatory phenomenon characterized by a combination of sensory (allodynia, hyperalgesia), autonomic, vasomotor and motor dysfunctions. The sooner treatment is instituted, the better the chance of avoiding severe complications. Moreover, the more CRPS progresses, the more refractory it becomes to sympathetic nerve blocks, conventional analgesics, antiepileptics and antidepressants" (*Chopra et al., 2013*).

CRPS-1 related to EDS

From our experience, shared with a few colleagues, came the impression that CRPS-1 is very frequently encountered in EDS patients. Conversely, we were convinced that most of the patients with CRPS-1 also had EDS. Since EDS also includes dysautonomia and MCAD in its description, it seemed essential to us to know whether CRPS-1 is more frequently encountered in EDS than in the general population, or demonstrates that it is a frequent EDS' complication:

I conducted a retrospective study of 344 patients with EDS. The patients could answer the two statements: "I have EDS and have had algoneurodystrophy" or "I have EDS and have never had algoneurodystrophy". They were also asked to mention a close family history of CRPS-1 (parents, siblings, children).

Results:

20.1% of the patients, all ages combined, presented with CRPS-1 during their lifetime. 15% of the patients had one or more close relatives who developed CRPS-1, irrespective of whether these patients themselves had developed CRPS-1 in their lifetime.

More interesting is the study of quartiles by age groups, separating respectively: patients under 20 years, 21 to 40 years, 41 to 60 years and over 60 years. The percentage of EDS patients who have previously had CRPS-1 (P), and the percentage of patients who have a family history of CRPS -1 (F) are as follows:

For those under the age of 20 (N=15):
The results are 13.3% (P) and 20% (F), respectively.

For those between the ages of 21 and 40 (N=132):
The results are 15.9% (P) and 16.7% (F), respectively.

403

For those between the ages of 41 and 60 (N=170):
The results are 23.4% (P) and 10.6% (F), respectively.

For those over the age of 60 (N=27):
The results are 29.6% (P) and 25.9% (F), respectively.

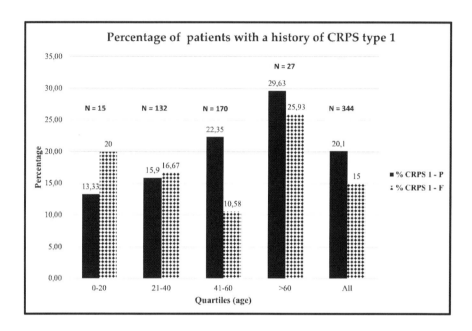

In 2017, I presented a poster with my findings at the third International University Colloquium, organized in Paris by Professor Claude Hamonet. The participants showed a great interest. I had the opportunity to speak with Dr. Pradeep Chopra. He told me that he thought the same as we did, and even more, he was convinced that Causalgia (CRPS-2) appears largely as related to Ehlers-Danlos Syndrome. We have exchanged a lot since then on this fascinating subject. He found similar figures to mine in an unpublished study of 307 patients with EDS.

Discussion:

The differences observed in the percentages obtained are probably due to biases related to the age of the patients, on the one hand, and to the time at which the patients were diagnosed, on the other hand:

1. The probability of having had an algodystrophy (CRPS-1) naturally increases with age.

2. The percentage of patients with a family history of CRPS-1 also varies with the age of the patients:

   ➤ For the younger patients, it is their parents, siblings, or even grandparents who have had CRPS-1.

   ➤ For the older patients, it is their children and grandchildren who have been affected.

   ➤ For the 41–60-year-olds, the percentage of family history drops. On the one hand, their children are still relatively young, and they have, for the most part, not had time to develop CRPS-1. On the other hand, they have older parents, for whom, in their time, there was little or no diagnosis of algoneurodystrophy (CRPS-1).

The prevalence of CRPS-1 is generally estimated to be 20.57 per 100,000 people (i.e., about 1/5000) (*Sandroni P et al. Pain., 2003*).[176] Its incidence is estimated to be about 1 in 4000 people per year in the general population.

In this study, more than 20% of patients with hEDS reported having had CRPS-1. Therefore, a considerable proportion of CRPS-1 may be related to having EDS or other connective tissue diseases.

Since mast cells and dysautonomia seem to play a role in the development of CRPS-1, it would be interesting to link these four conditions: EDS - MCAD – Dysautonomia – CRPS 1.

Conclusions:

♦ CRPS-1 appears to be a common complication of Ehlers-Danlos Syndrome. This is confirmed by other physicians specializing in this field.

---

[176] Sandroni P, Benrud-Larson LM, McClelland RL, et al. Complex regional pain syndrome type I: incidence and prevalence in Olmsted county, a population-based study. Pain. 2003;103(1-2):199-207.

♦ Future studies should be developed to establish a causal link between Causalgia (CRPS type 2) and Ehlers-Danlos Syndrome.

Perspectives and attitudes

- I think that all orthopedists, algologists, neurologists, rheumatologists, physical rehabilitation physicians and general practitioners should systematically test patients with algoneurodystrophy (or CRPS-1) for Ehlers-Danlos Syndrome. The results could be surprising and even explosive.

- With a better understanding of EDS, could we finally have discovered the main cause of CRPS-1?

- Furthermore, for any EDS patient who has a sprain or fracture (especially when in a cast) but also a functional surgery or a joint replacement surgery (shoulder, knee, and hip, mainly), preventative treatment of CRPS-1 should be given. Casts should be avoided as much as possible: removable and inflatable stabilization orthoses should be preferred.

- Specific treatments should be introduced as soon as possible (see below). [177,178,179,180]

[177] Taylor SS, Noor N, Urits I, et al. Complex Regional Pain Syndrome: A Comprehensive Review. Pain Ther. 2021. doi: 10.1007/s40122-021-00279-4.

[178] Molderings GJ, Haenisch B, Brettner S, et al. Pharmacological treatment options for mast cell activation disease. Naunyn Schmiedebergs Arch Pharmacol. 2016;389(7):671-94. doi: 10.1007/s00210-016-1247-1.

[179] Shim H, Rose J, Halle S, et al. Complex regional pain syndrome: a narrative review for the practising clinician. Br J Anaesth. 2019;123(2):e424-e433.

[180] Chevreau M., Romand X., Gaudin P., et al. Bisphosphonates for treatment of Complex Regional Pain Syndrome type 1: a systematic literature review and meta-analysis of randomized controlled trials versus placebo. J Bone Spine. 2017;84:393–399.

PRACTICAL TIP SHEET:
My treatments for CRPS-1

Treatments for acute CRPS-1:
To be initiated as soon as possible

➤ Type 1 antihistamines (e.g., Desloratadine 5mg twice daily and Rupatadine 10mg at noon) for 3 months.

➤ Type 2 antihistamines (example: Ranitidine 300mg or Famotidine 40mg at night) for 3 months (if commercially available).

➤ Anti-leukotrienes: Montelukast 10mg in the morning (it often gives nightmares if taken in the evening in EDS) for 3 months (beware of the psychological disorders induced).

➤ Vitamin C, from 1 to 3 grams per day, for 3 months.

➤ N-Acetylcysteine (NAC) 600mg, three times a day for one month; then once a day for two months (3 months total).

➤ Alendronate 70mg, three times a week for one month; then once a week for two months (3 months total).

➤ Calcium citrate 1000mg + 25-OH vitamin D 3000UI, once a day, with meal, in the evening (to avoid hypocalcemia on Alendronate intake) for 3 months.

➤ PPI in preventing esophagitis on Alendronate: e.g., Pantoprazole 20 to 40mg daily, for three months.

➤ Local injections of Lidocaine, at concentrations between 0.5% and 1%, could be tried.

➤ Physical, psychological, and occupational therapies.

➤ Mirror therapy and graded motor imagery.

Acute phase treatment may be extended to 6 months if effects are beneficial but incomplete.

Other available therapies: low-dose naltrexone, ketamine, and Botulinum toxin A (BTX-A); Amitriptyline or Gabapentin (neuropathic pain medications); Palmitoylethanolamide (PEA); NSAID or corticosteroids.

- Type 1 antihistamines (e.g., Desloratadine 5mg, twice daily, from D0 to D+15 relative to the event).
- Type 2 antihistamines (D0 to D+15), if commercially available.
- Anti-leukotrienes (Montelukast, from D0 to D+15).
- Vitamin C, 1 to 3 grams per day (to be given continuously in EDS).

If it is a scheduled orthopedic procedure: treatments can be started at D-15, for example.

Secondary prevention treatment of an EDS patient
(who has had algodystrophy in the past,
or a family history of CRPS-1)

- Same as primary prevention and add:
- Alendronate 70mg, once a week, from D0 to D+30.
- Calcium citrate 1000mg/day from D0 to D+30.
- 25-OH-Vitamine D, 3000 UI/day with meal.

If it is a scheduled intervention: start at D-15, for example.

Specific treatments for CRPS-1 and CRPS-2 in EDS

1. Low Dose Naltrexone (LDN):

Naltrexone is a competitive antagonist of certain opioid receptors: The Toll-Like Receptors-4 or TLR4 (sometimes called CD284, for cluster of differentiation 284).

TLR4s are present on macrophages and on certain adipocytes (pre-adipocytes and mature adipocytes), but also and especially, as far as we are concerned, on CNS microglia.

TLR4 are membrane receptors belonging to the family of pattern recognition receptors (PRR). The TLR4 gene is located on chromosome 9 and is admirably conserved throughout species' evolution (phylogenesis).

When activated by a ligand, they induce intracellular signals mediated by the NF-kB pathway. This leads to inflammatory cytokines production (such as inerleukin-1 and TNFα) and the innate immune system's activation.

Viral proteins, lipoproteins, β-defensins, antimicrobial peptides, heat shock protein (released under stress) and LPS (lipopolysaccharide, also called endotoxin) can bind to TLR4. LPS is present in various Gram-negative and Gram-positive bacteria (see dysbiosis in EDS patients).

Morphine is a TLR4 agonist: the release of inflammatory cytokines decreases opioid efficacy and increases tolerance; it also contributes to various adverse effects such as hyperalgesia and allodynia (central sensitization).

In the study by *P. Chopra and M.S. Cooper (2013)*[181], Low-Dose Naltrexone improved the painful symptoms of algoneurodystrophy (CRPS-1) and those of dystonic spasms and fixed dystonia related to CRPS-1.

Mode of action of naltrexone:[182]

It has been used for over thirty years in addiction. Naltrexone has a suppressive effect on glia and decreases the production of pro-inflammatory cytokines and neurotoxic superoxide.

Possible side effects:

Insomnia, headache at the beginning of treatment.

---

[181] Chopra P, Cooper MS. Treatment of Complex Regional Pain Syndrome (CRPS) using low dose naltrexone (LDN). J Neuroimmune Pharmacol. 2013;8(3):470-6. doi: 10.1007/s11481-013-9451-y.
[182] Trofimovitch D, Baumrucker SJ. Pharmacology Update: Low-Dose Naltrexone as a Possible Nonopioid Modality for Some Chronic, Nonmalignant Pain Syndromes. Am J Hosp Palliat Care. 2019;36(10):907-912.

Naltrexone 100 μg:
- 1 capsule, once a day for 2 days,
- 1 capsule, twice a day for 2 days,
- 1 capsule, 3 times a day for 2 days,
- 1 capsule, 4 times a day for 2 days,
- 2 capsules, 4 times a day for 2 days,
- 3 capsules, 4 times a day for 2 days,
- 4 capsules, 4 times a day for 2 days.

Then,

Naltrexone 500 μg:
- 1 capsule, 4 times a day for 2 days,
- Then, 2 capsules, 4 times a day (= 4mg/day) (or 1mg, 4x/day).

If the effect is achieved at lower doses, continue at that dosage.

No morphine, opioids, tramadol!

Try 6 months and see.

For the pharmacist: start with a 50 mg tablet and dilute to 100 μg (micrograms) per capsule, in a magistral. Produce 500 capsules of 100 μg for 1 tablet of 50 mg. Then make Naltrexone 1mg/capsule (x 300 capsules, magistral) for higher dosages.

Pathophysiological parenthesis concerning Naltrexone

I will focus on the Toll-Like Receptor-4 (TLR4) mechanism of action, as it will help us understand why opioids, morphine and its derivatives, are most often contraindicated in CRPS.

In CRPS, during neuroimmune activation, microglia glial cells (CNS immune cells) increase TLR4 receptor synthesis. TLR4 activation in microglia and CNS neurons results in the release of pro-inflammatory cytokines and neurotoxic superoxide via the NF-kB pathway. These substances mediate neuropathic pain, but not only. One cytokine, called BDNF (Brain-Derived Neurotrophic Factor), increases the excitability of the nociceptive network, leading to hyperalgesia or allodynia. Over time, TLR4 stimulation can cause neuronal damage. Naltrexone is a TLR4 receptor blocker and will decrease the release of pro-inflammatory cytokines (such as interleukin-1 or TNF-alpha) as well as superoxide anions from activated glial cells.

At another level, Naltrexone may indirectly inhibit NMDA receptor activity. It also ameliorates dystonic movements associated with CRPS (*Chopra et al., 2013*).

Naltrexone is used at doses 50 times lower than for morphine withdrawal among drug addicts. Significantly, Naltrexone, at low doses, does not interfere with opioid receptors μ (mu), allowing endogenous antinociceptive pathways, involving these receptors, to continue their actions.

> Opioids are agonists of TLR4 receptors.
> Giving morphine chronically in EDS increases
> central sensitization and worsens pain!

This is a crucial fact, given the number of EDS patients I see who consume morphine or its derivatives, which have been prescribed by certain colleagues.

It is also thought that the chronic release of cytokines, by activated glial cells, induces opioid tolerance, and will increase hyperalgesia and allodynia in patients taking morphine. On the other hand, if the use of Naltrexone, at low doses, inhibits TLR4 but not μ-opioid, it could have a beneficial influence on the analgesic effect of opioids in the long term, by decreasing the production of cytokines by glial cells.

Bibliography:

Bolton MJ, Chapman BP, Van Marwijk H. Low-dose naltrexone as a treatment for chronic fatigue syndrome. BMJ Case rep. 2020;13(1). Pii :e232502. Doi : 10.1136/bcr-2019-232502.

Metyas S, Chen CL, Yeter K et al. Low dose Naltrexone in the treatment of fibromyalgia. Curr Rheumatol Rev. 2018;14(2):177-180.

Toljan K, Vrooman B. Low-dose Naltrexone (LDN) – Review of therapeutic utilization. Med Sc (Vasel). 2018;6(4). Doi : 10.3390/medsci6040082.

Pattern DK, Schultz BG, Berlau DJ. The safety and efficacy of low-dose Naltrexone in the management of chronic pain and inflammation in multiple sclerosis, fibromyalgia, Crohn's disease, and other chronic pain disorders. Pharmacotherapy. 2018;38(3):382-389.

Bostick KM, McCarter AG, Nykamp D. The use of low-dose Naltrexone for chronic pain. Sr Care Pharm. 2019;34(1):43-46.

Sturn KM, Collin M. Low-dose Naltrexone: A new therapy option for Complex Regional Pain Syndrome type 1 patients. Int J Pharm Compd. 2016;20(3):197-201.

Chopra P, Tinkle B, Hamonet Cl, Brock I, Gompel A, Bulbena A, Francomano C. Pain management in the Ehlers-Danlos syndromes. Am J Med Genet Part C Semin Med Genet 9999C:1-8.

Chopra P, Cooper MS. Treatment of Regional Complex Syndrome (CRPS) using low-dose Naltrexone (LDN). J Neuroimmune Pharmacol. 2013 ;8 :470-476.

Non-exhaustive list of TLR4 agonist and antagonist substances:

Agonists:

Buprenorphine (Temgesic®, Transtec®), Carbamazepine (Tegretol®), Ethanol (alcohol), Fentanyl, Levorphanol, Lipopolysaccharides (LPS), Methadone, Morphine, Oxacarbazepine (Trileptal®), Oxycodone (OxyContin®, OxyNorm®), Pethidine (Pethisom®), Tapentadol (Palexia® ; both agonist and antagonist), etc.

Antagonists:

Lipid A, Amitriptyline (Redomex®), Cyclobenzapine, Ketotifen (Zaditen®), Imipramine (Tofranil®), Mianserin (Lerivon®), Ibudilast, Pinocembrin, Naloxone, LPS-RS, propentofylline, Tapentadol (Palexia® ; agonist and antagonist), etc.

2. Ketamine:

It is a noncompetitive and potent NMDA receptor antagonist that can decrease central sensitization. Ketamine also inhibits the reuptake of catecholamines by neurons, acts on the descending inhibitory system, inhibits cholinergic receptors of the muscarinic type, and is also an agonist of mu (μ) and kappa (κ) morphine receptors. It induces or reactivates the diffuse inhibitory controls of pain. Finally, it is known that Ketamine can facilitate the pain-relieving effect of opioids, decrease their tolerance, and decrease the painful crises of opiate withdrawal. It is also used as a general anesthetic.

It is administered intravenously, in low doses, and must be repeated (once a month, for example). Ideally, it requires a one-day clinic with monitoring (oximetry for oxygen saturation, heart rate and blood pressure, electrocardiograms) and repeated clinical examinations of the state of consciousness. It can also be used orally (e.g., taken between intravenous courses). The room should be quiet and dark.

In a study by *A. Néron et al.* of Montreal (2017)[183], 45 records of patients who received IV Ketamine infusions, for various pain conditions, were reviewed: 64% of patients (29/45) had at least a 30% decrease in pain intensity; 31% of patients (14/45) had at least 50% relief. However, this relief's duration was very variable: from a few hours to a few days (3 or 4 days), sometimes a few weeks (up to 6 weeks). The potential side effects are not negligible: headache, nausea, vomiting, profuse dreams, nightmares, hallucinations, euphoria, somnolence, dizziness, numbness of the lips and chin, diplopia, bradycardia, flushing, increased pain during infusion (cause unknown). There is an improvement in daily activities, a reduction in other treatments, and improved quality of life in about 85% of cases.

This does not always work and only in combination with other treatments, regular exercise, etc. (*P. Chopra, USA*). One might

---

[183] Néron A. et al. Perfusions intraveineuses de lidocaïne et de kétamine pour le traitement des douleurs réfractaires aux traitements conventionnels. Pharmactuel. 2017;50(4):227-233

think that a combination [Naltrexone + Ketamine] would be useful in some cases.

3. Antioxidants:

Free radicals (superoxide anions) attack cells, nerves, muscles, etc. Various well-known substances can slow down or prevent oxidation such as glutathione, N-acetylcystein, vitamin C, alpha-lipoic acid, coenzyme Q10 ubiquinol, vitamin E, β-carotene, polyphenols, flavonoids, turmeric, cranberry, etc.

Some molecules are remarkably interesting in the clinic:

➢ Alpha-lipoic acid (ALA) or Lipoate.

It is a sulfuric acid (formula $C_8H_{14}O_2S_2$) derived from cysteine. It is present in all the cells of our body and plays a key role in energy production. It is also a powerful antioxidant, active in water (water-soluble) and in fats (fat-soluble): it is called the universal antioxidant.

It can participate in recycling other antioxidants such as glutathione, vitamin E, and vitamin C (it increases their lifespan and therefore their effectiveness). It can trap heavy metals such as arsenic, cadmium or mercury. It is a potentially effective treatment for neuropathic pain, POTS, dysautonomia. It decreases insulin resistance (in diabetics, this can be useful). It may help relieve the *burning mouth syndrome* (burning and itching sensation in the mouth) that can occur in some EDS patients. Other trials suggest that it has positive effects in glaucoma, loss of smell or taste (to be tried in EDS or in certain infections such as Covid-19), and prevent migraines (in addition to riboflavin B2 at 400mg/day, for example).

Recommended doses of ALA are 600 to 1200mg per day, *per os* (it is sometimes given intravenously).

Precautions: monitor blood sugar levels and adjust hypoglycemic treatments. Monitor iron, of which ALA can be a chelator.

➢ Vitamin C: between 1 gram and 6 grams per day, is a powerful natural antioxidant.

➢ Dimethyl-Sulfoxide 50%:
  - It is a polar organo-sulfur solvent with the chemical formula C_2H_6OS. It has cytoprotective, anesthetic and antibacterial properties.
  - In the hot phase of CRPS-1: 5 times a day, for 3 months, in local applications.
  - In the cold phase of CRPS-1, it can be tried for one month and if it helps, it can be continued (in local applications).
  - It has been found to have properties in intra-vesical injections, for intractable interstitial cystitis.

➢ N-Acetylcysteine (NAC) is a non-essential amino acid (formula $C_5H_9NO_3S$), which stimulates the production of glutathione. It is then indirectly a powerful antioxidant. It is used, among other things, as a mucolytic (splitting of disulfide bridges of mucoproteins). It is a liver protector in cases of Paracetamol intoxication (intravenously). In psychiatric disorders, NAC has been tested against depression and bipolar disorders. It would decrease the symptoms of schizophrenia and would act in autism, and obsessive-compulsive disorders (OCD).[184] It also stabilizes mast cells. Doses: 600mg, 1 to 3 times a day.

➢ Coenzyme Q10 Ubiquinol in doses of 2 to 4 x 100mg/day. It has an important role in the Krebs' cycle of the mitochondria (the brain and muscles are the largest consumers of oxygen to produce energy, in the form of ATP). It is an antioxidant, increases the bioavailability of NO, and could decrease brain and peripheral cells' damage. We can also associate NAD+ (nicotinamide adenine dinucleotide), for fatigue, among others. Nicotinamide Riboside (or N-Ribosyl-Nicotinamide, NRN) is more easily given with coenzyme Q10. NRN is converted into NAD+ by NRN kinase[185].

---

[184] Smaga I, Frankowska M, Filip M. N-acetylcysteine as a new prominent approach for treating psychiatric disorders. Br J Pharmacol. 2021;178(13):2569-2594.
[185] Mancuso M, Orsucci D, Calsolaro V et al. Coenzyme Q10 and neurological diseases. Pharmaceuticals (Basel). 2009;2(3):134-149.

➢ Cannabidiol (CBD) is also an antioxidant (see below).

4. **For muscles and spasms:**

➢ Magnesium (*per os*, IV), oral electrolytes supplements.
➢ Baclofen (it is an agonist of the γ-aminobutyric acid receptors or $GABA_B$). It inhibits synaptic reflexes and promotes muscle relaxation. It may also have effects on spasms and chronic spasticity. It is believed to relieve hiccups (a common symptom in EDS).
➢ Diazepam 5 to 10 mg.
➢ Levodopamine (Prolopa®, Modopar®), also used in Parkinson's disease (but here in lower doses).
➢ Pramipexole.
➢ Naltrexone low dose.
➢ Cannabidiol (CBD) : see below.
➢ PEA (Palmitoylethanolamide).
➢ Treat dysautonomia and proprioception (fluid intake, salt, electrolytes, compressive garments, posture insoles, and more).
➢ Treat MCADs.
➢ Stabilize hyperlaxed joints.
➢ Treat anxiety, stress and hyperventilation (physiotherapy, osteopathy, relaxation, sophrology, Yoga, and more).

5. **Other treatments**, in case of failure or in addition to other medications:

➢ Gabapentin (Neurontin®), Pregabalin (Lyrica®): few effects here.
   • Gabapentin is a derivative of γ-aminobutyric acid (or GABA). It inhibits explicitly certain calcium channels. It has a role as an anti-epileptic, analgesic (neuropathic pain of diabetes and shingles), anxiolytic, and co-analgesic in association with morphine derivatives. It should be

interesting in alcohol withdrawal. It is also used as a recreational drug by some drug addicts.[186,187]

- Pregabalin is an analog of GABA (a gabapentinoid). It is used in neuropathic pain, epilepsy, and generalized anxiety disorders.

➤ Tricyclic antidepressants such as Amitriptyline (Redomex®) and Serotonin and Norepinephrine reuptake blockers (Venlafaxine - Efexor®, Duloxétine - Cymbalta®): they work quite well[188], decreasing (neuropathic) pain signals, but the side effects are not negligible. Amitriptyline, e.g., has antihistamine H1 blocking activity (it may be useful in the treatment of urticaria even when conventional antihistamines have failed). Side effects of amitriptyline: sedation, drowsiness, dry mouth, blurred vision, constipation, increased sweating, difficulty urinating, dizziness (drop of blood pressure on standing up, HOS), nausea, confusion, headache (hyponatremia), weight gain, heart rhythm disturbances. Anticholinergic/antimuscarinic side effects may occur in up to 50% of patients (elderly patients are at greater risk).

➤ Selective serotonin reuptake inhibitors (SSRIs), such as Fluoxetine (Prozac®) : they have little effect in this case.[189]

➤ Any interest in Aprepitant? See the chapter on MCAD.

➤ Adapted (and incredibly gentle) physiotherapy.

➤ Mirror therapy (graded motor imagery), such as that used for phantom pain in amputees.

➤ Sensory deprivation therapy (60 minutes per session): sounds increase pain in the CRPS.

---

[186] Serpell M.G. Neuropathic pain study group. Gabapentin in neuropathic pain syndromes: a randomised, double-blind, placebo-controlled trial. Pain. 2002;99:557–566.

[187] van de Vusse A.C., Stomp-van den Berg S.G., Kessels A.H., et al. Randomised controlled trial of gabapentin in complex regional pain syndrome type 1 [ISRCTN84121379] BMC Neurol. 2004;4:13.

[188] Brown S., Johnston B., Amaria K. A randomized controlled trial of amitriptyline versus gabapentin for complex regional pain syndrome type I and neuropathic pain in children. Scand J Pain. 2016;13:156–163.

[189] Barakat A, Hamdy MM, Elbadr MM. Uses of fluoxetine in nociceptive pain management: A literature overview. Eur J Pharmacol. 2018;829:12-25. doi: 10.1016/j.ejphar.2018.03.042.

➢ Hyperbaric oxygen treatment (HBOT): there are anecdotal cases, expensive, and have not shown long-term effects. More studies are needed.[190,191]

➢ The assistance dog: The Sedichien, in France. It helps patients in their daily tasks, as is the case for guide dogs.

6. Treatments to be avoided if possible (CRPS-1):

o Sympathetic nerve blocks.
o Transcutaneous Electrical Neurostimulation (TENS).
o Opioids and morphine derivatives (see above).
o Spinal cord stimulators: they already cause 25% to 50% of complications in non-EDS patients. They work well at first, but there seems to be little benefit after three years of use. Dorsal root ganglion stimulation has greater statistical pain relief (74.2% *vs* 53.0%) compared with the spinal cord stimulation[192].

Ali Z, Raja SN, Wesselman U et al. Intradermal injection of norepinephrine evokes pain in patients with sympathetically maintained pain. Pain. 2000;88(2):161-8.

Baron R, et al. 1999. Causalgia and reflex sympathetic dystrophy: does the sympathetic nervous system contribute to the generation of pain? Muscle nerve. 1999;22(6) :678-95.

Baron R, Fields HL et al. National Institutes of Health workshop: Reflex sympathetic dystrophy/Complex regional pain syndromes – state-of-the-science. Anesthesia & Analgesia. 2002;95(6):1812-1816.

Birklein F, Riedl B, Claus D et al. Pattern of autonomic dysfunction in time course of complex regional pain syndrome. Clin Auton Res. 1998;8(2) :79-85.

---

[190] Hájek M, Chmelar D, Tlapák J, et al. Hyperbaric oxygen treatment in recurrent development of complex regional pain syndrome: A case report. Diving Hyperb Med. 2021;51(1):107-110.

[191] Schiavo S, DeBacker J, Djaiani C, et al. Mechanistic Rationale and Clinical Efficacy of Hyperbaric Oxygen Therapy in Chronic Neuropathic Pain: An Evidence-Based Narrative Review. Pain Res Manag. 2021:8817504.

[192] Deer T.R., Levy R.M., Kramer J. Dorsal root ganglion stimulation yielded higher treatment success rate for complex regional pain syndrome and causalgia at 3 and 12 months: a randomized comparative trial. Pain. 2017;158:669–681.

Birklein F, Schmelz M. Neuropeptides, neurogenic inflammation and complex regional pain syndrome (CRPS). Neurosci Lett. 2008;6,437(3):199-202.

Celletti C, Camerota F, Castori M et al. Orthostatic Intolerance and Postural Orthostatic Tachycardia Syndrome in Joint Hypermobility Syndrome/Ehlers-Danlos Syndrome, Hypermobility Type: Neurovegetative Dysregulation or Autonomic Failure? Biomed Res Int. 2017;2017:9161865.

Chopra P, Cooper MS. Treatment of complex regional pain syndrome (CRPS) using low dose naltrexone (LDN). J Neuroimmune Pharmacol. 2013;8 :470-476.

De Mos M, De Bruijn AG, Huygen FJ et al. The incidence of complex regional pain syndrome: a population-based study. Pain. 2007;129(1-2): 12-20.

Dirckx M, Groeneweg G, van Daele PL, et al. Mast cells: a new target in the treatment of complex regional pain syndrome? Pain Pract. 2013;13(8):599-603.

Hakim A, O'Callaghan C, De Wandele I et al. Cardiovascular autonomic dysfunction in Ehlers-Danlos syndrome – Hypermobile type. Am J Med Genet Part C Semin Med Genet. 2017;175C:168-174.

Hakim AJ, Sahota A. Joint hypermobility and skin elasticity: the hereditary disorders of connective tissue. Clin Dermatol. 2006;24(6):521-33.

Hamonet C, Brock I et al. Syndrome d'Ehlers-Danlos (SED) type III (hypermobile) : validation d'une échelle somatosensorielle (ECSS-62), à propos de 626 cas. Bull. Acad. Natle Méd. 2017 ; 201, n°2 (séance du 28 février 2017)

Hamonet C, Ducret L, Baeza-Velasco CL et al. Ehlers-Danlos-Tchernogobov : histoire contrariée de la maladie. Hist Sci Med. 2016;50(1):29-41.

Hamonet C. Note d'information rédigée à l'intention des membres du groupe de travail « douleurs chroniques et rebelles » de l'Académie de Médecine. 17 avril 2017.

Morris SL, O'Sullivan PB, Murray KJ et al. Hypermobility and musculoskeletal pain in adolescents. J Pediatr. 2017;181:213-221.

Mulvey MR, Macfarlane GJ, Beasley M et al. Modest association of joint hyper mobility with disabling and limiting musculoskeletal pain: results from a large-scale general population-based survey. Arthritis Care Res (Hoboken). 2013;65(8):1325-33.

Seneviratne SL, Maitland A, Afrin L. Mast cell disorders in Ehlers-Danlos syndrome. Am J Med Genet Part C Semin Med Genet. 2017;9999C:1-11.

Thimineur M, Sood P, Kravitz E et al. Central nervous system abnormalities in complex regional pain syndrome (CRPS): clinical and quantitative evidence of medullary dysfunction. Clin J Pain. 1998;14(3):256-67.

Wen-Wu Li, Tian-Zhi Guo, De-yong Liang et al. Substance P signaling controls mast cell activation, degranulation, and nociceptive sensitization in a rat fracture model of complex regional pain syndrome. Anesthesiology. 2002;116:882-895.

CHAPTER X

Intense and Disabling Fatigue

By Dr. Stéphane Daens

Some patients may present to their family physicians or to the emergency department with intense fatigue; they feel empty of energy, a term often used by patients, and they feel without strength. Fatigue is, along with pain, the most disabling symptom in EDS. It is a chronic fatigue that is inextricably linked to Chronic Fatigue Syndrome (CFS). All patients diagnosed with CFS should be tested for EDS.

This can be a legitimate concern for emergency physicians and general practitioners.

Fatigue in EDS is multifactorial

1° Venous pooling in the lower extremities.

In EDS, the walls of arteries and veins contain altered collagen. The veins dilate, and the venous valves are incompetent. These elements promote blood stagnation in the lower parts. The blood is sequestered there, thus decreasing the circulating blood volume. This stagnation of blood, with an increase in pressure on the venous walls, also favors the development of varicosities of all kinds, such as hemorrhoids at the anorectal level and at the level of the uterus, the testicles (varicocele), or other organs of the abdomen. This secondarily aggravates the peripheral venous pooling.

Dysautonomia aggravates the lack of circulating blood volume. *Professor Jaime F. Bravo* very well describes this in his chapter. Dysautonomia is concomitant and closely related to EDS. Thus, chronic fatigue is favored by the relative chronic deoxygenation of the brain (the central nervous system or CNS). At the level of peripheral muscles, symptoms secondary to a local increase in the level of lactic acid and relative hypoxia can be observed: the appearance of cramps and spasms, even dystonia, mainly in the calves. There is also a chronic muscular weakness and a muscular fatigability. It should be remembered that the muscles are, along with the brain, the most important consumers of oxygen (to produce energy or ATP, and the Krebs' cycle may also be dysfunctional).

Reminders of the ANS reflexes in the healthy individuals

A. Baroreceptors are sensitive to the tension exerted on the arterial wall. They are located at the aortic and carotid level, at the carotid sinus and right atrium.

Innervation :
- The afferent nerves are the Vagus and Hering's nerves.[193]
- The cardiovascular center of the medulla oblongata.
- The parasympathetic and sympathetic reflex efferent nerves.

A drop in blood pressure (by venous pooling of the lower limbs, for example) provokes, by reflex, an increase in cardiac output and peripheral vascular resistance (a vasoconstriction with aggravation of phenomena evoking a Raynaud's syndrome, among others).

B. Voloreceptors are located in the walls of the low-pressure system. They respond to changes in volume, which are secondary to dehydration or hemorrhage, for example. The reflex is similar to the baroreceptors. They respond, in fact, to stretching produced by changes in circulating blood volume. So, if there is an increase in circulating blood volume, there is a stimulation of the voloreceptors that results in a decrease in

---

[193] Hering's nerve is bilateral and comes from the glosso-pharyngeal nerves. They end at the carotid sinus. They play an important role in the regulation of blood pressure. They are stimulated by the pressure exerted by the blood on the wall of the carotid arteries (baroreceptors). They are the first segment of a reflex arc that triggers, at the level of the medulla oblongata, a vasoconstrictive or vasodilatory vagosympathetic activation (the vasodepressor nerve). The goal is to restore normal blood pressure. H.E. Hering was an Austrian pathophysiologist (1866-1948).

cardiac output and peripheral vascular resistance, with a consequent drop in blood pressure.

C. Chemoreceptors are in the aortic and carotid corpuscles. They are sensitive to variations in blood oxygen (O_2) and carbon dioxide (CO_2) concentration, but also pH (acid-base balance). They stimulate the vasomotor center. To simplify: when there is a drop in blood pressure, there is a drop in oxygen levels experienced, an increase in CO_2 levels, and a drop in pH (the blood becomes more acidic), which leads to a stimulation of the vasomotor center and, ultimately, an increase in blood pressure.

D. The central ischemic response (in the brain). Cerebral ischemia leads to massive stimulation of the vasomotor center and thus to intense peripheral vasoconstriction with an increase in mean arterial pressure.

E. The medium-term release of adrenaline and noradrenaline (by the adrenal medulla). This release is ten times slower than the rapid nervous responses mentioned above. There is also a role for the renin-angiotensin system, which has a renal origin: the fall in blood pressure leads to an increase in renin and then angiotensin I and angiotensin II, increasing blood pressure. In the longer term, there is a secretion of aldosterone, which causes water retention (mainly due to sodium retention), an increase in circulating blood volume, and increased blood pressure.

Let us remember the properties of the connective tissue in which the various receptors and sensors are bathed. These alterations in the connective tissue would cause these structures to misperceive variations in circulating blood volume and blood pressure. The consequences: there are erroneous afferent influxes sent to the CNS and Dysautonomia. The brain is functional, the sensors and receptors are of good quality. But the brain responds to what is sent to it as a message, it responds either late or out of tune, as we commonly say.

2° Fatigue is often aggravated by EDS/MCA (mast cell activation related to EDS, see the dedicated chapter).

3° There is an alteration in the performance of the Krebs' cycle in the mitochondria (which are the little energy factories of our cells) which is used to form energy (ATP, adenosine triphosphate) from oxygen. However, the structures that consume the most oxygen, and therefore energy, are the brain and the muscles. Vitamin B1, B2, B3, B6, B9, B12, coenzyme Q10, NAD+, magnesium, vitamin C, and vitamin D are, among others, particularly useful for the Krebs' cycle.

4° Patients with EDS often have involuntary muscle contractions such as spasms, dystonia, and almost permanent muscle contractions to correct posture and proprioceptive inputs. This activity requires increased oxygen consumption by the muscles (at the level of the mitochondria) to produce energy. As muscles consume more oxygen on the one hand, and dysautonomia reduces cerebral oxygen supply on the other, the availability of oxygen for brain function will further decrease, thus aggravating patient fatigue. Reducing inappropriate or even parasitic muscle contractions will therefore improve the oxygen available to the brain. Management: posture re-education (GPR, muscle chains, fascia, etc.) and correction of proprioceptive input (insoles, orthoptics, occlusiodontics, speech therapy), magnesium supplements and other oral electrolytes, Baclofen or Diazepam, or possibly Levodopa.

5° In EDS, there is often an irritable bowel, a leaky gut, and an alteration of the intestinal microbiota: intestinal dysbiosis, often with an excess of fermentation and putrefaction flora and/or candidiasis, leads, among other things, to a decrease in tyrosine and tryptophan blood levels.

Tyrosine is a non-essential amino acid, made from phenylalanine. It is important to produce certain neurotransmitters such as dopamine, adrenaline, noradrenaline, and the synthesis of thyroid hormones. This causes, in addition to muscular disorders following the decrease in dopamine (see the symptoms of Parkinson's disease due to a decrease in dopamine): an aggravation of fatigue, energy crashes, a decrease in vigilance and reactivity.

Intestinal disturbances also aggravate EDS/MCA (via intestinal mast cells) and trigger immune reactions: our patients often report a chronic flu-like state (with fatigue and aches). These symptoms are probably the consequence of the stimulation of intestinal lymphocytes (60% to 70% of mature lymphocytes are in our digestive system).

All this finally gives reason to Hippocrates, who, about 2400 years ago, already postulated a major role for the digestive system in the emergence of human diseases. The intestine, often referred to as the second brain, would also play a role in developing autism, Alzheimer's disease, Parkinson, autism spectrum disorders, anorexia, autoimmune diseases, and more.

6° Deficiencies in vitamins, trace elements, etc.

7° Sleep disorders (see above):

➢ Obstructive sleep apnea (OSA) worsens fatigue. A CPAP can be considered (although it is very noisy and not always well tolerated in EDS, because of hypersensoriality).

➢ There is an altered day/night rhythm, with excess adrenergic (orthosympathetic) activity at night, often combined with decreased adrenaline and norepinephrine levels during the day (due to lack of tyrosine, among other things).

➢ There is often a restless legs syndrome (RLS). Prolopa® (or Modopar®) seems to me to be more effective than Pramipexole (Sifrol®) or Clonazepam (Rivotril®) on the long term in EDS. Pramipexole, remember, increases available dopamine. Besides, Prolopa® improves the quality of deep restorative sleep.

➢ In case of disturbing palpitations during the night: Bisoprolol, Nebivolol or Ivabradine can be prescribed for the evening, dosed between 1.25 and 2.5mg, depending on the blood pressure. β-blockers also improve, per se, the quality of sleep by decreasing the nocturnal adrenergic activity and consequently any micro-awakenings. Bisoprolol and Nebivolol rarely cause hypotension during the night: in the supine position, the diurnal venous pooling observed in the lower limbs and abdomen is redistributed to the whole body, resulting in an increase in circulating blood volume. In case of hypotension during the night, we prefer Ivabradine (more selective).

➢ In case of important nycturia, which is moreover aggravated by the redistribution of the venous pooling of the lower limbs in a lying position: one can try Solifenacin or Oxybutynin, at a rate of 2,5mg in the evening. It also reduces nocturnal sweating, if present.

8° Iron deficiency anemia:

➢ Look for the origin: upper or lower digestive, gynecological, repeated significant bruising, bleeding from the ENT or oral sphere, etc.

➢ Iron supplementation, *per os* or IV (Injectafer® 1000mg IV in 30 min).

➢ A blood transfusion of packed red blood cells, if necessary.

Complementary examinations to be performed immediately

➢ Complete biology (including various hormone levels, autoantibodies, iron, and more) + serology (CMV, EBV, Lyme, HIV, HCV, HAV, HBV, SARS-CoV-2, tuberculosis, parasites, and more).

➢ Rectal examination and stool blood test.

➢ Gynecological examination, if necessary.

➢ Abdominal ultrasound (to look for blood collections, tumors, etc.).

➢ Chest x-ray (front and side).

➢ Electrocardiogram (ECG) and transthoracic cardiac ultrasound if there are warning signs at this level.

➢ PET-CT scan (tumors, sarcoidosis, lymphoma, chronic infections, endocarditis, etc.): if necessary, on an outpatient basis.

What to do about severe fatigue in EDS?

➢ Do not misdiagnose fibromyalgia or isolated CFS.

➢ Do not wrongly psychiatrize these patients (depression, anxiety, cyclothymia, etc.). They are rather sad about their situation of fatigue and intense pain. While they would like to do many things, they cannot. They are very brave, but sometimes they give up.

➢ Do not misdiagnose a narcoleptic state.

➢ The most important thing is to reassure, encourage and explain the situation to the patient. It must be emphasized that this fatigue phenomenon is not due to a life-threatening disease, and will certainly improve with appropriate treatments. Their life is not over, as some patients sometimes think.

The role of caregivers is essential in this positive approach to the disease.

Treatments to start quickly in the Emergency Room

➢ Treat Dysautonomia: see this chapter.

➢ Continuous oxygen therapy, with nasal cannulas, at a flow rate of 3 to 5 liters per minute, unless there is chronic obstructive pulmonary disease - COPD. In this case, the flow rate is reduced to 1.5 to 2 liters per minute to avoid carbonarcosis (toxic increase of carbon dioxide in the blood, causing, among other things, a decrease in alertness and a respiratory acidosis).

For the GPs, who are required to see the patient quickly the patient after the visit to the Emergency Room

➢ The patient should rest as needed (prescribe an incapacity to work): do not force, rest and recharge (go for walks, see family and friends, etc.).

➢ Treat Dysautonomia: see this chapter.

➢ Introduce sequential oxygen therapy with a humidifier in a fixed station at home: a flow rate of 2 to 5 liters/minute, 20-to-40-minute sessions, with nasal cannulas. If there is pain and/or lesions of the nasal mucosa because of the cannulas: try neutral gel (as for intimate relations) or Vaseline, to be applied at the beginning of the nasal orifices (but this can obstruct the air inlet). If this does not work, you can try wearing a mask instead of a nasal cannula. The positive effects on fatigue are sometimes felt after a few days, but it takes three months of regular use to conclude whether this treatment is effective or not. It is preferable to start by renting the device for three months. Then, if the effects are positive, you can ask for a one-year lease from the oxygen company or buy a new device. Portable devices are available for work, school or college, travel, etc. The cost is not negligible, as oxygen therapy is not currently reimbursed in many countries for EDS. Oxygen therapy can also improve concentration, memory, and the occurrence of headaches. It also reduces certain muscular pains and even diffuse pains in EDS. The mechanism may, in whole or in part, be linked to the MCAD's decrease. Note: oxygen therapy has to be instituted after the correction of a possible circulating hypovolemia (see the chapter on dysautonomia).

➢ Levocarnitine: a dosage of between 2 and 6 grams per day is required (start with 2 to 3 x 1 g/day). Levocarnitine relaxes, reduces muscular pain, and even more diffuse pain. It decreases constipation and reduces intestinal bloating. It induces diarrhea at too high a dose (especially in case it is associated with MCAD, dysbiosis and leaky gut).

➢ Magnesium, among other electrolytes, *per os*.

➢ L-tyrosine: 500 mg, taken once in the morning and once around 1 p.m. (in any case before 4 p.m.). It reduces fatigue during the morning and afternoon (after correcting any circulating hypovolemia, see the chapter on dysautonomia).

➢ Vitamin C: 2 grams in the morning.

➢ 25-OH-Vitamin D: 3000 IU/day with food (it is a lipophilic, fat-soluble vitamin). To be taken continuously, all year round, in EDS.

- ➤ Probiotics and prebiotics (e.g. Bio-Floracare XL®, Probactiol plus®, Probiotical®, Arko Biotics Supraflor®, Inuline FOS ALTISA®, or another preparation): they reduce the flu-like condition that is often observed in EDS: aches and pains, muscle and joint pain, usually without fever but sometimes with an inflammatory syndrome - especially an elevated level of CRP - whose origin has not yet been determined.

- ➤ L-Glutamine 800mg can be added at a rate of 2 to 4 doses/day in case of leaky gut. It improves the tight junctions' quality of the small intestine.

- ➤ In case of EDS/MCA: e.g., add type 1 antihistamines, 2 to 4 doses/day + type 2 antihistamines in the evening (if available on the market) + vitamin C 2g/day + anti-leukotrienes in the morning (this is the basic quartet).

- ➤ Compression garments for the lower limbs: knee-high stockings (or long pants or leggings) reduce venous pooling in the lower limbs and stabilize the sensors and peripheral nerve endings (such as those of the ANS and proprioception).

- ➤ A correct nycthemeral rhythm must be re-established: Melatonin can be given at a rate of 3 to 6mg in the evening (to be taken 30 to 40 minutes before bedtime). You can take another dose if you wake up during the night, but not after 3 am.

- ➤ Depending on the nocturnal symptoms observed:
  - Palpitations: Bisoprolol/Nebivolol at 1.25mg, or Ivabradine 2.5mg.
  - Nocturia: Solifenacin or Oxybutynin 2.5mg.
  - Profuse sweating and nocturia: Solifenacin or Oxybutynin 2.5mg.
  - Restless legs syndrome (RLS) or dystonia during sleep: Prolopa® or Modopar® 31.25mg at night. Increase gradually if necessary.
  - If OSA: consider CPAP (continuous positive airway pressure) or even BiPAP (bi-level positive airway pressure). Studies are underway to determine what is most appropriate in EDS.

On a case-by-case basis, if necessary

- Riboflavin (vitamin B2): 50mg to 100mg (it improves migraines at higher doses: 400mg/day).

- Nicotinamide riboside (derived from vitamin B3, nicotinamide): 125mg, 3 times a day. It improves fatigue and, it seems, muscular performance via the Krebs' cycle. It is to be associated with the coenzyme Q10 Ubiquinol (at a rate of 200mg/day) to obtain an optimal effect at the cellular and mitochondrial level.

- Thiamine (vitamin B1): 100mg/day.

- Pyridoxine (vitamin B6): 300mg/week, minimum.

- Coenzyme Q10 ubiquinol: 200mg/day (it is also helpful in gingivopathies), in association or not with Nicotinamide riboside.

- Vitamin B12 with intrinsic factor (especially if taking proton pump inhibitors, after a bypass or sleeve gastrectomy).

- Folic acid (vitamin B9): 5 to 10 mg/day (if deficient).

- Iron supplementation (*per os, intravenous*) or blood transfusion of packed red blood cells (if severe iron deficiency anemia).

- Zinc, copper, or selenium supplementation, if necessary.

- Acupuncture, acupressure (shiatsu), dry needling: toning, stress management, sleep.

- Stress management, relaxation, hypnosis or self-hypnosis, meditation, sophrology, cardiac coherence, Yoga, etc.

- Thermalism, gentle physiotherapy, fascia therapy, osteopathy, hydrotherapy.

Levocarnitine (or 3-hydroxy-4-trimethyl-ammonio-butanoate, of gross formula $C_7H_{15}NO_3$) is biologically synthesized from two amino acids at the level of the liver and kidneys: methionine and lysine. At the cellular level, it participates in the transport of acyl chains of fatty acids from the cytosol to the mitochondria (acyl-carnitine). The acyl-chains are transformed into acetate by β-oxidation, thus helping the energy metabolism at the level of the

Krebs' cycle. For the record, it was discovered as a growth factor for mealworms. Only the left (levo-) form is active. Vitamin C is essential for the synthesis of carnitine.[194] Other positive effects of carnitine include an increase in osteoblast activity (the cells involved in bone formation), which may be useful to help prevent osteoporosis. It also has antioxidant properties, with potentially interesting effects on the heart and arterial vessels. A harmful role of carnitine has been suggested, via the intestinal microbiota of meat-eaters, in the development of atherosclerosis, but this remains controversial. Positive effects have been reported on spermatozoa [195], neuroinflammation [196], and neurogenesis[197]. Carnitine deficiency is often observed during pregnancy[198], and supplementation could be systematic in EDS women expecting a child.

[194] Dahash BA, Sankararaman S. Carnitine deficiency. In: SatPearls. Treasure Island (FL): StatPearls Publishing; 2021 Jan.2020 Aug 10. PMID:32644467.

[195] Lipovac M, Nairz V, Aschauer J, et al. The effect of micronutrient supplementation on spermatozoa DNA integrity in subfertile men and subsequent pregnancy rate. Gynecol Endocrinol. 2021;1-5. doi:10.1080/09513590.2021.1923688.

[196] Jamali-Raeufy N, Alizadeh F, Mehrabi Z, et al. Acetyl-N-carnitine confers neuroprotection against lipopolysaccharide (LPS) – induced neuroinflammation by targeting TLR4/NFkB, autophagy, inflammation and oxidative stress. Metab Brain Dis. 2021;36(6):1403.

[197] Fathi E, Farahzadi R, Charoudeh HN. L-carnitine contributes to enhancement of neurogenesis from mesenchymal stem cells through Wnt/β-caretin and PKA pathway. Exp Biol Med (Maywood). 2017;242(5):482-6.

[198] Ringseis R, Hanisch N, Seliger G, et al. Low availability of carnitine precursors as a possible reason for the diminished plasme carnitine concentrations in pregnant women. BMC Pregnancy Childbirth. 2010;10:17.

CHAPTER XI

Acute and Chronic Pain

By Dr. Stéphane Daens

« I suffer so much that my soul screams,
even if my mouth is silent,
for lack of imagining a suitable cry. »

> *« Cursed be the suffering! Without it,*
> *would we still be looking for a culprit? »*
>
> Amélie Nothomb, *Soif (Thirst), 2019.*

Pain management in EDS is a real challenge, as it can be so varied, multiple, multiform, and variable from one patient to another and from one moment to another. It is, therefore, necessary to know how to adapt to each patient by listening to him/her and questioning him/her in detail about:

- ➤ The location of the pain and its depth:
  - The skin level.
  - The muscular level.
  - The articular level.
  - The bone level (pain felt deeply).
  - Generalized pain (the asthenoalgic crisis).

- ➤ The moment of the pain: during certain movements, at rest, during efforts or at a distance from them, during the day or at night, after triggers, according to meals, etc.

- ➤ The feeling of pain such as burning, compression, stabbing pain, lacerations, tingling, painful numbness in certain areas, etc.

A. A typical day for a patient with Ehlers-Danlos Syndrome.

How do I explain it to you?

Patients wake up feeling like they have not slept, heavy, crushed as if a steamroller or heavy truck had passed over them. They wake up feeling like they have been beaten up or washed down. These are the most common expressions used. Then they get out of bed or passively fall out of bed because the pain and fatigue are so intense.

After about two hours, after taking a hot shower or bath, often a few coffees and painkillers, they start their day painfully.

Every moment of the day can become an unbearable calvary.

When they are on the move, they hold on as best they can. But if they must sit down and do a desk job, getting up afterward can become a real ordeal:
"Would gravity have tripled? "
"Would the earth have grown in the meantime? "
They might think.

They often feel tired, especially after meals (role of dysautonomia, food intolerances, histamine, MCAD, etc.).

At the end of the day, they are sometimes slightly better; they prepare the family meal and take care of their children, if necessary. However, in some cases, this is impossible or even illusory.

When they are alone, preparing the meal becomes a painful luxury. They hardly eat anything, or they buy ready meals. This is so much less painful than having to spend an hour on your feet preparing something healthy (watch out for junk food!).

In the evening, they are exhausted, but they cannot sleep; they cogitate or ruminate before going to sleep. They often have a fear of tomorrow, as I call it. That lump in their stomach and chest that they may not be able to do their daily tasks or work.

Every day is a struggle to exist in an ever-changing world.

They often wake up during the night, typically around two or three in the morning: they must urinate, they are sore in bed, they are sweaty, they have to get up, and they have trouble falling back to sleep.

In the morning, whether they have slept or not, the feeling is the same: they are physically and emotionally drained.

The pain and fatigue that patients feel are often unimaginable for those around them. However, they are full of courage. They are mothers or fathers who want to do so much for their partners and children that they struggle until they are exhausted. They do not like doing nothing, they hate feeling or being useless. They enjoy human contact, communication, and interaction with others.

Patients with Ehlers-Danlos Syndrome often say to me: "It would be enough for some people to spend even one hour in my body for them to stop judging me!"

This applies to the people around them as well as to some caregivers and to some medical advisors, from the health insurance companies or the disability services, who call them lazy or imaginary patients.

This is a day in the Life of an EDS patient, as I feel it. I hope this brief description can open some minds to caring, listening, and understanding.

B. Management of Pain, according to its location and type.

1. Cutaneous pain (paresthesias or superficial dysesthesias):

Complaints may appear odd to caregiver's uninitiated or unfamiliar with EDS. They may manifest themselves as tingling of a generalized type or affecting only a segment of the body. At other times, they are burning sensations, sometimes intense, suggesting neuropathic involvement of either the small pain fibers (Aδ and C) or the ANS. Sometimes, they evoke an attack on proprioception fibers (Aα) or touch (Aβ).

As a reminder, the skin contains different types of sensors:

➢ Tactile mechanoreceptors:
  • Meissner's corpuscles are found in the superficial layers of the skin (at the junction between the epidermis and the dermis). They are mainly present in the hairless areas (lips, fingers, etc.). Their reception field (which is the discrimination limit between two distinct points) is a few millimeters. They are activated by stimuli such as touch, light surface movements and slow vibrations.
  • Pacini's corpuscles (or Vater-Pacini's corpuscles) are in the dermis and in the subcutaneous tissue (hypodermis). Their reception field is wider (equivalent to a finger's width, or even more), and the limits are more blurred. These corpuscles have a lamellar shape (like onion flaps). They are activated during deformations and rapid vibrations.
  • Merkel's corpuscles are located at the junction between the epidermis and the dermis, in hairless areas. Their receptive field is a few millimeters. They are activated by light pressure and allow discrimination of shapes and textures.
  • The mechanoreceptors of Ruffini have a wide receptive field, with blurred limits, containing an entire finger. They have an elongated spindle shape and are sensitive to persistent stretching such as joint movements. They are present in the dermis, subcutaneous tissue, and joint capsules.

➢ Thermoreceptors are sensitive to temperature variations:
  • To heat (type C fibers, non-myelinated): from 30°C and especially beyond 45°C.
  • Cold (type Aδ fibers, myelinated): they begin to be activated between 35°C and 25°C. Then their activity decreases, to become null around 10°C (it is the cold anesthesia).

> The Pain receptors (nociceptors) are in the skin:
> - Mechanical nociceptors (mostly Aδ-fibers) are activated when the skin is pricked, pinched, or twisted. They provoke brief and precise sensations. They are in the epidermis and dermis.
> - Thermal nociceptors (C fibers).

For small fibers, no risk factor is generally found in these patients:

- Metabolic: diabetes, hyperlipidemia (especially hyper-triglyceridemia).
- Hereditary: familial amyloid polyneuropathy (FAP), Tangier disease (analphalipoproteinemia = lack of HDL), hereditary sensory and autonomic neuropathies (HSAN), Fabry disease.
- Autoimmune or infectious: vasculitis, hepatitis C, HIV, post-viral autoimmune reaction, Goujerot-Sjögren syndrome.
- Toxic: alcoholism, drugs.
- Other: vitamin toxicity.
- Idiopathic (i.e. without apparent cause): usually after the age of 60 (suspicion of a post-infectious or immune origin).

When the pain is generalized, it resembles Causalgia (CRPS-2), which moreover seems to be most often related to EDS (see chapter on CRPS-1 and CRPS-2).

Additional examinations:

- A complete blood test including ANA (antinuclear antibodies), ANCA (antineutrophil cytoplasmic antibodies), ACE (angiotensin converting enzyme), cryoglobulins, protein electrophoresis (in blood and urine), vitamin B12, hepatitis C serology, HIV serology, Lyme disease, and anti-Hu antibodies. Genetic tests should be performed depending on the situation (FAP, HSAN). Search for anti-gliadin, anti-transglutaminase (celiac disease), etc.
- Electromyography and peripheral nerve conduction velocities (for large fibers, with sensory or motor functions)
- The sympathetic skin response (SSR) studies sweating. SSR is the potential generated by sweat in response to different

stimuli. It allows: An evaluation of the SNA in Parkinson's disease, stroke, MSA, MS, ALS, etc. A search for axonal neuropathy of diabetic, amyloid, alcoholic, uremic origin, etc.[199,200]

- A skin biopsy may be performed to evaluate, under microscopy, the density of the small fibers.[201]
- The study of thermal sensitivity thresholds.
- Laser evoked potentials. They activate the nociceptors and the stinging/burning sensations.[202,203]

These tests will most often be within the normal range in EDS and will not explain the pain. One should not be too quick to label patients with idiopathic small fiber neuropathy. Here, the complaints result from erroneous afferent signals to the CNS or ANS (because the peripheral sensors are over- or under-stimulated) or of central sensitization, or even more often of these two mechanisms.

Suggested Treatments:

→ Patients should always be reassured that It is not in their head.
→ Sequential oxygen therapy, 3 to 5 liters/minute flow (for children: 1 to 2.6 l/minute, depending on age and weight). Sessions of 20 to 30 minutes, 2 to 6 times a day.
→ Compression garments on the areas affected by dysesthesia.
→ Gentle physiotherapy, fascia therapy, osteopathy, hydrotherapy, Thermalism, etc.
→ Stress management, heart coherence, hypnosis, self-hypnosis, sophrology, Yoga, and meditation.

[199] Gutrecht JA. Sympathetic skin response. J Clin Neurophysiol. 1994;11(5):519-24.
[200] Vetrugno R, Liguori R, Cortelli P, et al. Sympathetic skin response: basic mechanisms and clinical applications. Clin Auton Res. 2003;13(4):256-70.
[201] Devigili G, Rinaldo S, Lombardi R, et al. Diagnostic criteria for small fiber neuropathy in clinical practice and research. Brain. 2019;142(12):3728-3736.
[202] Sène D. Small fiber neuropathy: Diagnosis, causes, and treatment. Joint Bone Spine. 2018;85(5):553-559.
[203] Créac'h C, Convers P, Robert F, et al. Neuropathies sensitives des petites fibres : intérêt des potentiels évoqués laser [Small fiber sensory neuropathies: contribution of laser evoked potentials]. Rev Neurol (Paris). 2011;167(1):40-5.

→ Analgesic medication according to the intensity of the complaints:
- Paracetamol 1g, max 4x/day.
- Nefopam hydrochloride: 20mg/ampoule (to drink) or 30mg/tablet. Maximum dose between 3 and 6 doses/day (90 to 180mg).
- Cannabidiol (CBD) without THC (Δ^9-Tétrahydro-cannabinol), in a 10ml bottle. The concentration generally varies from 10% to 30%. Prescribe 2 to 5 drops per dose, sublingual, at a rate of 2 to 4 doses per day. This works quite well for this type of Pain. See the paragraph on CBD below.
- Low Dose Naltrexone (LDN): see the appropriate therapeutic regimen in the chapter dedicated to CRPS. It works well in generalized burning sensations evoking, wrongly, a neuropathic attack, or idiopathic Causalgias (CRPS-2).

→ Antioxidants, in simple or combined use:
- Vitamin C: 1 to 6 g/day.
- N-acetylcysteine (NAC): 600mg, 1 to 3 times daily.
- Alpha-lipoic acid (ALA): 600 to 1200 mg/day.
- Coenzyme Q10 improves the bioavailability of nitric oxide (NO) and is a powerful antioxidant. It has a major role in the cellular Krebs' cycle which produces energy.

→ Treat MCAD, if appropriate.

→ Acupuncture, acupressure (Shiatsu), dry needling (at trigger points).

→ Local injections of lidocaine, at concentrations ranging from 0.5% to 1% (at trigger points).

→ Essential oils: 100% pure, organic, and natural (beware of allergies).

→ If the pain is only present on one side: try mirror therapy.

→ Sensory isolation: this consists of reducing stimuli from other sense organs such as light, sounds, smells, and food.

2. Muscle pain:

They manifest themselves and are expressed by the patients in different ways: cramps, twists, spasms, involuntary movements, the impression of having been beaten up, and painful retractions.

These are phenomena of multiple and varied origins:

➤ In EDS, joint instabilities and laxity of the tendons (which are the extremities of the muscles) inevitably provoke muscular contractions of stabilization in a quasi-permanent way. This leads to contractures and spasms, with increased lactic acid production and mitochondrial depletion (due to the Krebs' cycle). Remember that the two most essential consumers of oxygen in our body are the muscles and the brain.

➤ Erroneous messages come from the peripheral proprioceptive sensors (located in the joint capsules, neuromuscular spindles, Golgi tendon organs, etc.) and are transmitted to the CNS. The consequence is proprioceptive dysfunction syndrome. See the chapter on posturology and proprioception.

➤ Peripheral and central sensitization: see this chapter.

➤ MCAD: see this chapter.

➤ Stress and anxiety are aggravating factors.

Suggested Treatments:

→ Custom-made compression garments.
→ Sequential oxygen therapy.
→ Physiotherapy, muscle chains techniques (Mézières, Busquet, Godelieve Denys-Struyf - GDS, MacKenzie, etc.), fasciatherapy, osteopathy, micro-physiotherapy, etc.
→ Hydrotherapy, balneotherapy, and Thermalism.
→ Proprioceptive re-education, global postural reeducation of P.E. Souchard (GPR), posture inserts, orthoptic reeducation, possible installation of prisms in glasses, etc.
→ Kinesio-taping (K-taping).
→ Acupuncture, Shiatsu, dry needling.
→ Local heat (infrared lamp, fango, heated gel or cherry pits): be careful not to induce burns to the skin, which is fragile in EDS.
→ Local injections of lidocaine, at concentrations of 0.5% to 1% (at trigger points).
→ Stress management: sophrology, hypnosis and self-hypnosis, meditation, Yoga, heart coherence, etc.

→ Essential oils: 100% pure, organic, and natural (beware of allergies).

→ Vitamins and coenzymes of the Krebs' cycle (vitamin B1, B2, B3, B6, B12, C, D, coenzyme Q10, NAD+, and more).

→ Antioxidants (NAC, ALA, Vitamin C, Coenzyme Q10 ubiquinol, and more).

→ Muscle relaxants:
  - Magnesium, electrolytes.
  - Baclofen from 10 to 25mg, maximum from 60 to 75mg per day.
  - Diazepam (Valium®) : from 5 to 10mg, max 3 to 4 times a day.
  - CBD without THC, from 10% to 30% concentration.
  - Levodopa + Benserazide (Prolopa®, Modopar®).
  - Palmitoylethanolamide (PEA).
  - Therapeutic Cannabis (with THC), in the future?

→ In case of dystonia (see the chapter on neuromuscular manifestations):
  - Prolopa® or Modopar® : 31,25mg then 62,5mg per dose, 1 to 3 times a day. Maximum dose: 125mg, 3 times a day (rarely more).
  - CBD without THC, from 10 to 30% concentration.
  - If unsuccessful: try LDN (see central sensitization).

→ Treat MCAD, if necessary : see this chapter.

→ Stabilize the most affected and/or symptomatic joints, which may trigger muscle contractures or reflex dystonia: resting or functional orthotics, Murphy's rings for fingers, cervical collar, tailor-made thoracolumbar belt with shoulder straightener, bespoke sacroiliacs and hips stabilization belt, etc.

3. Joint pain:

Joint and periarticular pain are of multifactorial in origin. The joint capsule, which encloses the joint, contains various sensors:

➢ Ruffini's corpuscles (see above).

➢ The free nerve endings, small diameter, myelinated type Aδ and non-myelinated type C. They are located in ligaments

441

and joint capsules. They are stimulated during forced movements.

> Polymodal nociceptors (C fibers) are sensitive to pain and temperature (more than 45°C and less than 10°C). They are in the muscles, tendons and joints.

In EDS, the joints are unstable and misaligned:

> On the one hand, the joint capsules and periarticular structures (such as ligaments and tendons) are too loose due to changes in the connective tissue.
>   • This also explains true dislocations.

> Secondly, because of erroneous messages sent to the CNS: the sensors and receptors located in the altered connective tissue potentially send information either too quickly, too late, or completely off the mark.
>   • For example, if the capsule sends a message to the brain that the knee joint is misaligned when it is correctly aligned, the brain (which is good and responds correctly to what is sent to it), moves the joint and eventually misaligns it, causing pain.
>   • Another typical example: if you make a movement and hear a crack, it is probably the consequence of a delay of information from the joint capsules to the brain, leading to a transitory subluxation of the joint. It is a back and forth movement of the joint components that becomes audible. Doctors from mutual insurance companies or health organizations often ask if there are subluxations: one can only answer "Yes", when faced with joint creaks.

According to Palmer W. et al (2020)[204]: "Joint subluxation is the malalignment of articular surfaces. Whereas dislocation refers to complete (100%) loss of articular overlap, subluxation refers to partial loss. Subluxation is usually trauma-related, but it can be congenital (developmental dysplasia of the hip) or atraumatic (Ehlers-Danlos syndrome, neuromuscular imbalance).

---

[204] Palmer W, Bancroft L, Bonar F, et al. Glossary of terms for musculoskeletal radiology. Skeletal Radiol. 2020;49(Suppl 1):1-33.

Traumatic subluxation is associated with ligamentous injury. Chronic subluxation suggests joint instability. Radiographs show articular incongruity. Subluxation may be mild (< 25% loss of overlap) or severe (> 75% loss of overlap). Provocative maneuvers and contralateral comparisons increase diagnostic sensitivity for subtle subluxation. CT better demonstrates occult (Lisfranc fracture–subluxation) and complex (Chopart fracture–dislocation) fractures. In the elbow, shoulder, and knee, post-reduction radiographs may be negative despite extensive soft tissue injury. MR shows patterns of bone marrow contusion and ligamentous injury that can clarify traumatic mechanism and help to differentiate transient subluxation from dislocation. Dynamic US enables stress maneuvers that provoke malalignment and prove joint instability".

Therefore, the treatments will either restore correct perceptions to the joint capsules and periarticular structures (through custom-made compression garments) or stabilize the joints (through flexible or rigid orthoses, custom-made silver stabilizing rings, etc.). Joint instability also leads to painful muscle contractions (cramps, contractures, retractions) or dystonia (see above).

We can also protect the articular cartilage by recommending supplements such as type 2 collagen, glucosamine or chondroitin sulfate, turmeric derivatives, etc. Periarticular and peri-muscular lidocaine injections can also be performed.

For the temporomandibular joint, physical treatments, a splint, or specialized devices can be prescribed (posturologist, occlusiodontist, orthodontist, stomatologist).

Hypermobile vertebrae can be stabilized by wearing a custom-made thoraco-lumbar belt (which has a stabilizing role and a proprioceptive function).

A custom-made sacroiliac and hip stabilization belt can be prescribed for the hips and sacroiliacs (even the pubis).

For the shoulders, there are custom-made or prefabricated shoulder slings and stabilizers. A figure 8 shoulder straightener can also be prescribed. Stabilization orthoses are also available for sternoclavicular and acromioclavicular joints. Beware, the placement of anterior bone blocks with bone graft is mostly contraindicated in EDS!

Mast cell activation disorder (MCAD) play a key role in muscle and joint pain (see the chapter wrote by Dr. N. Marcus).

4. Pain felt deeply:

Patients describe non-articular pain, located around just above the bone, or in the bone.

At the level of innervation:

➢ There are nerve fibers, both myelinated and unmyelinated, in the bone and at the periosteum. They are related to the arterial tree and to the sinusoidal capillaries. The fibers are of both of sensitive and autonomic origin.

➢ Sympathetic efferent fibers, are dedicated to the bone and come from the sympathetic ganglia. Sensory afferent fibers (to the CNS) come from the spinal and trigeminal ganglia.

➢ The nerve trunks of the bony diaphysis enter the medullary canal with the feeder's vessels, while the epiphyses' nerve fibers pass through the venous and arterial canals. These nerve fibers are very dense at the epi-metaphyseal junction (the growth plates in children and adolescents) and at long bones' metaphyses.

➢ At the level of the periosteum (the envelope of the bones), at multiple locations, the nerve fibers join together and create a richly developed nerve plexus. In this dense network, there are encapsulated nerve endings such as Meissner's corpuscles (mechanoreceptors), Vater-Pacini's corpuscles (mechanoreceptors), Krause's corpuscles (thermoreceptors or cold receptors), and Golgi's corpuscles (proprioceptive sensory receptors). There are also free endings, myelinated or not. The periosteum of the tibias, mandibles and skull is extraordinarily rich in nerve fibers. Some fibers can penetrate the cortical bone through Havers' or Volkmann's canals.

The pain experienced here can also be of multifactorial origin:

➤ Altered properties of the connective tissue in the periosteum and bone could result in hyper- or hypo-stimulation of receptors and sensory free endings. Incorrect information would then be sent to the CNS (afferent messages).

➤ The dysautonomia associated with EDS could play a role in the efferent messages from the ANS to the bone.

➤ The connective tissue of the dermis and hypodermis in EDS would facilitate the fact that a low pressure on the skin is exaggerated on the periosteum and bone. The thinner and/or looser connective tissue would therefore transmit superficial stimulation more easily.

➤ In the case of joint misalignments (see above), the pressures exerted on the bony and periosteal parts would induce pain by hyperstimulation of the free nerve fibers and the various receptors.

➤ The role of peripheral and central sensitization is potentially important (see above the role of TLR4 and NMDA receptors in the CNS).

➤ The role of mast cell activation disorders (MCAD).

Suggested treatments:

→ Custom made compression garments.
→ Sequential oxygen therapy.
→ Stabilization of unstable joints, posture inserts.
→ Physiotherapy, K-taping, RPG, fasciatherapy, muscle chains techniques, osteopathy, hydrotherapy, etc.
→ Simple analgesics (Paracetamol, etc.).
→ Nefopam Hydrochloride, Tramadol, Ibuprofen 200 to 400mg, etc.
→ CBD without THC, 10% to 30% concentration.
→ Local injections of Lidocaine 0.5% to 1% (at trigger points).
→ Acupuncture, Shiatsu, Dry Needling.
→ Try MCAD treatment if other typical signs and symptoms are present.

→ Treat associated muscle contractures and dystonia (see above).

→ In case of central sensitization: Naltrexone Low Dose, antioxidants (vitamin C, NAC, ALA), Ketamine IV, Lidocaine IV, etc.

Lidocaine is well known as a local analgesic for loco-regional surgery or injections in EDS. It can also be used intravenously. It alters the trans-membrane cationic conduction potentials of neurons and myocytes (these are the muscle cells). Their classical targets are sodium channels. It has also been described as favoring a reduction in the hypersensitivity of action potentials in the spinal cord (the *wind-up* phenomenon). It could thus lead to a reduction in allodynia, hyperalgesia, spontaneous pain, and dysesthesia.

5. Generalized pain or astheno-algesic attacks, pain debts after an effort, and diffuse pain present on waking up or on starting up:

As much as exercise, in the long term, improves the symptomatology of the disease (role of epigenetics? Role of joint protection via better trained muscles?). But, at the beginning of a resumption of regular physical exercise, one may feel pain or even a diffuse astheno-algesic crisis. Mast cells activation might play a key role here.

After sitting (at work or after rest) or lying down for a long time (waking up in the morning), the start of exercise can generate pain. These pains, which are well known to patients suffering from Ehlers-Danlos syndrome, often lead to kinesiophobia (the fear of moving and getting going, the fear of being in pain when moving). It is a vicious circle that must be broken as quickly as possible.

It is often difficult to make patients understand that regular physical exercise and a return to social life are essential for the disease's long-term evolution.

In addition to the treatments previously mentioned, I would give some additional advice:

➢ For physical exercise: start slowly and according to your pain. Do not force yourself. You must learn to listen to your body. Do gentle stretching before and after exercise. Do not forget the vitamins and molecules that help the Krebs' cycle and drink enough (at least 2 liters/day). Put on your orthotics, postural inserts, and compression garments when exercising. Stop telling patients that orthotics and compression garments are harmful and weaken the muscles: this is not true.

➢ For physiotherapy and osteopathy sessions, start with gentle treatments: gentle massages, micro kinesis, muscle chains techniques, global postural rehabilitation (GPR), fasciatherapy, cardiac coherence, rib raising techniques (RRT), neural therapy, cranio-sacral therapy (CST), and more. One should not immediately try to reeducate to the effort, to resuscitate excessively, etc. On the one hand, reinforcing a patient who is askew makes things worse and, on the other hand, it often discourages your patients, who will then stop their physiotherapy treatment.

➢ During physiotherapy sessions, it is necessary to put on compression garments, certain stabilizing or protective orthoses, and plantar orthoses or even splints. The goal is to give back good information to the CNS. The CNS must be retrained to receive good peripheral messages.

➢ Before and after exercise, do a sequential oxygen therapy session (10 to 30 minutes) to reduce the astheno-algesic debt, which can last several days (same for outings with friends or walks, exhibitions, openings, etc.).

➢ Treat MCAD.

➢ Besides the advice given above, for sleep, opt for a mattress, a mattress topper, and firm memory foam pillows (neither too soft nor too hard). This avoids incorrect joint positions and crushing of certain parts of the body during sleep.

➢ When you wake up, if necessary, take your painkillers directly. Then wait 30 to 40 minutes before getting up. Set your alarm a little earlier and stay in bed, until medications are beginning to take effect. If you have a fixed oxygenator with a humidifier near your bed, do a session before getting up.

➢ Do gentle stretching exercises, as recommended by your physiotherapist, before going to sleep and upon waking.

➢ If possible, and if there is no severe orthostatic hypotension (dysautonomia), take a hot shower or a hot bath. In the bath, you can put either essential oils (if there is no allergy or olfactory hypersensitivity) or Epsom salt (magnesium-based). If you have time, put on soft, relaxing music.

➢ If you work, prefer a staggered schedule: do not start too early in the morning, knowing that you need about two hours to be relatively operational. Work from home: you can work at your own pace, take breaks, sit down, and get up at your convenience, all with less stress.

➢ Take time for yourself (even if it is just one evening a week) and work on *letting go*, with the help of a therapist, if necessary.

➢ In the case of diffuse and chronic astheno-algesic state, the possibility of a central sensitization phenomenon and/or MCAD must be considered. Appropriate treatment should then be started:
  • Central sensitization: low-dose oral naltrexone, oral antioxidants, IV or oral ketamine.
  • MCAD: type 1 antihistamines, type 2 antihistamines (if available on the market), anti-leukotrienes, NAC, antioxidants, sodium Cromoglycate, etc.
  • Intravenous lidocaine and magnesium sessions could be tried.

➢ Virtual Reality could be a therapeutic option. The goal is to immerse the patient in sounds and images that will divert his attention from the pain via the anterior cingulate gyrus. This is called *active distraction*. This leads, in fine, to an analgesic effect.[205]

---

[205] Gold JI, Belmont KA, Thomas DA. The neurobiology of Virtual Reality Pain Attenuation. Cyberpsychology & Behavior 2007;10(4):536-544.

> Hyperbaric oxygen therapy (HBOT): some therapeutic trials have been carried out in chronic pain and fibromyalgia. Patients were able to reduce their other analgesic medication. Hyperbaric oxygen therapy would have an anti-inflammatory action and an oxygenation action of the tissues. In fibromyalgia, a decrease in cerebral activity in the posterior cortex has also been noted, but an increase in activity in the frontal region, the cingulate region, the middle temporal region, and the cerebellum[206,207]. Further Studies are still needed in Ehlers-Danlos Syndrome.

> In all cases, bio-psycho-social care is recommended.

After this chapter, I dare to hope that this sentence heard *ad nauseam*, "Ehlers-Danlos Syndrome never hurts!", will be banished from some caregivers' vocabulary because it is full of villainy towards the patients.

Before detailing some of the specific treatments, fortunately, or unfortunately, used in the management of EDS, we have to remind the pain pathways.

It should be emphasized that the structure of opioid and cannabinoid receptors have significant structural similarities and belong to the same family, the G protein-coupled receptors. Through these receptors, therapeutic molecules can modulate many intracellular substances, substances that have various functions.

These two families of substances (opioids and cannabinoids) are also confronted, by this means, with a major problem: tolerance during long-term treatment. Receptor desensitization is one of the main causes of this tolerance to the drugs used. A better understanding of the mechanisms of tolerance to opioids and cannabinoids will allow us, in the future, to design more effective medications over time.

---

[206] Sutherland AM, Clarke HA, Katz J, et al. Hyperbaric oxygen therapy: a new treatment for chronic pain? Pain Pract. 2016;16(5):620-628.

[207] Barilaro G, Francesco Masala I, Parracchini R, et al. The role of hyperbaric oxygen therapy in orthopedics and rheumatological diseases. Isr Med Assoc J. 2017;19(7):429-434.

C. Pain pathways.

Pain receptors, stimulated in the periphery, send messages via nociceptive pathways to the spinal cord and the CNS. Two neurons are essential in this transmission: the first afferent neuron transmits the painful information from the receptor to the spinal cord (via electrical signals). These neurons discharge, at their synapses, neuromodulators that activate, in turn, other neurons in the spinal cord. These neurons send this information to higher level neurons in the cerebral cortex. These signals are translated into painful perceptions in the brain. This is the *ascending pathway of Pain*.

The brain, by reflex, tries to counter these nociceptive afferences by sending other signals, opposite and descending, towards the spinal cord. This is called the *inhibitory descending pathway of Pain*. These signals counteract the ascending pain pathway and ultimately decrease the pain perceived by the CNS. This phenomenon is linked to the release of endogenous opioid substances, the endorphins.

The work of Professor Clifford Woolf, a scientist of South African origin, professor of neurology and neurobiology in the USA (at the *Boston Children's Hospital F.M. Kirby* and at *Harvard Medical School*), has been vital in the understanding of Pain mechanisms. He also described the notion of central sensitization. In this case (see the dedicated chapter), researchers, including Woolf, noticed that a unique mechanism was set up during repeated painful stimulations on an area of the skin. This mechanism was such that the simple fact of touching the area of skin in question could cause disproportionate pain to the stimulus. As a result of these repeated stimulations, there was a phenomenon of central sensitization of the pain neurons. This sensitization can occur following a triggering injury and without any underlying injury (basically, the system goes haywire). These neurons may even remain sensitized after the injury in question has healed. In this case, the pain experienced is no longer simply a pain among others, but becomes a disease generated by a failing CNS.

Researchers have also shown that the emotional state of patients can modify or influence the perception of pain. Stress management techniques (such as mindfulness meditation, hypnosis, and virtual reality) have a potentially remarkably interesting role in pain management. This is one reason why some patients with Ehlers-Danlos Syndrome are referred to specialists in psychology and stress management.

Some have even proposed very advanced *deep brain stimulation techniques* that target the emotional component of pain.

The central perception of pain is extremely complex. There are several centers, or regions, that activate in response to a peripheral pain stimulus, including areas involved in emotions (such as anxiety and sadness), memory (pain perception may vary depending on whether the patient has experienced similar pain in the past, such as a burn), and decision making (such as *Fight or Flight*, see the Porges' Theory). Chronic pain can lead to anxiety and distress, worsening pain perception and/or decreasing pain's descending inhibitory pathway.

Therapeutic opioids and cannabinoids are derived from plants, *Papaver Somniferum*, and *Cannabis Sativa*. They act on heterotrimeric G-protein coupled receptors (GPCRs).

Opioids are placed on three specific types of receptors (mainly $G_{i/o}$ receptors): δ (delta), κ (kappa) and μ (mu) receptors. The endogenous opioids are mainly represented by β-endorphins (which are on μ and δ receptors), the enkephalins (on μ and δ receptors), and the dynorphins (on κ receptors). Morphine (such as etorphine, DAMGO, buprenorphine, and methadone) is located on the μ receptors. GPCRs are located at the central and peripheral levels.

The coupling of these molecules to their receptors results in various intracellular messages: the decrease in the activity of adenylate cyclase (which synthesizes cyclic AMP or cAMP), the activation of potassium channels, the mitogen-activated kinase pathway (MAPK), the inhibition of calcium channels, or the mobilization of intracellular calcium channels. Some of these messages result in decreased release of specific neurotransmitters at the synapse (the synapse is the place where information is exchanged between neurons).

While the messages generated by opioid receptors ultimately reduce pain perception, they also promote respiratory depression, potential respiratory arrest, and sometimes death in some individuals (this is how opioid addicts die of overdose).

Activation of opioid receptors also leads to feelings of euphoria and pleasure. This can lead to more and more use of these substances, and thus addiction.

D. Mechanisms of receptor desensitization and tolerance to opioids (the morphine derivatives).

Tolerance is characterized by a decrease in the expected effect of certain substances used over a long time. How do this desensitization and tolerance develop?

The best studied mechanism is mediated by a decrease in adenylate cyclase activity, an enzyme that allows the cyclic adenosine monophosphate (cAMP) production. The cAMP is one of the so-called second messengers, see the works of Earl W. Sutherland Jr (1915-1974). Sutherland was an American physiologist, chemist, biochemist, physician, pharmacist, and pharmacologist (researcher at the University of Washington). He was awarded the Nobel Prize in Physiology and Medicine in 1971.

Cyclic AMP is produced from ATP (adenosine triphosphate). This enzyme [208] is activated or repressed depending on the binding to a ligand-receptor (a substance that binds to a receptor such as an opioid or a cannabinoid).

The receptor in question is a transmembrane protein (it is in the membrane, with a part outside and inside the cell). This receptor is bound or coupled to a G protein (GPCR). If this G protein has an αs subunit, the enzyme adenylate cyclase is activated; on the other hand, if the G protein has an αi subunit, it is inhibited and

---

[208] An enzyme is a protein with catalytic properties.

decreases its enzymatic activity (which is the case for the opioid and CBD receptors).

Diagram:

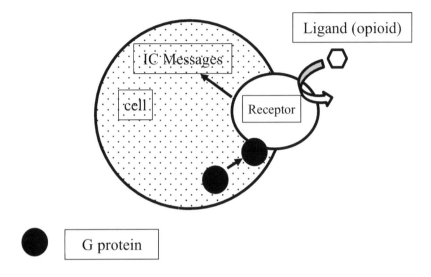

A group of enzymes, called the kinases, is involved in the mechanism of GPCR desensitization and drug tolerance. Various groups of kinases emerge in these mechanisms: the G protein-coupled receptor kinase (GRK) are the most important. Other kinases have a secondary role: protein kinase A (PKA, dependent on AMP cyclase), protein kinase C (PKC), CaM kinases, and tyrosine kinases.

GRKs play a key role in phosphorylating the receptor activated by its ligand and thus desensitizing it. They belong to the serine/threonine kinases. The GRKs phosphorylate the activated receptor. When the activated receptor is phosphorylated, specific proteins, called β-arrestins, will cause the receptor to uncouple from these G proteins and to be internalized in the cell, thus decreasing the total number of receptors available at the cell surface and thus the number of receptors accessible to specific ligands. The receptor is also degraded in special purification centers, the lysosomes. These two mechanisms contribute to the desensitization of the receptors.

The β-arrestins are also thought to play a role in the recycling of specific receptors, that have been dephosphorylated, in endosomes to the cell membrane, thus slowing down desensitization.

As fewer receptors are found on the cell surface, a higher dose of the drug will be needed to saturate as many of the remaining receptors as possible to achieve the same analgesic effect (or euphoric effect for morphine addicts). Many other mechanisms are involved in this desensitization dynamic, but GRKs are involved in essential mechanisms that open, via β-arrestins, new therapeutic pathways that are currently the subject of many publications.

Biased agonism:

Recent findings have shown that GPCRs can have different conformations. These particular conformations may induce different messages in the cell (*Kenakin, 2011*). As different ligands do not induce the same conformational state of the receptors, the intracellular messages will vary, ultimately resulting in different effects. Medical research aims to find specific ligands that stimulate one intracellular pathway over another to increase the desired effects while decreasing potential side effects.

Allosterism and allosteric ligands:

Allosteric ligands are molecules that can bind to sites on receptors other than those where endogenous ligands (called orthosteric ligands) bind. They can also influence the conformation of the receptors, and thus modify their cellular messages. They can be used alone or in synergy with orthosteric ligands. These mechanisms are being studied more and more and will allow the marketing of safer drugs with long-term therapeutic effects and fewer side effects.

In my reading, some publications talk about epigenetics in the modulation of certain receptors. Here we go again!

N. Marie. Mécanismes moléculaires de la tolérance aux opiacés et aux cannabinoïdes. Réanimation. 2009; 18: 626–632.

Thompson GL, Kelly E, Christopoulos A, et al. *Novel paradigms at the µ-opioid receptor. Br J Pharmacol. 2015;172(2):287-296.*

Madariaga-Mazon A, Marmolejo-Valencia AF, Li Y, et al. *Mu-opiod receptor biased ligands; a safer and painless discovery of analgesics? Drug Discov Today. 2017;22(1):1719-1729.*

Wooten D, Christopoulos A, Marti-Solano M et al. *Mechanisms of signalling and biased agonism in G protein-coupled receptors. Nat rev mol Cell Biol. 2018;19(10):638-653.*

E. Some selected treatments.

1. Cannabidiol (CBD) and Therapeutic Cannabis (with Δ^9-tetrahydrocannabinol or THC).

CBD (*cannabidiol*) is present in the *Cannabis Sativa* plant. This plant contains many substances (about 144 substances divided into 11 chemical classes) called *cannabinoids*. CBD is probably the best-known substance, next to THC (Δ^9 - *tetrahydrocannabinol*). CBG (*cannabigerol*) is also promising, alone or in combination with CBD.

Many articles have been published in recent years regarding the potential role of cannabinoids in pain relief. There is a strong patient demand for these derivatives, and I personally regularly prescribe CBD without THC with varying success from patient to patient. Legally, the tolerated concentration of THC is < 0.2 to 0.5% (in Belgium, France, and more).

In the scientific literature, studies are mainly focused on chronic pain such as neuropathic pain, chronic non-cancerous and cancerous pain, fibromyalgia, low back pain, migraines, rheumatoid arthritis and osteoarthritis. There are also data on preventing nausea and vomiting in chemotherapy, treatment-resistant epilepsy, asthma, multiple sclerosis, etc. Research topics abound on cannabinoids. Some studies do not show efficacy, others have contradictory conclusions.

However, cannabis is available for medicinal use in 33 US states and for non-medicinal purposes in 10 states. In Canada, its non-medicinal use was approved in October 2018. The WHO has even proposed that legal attitudes towards cannabis be reviewed internationally, as more and more therapeutic indications emerge. Products exist in both natural and synthetic derivative forms.

Natural forms:

- Sativex®, for therapeutic use (e.g., for pain related to multiple sclerosis). It contains CBD and THC in a ratio [1:1]. It is available in 29 countries including the UK, Israel, Canada, Brazil, Australia, France, etc.
- Epidiolex®, an oral CBD, has been approved in the US to treat two rare forms of childhood epilepsy: Lennox-Gastaut syndrome and Dravet syndrome.

Synthetic forms:

For medicinal use, Dronabinol® and Nabilone® produce effects similar to THC. They are authorized in some countries (USA, Netherlands, Germany, Austria, Croatia) for the treatment of significant weight loss (they stimulate appetite) in HIV patients or cancer patients undergoing chemotherapy (with significant nausea and vomiting). By extension, they would be interesting in severe anorexia. As for synthetic CBD derivatives, they abound on the internet in free access (without THC) or in some stores that are starting to open. in EDS, they could be interesting in certain eating disorders inducing weight loss.

It is necessary to be interested in these compositions and modes of action to understand the therapeutic openings which are possibly offered to us as well as their limitations:

Cannabis Sativa L. is a plant belonging to the *Cannabaceae* family and is present throughout the world. It has been used for thousands of years for its psychoactive properties, its medicinal qualities or to make textiles.

There are three types of cannabis plants:
- *Cannabis Sativa L.* is a fibrous type (fiber-type, hemp).
- *Cannabis Indica Lam.* is characterized by its high levels of the most psychoactive compound, Δ^9-THC (*drug-type*).

- *Cannabis Ruderalis Janisch* has intermediate properties.

However, due to the large number of mixed subtypes, it is best divided into chemotypes:
- Chemotype I includes a preponderance of Δ^9-THC (*drug-type*).
- Chemotype II has intermediate characteristics.
- Chemotypes III and IV contain little Δ^9-THC, but more non-psychoactive substances (*fiber-type*).
- Chemotype V contains no cannabinoids.

Fiber-type is used more in food or textiles, while *drug-type* is used as a medicinal form.

The most important cannabinoids are:
For *drug-type* :
- Δ^9-tetrahydrocannabinolic acid (Δ^9-THCA)
- Tetrahydrocannabinol (Δ^9-THC)

For *fiber-type* :
- Cannabidiolic acid (CBDA)
- Cannabigerolic acid (CBGA)
- Cannabidiol (CBD)
- Cannabigerol (CBG)

Minor forms include:
- Cannabichromenic (CBCA)
- Cannabichromene (CBC)
- Canabinolic acid (CBNA)
- Cannabinol (CBN)

We have two types of natural cannabinoid receptors, CB1 and CB2. The cannabinoid receptors, transmembrane, are of the same family, but different, from opioids. They are G protein coupled receptors (GPCR). Endogenous substances, the endo-cannabinoids, present in our body, can bind to them. Anandamide (its name comes from the Sanskrit, *Ananda*, the goddess of eternal sweetness), isolated in 1992, has a high

457

affinity for CB1 receptors (discovered in 1988). The latter have euphoric effects. Anandamide's mode of action is remarkably close to that of Δ^9-THC, even if they have different chemical structures. 2-Arachidonoyl Glycerol (2-AG) and 2-AG ether were then discovered. The 2-AG has an affinity for both types of CBD receptors, types 1 and 2. There are probably about ten different endogenous cannabinoids.

The endocannabinoids have quite particular characteristics:
➢ They are produced in small quantities.
➢ They have a short life span and are rapidly eliminated.
➢ They are synthesized on demand, unlike other neuro-transmitters that are produced continuously.
➢ They are not stored as vesicles, but diffuse freely.

CB1 receptors (CB1R) are mainly located in the central nervous system, but also, in small quantities, in the peripheral nervous system:

The central CB1R participates in essential functions such as brain development, learning, and memory, motor behavior, regulation of appetite and body temperature, perception of pain and inflammation. They would be involved in neurological and psychiatric diseases. They induce the euphoric, analgesic, and anticonvulsant effects of cannabis because there are receptors in the hippocampus, associative cortex, cerebellum, basal ganglia of the brain, and spinal cord. There are also receptors, in lesser quantities, in the hypothalamus, thalamus, and brainstem.

CB1Rs are found in the lungs, gastrointestinal system, uterus, and testicles at the peripheral level. These receptors are mainly presynaptic receptors. The synapse is the place of communication between the efferent end of one neuron (the axon) and the afferent part of another (the dendrite). Therefore, the receptors are located at the end of the axon of the former, in a transmembrane position.

CB2 receptors (CB2R) are in various regions of our immune system: in the spleen and in certain immune cells such as monocytes, macrophages, basophilic cells, lymphocytes, and dendritic cells.

Δ^9-THC exerts its analgesic effects via CB1R, and its immunomodulatory effects via CB2R.

CBD (cannabidiol) has less affinity for the CB1R and CB2R than Δ^9-THC. CBD is not psychoactive (euphoric). However, CBD has antioxidant, anti-inflammatory (by decreasing cytokines at the peripheral and central level), antibiotic, anxiolytic, neuro-protective, and anticonvulsant properties, via the CB2R.

With the use of CB1R orthosteric agonists and antagonists, in studies conducted in the treatment of obesity and pain management, authors realized that stimulating CB1Rs provoked episodes of psychosis and panic attacks, while inhibiting them favored depressive symptoms and anxiety. Activation of CB1Rs also produced a negative oxidative effect and a pro-inflammatory response. Given the significant side effects of these orthosteric ligands, one wondered why CBD acted so positively when it was also bound to the CB1R.

CBD is, in fact, a negative allosteric modulator of CB1Rs and an agonist of CB2Rs (see paragraph on opioid receptors and allosteric ligands). The agonist effect of CBD on CB2Rs ultimately leads to a decrease in pro-inflammatory reactions and oxidative stress. The action of CBD on the two receptors would thus go in the same direction. Research is trying to synthesize other negative allosteric ligands than CBD, but with higher affinities for this or that type of cannabinoid receptor.

CBD has shown interesting properties in the treatment of several pathologies such as inflammatory bowel diseases (Crohn's disease or ulcerative colitis), certain neurological diseases (Alzheimer's or Parkinson's disease), dermatological diseases (atopic dermatitis, psoriasis, etc.), and asthma. Its interest in cancer, by its action of relieving pain and anxiety, and its possible effects on cell proliferation could be fascinating.

CBD also has affinities for other receptors (TRP receptors, PPARγ receptors, GPR receptors, S-HT1A receptors, Adenosine A2A receptors). Studies are underway on this subject and could lead to other medical uses of cannabinoids and various synthetic derivatives.

CBD has a particular property: it counteracts the effects of THC on CB1 receptors by interacting with other receptors (among those named above). This could reduce some of the side effects of THC such as tachycardia, anxiety, fatigue, and bad mood.

CBG (cannabigerol) has anti-inflammatory, antimicrobial, and analgesic effects.

CBD, therefore, has potentially positive effects on EDS, but one must be careful about the quality of the product used. It is, however, well-tolerated and is not toxic to organs such as the gastrointestinal tract, liver, and kidneys at the doses used in our practice. However, caution should be exercised if it is administered with other potentially hepatotoxic medications. It should be started after having tried first and second-line analgesics and/or in case of intolerance or toxicity to the latter substances (Paracetamol, Tramadol, Nefopam, opioids, etc.). In the future, synthetic compounds, more specifically, will certainly see the light of day to increase the beneficial effects and to decrease the possible side effects of CBD.

I usually prescribe CBD (<0.3% of Δ^9-THC) in sublingual drops. The concentrations vary according to the bottles and the brands: in general, one sees noted on the bottles of CBD of the percentages such as 2.5%, 5%, 10%, 20%, 24%, 25% or 30%. For 10%, it means that in 10ml of product, there is 1000mg of substance. It is important to know that 20 drops of aqueous solution are equivalent to 1ml, or 100mg of product. I recommend between 2 and 5 drops per dose, from 2 to 4x/day. The price is relatively high in Europe, and it is usually not subject to reimbursement or coverage by social security. It is necessary to count approximately 70-85 USD for a bottle of 10ml with 10% of CBD and approximately 120-144 USD for 20%. It also exists in other oral forms (capsules, tablets) or in electronic cigarettes (only recommended for active smokers who do not want to stop smoking).

Some patients take 10% as a routine, and if they are planning an outing or a meal with friends, they take 20% to avoid a painful debt. Everyone has to find what works best for them. The doses of CBD used here are relatively low: between 50mg and 75 mg/day. In various studies carried out in the context of other diseases, the doses used are often higher: between 150mg and 1500mg/day.

Occasionally, I suggest using a pre-packaged mixture of [CBD 5.5% + CBG 8%], available, for example, in sublingual oil. The dosages of each compound are lower and this combination is sometimes better tolerated by sensitive subjects.

Capano A, Weaver R, Brukman E. Evalation of the effects of CBD hemp on opioid use and quality of life indicators in chronic pain patients: a prospective cohort study. Postgrad Med. 2020;132:1:56-61.

Freeman TP, Hindocha C, Bloomfield MA. Medicinal use of cannabis based products and cannabinoids. BMJ. 2019;365:l1141 doi:10.1136/bmj.l1141

Pellati F, Borgonetti V, Brighenti V et al. Cannabis sativa L. and nonpsychoactive cannabinoids: their chemistry and role against oxidative stress, inflammation and cancer BioMed Research International. 2018. doi:10.1155/2018/1691428.

Chung H, Fierro A, Pessoa-Mahana CD. Cannabidiol binding and negative allosteric modulation at the cannabinoid type 1 receptor in the presence of delta-9-tetrahydrocannabinol: an in Silico study. PLoS ONE 14(7):e0220025

Atalay S, Jarocka-Kaprowicz I, Skrzydlewska E. Antioxydative and anti-inflammatory properties of cannabidiol. Antioxydants. 2020 ;9:21; doi:10.3390/antiox9010021.

2. Nefopam Hydrochloride (Acupan®).

Nefopam is a central painkiller (it acts on the CNS) of stage II, derived from benzoxazocine. It was developed a long time ago, in the 1960s. Fenazocin was renamed Nefopam in 1970. Its structure resembles that of an orphenadrine and diphenhydramine antihistamine.

It is not an opioid, and it is not a non-steroidal anti-inflammatory drug. It has a particular structure that is different from that of the most commonly used analgesics.

In vitro, there is an inhibition of catecholamines' reuptake (noradrenaline, dopamine) and serotonin: therefore, their levels increase as for antidepressants. In vivo, in animal studies,

Nefopam has shown antinociceptive properties (painkillers). It was also noted that it had a central anti-hyperalgesic activity: a decrease in central sensitization was observed, as Nefopam had an inhibitory action on NMDA receptors. The mechanism is not completely understood, but it could activate descending serotonergic inhibitory pathways and act on ATP-sensitive potassium channels that modulate allodynia.

The doses used vary from 30mg to 180mg/day (divided into 3 to 6 doses/day).

It decreases postoperative shivering and has been used as an analgesic after surgery. It has no antipyretic effect. There is no depression of the respiratory function, and it does not slow down the intestinal transit (contrary to opioids or Tramadol). It also has an anticholinergic action: it could perhaps improve specific symptoms of dysautonomia (e.g., pollakiuria), but it can worsen the sicca syndrome which is often present in EDS. Side effects may include transient and moderate increases in heart rate and blood pressure, nausea, vomiting, and sweating.

Nair AS. Nefopam : another pragmatic analgesic in managing chronic neuropathic pain. Indian J Palliat Care. 2019;25(3):482-483

Koh Wu, Shin JW, Bang JY et al. The antiallodynic effects of nefopam are mediated by adenosine triphosphate-sensitive potassium channel in a neuropathic pain model. Anesth Analg. 2016;123(3):762-770.

Sanga M, Banach J, Ledvina A et al. Pharmacokinetics, metabolism, and excretion of nefopam, a dual reuptake inhibitor in healthy male volunteers. Xenobiotica. 2016;46(11):1001-1016.

Girard P, Chauvin M, Verleye M. Nefopam analgesia and its role in multimodal analgesia: a review of preclinical and clinical studies. Clin Exp Pharmacol Physiol. 2016;43(1):3-12.

3. Tramadol.

It is a centrally acting analgesic of stage II. Its pharmaceutical presentations are numerous: Tradonal®, Tramadol®, Zaldiar®, Algotra®, Contramal®, Zomudol®, Monoalgic®, Monocrixo®, Biodalgic®, Takadol®, Zumalgic®.

It acts on two levels, in synergy:

➢ An opioid effect (like morphine): it binds to μ (mu) type morphine receptors.

➢ A central mono-aminergic effect, due to an inhibition of the reuptake of serotonin and noradrenaline (which are involved in the control of pain transmission to the CNS).

It has antitussive properties (against coughing). It has little action on intestinal transit in moderate doses. It has effects of respiratory depression, tolerance, and dependence, but less than those observed with morphine.

4. Palmitoylethanolamide (PEA).

PEA (Palmitoylethanolamide) is an endogenous fatty acid amide with anti-inflammatory, antinociceptive, neuroprotective, and mast cell stabilizing properties.

PEA supplements are increasingly being studied and used in Medicine for various indications, including fibromyalgia, Parkinson's disease, Alzheimer's disease, multiple sclerosis, amyotrophic lateral sclerosis, autistic spectrum disorders, acute and chronic pain (improvement of fracture regeneration and antinociceptive effect), sciatic nerve injury, neuropathic pain, and diabetes mellitus.

Neuroinflammation is defined as "*any inflammatory process, acute or chronic, that affects the central or peripheral nervous system*" (*Boche D et al., 2013*) (See the chapter on central sensitization). Immune cells such as mastocytes, microglia, and astrocytes are all involved in these inflammatory mechanisms.

PEA is natural in mammals and is produced on demand by various immune cells to restore homodynamic balance in a variety of pathological situations. Endogenous PEA production is frequently insufficient to compensate for neuroinflammation; oral PEA supplementation appears to be an effective aid in reducing central and peripheral neuroinflammation, pain, and mast cell activation, including in EDS.

Additionally, it may act synergistically with other medications and/or reduce the doses of other medications used in patients with chronic pain.

The recommended dose is 10mg/kg of body weight (from age 6), preferably in micronized form (PEA-m, with a particle size of 2-10mm) or ultra-micronized form (PEA-um, in a 0.8-6mm range). The naive PEA has a particle size distribution of 100–700mm and has a lower diffusion and distribution. Adults should take 600mg bid for 2-4 weeks, followed by 300mg bid (for 3 months or more).

PEA can be used in conjunction with polyphenolic antioxidants derived from plants, such as luteolin (formula $C_{15}H_{10}O_6$; inhibitor of phosphodiesterase-4 or PDE-4; flavonoid), Quercetin (formula $C_{15}H_{10}O_7$; flavonoid) or Polydatin (or Piceid, formula $C_{20}H_{22}O_8$; natural precursor and glycoside form of resveratrol with a monocrystalline structure). Additionally, it is frequently associated with alpha-lipoic acid (ALA, the universal antioxidant), vitamins (B1, B6, B12, C, D, and others), and probiotics, and more.

PEA is a molecule that appears to have a benign safety profile and no evidence of toxicity. PEA is actually classified as a *Food for Special Medical Purposes* (FSMP), under *European Union Regulations*. Nobel prize (Physiology or Medicine, 1996) Rita Levi-Montalcini (1909-1912) wrote: "The observed effects of Palmitoylethanolamide appear to reflect the consequence of supplying the tissue with a sufficient quantity of its physiological regulator of cellular homeostasis".

Levi-Montalcini et al. A nerve growth factor: from neurotrophin to neurokine. Trends Neurosci. 1996;19:514-520)

Boche D, Perry VH, Nicoll JAR. Review: activation patterns of microglia and their identification in the human brain. Neuropathol Appl Neurobiol. 2013;39:3-18.

Petrosino S, Moriello A. Palmitoylethanolamide: a nutritional approach keep neuroinflammation within physiological bounderies – A systematic review. Int J Mol Sci. 2020;21(24):9526. doi: 10.3390/ijms21249526.

D'Aloia A, Molteni L, Gullo F, et al. Palmitoylethanolamide modulation of microglia activation: characterization of mechanisms of action and implication for its neuroprotective effects. Int J Mol Sci. 2021;22:3054. doi: 10.3390/ijms22063054

Del Giorno R, Skaper S, Paladini A, et al. Palmitoylethanolamide in Fibromyalgia; results from prospective and retrospective observational studies. Pain Ther. 2015;4:169-178.

Schweiger V, Martini A, Bellamoli P, et al. Ultramicronized palmitoylethanolamide (um-PEA) as add-on treatment in Fibromyalgia syndrome (FMS):Retrospective observational study on 407 patients. CNS Neurol Disord Drug Targets. 2019;18:326-333.

5. Local injections of lidocaine and Acupuncture in EDS.

By Dr. Daniel Grossin

Pain is one of the major symptoms of Ehlers-Danlos Syndrome. Its intensity, sometimes considerable, is responsible for many situations of disability. Resistance to painkillers is common. On the other hand, it is often accessible to local treatments: heat, orthoses, TENS, etc. It is therefore coherent to favor peripheral pain treatments.

Local injections of lidocaine:

Unfortunately, local injections of lidocaine are often criticized by people who have either never benefited from them or have never performed them. They have, therefore, never been able to see the benefits. Some people hide behind extremely rare and/or minimal side effects in the face of major and proven therapeutic benefits. The action of these injections can be spectacular and lasting.

Janet G. Travell (1901-1997) wrote her first article on this subject in 1942 in the *Journal of the American Medical Association* (JAMA), an internationally renowned medical journal. She described the type of injections that her father, a physician, gave her for shoulder-hand syndrome.

The injections are performed on a set of points that she would later call trigger points. Cardiologist, orthopedist, pharmacologist, teacher, and researcher, Janet Travell was President J.F. Kennedy's physician. She was incredibly passionate about chronic myofascial pain, which led to the publication of a reference book in 1983 with Dr. David Simons: "*Myofascial Pain and Dysfunction - The Trigger Point Manual*".[209]

Manual therapy, dry needling, and traditional acupuncture can be performed on these same trigger points. 70% of the trigger points overlap with known acupuncture points. Local injections of lidocaine are indeed the simplest, longest-lasting, and most effective way to treat these chronic myofascial pains.

Lidocaine (Xylocaine®), with no added product (neither adrenaline nor preservative), is available in three concentrations: 0.5%, 1%, and 2%. We usually use the lowest concentration, but some of our knowledgeable colleagues use a higher concentration.

However, it seems to us that the identification of trigger points and the injection site's recognition are more important than the quantity of product used. A few years ago, lidocaine was present and used daily in all medical practices. It was THE essential molecule for local anesthesia for any minor surgery, in the office. This shows the hindsight we have on this molecule, both in its daily use and age (1949)[210]. A 20-milliliter bottle costs less than 3.55 USD, making it a very accessible molecule for all patients.

For the rest of the material to be provided: syringes of 10 or 20 ml, needles of 10 to 40 mm in length and 0.3 to 0.6 mm in section, hand washing with hydro-alcoholic gel and a disinfectant solution for the skin (70° alcohol).

Stitches should be located and noted before the first injection. The search must be careful, by attentive and very cautious

---

[209] Travell J. Basis for the multiple uses of local block of somatic trigger areas; procaine infiltration and ethyl chloride spray. Miss Valley Med J,1949;71(1):13-21.
[210] Lozier M. The evaluation of xylocaine as a new anesthetic. Oral Surg Oral Med Oral Pathol, 1949;2(11):1460-8. doi: 10.1016/0030-4220(49)90095-x.

palpation, to not trigger lasting pain for the patient with Ehlers-Danlos Syndrome.

The injection must be done where the pain is the most acute. There are two types of points: *remote trigger points* and *strictly local points*. Sometimes conventional trigger point injections may be sufficient, and other times they must be supplemented with strictly local points.

The skin crossing can be harrowing because of the skin's hyperesthesia, which is frequent in EDS. One can use the *touch and prick technique*: the patient is told verbally, "I am touching you", and then the surface of the skin is touched but not pricked (one simply warns where the injection is to be made). Then the patient is told, "I am pricking you", and the needle is inserted. This way of proceeding, acquired through experience, gives excellent results on the experience of the injection for the patients and avoids the surprise, which often generates sudden movements.

Then, the product is injected very slowly, and we stop immediately if the slightest pain is reported. The volume of the injections ranges from a few drops to 5 ml per point. One to ten injections are performed per session for a maximum total volume of 20 ml.

Sometimes a point can be hyperalgesic. It is then preferable not to insist, withdraw the needle, and, possibly, return to it after carrying out other injections in the same area.

The first session must be well received by the patient, who is often very anxious. It is better to have a less immediate effect than to jeopardize further sessions.

On the next page: The essential points

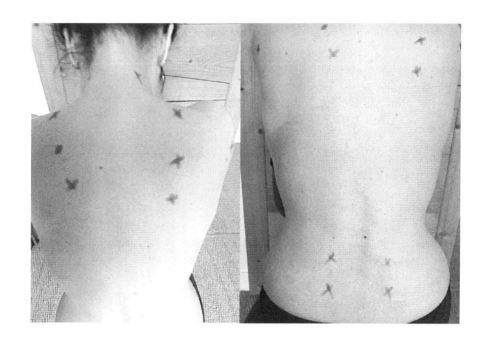

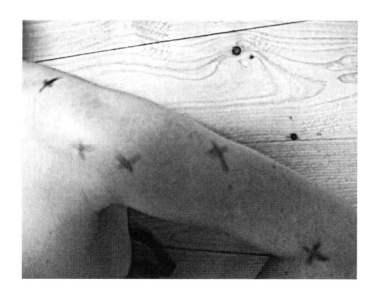

468

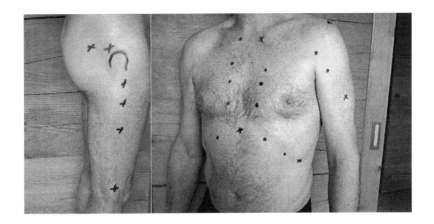

A single session can be enough to erase chronic and old pains, other times it is a complete failure, despite repeated sessions. However, in most cases, a good result is obtained, which generally does not last long, but gradually increases in duration with each session. Allergies are extremely rare. A reaction of fatigue and/or drowsiness sometimes accompanies lidocaine injections. There is no limitation in the frequency of injections. However, there is at least two days between each session. The effect usually lasts several days, sometimes several weeks or months.

The hypothesis of these local injections' action would be to disrupt, or even interrupt, a reflex loop that is self-sustaining and at the origin of the chronic pain. Lidocaine's duration is very short, between 60 and 120 minutes on average, since its initial plasma half-life is less than 30 minutes and its elimination half-life is one to two hours.

If a therapeutic effect exceeds one day, this verifies this pathophysiological theory of a reflex loop that has been disrupted or stopped by a simple brief local anesthesia.

These injections are, therefore, relatively easy to perform. Too much, perhaps? Many caregivers do not want to have the doubt and/or curiosity, however essential in Medicine, to try these injections and then be convinced. It is a prodigious tool at our disposal for all chronic pain, and in our case, for EDS. Easy and inexpensive, with few side effects and over 70 years of experience, the risk/benefit balance of lidocaine in the local injection is unquestionable.

Acupuncture in the treatment of EDS:

Acupuncture is a Traditional Chinese Medicine (TCM) which, by pricking needles and stimulating certain points on the skin (simple pricking, pricking-turning), makes it possible to rebalance and reinforce energies, as well as to eliminate specific blockages in the circulation of Energy (the *Chi*) or Blood (the Blood of TCM or *Xue*).

The UNESCO definition is: "Traditional acupuncture is a therapeutic art that bases its diagnostic and therapeutic reasoning on an energetic Taoist vision of man and the universe."

For a long time, I treated patients with acupuncture, many of whom had Ehlers-Danlos Syndrome. Of course, I did not know at the time that these patients were carriers of this complex disease. I treated them for DIPS (Diffuse Idiopathic Polyalgic Syndrome, as described by Professor M.F. Kahn) or Fibromyalgia. Acupuncture has been of great help to them.

Nowadays, knowing the wide range of therapies available in EDS, I think that all the classical means, defined previously in this book, should be used first, before considering acupuncture, at least if there are still troublesome symptoms for the patient.

Acupuncture has, for me, two pitfalls:

➢ The first one is the difficulty, in EDS, to make a symptom disappear radically. It takes several sessions, from three to five, to improve a symptom, and it is often necessary to repeat the acupuncture sessions in a period of time that is often too short for a chronic disease (which is defined as persistent for more than three months).

➢ The second is its cost, which is often high and not covered by social security in most cases. Moreover, it is preferable to find an acupuncturist who knows about EDS, it is better, but it is rare.

Acupuncture should be considered in indications that are resistant to classical therapeutic lines.

We can then quote as indications:

♦ Localized pain such as joint, tendon and muscle pain. For example, mixed pain of the temporomandibular joints, tendonitis of the gluteus medius, or pyramidal gluteus.
♦ Sleep disorders.
♦ Stress and anxiety.
♦ Chest, abdominal, digestive or pelvic pain.
♦ Headaches, tinnitus.
♦ Heart palpitations.
♦ Urinary or gynecological disorders.
♦ Problems related to pregnancy such as nausea (caution with certain points).
♦ Stopping smoking or other addictions.
♦ A request for general rebalancing, although it is part of an acupuncture session.

The side effects are, especially for EDS patients, pain caused by needle puncture, vasovagal discomfort, redness, hematoma, or asthenia occurring after a session (be careful with driving).

Bibliography:

Tewari S, Madabushi R, Agarwal A et al. Chronic pain in a patient with Ehlers-Danlos syndrome (hypermobile type): The role of myofascial trigger point injections. Journal of Bodywork and Movement Therapies. 2017; 31(1):194-196.

Lugo LH, Garcia HI, Rogers HL et al. Treatment of myofascial pain syndrome with lidocaine injection and physical therapy, alone or in combination: a single blind, randomized, controlled clinical clinical. BMC Musculoskelet Disord. 2016;17:101.

Borg-Stein J, Laccarino MA. Myofascial pain syndrome treatments. Clin N Am. 2014;25(2):357-374.

Money S. Pathophysiology of trigger points in myofascial pain syndrome. J Pain Palliat Care Pharmacother. 2017;31(2):158-159.

Machado E, Machado P, Wandscher VF et al. A systematic review of different substance injection and dry needling for treatment of temporomandibular myofascial pain. Int J Oral Maxillofac Surg. 2018;47(11):1420-1432.

Ahmed S, Subramaniam S, Sidhu K et al. Effect of local anesthetic versus botulinum toxin-A injections for myofascial pain disorders: a systematic review and meta-analysis. Clin J Pain. 2019;34(4):353-367.

Parthasarathy S, Sundar S, Mishra G. Assessment of predisposing factors in myofascial pain syndrome and the analgesic effect of trigger point injections – A primary therapeutic interventional clinical trial. Indian J Anaesth. 2019;63(4):300-303.

6. Endermotherapy and EDS.

By Mr. Dominique Ouhab

We know that edemas are very frequent in patients with EDS. They can be superficial, in the extremities of the limbs with soft swellings or of firm consistency, evoking rather a lymphedema, which is at the origin of certain night pains, at the level of the lower limbs.

One of the main characteristics of lymphedema is the retention of high molecular weight proteins in the interstitial environment. This results in an accumulation of water and bacteria. The proteins lead to progressive fibrosis, which in turn affects tissue nutrition. The retention of germs leads to infectious outbreaks during which macrophages and fibroblasts release their mediators, worsening fibrosis.

Several studies have shown that Endermotherapy (LPG® technique, using Cellu M6 Alliance) directly stimulates fibroblasts by increasing elastin and collagen fibers' synthesis. This concentration of technology, combining depression with mechanical palpation and rolling, causes a lasting increase in arterial and venous microcirculatory flow and activation of adipocytes.

Its action extends beyond the dermis and hypodermis to the muscular aponeuroses, whose role in venous hemodynamics is crucial.

Based on these observations, I thought it would be interesting to include Endermotherapy in the physiotherapy treatment of patients with Ehlers-Danlos Syndrome.

On the one hand, this technique is a valid alternative to manual lymphatic drainage because it has the advantage of acting on both the fibrosis and the functional recovery of the edematous limb. On the other hand, it allows a spacing of the treatment sessions (2 or 3 sessions per week maximum, instead of the usual five sessions of physiotherapy) as well as a lightening of the maneuvers of contention - compression, for the greatest satisfaction of the patients who are already subjected to a handicapping chronic affection and to a demanding treatment.

Endermotherapy can also be performed directly on compression garments, whose effectiveness on venous return has been proven.

7. Thermalism and its benefits in EDS

By Dr. Michel Horgue

7.1. A bit of History.

Thermalism, as a therapeutic tool, has developed in France since the 19th century. It is not an exclusively French fact but also European. If the Anglo-Saxon and Scandinavian countries are not extremely interested in Thermalism, the annual number of curists is important in Italy, Slovakia, Germany, and Russia. Thermal cures are based on the use of natural waters (called mineral waters) for therapeutic purposes: either by particular physical characteristics, such as temperature or by their singular chemical structures. Therefore, in France, at least, it is agreed to call mineral waters, natural springs endowed with therapeutic properties, whether by their physical character or mineralization. For this reason, the hygiene, conservation, and control of mineral waters, from their source of emergence to their use in the spa, is strictly regulated by the authorities. The research of the therapeutic virtues of thermal waters started incredibly early in France, as early as 1910, to identify their indications. France's thermal heritage is exceptional: there are more than 1,200 listed and controlled springs, more than 100 thermal spas, some of which are internationally recognized for their therapeutic values, their reputation, and the quality of their facilities.

7.2. Therapeutic indications.

A spa can develop its indications in two ways: the first, called Central European, insists on the versatility of the treatments. The second one comes more specifically from France and emphasizes a specialty of Medicine, this since the end of the 19th century.

The recognized therapeutic orientations are the following:

RH	Rheumatology and after-effects of osteoarticular traumas.
VR	Respiratory tract and ENT.
AD	Digestive tract and metabolic diseases.
GYN	Gynecology.
DER	Dermatology.
AMB	Diseases of the oral and lingual mucous membranes.
PHL	Phlebology.
PSY	Treatment of psychosomatic conditions.
TDE	Childhood Developmental Disorders (Growth Disorders).
NEU	Neurology.
MCA	Cardio-arterial diseases.
AU	Urinary tract and metabolic diseases.
And a new indication: Fibromyalgia	

Within the framework of hypermobile Ehlers-Danlos Syndrome (hEDS), the useful indications are: Rheumatology (RH), respiratory tract (RV), fibromyalgia (because people living with fibromyalgia are frequently undiagnosed Ehlers-Danlos Syndrome).

Because of the quality of their thermal waters, French spas often have several indications. For example, for the DAX spa[211], these are Rheumatology and Phlebology (and fibromyalgia, since 2008); for the Mont DORE spa[212], these are Respiratory Tract and Rheumatology. In France, the spa treatment is covered by social security for cures of three consecutive weeks, with a requirement to practice four treatments per day in the first indication prescribed (RH) and two treatments per day in the second indication (PHL). The double indication is rarely practiced in EDS because of the chronic fatigue and the fatigue induced by the cure, which is very often present. Most thermal cures are therefore done with only one indication.

7.3.   Teaching and Research.

Thermal medicine is taught at the Faculty of Medicine in France and is the subject of a two-year Diploma of Capacity of Hydrology and Medical Climatology for more than 50 years. Created on May 18, 2000, by the French Ministry of Education, the DAX Thermal Institute has become an essential tool for the whole thermal profession. Its missions of Research and Training, supported by the availability of a documentary pole and the development of international exchanges, are at the heart of the scientific, medical, and socio-economic stakes related to the field of water and Health. Besides, there is a Thermal Hospital in the spa town of Dax where cures can be carried out during hospitalization for the most severe cases. Within this hospital service, there is a consultation dedicated to Ehlers-Danlos syndrome. To date, it is the only hospital department in France that offers an inpatient spa treatment. These inpatient cures are subject to a request for prior agreement from the social security system to be covered.

7.4.   Contraindications of spa treatments.

♦ Acute progressive diseases: infectious, neoplasia, inflammatory. Crenotherapy is traditionally reserved for the treatment of chronic diseases, except for eczema.

---

[211] https://www.thermes-dax.com
[212] https://www.chainethermale.fr/le-mont-dore

♦ Decompensated heart failure, severe high blood pressure, recent stroke.
♦ Recent venous thrombosis.
♦ Immunosuppression.

7.5.   The prescription.

The prescription of the thermal doctor includes:

1. The therapeutic use of thermal water, with its different techniques which will be detailed later.
2. Physiotherapy in the form of massage, mobilization, motor rehabilitation in a hot water pool, and respiratory rehabilitation.
3. Rest: avoid excesses, fatigue, late bedtime.

It can also include elements not covered by social security:

4. Physical activity treatment, or getting back in motion, physical education.
5. In some cases, for physiotherapy: heliotherapy, thermotherapy, short waves, electrotherapy, etc.
6. Therapeutic patient education with practical workshops.
7. Dietetics, for digestive, renal, metabolic indications, hEDS.

Among the multitude of French spas, two of them have taken an interest in the treatment of EDS:

• The MONT DORE :

The specific EDS (and HSD) cure has been organized for several years within the framework of a partnership between the medical-thermal establishment of Mont Dore and the SED1+ patients' association[213], with the participation, at the beginning, of Professor Claude Hamonet.

In April, the specific cure takes place to benefit from the specific support offered by the SED1+ association, detailed in the following developments.

---

[213] http://www.assosed1plus.com

Some characteristics of the station:

➤ The resort is located in the Puy de Dôme, at an altitude of 1000 meters, at the Puy de Sancy foot.

➤ The thermal treatments are based on thermal gases and thermal waters (hydrotherapy).

➤ The relief of Mont Dore is mountainous.

➤ The presence of permanent elevation changes can be difficult for EDS patients to walk around, often out of breath on the slightest slope.

➤ The springs, very abundant and hot (from 34°C to 44°C), are characterized by:
  • Their richness in carbonic gas.
  • Their sodium bicarbonate, carbo-gaseous, and siliceous mineralization.
  • The presence of arsenic (at rate of 1 mg/liter).
  • The main properties of Mont-Dore's thermal water are relaxing, analgesic, sedative, anti-inflammatory, and decongestant. It cleanses and strengthens the mucous membranes, acting as a barrier to the penetration of allergens.

1° The possible care for the Respiratory Tract:

➤ Spraying (VR care): a thread-like jet of thermal water is broken by a sieve and is absorbed by the patient, mouth open. The droplets of thermal water settle and bathe the throat, tonsils, and pharynx.

➤ The steam shower (RH or VR treatment): these are local steam affusions targeted by the thermal doctor. It is a relaxing treatment with a vasodilatory effect that improves the irrigation of the treated area.

➤ Sonic aerosol (VR care): the sonic vibrator, an infrasound device, is coupled to an individual aerosol. It transmits a certain energy to the particles that allow them to reach areas of the respiratory system that are not easily accessible, such as the sinuses. This treatment is particularly interesting for treating sinuses, otitis, but also bronchitis with significant congestion.

- Individual aerosol (VR care): at the exit of the mask, particles of 2 to 5 microns of thermal vapors are emitted, reaching the upper and middle respiratory tract in depth.

- Nasal irrigation (VR care): using a cannula with a continuous low flow of thermal water, the patient performs a real shower of the nasal cavities. The result is an effective drainage of mucus and purification of the nasal filter.

- Humming: the patient inhales a warm mist of fine droplets of thermal water at the exit of a mask. Fine particles of thermal water are deposited on the mucous membrane of the nasal cavity and throat.

- The gaseous nasal shower: the thermal gases come from the springs and cracks in the mountain. The curist passes them through his nose with the help of a cannula which is placed, alternately, at the entrance of each nostril.

- The collective aerosol: the water inhaled in the form of exceptionally fine particles, passes through the upper and lower respiratory tracts. It is sometimes called *dry fog*.

- Respiratory re-education (VR care): respiratory gymnastics aiming at seeking, in the asthmatic and chronic bronchitis patient, a normal respiratory cycle from a directed ventilation, by insisting on the abdominal and diaphragmatic work.

- The Proëtz Method: this method ensures the penetration of thermal water inside the sinus cavities, using a pump system.

- Collective inhalation (VR care): in a dedicated room, excellent and abundant aerosols are emitted with the help of ultrasound, which allows the thermal water to be diffused deep into the respiratory tract during inhalation.

- The general jet shower (VR or RH treatment): the shower is administered at a variable distance, using a lance that propels a jet of thermal water under pressure of between 1.5 and 2 bars. The jet is modulated and directed on the parts of the body indicated by the doctor.

- Pharyngeal shower: this shower is applied by the doctor using a water gun. It is the method of choice because of its pressurized, thread-like jet that has a scouring action on the tonsil crypts and the pharyngeal wall and local trophic action on the tissue.

> Eustachian tube insufflation: this technique is essential in ENT medicine. The doctor himself introduces the thermal gases into the Eustachian tube with the help of a probe gently introduced along the floor of the nasal cavity. The probe is connected to the thermal gas generator.

2° Possible treatments for Rheumatology:

> Cataplasms (RH treatment): five bags of white clay cataplasms are applied to the painful areas, joints, or muscles, defined by the thermal doctor.

> Aero bath (RH treatment): this is a thermal water bubble bath accompanied by air microbubbles. In the case of EDS, the hyperesthesia of the skin may be difficult to tolerate, so the power of the jets must be set to a minimum.

> The general steam room (RH treatment): the patient enters a chamber and sits on a bench pierced with holes that allow the heat to envelop him or her; the head emerges into the open air, and the hot thermal gases arrive at the base.

> The local steam bath (RH care): the loco-regional steam bath allows two or four limbs (hands or feet) to be treated on the same principle as the general steam bath.

> The general penetrating shower (RH treatment): the patient lies on a treatment table, the thermal agent directs the multiple jets of an oscillating shower ramp, oriented perpendicularly to the body, to make them travel through the area defined by the thermal doctor.

> The mobilization pool (RH care): this technique is performed in a thermal water pool under the direction of a state-qualified physical therapist. Rehabilitation medical-gymnastics movements are prescribed to the curists according to their pathologies.

> Immersion in the pool (RH care): this technique is carried out in a thermal water pool: each station is equipped with automatically integrated jets to massage the areas of the body specified by the Thermal Physician.

> Thermal gas injections (RH care): the doctor carries out this treatment in the thermal establishment. The injections are made around the painful joint area by subcutaneous multi-punctures. The amount of gas varies depending on the type of joint or area to be treated. A vasodilator effect improves the punctured area and causes a neo-vascularization with a local anti-inflammatory reaction.

3° Specific SED1 + support:

This specific accompaniment is offered in April and is organized by both volunteers and professionals.

> Accompaniment by volunteers:
> ♦ A breathing yoga workshop, a writing workshop, creative leisure workshops, a luminous and 3D card workshop, a papercraft workshop, a sewing workshop, and a knitting workshop.
> ♦ The Café parole: three workshops over the three weeks.
> ♦ The workshops are conducted by volunteers who offer their time and professional skills to patients.

> The professionals' offer:
> ♦ A QI-Gong workshop.
> ♦ An orthotist consultation.
> ♦ A horseback riding workshop for children and adults.
> ♦ Lidocaine injections performed by the thermal doctor.

4° The results of the follow-up of the cures:

The thermal agents, as well as the thermal doctors, were sensitized to the hEDS and its specificities of care:

> The VR treatments are efficient for the hEDS on their congestion and their bronchial affections.

> Gas injections, for those who wish to perform them, carried out like mesotherapy, have a real effectiveness on the pains and on a duration which can go until 8 months for certain patients.

➢ In the various RH treatments, the properties of hot thermal water are remarkably effective on aches and pains, and contractures.

➢ The care that is carried out by the vast majority of patients is:
  ♦ RH: penetrating shower, swimming pool (mobilization), hydroxyurea (bubble bath) and classic bath, hand/foot dryer, steam shower, cataplasms (mud plasters). Underwater massages by trained physiotherapists, as well as gymnastics in the hot water pool, are beneficial.
  ♦ VR: humming, cannula.

  • The DAX station

The spa of DAX is the first rheumatological spa in France by its attendance: 47,458 curists in 2017, not counting curists from Saint Paul Les Dax, the neighboring resort with the same care, which received 14,130 curists in 2017. The thermal spa of Dax treats by hydrotherapy and by peloid. Its geographical/topographical location in wooded plains and its many health trails make it a favorable environment for getting hEDS patients back into motion. The medical indication for fibromyalgia, since 2009, also brings specificity to the care.

The thermal resources of Dax:

There are 3 types of thermal water:
- Hyperthermal water.
- Sodium chloride water.
- The natural Thermo-vegeto-mineral mud, or Peloid.

The Peloid:
  ♦ Its mode of formation did not change practically through the ages. It was born spontaneously on the banks of the Adour (a river in the South-West of France), in the natural craters from which thermal water emerged.
  ♦ The grafts were periodically submerged at the time of the floods of the river. The silt was deposited in these cavities when the water receded.
  ♦ The algae found there the best conditions to develop: mineral salts, heat, and especially the light.

- ♦ It is undoubtedly a seaweed that also provides the analgesic virtues of this pelotherapy.

Hygiene and Safety:
- ♦ The *Régie des Eaux* ensures the control of the mud and the thermal water during the production and the delivery.
- ♦ It ensures the management of the thermal water.

Qualitherme:
- ♦ The *Syndicat des Établissements Thermaux* de Dax (*Dax Thermal Establishments Union*), concerned with guaranteeing thermal treatments' sanitary safety, has created a quality charter called *Qualitherme*.

Aquacert Thermalism:
- ♦ This is a quality approach of the thermal establishments.
- ♦ From now on, all the resort thermal establishments are committed to a quality approach in order to obtain an AQUACERT Thermalism, or ISO 9000 certification.

Rheumatology Care:

➢ Pelotherapy: this consists of the application of thermal mud to the joints designated in the medical prescription (lasting 15 minutes, at a temperature of between 40°C and 42°C), followed by a shower with a thermal water jet and, depending on the case, a sweating session in an individual cabin which continues the vasomotor action of the mud. Its effects are analgesic and anti-inflammatory.

➢ Mobilization in the pool: immersed in a pool of thermal water, the curist works all his joints and the three segments of the spine through exercises led by a physiotherapist. These exercises are relaxing and improve joint mobility.

➢ The turpentine shower: a mixture of thermal water and components from pine trees is sprayed on the skin for 3 minutes at a temperature of 38°C. This local treatment is analgesic and anti-inflammatory.

➢ The local steam bath: this is a local thermal water steam bath for the hands or feet, between 35°C and 45°C. It has an analgesic action and improves mobility.

- Hydro-massage: this is a thermal water bath with numerous water jets of varying pressure. Its effects are relaxing, toning, and draining. Because of the hyperesthesia of patients' skin with EDS, the thermal agents of certain establishments reserve a low-pressure bath for them.

- Physiotherapy: massages based on thermal balsam allow for a softening of the tissues and reduce edema.

- Aero bath: this is a thermal water bath at 32°C with compressed air bubbles. It is a relaxing and draining treatment.

- The high-pressure shower consists of an underwater jet, with variable direction and pressure, performing a deep massage of the muscles and joints. Its effects are relaxing and analgesic. It is rarely prescribed and tolerated by patients with EDS.

- The general jet shower: this is a variable pressure jet that provides postural toning.

- The underwater shower: it is performed in a bathtub or swimming pool by a thermal agent. This treatment has an analgesic and relaxing effect. These pool showers are interesting in EDS: the thermal agent reduces the pressure of the jets for hEDS patients who can direct the jets themselves and thus reduce the pressure by managing the body/jet distance.

- Massage: this is a relaxing treatment carried out by a physiotherapist.

Phlebology treatments:

- Aero bath : a thermal water bath between 28 and 32°C, with compressed air bubbles. Relaxing and draining treatment.

- The carbon dioxide bath: immersion of the lower limbs in a bathtub in thermal water between 28 and 29°C, charged with carbon dioxide. This treatment aims to reduce edema, improve tissue trophicity and arterial microcirculation.

➤ Drinking cure: from 1 to 4 glasses per day, thermal water is used for its diuretic, laxative, and detoxifying action, as well as for its richness in trace elements.

➤ Hydro massage: a thermal water bath between 28 and 32°C, with numerous water jets of varying pressure. Relaxing, toning and draining effects.

➤ Lower limb massage: performed by a physiotherapist, this treatment softens the tissues and reduces edema.

➤ The walking course: a walk in a thermal water pool, lower limbs immersed in water between 26 and 29°C. The floor, covered with asperities, massages the arches of the feet, and jets of compressed air provide a light massage. This treatment stimulates venous return and is invigorating.

➤ The spraying of the lower limbs: it is a thread-like shower directed on, the lower limbs. It improves functional disorders (heavy legs and tingling) and reduces cellulite infiltration.

Complementary care proposed:

They are sometimes at the patient's expense (in the framework of Fibromyalgia) but are interesting in the hEDS:

♦ Sophrology.
♦ A consultation is possible at the Thermal Hospital for EDS follow-ups during the cure.
♦ Orthopedic consultation is possible at the *Orthopédie Landaise*, trained in EDS treatment (compression garments, orthoses, etc.).
♦ Soft gymnastics: Fibrotherapy.
♦ Free health courses.
♦ Conferences and workshops focused on health.
♦ Discussion groups.

Satisfying points:

For the curists who regularly come for a cure, the results are globally satisfactory and long-lasting.

- The cures' satisfaction carried out results essentially from the care, especially concerning the peloids.
- The underwater shower in the pool, the turpentine shower, and the hot water pool's rehabilitation are highly appreciated. For the bathtubs, one must pay attention to the pressure settings by the thermal agent.
- Underwater massages are also appreciated when the hyperesthesia of the skin makes them possible.
- It is possible to prescribe breaks between treatments to manage the fatigue linked to the cure.

Inconvenients:

- Skin tolerance on skin that is often atopic and easily irritated.
- Urinary incontinence, sometimes aggravated by hydrotherapy.
- Fatigue induced by 18-day care, which counter-indicates most often a double indication.
- Prefer establishments where travel between treatments is limited and where the thermal agents are aware of the EDS.

Conclusions concerning the thermal cure:

The thermal cure is thus beneficial in the management of the patient suffering from Ehlers Danlos Syndrome. He can expect a lasting improvement of his clinical condition by regularly practicing the cures. Only two thermal spas are interested in this pathology of EDS, with sensitized thermal agents. However, given the benefits observed, any hot water spa with a rheumatology indication can accommodate an EDS patient, especially if it is closer to the patient's home. The patient's condition will improve with a hot water hydrotherapy treatment, massage, and mobilization in a hot water pool. If the Fibromyalgia indication is also chosen in this station, it will be even more indicated. The lack of knowledge on the part of doctors and thermal agents regarding EDS's specificities is the main obstacle to the correct implementation of the cure.

However, this book is here to remedy this!

CHAPTER XII

Neurological and ENT Manifestations
Oral Care

1/ Neurological and pseudo-neurological manifestations

By Dr. Stéphane Daens

Neurological or pseudo-neurological manifestations are common in EDS and are of extreme concern, often justifiably so, to both patients and caregivers. The anxiety reaction generated is frequently exaggerated. It is often the consequence of a collective unconscious concerning the brain and its irremediable lesions:

"My grandmother was paralyzed by a stroke!"

"My grandfather died of a sudden brain aneurysm!"

"Remember that young footballer who died suddenly of an aneurysm during the game a year ago?"

Prompt action should calmly take place when faced with signs that suggest central nervous system involvement. Naturally, adequate tests are advisable to rule out urgent and severe conditions such as a stroke, aneurysm (carotid aneurysm, cerebral aneurysm), arterial dissection (carotid dissection, vertebral dissection), cerebrovascular malformation, and subdural or extradural hematoma[214]; or chronic degenerative diseases such as Parkinson's disease, Alzheimer's disease, epilepsy, or myopathies. After ruling out an urgent organic cause, one must keep in mind specific EDS manifestations that could mislead patients and caregivers.

---

[214] Kim ST, Cloft H, Flemming KD, et al. Increased Prevalence of Cerebrovascular Disease in Hospitalized Patients with Ehlers-Danlos Syndrome. J Stroke Cerebrovasc Dis. 2017;26(8):1678-168.

They can be intense and disturbing. A stroke or aneurysm is quickly thought when having EDS. It may be accurate, but in practice, it is still relatively rare. In all cases, additional targeted examinations (such as cerebral MRIA, encephalogram, evoked potentials, lumbar puncture with cautions) should be performed if the headache occurs suddenly and is very intense; This is especially true if the headache is atypically localized and accompanied by other peripheral clinical signs.

In EDS, headaches are of multiple, varied, and often multifactorial origins: [215] in addition to the front headaches related to hypovolemia (see chapters dedicated to dysautonomia and cardiology), to chronic cerebral deoxygenation (venous pooling and dysautonomia) and to MCAD, here are the leading causes to be mentioned in EDS and the attitudes to adopt on a case-by-case basis:

A. **Cranio-cervical instability and imbalances in the cervical structures. Tension headaches.**

In EDS, the fibrous, ligament, and tendon structures are altered by the connective tissue's unique properties. These alterations lead to instability between the skull and the cervical region, and protective reflex muscle contractures of the surrounding structures.

The anatomical reminder of this vital and complex region:

The nuchal ligament (*ligamentum nuchae*) is several fibrous membranes that contain a large amount of collagen. It is the superior extension of the supraspinatus ligament, located at the underlying vertebrae. This nuchal ligament extends from the external occipital protuberance to the spinous process of the 7th cervical vertebra. It is a kind of partition that separates the muscles on either side of the neck. The head's *trapezius* and

---

[215] Castori M, Morlino S, Ghibellini G, et al. Connective tissue, Ehlers-Danlos syndrome(s), and head and cervical pain. Am J Med Genet C Semin Med Genet. 2015;169C(1):84-96.

splenius muscles are attached to this nuchal ligament, which is too loose or too elastic in EDS, and then stretching too much. The occiput is located at the posterior base of the skull. One can effortlessly feel it with fingers like a hard protrusion. It allows the head to move up and down, helps support the head through the ligaments, and protects the brain. The occiput is the *inion* seat, which is at the nuchal lines' union where the different muscles are inserted. In the center of the occiput is the foramen magnum (or occipital hole) where the cervical spine is inserted, thanks to the two occipital condyles with which the Atlas (the first cervical vertebra) is articulated.

The essential muscles that fit over the occiput and at the base of the skull are:

1. The *sternocleidomastoid* muscle
2. The *trapezius* muscle
3. The *rectus capitis anterior* muscle
4. The *longus capitis* muscle
5. The *longissimus capitis* muscle
6. The *splenius capitis* muscle
7. The *spinalis capitis* muscle
8. The *semi-spinalis capitis* muscle
9. The *rectus capitis lateralis* muscle

The muscles that inserted in the cervical vertebrae and the nuchal ligament are:

1. The sternocleidomastoid muscle
2. The trapezius muscle
3. The anterior scalene muscle
4. The middle scalene muscle
5. The posterior scalene muscle
6. The *rhomboideus minor* muscle
7. The *levator scapula* muscle (the scapula).
8. The *longus colli* muscle
9. The *rectus capitis posterior major* muscle
10. The *rectus capitis posterior minor* muscle
11. The *obliquus capitis superior* muscle
12. The *obliquus capitis inferior* muscle
13. The *interspinalis cervicis* muscles
14. The *spinalis cervicis* neck muscles

15. The *semi-spinalis cervicis* muscle
16. The *longissimus cervicis* muscle
17. The posterior inter-transverse muscles of the neck
18. The anterior inter-transverse muscles of the neck
19. The *splenius cervicis* muscle
20. The *serratus posterior superior* muscle
21. The *musculi rotatores cervicis*

There is a fullness of ligaments between all the cervical and cranial structures, composed of connective tissue that are potentially altered in EDS. They may induce or aggravate cranio-cervical and cervical instability and may be the source of posterior headaches. As seen, it is an extraordinarily complex and diverse region. There are many possibilities of imbalance related to muscular tensions, and too loose ligaments or tendons. This hypermobility leads to spondylosis (degenerative damage to the spine) which aggravates the cervical pain.[216]

Cranio-cervical instability (in which the skull moves too much concerning the axis of the cervical spine) causes so-called tension headaches. Typically, they are headaches that start at the skull base and extend helmet-style forward to the frontal region. They are bilateral and non-pulsating, unlike most true migraines.

Tension headaches are aggravated by stress and anxiety. Sometimes they are triggered or aggravated by trauma (e.g., whiplash) or falls (EDS patients have dysproprioception and frequently fall). Tension headaches can be primary, secondary or both. They are common in the general population: 30 to 78% of individuals present them during their lifetime.

Wrongly considered psychogenic in the past, some studies have considered the neurobiological hypothesis, at least for the most severe forms.[217] Muscle tissue and fascia may send prolonged nociceptive impulses to the CNS. It can lead to central

[216] Malhotra A, Pace A, Ruiz Maya T, et al. Headaches in hypermobility syndromes: A pain in the neck? Am J Med Genet A. 2020;182(12):2902-2908.
[217] Bhoi SK, Jha M, Chowdhury D. Advances in the Understanding of Pathophysiology of TTH and its Management. Neurol India. 2021;69 (Supplement):S116-S123.

sensitization. This central sensitization is the hyperexcitability of neurons and glial cells in the CNS. The release of various neurotransmitters and neuromodulators such as nitric oxide (NO), substance P, neuropeptide Y, calcitonin gene-related peptide (see the chapter on central sensitization) is observed.

The attitude of care and treatment:

If the pain is very severe and brings the patient to the emergency department, it is preferable to do an MRI of the posterior fossa to rule out a tumor, an Arnold Chiari syndrome, a ventral compression of the brainstem or spinal cord, an aneurysm, etc.

If the clinic and MRI are reassuring:

➢ Comfort, inform, and reassure the patient.
➢ Muscle relaxants: prefer Baclofen (Lioresal®), between 10 and 25mg per dose, between 60 and 75mg/day if well tolerated (in several doses).
➢ If there is muscular spasticity : try Levodopa (Prolopa® or Modopar®): 31.25mg, one to three times a day. Then gradually increase the doses according to clinical results and if well tolerated.
➢ For pain: Paracetamol *per os* or IV, Paracetamol codeine, Tramadol 50-100mg *per os* or IV, Ibuprofen 200-400mg (analgesic and not anti-inflammatory doses), etc.
➢ If the pain is severe: try Nefopam hydrochloride (Acupan®), either per os at 30mg, or in ampoules at 20mg (intravenous, intramuscular, or drinkable). Maximum dose: 3 to 6 doses/day, depending on tolerance and potential drug toxicity.
➢ Amitriptyline (Redomex®), then Venlafaxine (Efexor®) and Mirtazapine (Remergon®), possibly Duloxetine (Cymbalta®) can be considered. Many of these products make patients gain weight.
➢ CBD from 10 to 30%, without THC. Two to five sublingual drops per dose, 3 to 4 times a day.
➢ Consider low dose Naltrexone (LDN) for central sensitization.
➢ Botulinum toxin A therapy could be tried (controversial).

- Avoid over a long period: non-steroidal anti-inflammatory drugs (NSAIDs), morphine, and glucocorticoids (Medrol®). They are generally discouraged in EDS. Also, avoid triptans, if possible.
- Local application of heat (by a cherry pit cushion, heated gel, or a *hot pack*).
- Put on a cervical collar, neither too soft nor too stiff. To be worn for a maximum of 4 hours/day, once or several times. It can also be worn at night, with no time restriction (given the absence of gravity in a lying situation). It limits potentially inappropriate or painful positions, supports the skull, and relieves the cervical spine of its weight.
- Establish adapted physiotherapy: insist on global postural rehabilitation (G.P.R.), a method of treatment of muscle chains (e.g., Mackenzie, Sohier, GDS, Mézières, or Busquet), and fasciatherapy.
- Stress management and relaxation techniques: sport, sophrology, yoga, meditation, holistic osteopathy, Pilates, heart coherence, Tai-Chi Chuan, biofeedback, cognitive-behavioral therapy, hypnosis and self-hypnosis, hydrotherapy, Thermalism, and more.
- Concerning osteopathy sessions: be careful to limit the cervical rotations to a maximum of 30° to avoid lesions of the vertebral arteries. Beware of CNS damage following cervical manipulation in cases of Arnold-Chiari syndrome not yet diagnosed by adequate MRI examination.
- In case of failure, treat possible central sensitization (see dedicated chapter): antioxidants (NAC, ALA, vitamin C, and more), possibly low dose Naltrexone, or other TLR4 and /or NMDA receptor antagonists.
- Ultimately, cranio-cervical surgical fixation could be performed.[218]

---

[218] Ramírez-Paesano C, Juanola Galceran A, Rodiera Clarens C, et al. Opioid-free anesthesia for patients with joint hypermobility syndrome undergoing cranio-cervical fixation: a case-series study focused on anti-hyperalgesic approach. Orphanet J Rare Dis. 2021;16(1):172.

B. Arnold's neuralgia (the occipital large nerve).

Its name comes from the German anatomist Friedrich Arnold (1803-1890), professor at the University of Heidelberg, in Germany. This nerve comes mainly from the roots (C1), C2, and C3. The pain usually comes from its chronic irritation induced by cranio-cervical instability. There is a nerve on the right and a counterpart on the left. The path is typical: it starts about an inch wide inside the mastoid processes (the pressure is painful) and then follows a straight line to the eye on the same side. These are often chronic pains with sometimes disabling paroxysms.

Proposed treatments:

➤ Cervical collar.
➤ Muscle relaxants (Baclofen type).
➤ Analgesics (Paracetamol, Tramadol, Nefopam hydro-chloride).
➤ Possibly an injection of corticosteroids around the nerve at its occipital level (it is often swollen and excruciating under pressure).
➤ Try Acupuncture, dry needling.
➤ Kinesitherapy, muscle chains techniques, fascia therapy, cranio-cervical osteopathy, and more.
➤ Stress management, heart coherence, relaxation, and more.

C. Arnold-Chiari syndrome or malformation (ACS).

ACS was described by the Austrian pathologist Hans Chiari (1851-1916) in 1891[219] and by the German pathologist Julius Arnold (1835-1915) in 1894.[220] A similar case was described earlier by the British anatomist John Cleveland (1835-1925), in 1883.[221] Because of the connective tissue properties that make up the brain's envelopes, the lower part of the cerebellum

---

[219] H. Chiari. Über Veränderungen des Kleinhirns infolge von Hydrocephalie des Großhirns. Deutsche Medizinische Wochenschrift. 1891;17:1172-1175.

[220] J. Arnold. Myelocyste, Transposition von Gewebskeimen und Sympodie. Beiträge zur pathologischen Anatomie und zur allgemeinen Pathologie. 1894;16:1-28.

[221] J. Cleland. Contribution to the study of spina bifida, encephalocele and anencephalus. Journal of Anatomy and Physiology. 1883;17:257

(especially the cerebellar tonsils) may descend into the occipital hole (the foramen magnum).

The consequences can be severe! Cerebellar tonsils can interfere with the proper flow of cerebrospinal fluid (CSF) and increase pressure in the brain (called intracranial hypertension or ICH) and the upper spinal cord. It can lead to hydrocephalus and hydrosyringomyelia: with the increased pressure, the CSF can abnormally infiltrate the spinal cord and form a cavity called a *Syrinx*.

Arnold-Chiari syndrome (ACS) is classified according to its anatomical consequences on the brain or spinal cord as type I, II, III, and IV.

Symptoms of ACS are many and varied, with, for example:

- Tinnitus, visual disturbances.
- Numbness in the limbs or face.
- Jerky, involuntary movements of the eyeballs (nystagmus).
- Disorders of coordination and balance (cerebellar ataxia), dizziness.
- Dysphagia (trouble swallowing).
- Paresthesia (tingling sensations) in the limbs.
- Progressive and ascending amyotrophy (muscle wasting) of the upper limbs (from the hand to the shoulder), thermo-algesic anesthesia *suspended in pilgrimage*, and tendinous areflexia (it is a triad).
- Dysesthesia, hyperesthesia, or hypoesthesia.
- Neck stiffness and aggravation during the Valsalva maneuver: coughing, defecation or sneezing.
- Deep, bone-level pain.
- Speech disorders (dysarthria).
- Digestive disorders (intestinal meteorism), sphincter control disorders (anus, urinary tract), sexual disorders.

Treatment: In type I, surgery is not always necessary, but MRI monitoring and controls are essential. The treatment of advanced forms is very specialized (surgery and CSF shunt) and should be left in the hands of neurosurgical specialists who are familiar with EDS. Indeed, the risk of post-CSF puncture or post-surgical breaches is more frequent. They then require a Blood patch.[222]

D. **Sinusitis (often chronic) is mainly related to MCADs (mast cell activation disorders).**

MCADs appear to be present in more than 80% of EDS patients; we have called it EDS/MCA, the mast cell disorder related to EDS (see this chapter).

As mast cells are located in the sinuses and airways, they release their substances (histamine and pro-inflammatory substances) excessively into the sinuses and airways, causing blocked or runny noses, but also chronic sinusitis. These sinusitis cause aggravated anterior headaches, typically by tilting the head forward, such as tying one's shoes.

The sinus points are painful under pressure or percussion (most easily appreciated over the frontal or maxillary sinuses). An MRI or CT scan of the sinuses may be helpful. A blood test should be taken to insure that it is not purulent bacterial sinusitis that would require treatment with specific antibiotics. Fluoroquinolones in EDS should be avoided as these antibiotics potentially weaken tendons and increase the risk of aneurysm.

Treatments:

➤ Treat MCADs: type 1 antihistamines (Desloratadine, Rupatadine, Levocetirizine, and more), 2 to 3 tablets daily, and vitamin C, 1 to 3 grams per day. Vitamin C stabilizes mast cells and is a natural anti-infective. Montelukast 10mg daily could be added (in the morning).

➤ Add N-Acetylcysteine (NAC), 600mg, 1 to 3 times daily, especially if there is a rear discharge with sticky mucus at the back of the throat. NAC also stabilizes the mast cell walls and is a strong antioxidant.

➤ Washing the nose and sinuses with hypertonic saline solutions: this creates an osmotic call for water, and clears the sinuses.

---

[222] Blood patch is the injection of autologous blood into the epidural space.

> Avoid the use of long-term corticosteroid-based sprays in EDS, which further potentially weaken the nasal mucosal membranes: this adverse event is controversial in the general population[223], but cautions may be necessary in EDS due to the altered connective tissue properties.

Exclude also, in case of atypical headaches:

E. **Tumors in the posterior fossa: MRI and see a neurosurgeon.**

F. **Migraines with or without aura: see a neurologist.**

G. **Cerebrospinal fluid leak (CSF leak): see a neurologist.**

H. **Arterial and carotid-cavernous aneurysms: MRI and see a vascular surgeon.**

I. **Stroke: MRI and see a neurologist.**

Pseudo-paralysis of one or more limbs

We meet, a few times a year, patients who have paralysis or paresis of one or more members. They are often brutal and occur from a distance of a particular event: stress, emotional shock, road accident, mistreatment, post-traumatic, post-operative.

For some unknown reason, the brain cuts the motor skills of a part of the body (e.g., hemiparesis, hemiplegia), of an upper limb, lower limb, or even both legs or two arms (suggesting paraparesis or paraplegia). We encountered these various situations in consultation. In all these cases, the patients, in good faith, presented themselves in a hospital emergency department. Additional examinations were performed and were all found normal. Unfortunately, all patients, without exception, were considered as Psychiatric faced with the dissociation between clinical signs and symptoms and the normality of additional examinations. Caregivers have labeled them as conversion hysteria or Münchhausen syndrome, simulators, madmen and

---

[223] Verkerk MM, Bhatia D, Rimmer J, et al. Intranasal steroids and the myth of mucosal atrophy: a systematic review of original histological assessments. Am J Rhinol Allergy. 2015;29(1):3-18.

have been sent home without any treatment. Some patients did not yet have an established diagnosis of Ehlers-Danlos Syndrome. Some were diagnosed, but caregivers told them said: "EDS does not hurt, does not give paralysis, this is people who make the circus, it is the fashionable disease". What mistreatment! Faced with the dismay of these patients, fortunately, family physicians have given them to us urgently addressed.

Additional examinations must naturally be carried out in all cases and chosen according to the events clinical:

- ◆ Complete neurological examination.
- ◆ Brain MRI.
- ◆ Spinal cord MRI.
- ◆ Evoked potentials (sensory, motor, laser).
- ◆ Nerve conduction velocities and electromyography (EMG).
- ◆ Ophthalmologic examination (in MS, exclude an optic neuritis).
- ◆ Lumbar puncture (LP). Watch out for meningeal breaches.
- ◆ Electroencephalogram (EEG).

Treatments should be initiated without delay in the face of these pseudo-paresis or pseudo-paralysis:

- ➤ Listen, examine, understand, and reassure patients (this may seem elementary, but vital).
- ➤ Sequential oxygen therapy (a fixed station with humidifier): 5 liters per minute flow rate, 3 to 6 sessions per day of 60 minutes.
- ➤ Have custom-made compression garments made by an orthotist specialized in EDS. While waiting to be made, cycling type clothing can be bought in supermarkets, or a sports store. Take half a size or one size below the current one, as it should be a little tight.
- ➤ Physiotherapy, osteopathy, Thermalism, sophrology, relaxation, and more.
- ➤ Mirror therapy could be useful.
- ➤ In case of muscular contractures or dystonia:

- Magnesium (e.g., Métarelax®, Stresspure®, D-Stress®, etc.)
- Baclofen, from 10mg to 25mg (Lioresal®), in case of muscle contractures and/or dystonia.
- If dystonia are present: add Levodopa + Benserazide (Prolopa® or Modopar® 100mg/25mg) at 31.25mg/dose, three times daily. Doses to be gradually increased according to tolerance and possible adverse effects.
- One can add substances intervening in the Krebs' cycle at the level of mitochondria and vitamins: vitamin C 1g, vitamin D 3000 IU/day at mealtimes, a vitamin B1-B2-B6-B12 complex (e.g., Befact forte®, Mannavital B complex platinum®), Nicotinamide riboside (125mg, 3x/day), coenzyme Q10 ubiquinol 100 to 200mg.
- Antioxidants (NAC, ALA, vitamin C…)
- Treat MCAD and central sensitization, if necessary.

Loss of sensation in limbs, trunk, or face

They are frequent in consultation, and worry the patients. They exhibit localized numbness, and loss of feeling in a limb or part of a limb (e.g., only fingers or forearm, tibia or part of the thigh). They usually do not follow any specific truncal or root nerve topography. These sensitivity losses can affect the limbs asymmetrically (for example, a right arm, and the front of the left patella). Sometimes they affect an unilateral part of the face (forehead, face or mandibular region, lips) or the trunk. These sensations are most often temporary and/or intermittent, rarely constant.

Their origin is unknown, but probably lies in the erroneous afferent sensory messages sent to the CNS. Additional neurological examinations are usually regular. Recovery is improved by sequential oxygen therapy.

Dysesthesias and paresthesias, false neuropathic pain (see the chapter on Pain).

Alcock canal syndrome or Pudendal neuralgia

Pudendal pain is an excruciating pain of undetermined origin in most cases. The criteria were established in Nantes in 2008.[224] They cause pain, tightness, burning, and numbness between the clitoris (or penis) and the anus. They are more critical during the day and in a sitting position, but they are less important at night when lying down. They are often focused on one side, and sometimes there is an impression of a foreign body in the vagina or rectum. There is no loss of sensation in the perineum and no disturbance of urination, defecation, or gas emission. Injecting Lidocaine into the path of this pudendal nerve reduces the complaints. In EDS, they appear to be more frequent and related to central sensitization and/or joint hypermobility (sacroiliac and hips joints). Significant contractures of the muscles surrounding the pudendal nerve may play a role (as in false sciatica, induced by the hypermobility of the sacroiliac and hip joints, which generates contractures of the piriformis and gluteus' muscles).

Recommended treatments for pudendal pain in EDS:

➤ Try, if supported, compression shorts or leggings ¾ to restore relevant sensations to the subcutaneous tissues.
➤ Custom-made hip and sacroiliac stabilization belt.
➤ Buoy type cushions on seats.
➤ Non-opioid analgesics (Paracetamol, Nefopam).
➤ Injections of Lidocaine 0.5% to 1%, at the trigger points.
➤ Treat MCAD, if necessary.
➤ Try sequential oxygen therapy.
➤ Antioxidants (NAC, ALA, vitamin C).
➤ Muscle relaxants (magnesium, Baclofen, Levodopa).
➤ Stress management, relaxation, mindfulness meditation, cognitive-behavioral therapy.
➤ Physiotherapy, muscle chains' techniques (piriformis muscles, obturator internus muscle), fascia therapy, osteopathy.
➤ Acupuncture or dry needling can be tried.

---

[224] Labat JJ, Riant T, Robert R et al. Diagnostic criteria for pudendal neuralgia by pudendal nerve entrapment (Nantes criteria). Neurourol Urodyn. 2008;27:306-310.

> In recalcitrant cases:

- Low dose Naltrexone (see above, treatment of central sensitization), as an TLR4 antagonist.
- Intravenous Ketamine (Ketalar®) to inhibit NMDA receptors.
- Pregabalin, Amitriptyline, Venlafaxine, Duloxetine.
- Botulinic toxin injections.
- Avoid surgery in the EDS. If the surgical treatment: prevention of bleeding, and instructions for anesthesia and healing.

Generalized tremors or tremors of the extremities: the false-Parkinson.

Several patients with EDS have tremors of the limbs or disturbances in the adjustment of positions (hands, wrists, fingers). Some patients are also prone to generalized tremor attacks (falsely suggesting epileptiform or hysterical seizures). In EDS, it seems that dysautonomia, dysfunction of the Krebs' cycle, and dysproprioception are the cornerstones of these phenomena.

The movements observed in EDS are not typical of Parkinson's disease. The disease was described in 1817 by James Parkinson (1755-1824), a British physician, neurologist, botanist, pharmacist, surgeon, paleontologist, geologist, and politician. It is a chronic neurodegenerative disease, schematically characterized by the progressive loss of neurons in the *pars compacta of the locus niger* and an impairment of the nigro-striated fascicles. The dopaminergic neurons are severely affected. It usually begins between 40 and 75 years of age and is typically an extrapyramidal syndrome with:

> A slow, steady resting tremor of the extremities, increased when attention is diverted (not the case in EDS);

> A hypertonia (rigidity) known as plastic (as opposed to the spastic state of the pyramidal syndrome) which gives way in a jerky manner: we evaluate the sign of the cogwheel, Froment's maneuver (or the frozen wrist test), or other extrapyramidal signs. It is also not the case in EDS.

- Hypokinesis (oligokinesis, bradykinesias, akinesias): rare and slow movements (a bit like lazy monkeys, the aïs).

Recommended treatments for tremors in EDS:

- Try a beta-blocker at exceptionally minimal doses: for example, 1.25mg of Bisoprolol or Nebivolol, once or twice a day + magnesium.
- Treat dysautonomia (see previously): fluid intake, salt and electrolytes, compressive garments, etc.
- Put on compression gloves (they improve proprioception by stabilizing the sensors).
- In case of failure, try Levodopa at a low dose (31.25mg per dose, then gradually increase).
- Sequential oxygen therapy (see above).
- Systematically:
  - Antioxidants (vitamin C 1 to 2g, coenzyme Q10 ubiquinol 100 to 200mg, N-acetylcysteine 600mg) are added to protect against potential cell damage induced by superoxide anions.
  - An aid to the Krebs' cycle (coenzyme Q10 ubiquinol 100mg to 200mg, a complex of vitamin B1 B2 B3 B6 B12). Tremors deplete oxygen and energy from agonist/antagonist muscles, which can trigger or accentuate muscle cramps.

2/ Ear, Nose, and Throat (ENT) Events

By Dr. Stéphane Daens.

With the participation of Dr. Georges VEROUGSTRAETE
Otorhinolaryngologist, Brussels, Belgium

Ears: hearing and balance

We will successively approach the outer ear, the middle ear, and the inner ear. From the outside to the inside, we find successively:

- The external ear canal leading to the eardrum (the tympanic membrane) (1). The eardrum is a taut membrane that separates the outer ear from the middle ear (2). It vibrates with noises, sounds, or voices.

- The middle ear contains the three ossicles (3): the malleus, the incus, and the stapes. The malleus handle is integrated into the tympanic membrane and vibrates with it. These vibrations are then conducted via the incus and then the stapes; the three ossicles being articulated between them. The footplate of the stapes propagates vibrations to the inner ear via the oval window (a membrane) (4). The middle ear communicates with the pharynx through the eustachian tube (5).

- The inner ear contains the cochlear system (the seat of hearing) and the vestibular system (the seat of balance). They are often confused and misunderstood in the general population, and this is quite normal: it is a too complex system. The inner ear is potentially the site of numerous alterations that can induce various clinical signs and symptoms. The inner ear is in the petrous pyramid of the temporal bone. It is a bony labyrinth containing, in its anterior part, the cochlea (hearing) (6) and, in its posterior part, the three semicircular canals and the vestibule (balance) (7). This bone sheath is filled with a substance that protects the membranous labyrinth: the perilymph.

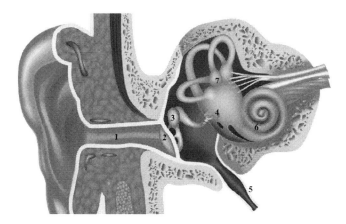

The membranous labyrinth, which fits perfectly with the bone labyrinth, is composed of two parts. An anterior part or cochlear canal, and a posterior part composed of the utricle (which is more extensive and in continuity with the semicircular canals), the saccule (which joins the cochlea) and the semicircular canals. The utricle and saccule float in the vestibule and are joined by a duct. These structures' walls line up with an epithelium consisting of support cells on the one hand, and sensory cells with eyelashes on the other.

For the vestibular system, stereocils (long microvilli) penetrate the otolith membrane, a gelatinous structure containing calcium carbonate crystals: the otoliths. Depending on the head's position, these otoliths press firmly on the stereocils of the sensory cells. A message is then sent to the CNS via the vestibular nerve. The vestibular system informs the CNS of the head's position and movements, allowing body movement coordination. The inner ear is part of the postural control system (PCS) and is one of its exosensors.

The ciliary mechanism is identical in the cochlea. Depending on the sound vibrations, these hair cells transmit information to the CNS via the auditory nerve. In EDS, the hair cells are intact, but they rest on an altered connective tissue, disrupting their function.

The consequences of connective tissue alteration in EDS are many and varied, and can affect all parts of the ear structures:

- In the outer ear: the tympanic membrane contains collagen, and its properties may be altered in EDS. Too loose, it could vibrate more and induce tinnitus or even transmission deafness. Too fragile, the membrane could be punctured.

- In the middle ear: the ossicles are articulated with each other. In EDS, they could be hypermobile with multiple consequences ranging from tinnitus to balance disorders. The eustachian tube, which is too loose and too dilated, can induce repeated otitis media, especially in children. One article even described a case of EDS with conductive hearing loss secondary to otosclerosis, and abnormal scars due to after-effects of otitis media.[225]

- In the inner ear: the various structures contain connective tissue, potentially altered by EDS, which can disrupt their roles

---

[225] Miyajima C, Ishimoto S, Yamasoba T. Otosclerosis associated with Ehlers-Danlos syndrome : report of a case. Acta Otolaryngol Suppl. 2007 ;(559) :157-159.

and functions. Otoliths or sensory cells may be involved, leading to disturbances in their balancing functions (dizziness and balance disorders for vestibular cells) or hearing (hearing loss or tinnitus for cochlear cells).

Two recent articles report temporal bone damage that has resulted in a third window in the inner ear (In addition to the round and oval physiological windows), with dehiscence of the upper canal. All patients had auditory and vestibular damage.[226,227]

Definitions:
- Conductive hearing loss occurs when the ear's ability to transmit sound from the outer ear to the inner ear is diminished or lost. For example, if there is a plug of earwax in the external ear canal, the transmitted sound will be altered. The same is true in the case of ear infections, ossicles lesions, and more. As a rule, this deafness mainly affects low, soft sounds such as low voices or whispers.
- Sensorineural or sensorineural hearing loss: this is the result of a dysfunction of the inner ear, the hair cells of the cochlea, or the nerve pathways of the auditory nerve.

Hypersensoriality.

In EDS, some patients have a hyper-sensoriality that can interfere with their daily life. They may have severe noise intolerance.

- *The sign of the hubbub*: this hypersensoriality can lead to circumstantial hearing loss. When several people speak simultaneously, patients either cannot follow the conversation or cannot hear anything.
- *An advantage?* Patients can also develop a musical ear or even a perfect ear. They often have extraordinary hearing acuity.

---

[226] Preet K, Udawatta M, Duog C et al. Bilateral superior semicircular canal dehiscence associated with Ehlers-Danlos syndrome: a report of two cases. World Neurosurg. 2019;122:161-164.
[227] Chung LK, Lagman C, Nagasawa DT et al. Superior semicircular canal dehiscence in a patient with Ehlers-Danlos syndrome: a case report. Cureus. 2017;9(4):e1141

They hear very low real noises that other people do not perceive.

Stereophony.

Some patients have stereophony's disturbances, with difficulty locating noises and sounds in space. They can suffer from real auditory sensory dyspraxia. Proprioceptive inputs being disturbed, we may encounter some cases of visuospatial dyspraxia.

Proprioception.

From 3.7% to 7.0% of tinnitus find their origin in a malfunction of the manducatory apparatus. In posturology, trigeminal nerve branches connects the eye, the manducatory apparatus, and the muscle tensor tympani. Tinnitus often accompanies teeth clenching (or parafunctions) and bruxism (teeth grinding). Tinnitus is caused here by myoclonia of the muscle tensor tympani. In these particular cases, the processing is based on orthodontics, occlusiodontics, posturology, speech/language therapy, ENT physiotherapy, and exceptionally surgery. Stress aggravating these mechanisms, bio-psychosocial care is often useful. Treatment may include cognitive behavioral therapy and stress management (e.g., relaxation, hypnosis, mindfulness meditation, and more).

Treatments:

> Treat ear infections with caution (especially in children). Be careful in the application of drains.
> It is necessary to be very vigilant in the transplants of the eardrums and tympanoplasties.
> If there is a severe pathology of the ossicles, we can perform reconstructions or even prosthetic replacement of ossicles.[228,229]

[228] Ziąbka M, Dziadek M, Królicka A. Biological and Physicochemical Assessment of Middle Ear Prosthesis. Polymers (Basel), 2019;11(1):79.
[229] Ziąbka M, Malec K. Polymeric middle ear prosthesis enriched with silver nanoparticles - first clinical results. Expert Rev Med Devices, 2019;16(4):325-331.

♦ For tinnitus:
- TMJ examination and reeducation (see above).
- Sensory isolation is not advisable. They have to get used the noises more than exclude them. One can try *habituation sound therapy*, using white noise, pink noise, speech noise or the high tone.[230]
- Stress management, relaxation, breathing, sophrology, sleep hygiene, cognitive-behavioral therapy, mindfulness meditation, hypnosis, self-hypnosis, and more.

♦ For vertigo of labyrinthine origin:
- Vestibular physiotherapy.
- Betahistine up to 3x32 mg/day in acute phases. Then take 16mg, one to three times a day.
- Sensory isolation is not advisable.
- Stress management, relaxation, breathing, sophrology, sleep hygiene, cognitive-behavioral therapy, mindfulness meditation, hypnosis, self-hypnosis, and some more.

♦ Hearing hypersensoriality (hyperacusis):
- Hearing overprotection is not advisable. There are however hearing protectors that filter out certain sounds.
- A gradual desensitization program can be undertaken with an audiologist.
- Try to enrich the sound environment. It is necessary to gradually be surrounded with sounds that are not annoying, such as relaxing music at low volume, the radio or television, the sound of a fan on or of a water fountain. The goal is to tolerate gradually outside sounds.
- There are noise-generating hearing aids. They produce continuous sounds.
- Stress management, relaxation, breathing, sophrology, sleep hygiene, cognitive-behavioral therapy, mindfulness meditation, hypnosis, self-hypnosis, and more.

---

[230] Mondelli MFCG, Cabreira AF, Matos IL, et al. Sound Generator: Analysis of the Effectiveness of Noise in the Habituation of Tinnitus. Int Arch Otorhinolaryngol. 2021;25(2):e205-e212.

The nose and sinuses

See the chapter on MCADs for associated symptoms and their treatments: stuffy or runny noses, sinusitis, and more.

Hyperosmia.

Odors can be unpleasant and interfere with everyday life. Pollution, animal odors, the scent of flowers or perfumes can cause headaches and nausea. It is the same for diffusers of essential oils or synthetic perfumes, body odors, or toilets. Smells are everywhere and surround us. Some patients come to isolate themselves completely, windows closed. They lock themselves in their house, without any social life. For others, it is a blessing: they are noses in perfumery or enology.

The treatment is case by case, and there are only a few solutions: odors that disturb them should be avoided, possibly mask them with mint chewing gum (if tolerated), wear a surgical mask when traveling in town transport public or stores. Consider stress management, relaxation, sophrology, cognitive-behavioral therapy, mindfulness meditation, hypnosis, self-hypnosis, and more.

Hyposmia or anosmia.

Many of these patients pass by depressive episodes, sometimes severe. A strong bond exists between smell and memory: some memories can even disappear.

We must try to submit to *olfactory training*. We thus voluntarily expose ourselves to known odors that could, according to some studies, promote at least partial recovery of smell. For example, we can enter a cheese factory, a forest, smell flowers, and more. It is necessary to re-habituate the olfactory cells, and therefore the brain, to simple smells. The results are mixed, but, in the EDS, there is no destruction of the olfactory cells or nerve damage. The connective tissue on which olfactory cells rest is altered, but the rest is viable and intact. There is, therefore, the hope of partial recovery thanks to the rehabilitation.

The larynx and the trachea

Laryngeal and tracheal pain:

➤ Rule out gastroesophageal reflux (with or without hiatal hernia).
➤ Rule out MCAD (local inflammation due to mast cells activation).
➤ Post intubation's laryngotracheal pain and dislocation.

Tracheomalacia or tracheobronchomalacia:

In this condition, the trachea and bronchi relax, and pulmonary oxygenation is insufficient. The expiration is difficult and loud; a hissing sound can be heard. The patient is short of breath on exertion, and fatigue worsens. The tracheal lumen decreases sharply in exhalation. The secretions stagnate and cause repeated infections. In EDS, connective tissue damage predisposes to this kind of pathology, but it remains relatively rare. It occurs mostly in newborns. Treatment: physiotherapy, CPAP, oxygen therapy (sequential or continuous).

Laryngoscopy images: A. In exhalation, B. In inspiration.

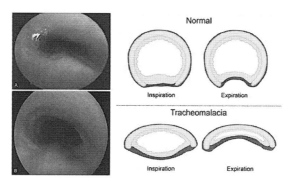

Stenosis and tracheal ruptures:

These are rare complications. They can be spontaneous or be the consequence of technical acts (intubation) and surgery.

- One case of 80% tracheal stenosis, idiopathic: *Guiraudet P, Morel S, Dhouib F et al. Subglottic tracheal stenosis associated with Ehlers-Danlos syndrome, hypermobile type. Respir Med Res. 2019;76:19-21.*

- One case of post-intubation rupture: *Besselink-Lobanova A, Maandag NJ, Voermans NC et al. Trachea rupture in tenascin-X-deficient type Ehlers-Danlos syndrome. Anesthesiology. 2010;113(3) :746-749.*

Chronic cough:

➢ MCADs (see above).

➢ Dry mucous membranes and/or sticky mucus. Treatment: physiotherapy, breathe humidified air, N-acetylcystein.

➢ Mounier-Kuhn Syndrome (or tracheobronchomegaly, TBM) may be associated with EDS. It is a rare disease, of unknown cause. It provokes an increased flaccidity and a collapse of the trachea on exhalation. In Mounier-Kuhn syndrome, naso-sinusal polyps are often associated. This syndrome involves a chronic cough, often cavernous, and bronchial superinfections. It can progress to tracheomalacia and chronic respiratory failure. The CT scan is the exam of choice at the complementary exams: the tracheal walls are enlarged (more than 25mm) and irregular, especially in their intra-thoracic portions. Musculomembranous hernias can be found between the cartilage rings. Respiratory function tests (RFTs) confirm an obstructive syndrome. Treatment: tracheobronchial drainage physiotherapy and antibiotics, if necessary. In the most severe cases, continuous positive pressure ventilation or even a bronchial stent placement should be considered.[231,232,233]

➢ Dysautonomia and decreased vagal brake (see Polyvagal Theory).

---

[231] Fraser RG, Pare, Pare PD et al. Tracheobronchomegaly. In Fraser RG, Pare JA, Pare PD, Fraser RS, Genereux GP. Wb Saunders diagnostisis of the diseases of the chest, third edition, 1990:1995-6.
[232] Girit S, Senol E, Cag Y et al. Ehlers-Danlos type IVB and tracheobronchomegaly. J Bronchology Interv Pulmonol. 2018;25(1):70-72.
[233] Barakat J, Belleguic C, Le Garff G. Treatment of tracheobronchomegaly with an Unflex prosthesis. A case report. Rev Pneumol Clin. 2002;58(1):19-22.

The voice changes (aphonia, dysphonia).

In EDS, causes are of multifactorial origin: MCAD, gastroesophageal reflux disease (GERD), dysproprioception, altered connective tissue properties (incoordination or hypermobility of the vocal cords, reduced mobility of the cricoarytenoid joint, loss of mucosal wave[234], and more).

In the survey reported by *Hunter et al (1998)*, 28% of adults and 48% of children had difficulty with sustaining their voice and with speech and language.[235]

Some patients have paresis of one or both vocal cords. It might be equivalent to the limbs' pseudo-paralysis attacks, as discussed in the chapter on neurological manifestations. Speech and language therapy sessions are essential here. It also takes much patience, and this situation is often discouraging; these people are even more isolated patients from their loved ones.

Some patients may have laryngospasm which can be very distressing; it is the consequence of a sudden inability of the vocal cords to open.

The pharynx

Swallowing pain (dysphagia).

According to the recent study by *J. Nee et al.* (2019) involving 1,804 EDS patients (of various variants or subtypes) and 600 patients with Marfan syndrome: 28.5% of EDS patients had dysphagia (compared to 18.3% in Marfan, p<0.001). In this study [236], it is interesting that the prevalence of digestive

---

[234] Birchall MA, Lam CM, Wood G. Throat and voice problems in Ehlers-Danlos syndromes and hypermobility spectrum disorders. Am J Med Genet C Semin Med Genet. 2021 Dec;187(4):527-532.

[235] Hunter A, Morgan AW, Bird HA. A survey of Ehlers-Danlos syndrome: hearing, voice, speech and swallowing difficulties. Is there an underlying relationship? Br J Rheumatol. 1998;37(7):803-4.

[236] Nee J, Kilaru S, Kelley J et al. Prevalence of functional GI diseases and pelvic floor symptoms in Marfan syndrome and Ehlers-Danlos syndrome: a national cohort study. J Clin Gastroenterol.2019;53(9):653-659.

problems in EDS is independent of EDS subtypes. It once again goes back to the Global Vision of EDS.

Castori M, Morlino S, Pascolini G et al. Gastrointestinal and nutritional issues in joint hypermobility syndrome/Ehlers-Danlos syndrome, hypermobile type. Am J Med Genet C Semin Med Genet. 2015;169C(1):54-75.

Fikree A, Aziz Q, Sifrim D. Mechanisms underlying reflux symptoms and dysphagia in patients with joint hypermobility syndrome, with and without postural tachycardia syndrome. Neurogastroenterol Mobil. 2017;29(6). doi: 10.1111/nmo.13029.

The causes of this dysphagia are multiple and varied in EDS:

➢ The fragility of the mucous membranes can induce lesions in the passage of food.
  - Take a teaspoon of lidocaine gel before eating: swallow quickly to avoid anesthesia that would promote wrong routes.
  - For added safety, swallow a viscous gel containing lidocaine, such as a gel usually used after radiation therapy. Syngel®, for example, contains, for one teaspoon (5ml): 200mg magnesium hydroxide, 125mg magnesium carbonate and aluminum hydroxide (cotried gel), 125mg magnesium trisilicate, and 12.5mg lidocaine hydrochloride.
➢ Alterations in proprioceptive and nociceptive impulses, caused by the alteration of the connective tissue in which the sensors and free terminations are located. Do speech/language therapy sessions.
➢ Motility disorders of the upper digestive tract (role of dysautonomia, dysproprioception and/or MCAD) and the upper respiratory tract (larynx, trachea).
➢ Lesions of the epiglottis such as vallecular cysts. They are theoretically rare, but cysts are potentially more common in EDS. Symptoms: dysphagia and often dysphonia. Treatment is surgical with cautions.
➢ Patients often complain of sticky secretions in the back of the throat that interfere with swallowing. It includes a probable posterior throwing, within MCAD and a relative dryness of the tracheobronchial mucous membranes play a role. They are improved by N-acetylcysteine (NAC) at a rate of 600mg, once or twice per day.

Swallow the wrong way.

Food passes through the airways rather than the esophagus. They are common in EDS, due to laryngopharyngeal hypotonia and dysproprioception of the manducatory apparatus. A complete posturological examination (with examinations of the exosensors of the postural control system) and speech/language therapy are required.

Symptoms and possible consequences:

- A cough when swallowing solids, medicines, fluids, and even his saliva. Beware there may have a decrease in the cough reflex in the EDS patient or, on the contrary, hypersensitivity.
- Throat clearing.
- Lengthening of mealtimes.
- Breathlessness, asthma.
- Weight loss, refusal to eat, anorexia.
- Anxiety when approaching meals.
- Fatigue during meals.

Dangers of wrong ways:

- Choking, coughing fit.
- Bronchopulmonary infections (typically from right lung, because of the almost vertical of the right mainstem bronchus).
- Dehydration, weight loss, nutritional deficiencies, and more.

Treatments suggested:

- Improve proprioceptive inputs, do sessions speech/language therapy. Swallowing physiotherapy.
- Possibly: cognitive-behavioral therapy, relaxation, sophrology, mindfulness meditation, hypnosis and self-hypnosis.
- The position of the head when swallowing is also important. For example, we can bring the chin closer to the rib cage's top to improve the passage.

- Some people advise focusing on swallowing, and not to do several things at the same time, in order to not be distracted.
- Other patients would say that it is best not to overthink the drugs that should be taken instead of thinking about something else to avoid being blocked by the wrong route's anguish.
- Still others swallow their medication with a liquid and move their head backward to propel the drugs to the bottom of their throat.
- To conclude, there are several methods, and it is necessary to find the appropriate method depending on the circumstances or what is ingested.
- It seems that singing is an excellent exercise to strengthen the oropharynx and larynx muscles, and improve proprioception (the perception of the passage of air).

3/ Dentistry and Somatology

By Dr. Stéphane Daens

There is frequent damage to the teeth and gums in the EDS. The reasons are:

➢ The palate is often high and / or narrow (this is often an ogival palate), which promotes dental misalignment, dental overlays (especially of the jaw lower), and often requires the wearing of braces from childhood or adolescence. Regularly, the teeth misalign again after stopping the device port dental.

➢ Proprioceptive dysfunction syndrome, associated with EDS, may promote teeth clenching or parafunctions, with an increased risk of tooth wear. Teeth can also break, fracture, or have cracks, the enamel being fragile. Masseter muscles often present painful contractures on waking. There is an observation of temporomandibular joints' repeated subluxations, and their menisci regularly present a dislocation with signs of degeneration. Bruxism during sleep and while awake is very ordinary. Patients regularly complain of headaches radiating from the jaw to the temporal and cervical regions.

- Posturological and orthodontic treatment is essential.
- Look for alterations in ocular convergence and for tinnitus. In posturology, there is a close link between the manducatory apparatus, the eyes and the eardrum (via the trigeminal nerve).
- Bio-psycho-social care is useful, as stress aggravates these phenomena.

➢ Misalignments of the upper and lower teeth are often observed (bite disorders).
  - Treatment by an orthodontist and occlusiodontist.

➢ The mucous membrane is fragile in EDS. There is a lot of gingivitis, bleeding gums, and receding gums.
  - Coenzyme Q10 ubiquinol can help in some cases at a dose of 100 or 200mg per day.
  - Dental scaling is also recommended, at least twice a year.
  - Use toothpaste for sensitive teeth and gums.
  - The use of soft interdental brushes is desirable.
  - Finish your daily care with an alcohol-free mouthwash.

➢ Hypersensitivity of the mucous membranes can lead to brushing pain, cough reflexes (primarily via stimulation of the palate veil), nausea, and vomiting. Dental care can be challenging under these conditions of hypersensitivity (due to tissues' fragility, dyssensoriality, dysproprioception, and dysautonomia) . It may result in impaired oral health in some patients.
  - One option is using a minimal amount of lidocaine gel on the gums before brushing or before scaling by the dentist.
  - A lidocaine spray can also be used during the care of the posterior teeth to avoid nausea or cough reflexes (beware swallowing wrong ways aftercare).

➢ Dry mouth is expected in EDS, as with all mucous membranes and skin. There is a need to stay hydrated naturally. Some sprays or gels improve lubrication, such as those used in the sicca syndrome accompanying Sjogren's disease.

➢ Alpha-lipoic acid helps in case of burning tongue syndrome, at a rate of 600 to 1200mg/day.

CHAPTER XIII

Muscular Manifestations in EDS

1. Clinical Aspects and Emergencies

By Dr. Stéphane Daens

We will look at severe dystonia that sometimes take the form of chorea, athetosis, or hemiballismus. These are emergency cases, to the point of preventing patients from eating, grooming themselves independently, and simply living. They may be continuous or discontinuous. In any case, it is crucial to keep in mind that we can help these patients in distress.

There is also pseudo-paralysis in the limbs or localized or locoregional losses of sensitivity (see the chapter on neurological manifestations).

Severe dystonia

Chorea is an arrhythmic, rapid, erratic, non-suppressive, and involuntary movement. It mainly affects the distal muscles of the hands and feet, as well as the face.

Athetosis is slow-acting chorea with non-rhythmic, creeping (like a snake), involuntary, uncontrollable, uncoordinated (with alternating contractions of agonistic and antagonistic muscles of the same segment), sinuous, and of great amplitude movements. It mainly affects the distal muscles and often alternates with abnormal postures of the limbs' proximal parts. The limbs, trunk, and face are the most affected. Athetosis does not allow any muscular rest, which leads to a depletion of local oxygen reserves (Krebs' cycle).

515

Hemiballismus is a unilateral, sudden and rapid, non-rhythmic, and non-suppressible movement. It mainly affects the proximal parts of an arm and leg. These movements are rarely bilateral (ballism). It can be considered as a severe form of chorea.

It will be necessary to exclude, above all, other pathologies:

➢ Chorea and athetosis occur in Huntington's Chorea, a degenerative, hereditary disease.
➢ Sydenham's chorea (also called *Saint Guy's dance* or Sydenham's disease).
➢ A complication of acute rheumatic fever (it is a complication of a child's infection due to certain streptococci). It can lead to uncontrollable jerky movements that can last for several months.
➢ Pregnancy can lead to a condition called pregnancy chorea. It appears during the first trimester of pregnancy, but disappears quickly and spontaneously after delivery.
➢ Rarely after taking oral contraceptives.
➢ A manifestation of systemic lupus erythematosus.
➢ In the case of an overactive thyroid gland (hyperthyroidism).
➢ In case of high blood sugar levels (hyperglycemia from diabetes mellitus).
➢ A tumor or a stroke affects a part of the base's nuclei: the caudate nucleus.
➢ Following the use of certain drugs and medications such as Levodopa, Phenytoin, and cocaine.
➢ In a limited number of people, antipsychotic medications can cause chorea, called tardive dyskinesia. It is characterized by lip and tongue wrinkling or choreoathetosis. Domperidone (Motilium®) and Metoclopramide (Primperan®) rarely cause tardive dyskinesia (see treatment for gastroparesis).
➢ Chorea sometimes develops in the elderly without apparent cause. This chorea, called senile chorea, mainly affects the muscles of the oral region.
➢ Hemiballismus is usually caused by a stroke that affects a small brain area below the base nuclei: the subthalamic nucleus. This structure helps to control voluntary movements.

There are many other causes of severe dystonia of hereditary, congenital, infectious, or metabolic origin. A neurologist must be consulted and must carefully exclude these pathologies. Once these causes have been ruled out, EDS can itself cause forms of pseudo-chorea, pseudo-athctosis, and pseudo-hemiballismus.

In EDS, let us remember that altered peripheral messages reach the brain, and are generally correctly interpreted, but what is sent is distorted. EDS patient's brain is a good brain, but tired.

The main reasons for this are:

➢ Chronic deoxygenation by venous pooling in the lower limbs.

➢ Dysautonomia means that the reflexes that should bring enough oxygen to the brain only do so awkwardly. Patients are like half-full bottles: there is not enough liquid in the upper parts when they are sitting or standing (and therefore not enough oxygen). See the chapter on dysautonomia, by Prof. J.F. Bravo.

➢ There is also an alteration of the Krebs' cycle. This cycle creates energy (ATP) from oxygen in the mitochondria (in all the cells of our body). The main consumers of oxygen are the brain and the muscles, but here they are chronically short of it.

Central sensitization (see the chapter on this particular topic) and mast cell disorders (see the chapter on MCDs) may play a role in these muscle manifestations.

Emergency treatment for severe dystonia:

➢ Begin continuous oxygen therapy (with humidifier) in severe cases, with 3 to 5 liters/minute (nasal cannulas). In moderate cases, sequential oxygen therapy may be sufficient, 4 to 6 sessions per day, each lasting 30 to 60 minutes.

➢ Put on compression garments (if possible, made to measure). The goal is to bring adequate information to the brain, by stabilizing the afferent peripheral messages.

➢ Introduce Levodopa (Prolopa®, Modopar®): start with the smallest possible dose: 31.25mg/day (= ¼ of 125mg tablets, in dispersible tablets), 3x/day. Then gradually increase the doses every two days. As a general rule, in severe forms, 3 x 125mg per day is sufficient. Finally, we need to reduce gradually increasing doses just above the threshold dose at which symptoms reappear.

➢ In MCAD, introduce type 1 and 2 anti-histamines, anti-leukotrienes, NAC, and vitamin C.

➢ Magnesium supplements (per os or IV).

➢ Baclofen at 10mg (1 to 6/day) or 25mg (1 to 3/day), if necessary.

➢ Antioxidants (ALA, NAC, vitamin C, and more): as cell protectors.

➢ CBD from 10% to 30% (without THC) or even therapeutic cannabis can be tried (see the chapter on Pain).

➢ A progressive regimen of low dose Naltrexone (LDN) can be instituted if there is a failure: see the chapter on central sensitization.

Case report

Catherine, 41.

One day in February 2019, two ladies came to my medical practice. The first, hEDS diagnosed earlier in Paris, did not come for herself. Having learned that she had a half-sister, Catherine, she had come to meet her by visiting her. Catherine was staying in a para-hospital service in Brussels, Belgium. Seeing the state she was physically and mentally, this lady insisted on coming in for a consultation to find out if Catherine did not also have a form of EDS. Catherine's diagnoses were unknown in this institution. She was taking antiepileptics, and only comfort care was given to her. This lady had taken care of everything: she had brought her half-sister to me with the strength of her arms, helped by a caretaker. Catherine was moaning and complaining. Her gaze was absent, her face expressionless, amimic, and sometimes tortured like a painting by Jerome Bosch (1450-1516). Her body showed slow and tense movements, muscles were extremely contracted. Her hands and feet took dystonic positions with slow creeping (like a snake) and athetotic movements. At first glance, she suffered from a severe autism spectrum disorder, and communication was impossible. She had self-harm movements (e.g., she was trying to bite her forearms). Her Beighton's score was 5/9. Her hips, ankles, and shoulders were also hypermobile. She had signs of skin allergy, her nose was congested, and she had digestive problems (bloating, abdominal pain, diarrhea): these are typical signs of MCAD. Her skin was stretchy up to 2 to 3 cm at the neck and at the back of the elbows. Skin biopsy was performed, and the ultrastructural changes (TEM) were compatible with a classical EDS variant (cEDS) with large *flower-like* collagen fibrils: many of these fibrils had a transverse diameter of 5 to 6x the diameter of the adjacent normal collagen fibrils.

Catherine' pictures (private collection):

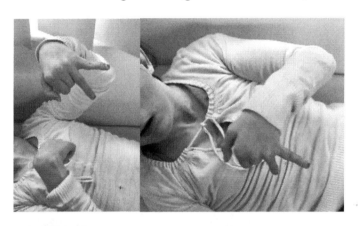

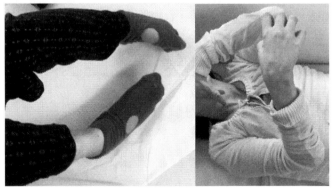

Photos: dystonic and athetotic movements, mainly affecting the extremities. Intense contractures of the neck and leg muscles.

Specific treatments were added immediately after the first consultation:

- Sequential oxygen therapy, 5 liters/minute, 4 to 6 times 30 minutes per day.
- Complete custom-made compression garments: long-sleeved vest, full leggings, gloves, and socks.
- Baclofen 10mg, three times a day.
- Magnesium per os.
- Prolopa® (or Modopar®) 31.25mg - three intakes per day.
- Physiotherapy, osteopathy, fasciatherapy, and hydro-therapy.
- Desloratadine 2x5mg/day.
- Montelukast 10mg, in the morning.
- Vitamin C 1 gram, in the morning.
- Pantoprazole 20mg, at night.

Catherine was seen again after four weeks of treatment. Her condition had improved rapidly. We notice a reduction in dystonia, spasms and she had much less self-harm behavior. Her face was relaxed; she no longer groaned and seemed to have less pain. There was also a marked improvement in MCAD.

Please note: patients have good brains and "It is not in the head"! Above all, these patients must not be labeled hysterical conversion or over-psychiatrized in the face of atypical neuromuscular symptoms: the abuse they suffer is already significant enough!

2. The Role of Muscle Dysfunction in Pain and Mobility in EDS

By Dr. Norman Marcus

Note: the chapter will focus on muscle although it is acknowledged that soft tissue represents muscles, ligaments, tendons, and fascia, all of which may be sources of pain

Pain is frequently reported in patients with EDS. Multiple explanations are offered (1-4); however, successful treatments remain a challenge. Without clear specific pain mechanisms, generic analgesic medication is often prescribed (3). The lack of a unifying hypothesis to link the ubiquitous presence of diffuse pain, stiffness, clumsiness, and poor coordination leads to the often-mistaken conclusion that multiple disparate etiologies are responsible for symptoms that could be the result of muscle dysfunction. Although *Wall and Woolf* (5) observed that a brief stimulus from a muscle nociceptor caused more long lasting excitation in dorsal horn neurons than cutaneous stimulation, muscle generated pain has not inspired wide interest.

Although EDS is relatively rare, common clinical pain syndromes such as chronic low back and neck pain which frequently occur in EDS, are also sub-optimally understood and treated, and it is suggested that although EDS patients are unique, related to dysfunctional connective tissue and hypermobility of joints, the same pathophysiological mechanisms of muscle pain are present in patients with and without EDS. Since there is little literature on the pathophysiological mechanisms of muscle pain in EDS, studies of populations not specifically identified as EDS and animal studies on muscle pain pathophysiology will be cited to explain and support the hypothesis that muscle is a key factor in EDS-related pain phenomenon.

Nomenclature confounds Epidemiology.

Muscle pain as a cause of or co-existing with other sources of pain:

Although EDS patients will often endorse spine and shoulder related pain which are common in the general population and often caused by soft tissue dysfunction (6,7), their records would not identify the pain complaint as muscular. Body region or specific joints will often be identified as the putative pain generator and ignore the surrounding soft tissue which may be important in the total pain presentation, e.g., epicondylitis may begin with inflammation involving the epicondyle but often persistent pain is generated by the muscles attaching to the epicondyle (8,9). Tension type headache may be related to muscle generated pain (10). Non-specific low back pain (NSLBP) is defined as sprains and strains of soft tissue (6,7). Sixteen muscles move the shoulder; if specific muscle(s) can be a source of pain, any of the 16 could be a contributing cause of shoulder/neck pain and dysfunction. Various (11) authors mention the role of musculoskeletal pain in EDS but interestingly never discuss muscular pathophysiological mechanisms as a source of the ongoing pain.

Why is muscle overlooked by clinicians as a source of pain or a target of treatment?

Clinicians and patients have a narrow view of the sources of pain. Arthritic joints and herniated discs are compelling explanations for pain complaints but are often not the source of pain (12). We cannot see biochemical changes in muscles and their nerves that cause pain and associated dysfunction.

Education on the mechanisms of muscle pain is not part of the pre and post graduate medical curriculum. Without an understanding that a muscle can be a pain generator, the search for the source of pain focuses on joints and the nerves exiting the spine and muscle pain often is considered secondary to these tissues.

In surveys of large ambulatory populations, the most common (70-85%) diagnosis of low back pain is Non-specific or Idiopathic Low Back Pain (NSLBP, ILBP), defined as strains and sprains of soft tissue (6, 7). A retrospective analysis at NMPI[237] of the incidence of muscle pain in 358 patients with and without EDS found an approximately 12-fold incidence in the number of muscles identified in EDS patients.

EDS Related Pain in Childhood:

EDS patients are born with a genetic alteration of their collagen which produces excessive stretching of the tissues that holds joints together (ligaments and tendons). The looseness of joints is typically present from birth, often enhancing abilities in sports,

---

[237] Norman Marcus Pain Institute

dance, and playing an instrument. However, joint instability may be associated with pain as well.

Children with EDS often complain of pain. In a retrospective study of 205 children diagnosed with EDS attending sports medicine or orthopedic clinics at a large pediatric hospital (13), knee, back, shoulder, ankle and hip pain were most often reported. 96 patients did not have a specific etiology, receiving a general diagnosis of pain. The initial event may have begun in a joint (sprain, subluxation, dislocation). The joint is assessed often without evaluating the surrounding muscles as a potential source of ongoing pain. The child is often told that absent any pathological findings, they have "growing pains" (14). They are told not to worry, that they are anxious, or worse, that they are making it up. Many EDS patients stop complaining about their "usual pain" feeling that they will not be understood by physicians and family. When they seek help for a new severe pain compliant, they often may not mention their longstanding pains.

Joint Instability Affects Periarticular Muscles:

The body responds to joint instability by tightening the muscles surrounding the (loose) joints (peri-articular muscles) which creates the strange paradox of being flexible and at the same time experiencing joint and muscle stiffness. The persistent tightening of the periarticular muscles results in diminished blood flow with decreased oxygen resulting in sensitization of the muscle.

Muscle Pain and Neuroplasticity:

Chronic irritation of muscle tissue, hypoxia and acidic milieu may all cause muscle nociceptors to become sensitized (*see below-Continued stimulation of nociceptors produces sensitization*). Sensitized nociceptors stimulate and sensitize dorsal horn neurons (DHNs). Sensitized DHNs open previously ineffective pathways resulting in stimulation of DHNs at other levels of the spinal cord, producing referred pain patterns. Impaired descending inhibitory pathways and referred pain from other tissue (nerve, joint, viscera) may result in chronic self-sustained muscle pain and a confounded clinical presentation.

Muscles may entrap nerves producing apparent nerve related pain.

A sensitized, partially contracted muscle may compress a nerve passing through or around it producing pain thought to be radicular or neuropathic without considering an underlying muscular etiology. The piriformis syndrome is only one such example (15).

How muscles generate pain?

The following pathophysiological and functional explanations of muscle pain are largely derived from the chapter Muscle Pain: Pathophysiology, Evaluation, and Treatment, by Marcus and Mense (16). Most of the cited studies are in laboratory animals.

Neuroanatomy and physiology of muscle pain pathways.

Muscles are innervated by sensory nerves that inform us about motion, touch, pressure, and temperature. When the sensation is so strong that it can be damaging to the muscle tissue, specialized nerves called nociceptors are activated. These are thinly (type III) or non-myelinated (type IV) nerves.

The density of free nerve endings in the rat is much higher in the tissue surrounding the tendon than in the gastrocnemius-soleus's muscle (17). This is consistent with the clinical finding of increased tenderness in musculo-tendinous attachment sites.

Nociceptors are sensitive only to strong stimulation and therefore they are referred to as high threshold neurons. The types of stimulation that cause them to be activated (fire) are mechanical (trauma, strong pressure) and chemical (low oxygen, acidity) so they are referred to as high threshold mechanoreceptors and chemoreceptors, but most nociceptors respond to both mechanical and chemical stimuli and are referred to as polymodal nociceptors. Normal stimulation such as motion, touch, pressure, moderate heat, and cold are not potentially damaging to tissue and such stimulation would not be strong enough to cause the nociceptor to fire. Only those stimuli strong enough to threaten tissue damage or to have already caused tissue damage will activate the nociceptor.

Neuroanatomy of Muscle Nociceptors and Their Afferent Fibers.

Histologically, nociceptors are lightly myelinated (type III) or non-myelinated (type IV) fibers (18) analogous to cutaneous A-delta and C fibers. The usual structure sensing and mediating muscle pain is the free nerve ending (19) which refers to the absence of any receptive structure attached to the nerve fiber when viewed under a light microscope. The nociceptor is stimulated by potential or actual tissue damage and is not a pain receptor per se. The pain experience is a cortical distillation of nociception, emotional factors, and history of prior pain experiences.

Neuropeptide Content of Free Nerve Endings.

Substance P (SP) and Calcitonin Gene-Related Peptide (CGRP) are released from varicosities on the nerve fiber when the nociceptor is excited. SP causes vasodilatation and increases vascular permeability of the vessels adjacent to the stimulated nerve ending. SP in muscle nociceptors is at a lower concentration than in cutaneous nociceptors, perhaps to minimize swelling from increased vascular permeability, which would be deleterious to the muscle.

Physiological properties of muscle nociceptors (20,21).

SP increases permeability of the blood vessel resulting in seeping of plasma into the interstitial tissue and the depositing of neuro-active substances that sensitize the nociceptor (i.e., lower its threshold to fire). Bradykinin (BKN) is cleaved from a plasma protein, serotonin (5-HT) is released from platelets, prostaglandin (PGE2) is released from the lining of the blood vessels, and histamine is released from mast cells. Thus, the product of stimulation of the nociceptor is an edematous, neuro-vasoactive soup that facilitates production of an action potential in the nerve fiber. The action potential of the afferent nerve can travel back to the spinal cord producing neuropathic pain. SP and CGRP, with persistent stimulation of the peripheral nerve, act as neuro-modulators, enhancing the effect of glutamate on DHNs (22).

Sequence of events in the stimulated nociceptor (Figure 1).

The nociceptor is located close to an arteriole. Harmful stimuli excite the nociceptor causing the release of neuropeptides, such as substance P (SP), calcitonin gene-related peptide (CGRP), and somatostatin (SOM) from varicosities on the fiber. Substance P degranulates mast cells releasing histamine which, along with SP and CGRP, cause vasodilation and increased capillary permeability in the small blood vessels in the vicinity of the nerve ending. The action potential that is generated travels back to the spinal cord and can ultimately produce myogenic pain.

In contrast, compression of the afferent fiber close to the spinal cord (e.g., from disc herniation or degenerative changes in the bony spine) may initiate:

1. An action potential traveling toward the spinal cord in an anterograde fashion which would be experienced as neuropathic pain.
2. An action potential traveling in a retrograde fashion (against the normal direction of propagation) towards the nerve ending in the muscle, exciting the nerve ending (neurogenic inflammation) and causing release of SP and CGRP initiating the same reactions as with myogenic pain.

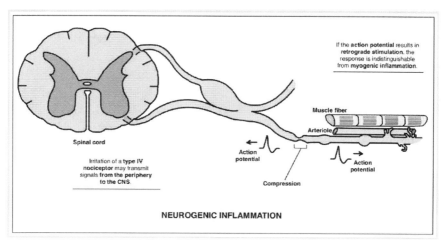

Figure 1a. Sequence of Events in a Stimulated Nociceptor during Neurogenic and Myogenic Inflammation. © Norman Marcus

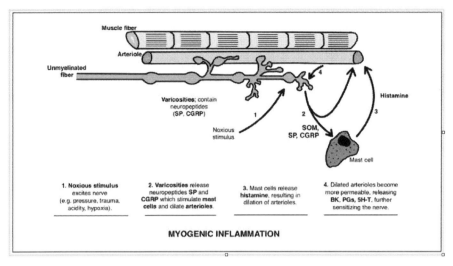

Figure 1b. Sequence of Events in a Stimulated Nociceptor during Neurogenic and Myogenic Inflammation. © Norman Marcus

Substances that Stimulate Nociceptors.

The transient receptor potential vanilloid subtype one (TRPV1) is stimulated by capsaicin (responsible for the heat you experience when eating chili peppers). The endogenous stimulus for TRPV1 is H^+ ions. Strenuous exercise increases the acidity of muscle tissue. The increase in H^+ ions sensitize the nociceptor through stimulation of TRPV1. Small decreases in pH may stimulate TRPV1 so that normal body temperature would be enough to cause pain (23). The diffuse pain accompanying a fever may be the result of stimulation of TRPV1. Human nociceptors are stimulated by capsaicin injections (24) consistent with the presence of TRPV1.

Mechanical stimuli.

TRPV4 is a receptor that response to both weak and strong local pressure (25), suggesting that it may be the major receptor for pain resulting from mechanical stimuli.

Substances that initiate an action potential:

Many substances sensitize the nociceptor, but only H^+ and ATP initiate an action potential.

Hydrogen Ions (H+)

Almost all pathological alterations in muscle tissue, for example exhausting exercise, ischemia, and inflammation (i.e., myositis), are accompanied by an increase in the concentration of H^+. Protons bind to Acid-Sensing Ion Channels (ASICs), with ASIC3 being most important in pain states (26, 27).

Adenosine Triphosphate (ATP)

ATP is present in all tissue cells and at a high concentration in muscle cells (28). It is released with tissue damage. ATP binds to the purinergic receptor P2X3 (29). ATP injected into human muscle causes pain.

Sensitizing molecules lower the threshold to excite the nociceptor, but do not initiate an action potential:

Nerve growth factor (NGF)

NGF is unique in that it sensitizes only nociceptors with no effect on non-nociceptive free nerve endings (30). It binds to tyrosine kinase A receptors (31). NGF synthesis is increased in the presence of muscle inflammation (32).

Bradykinin (BKN)

BKN is produced by the breakdown of plasma proteins. It binds to its receptor B_2 in healthy tissue, but under pathological conditions it binds to B_1 (33). This is an example of neuro-plasticity in the periphery.

Serotonin (5HT3)

It is released from platelets. It binds to the 5HT3 receptor in the periphery.

Prostaglandin E2 (PGE2)

Derived from endothelium, PGE2 binds to the prostanoid receptor EP2 (34).

Glutamate

NMDA receptors on the peripheral nerve respond to glutamate (35). Interestingly, in rat studies, female rats responded more to glutamate than male rats demonstrating gender differences in pain response in the periphery (36).

Potassium ions (K^+)

K^+ is released when muscle cells are damaged. K^+ can excite the nociceptor by directly depolarizing the membrane's potential to threshold.

Muscle Nociceptors synapse with DHNs

The DHN responds to stimuli from the nociceptor and produces a signal that travels up to the brain and may be perceived as pain. When the nociceptor stimulus is gone (when the irritation or damage heals) the DHN no longer fires, and the pain sensation may disappear.

With brief noxious stimulation (for example, blunt trauma, aggressive physical work, or exercise), glutamate, which is released into the synapse with the DHN, binds only to AMPA/Kainate receptors and not to NMDA receptors.

Continued stimulation of nociceptors produces sensitization:

In EDS, hyperextensible joints may cause continuous or intermittent stiffening of surrounding muscles with resultant reduced oxygen and recurrent release of inflammatory substances from the nociceptor, arterioles, and mast cells. Persistent stimulation of the peripheral nerve lowers the threshold to cause the nerve to fire. Now instead of only firing when a strong stimulus is present, the nociceptor will respond to normally non-painful stimuli such as simple movement or touch. With the muscle nociceptor being more easily stimulated, it is referred to as being sensitized (peripheral sensitization or PS).

Effects of PS

When the muscle nociceptor is sensitized, normal activity becomes painful.

1) More movement may be uncomfortable. This is referred to as mechanical or muscle allodynia. Allodynia means pain to a non-painful stimulus. Moving your muscles should not be painful.
2) Painful events become exaggeratedly painful, defined as hyperalgesia.
3) Pain may occur at rest from spontaneous firing of a nociceptor.

Now, usually nonpainful stimuli can cause pain. Almost as soon as this occurs in the peripheral nerve, the DHN to which it connects will also be altered. Sensitization in the periphery will cause the release of SP into the synapse which initiates the process of central sensitization (CS). Glutamate, in the presence of SP, will now bind to NMDA receptors with resultant alteration (phosphorylation) of the receptors on the DHN, causing an influx of cations (Ca^{++}, Na^+). The increased sensitivity in the DHN produces multiple changes in the central nervous system (CNS), which include referral patterns of pain and microglial activation. If CS persists, the DHN may remain sensitized independent of traumatized muscle (37).

Effects of CS

Pain in EDS often begins in a specific area and often spreads diffusely.

Referral of Pain

An unusual property of muscles is the referral of pain from one muscle to nearby or distant muscles. This is facilitated by two mechanisms.

1) In CS there is an opening of ineffective connections in the CNS. Most connections in the CNS are inactive (38,39). However, when central sensitization occurs, many of these closed connections open, thereby allowing a stimulus from one level of the spinal cord to travel to another level of the

spinal cord resulting in pain generated in one muscle being experienced in another muscle as well.

2) Convergence: Even without CS, pain referral can occur without sensitization when two muscles share an afferent nerve. This is called convergence.

Pain may also be referred to other tissue, such as joints. This is termed hetero-synaptic facilitation.

CS results in activation of microglia (40):

The nervous system is composed of cells that transmit information-sensory nerves that allow us to experience physical sensations, and motor nerves that allow us to move our muscles. 90% of CNS cells, however, do not transmit information. They are structural cells, called glia, and are the physical foundation of the nervous system. One type of glia important in pain production is microglia. Sensitized dorsal horn neurons stimulate a receptor on microglia called Toll-like receptor 4 (TLR4)(41). When TLR4 is stimulated, substances are released that sensitize DHNs. Pro-inflammatory cytokines, such as Interleukin 1B (IL-1B) and Interleukin-6 (IL-6), are released, causing *illness behavior* and *hyperalgesia.*

1/ Illness behavior

IL-1B is associated with fatigue and feeling ill. Pain elicits production of interleukin 1B, which may cause the sensation of wanting to be alone and wanting to rest. An EDS patient may say "I don't feel like talking; I don't want to go out; I'd rather be alone and rest; I'm tired." Their behavior could be seen as the body responding to pain by interpreting the pain as a signal that damage has occurred, and therefore energy needs to be conserved to facilitate healing. (There are other reasons for fatigue that are addressed in other chapters in this book.)

2/ Hyperalgesia

IL-6 can cause diffuse generalized pain and increased pain to mildly uncomfortable stimuli such as being bumped or strongly touched. This can also be seen as promoting the body's misunderstood need for "healing" and avoiding physical activity to conserve energy.

Microglia are stimulated by Mast Cells (42)

Microglia are also activated by mast cells. Overactive mast cells, referred to as Mast Cell Activation Syndrome (MCAS/*AN: or MCAD*) (43) produce pro-inflammatory cytokines that stimulate TLR4 on microglia. (See chapter on mast cells). If Mast Cell Activation Syndrome is present as it often is in EDS patients, it may result in further stimulation of microglia. Mast cells and microglia are thus fundamental as contributors to central pain- pain originating in the nervous and immune systems in contrast to peripherally generated pain from muscles and joints.

Pain sensations result from central and peripheral mechanisms

Sometimes addressing central pain by inhibiting products of microglia and mast cells may diminish pain. It is important therefore to address CS when suspected. If the central pain is not first addressed (if possible), successfully treating peripheral pain generators, such as muscles, may not be fully appreciated. Pain generated centrally may still be causing discomfort and the patient may interpret this as failure of treatment. The role of CS in chronic pain is gaining more awareness in the literature although the potential contribution of muscle pain pathophysiology is generally not appreciated (44).

Other centrally produced modulating effects:

Diffuse Noxious Inhibitory Control (DNIC) / Conditioned Pain Modulation (CPM).

Pain Adaptation Model (PAM)

CS is essentially pain causing more pain. Pain stimuli can also inhibit pain. Strong pain may inhibit the awareness of lesser pain. It is thought to be a survival mechanism. With a displaced bone fracture and a painful cut, one would be best served by first addressing the more serious bone fracture and when it was stabilized and causing less pain, become more aware of the cut. This phenomenon has been known as DNIC, currently as CPM.

It is facilitated by nerves originating in the brain and travelling down the spinal cord called tonic descending inhibitory pathways. It has been shown that these pathways are impaired in EDS (45) and other chronic pain states such as IBS, temporomandibular joint dysfunction, and fibromyalgia syndrome (FMS)(46-48). Many patients with EDS are often concurrently diagnosed with FMS. Conversely, many patients treated for FMS may have unrecognized hypermobility (49, 50).

Since a pain producing muscle may increase (CS) or decrease (CPM) pain in other muscles, pain treatment that successfully reduces or eliminates pain in any muscle will potentially decrease or increase pain in previously identified pain generating muscles. Therefore, during treatment of painful muscles, regular reassessment is necessary. Muscles initially identified as a source of pain may no longer appear to be a source during treatment. On the other hand, unidentified muscles initially may, throughout treatment, be found to be pain generators.

Pain Adaptation Model (PAM) (51)

James Lund in 1991 demonstrated that a pain generating muscle will be inhibited from maximum voluntary contraction whilst its antagonist may have increased electrical activity resulting in spasm and pain. For example, if your biceps brachii muscle is causing pain, it will feel weak as in doing a biceps curl because the body will not allow maximum contraction; at the same time, the muscle on the opposite side of your arm, the triceps muscle, will be stimulated possibly producing increased firing with spasm, stiffness, and pain, further limiting the movement initiated by the biceps. This phenomenon is called PAM. When examining muscles for tenderness and spasm, one must be aware that the muscle in spasm may not be the source of the pain and spasm.

PAM mechanism

A pain generating muscle activates a dorsal horn neuron, which in turn stimulates an intermediary neuron in the spinal cord which electrically inhibits the homonymous muscle that is the source of pain and stimulates another intermediary neuron which connects to and increases the electrical activity in the antagonist muscle. This phenomenon may be a contributing factor to the clumsiness experienced by EDS patients. An intentional movement of a body part by an EDS patient may not produce a clear coordinated contraction of a functional muscle group. This will interfere with the brain's ability to estimate the target of the intended motion.

Proprioceptive dysfunction

PAM may interfere with the sense of the position of body parts. Proprioception is the awareness of your body parts in space. For example, tripping, not knowing where your foot is in relationship to the pavement; the precise position of your hand when you put a glass on a table; knowing where your body is in relation to a doorway through which you wish to pass and bumping into the frame.

Altered Muscle Tissue:

The paradox of hypermobility and subjective stiffness

Although EDS patients have hypermobility, they also often complain of subjective stiffness, feeling drawn to yoga and often performing stretching on themselves. This phenomenon can be understood as a response of the body to instability in joints, which prompts the muscles surrounding the joint to tighten up and limit motion. Although the patients still will test as being hypermobile, they experience stiffness.

A majority of 232 EDS patients were found to have measurable muscle stiffness whilst still presenting with hypermobility in various joints (52).

Muscle stiffness affects blood flow

A muscle that cannot fully relax compresses its blood supply. Compressed vessels allow less blood to be delivered to parts of the muscle resulting in hypoxia in various parts of the muscle tissue.

Effects of muscle hypoxia

Hypoxia produces sensitization of nociceptors (53). An example is an arm within an inflated blood pressure cuff is not painful at rest but is painful with movement of the hand or arm.

Trigger points (TrPs)

TrPs are defined as palpable tender nodules in painful muscles that refer pain or discomfort to adjacent or distant muscles. EDS patients often experience tender areas in their muscles and physical examination often identifies TrPs. Studies of the chemical milieu in the TrP have shown an increase in inflammatory substances and H^+ ions (54).

TrPs are present in muscle tissue but equally important in the muscle attachment sites (55). Without knowing the specific muscle in which a tender nodule is found, it is not possible to identify and treat the ends (origin and insertion) of the muscle where the highest concentrations of nociceptors may be found (17) (see trigger point section below).

Clinical applications:

Spasm/Cramps

Spasm is defined as an involuntary long-lasting contraction of a striated muscle with increased EMG activity with or without associated pain. Cramps are brief self-limiting and generally painful muscle contractions accompanied by increased EMG activity.

The classical explanation of muscle spasm, the pain-spasm-pain cycle, has been disproven (51). Muscle spasm does produce muscle ischemia and pain; however, the pain produced does not reflexively cause muscle spam. On the contrary, a painful muscle inhibits its electrical activity while at the same time, increasing the electrical activity of the antagonist (56). The true source of pain is often not the painful tight muscle but rather another muscle often the antagonist, a joint moved by the muscle, a nerve, or an internal organ. An example of an antagonist would be pain in the region of the Vastus Lateralis/ITB reflecting pain actually originating in the Adductor Magnus. The rigid abdomen in appendicitis is an example of a spasm from a painful internal organ.

Cramps in EDS patients were reported in childhood in 43 of 100 patients (57) in contrast to the non-EDS population where cramps generally occur after age 60, generally at night in the lower extremities, but are also reported in children who exercise (58). Amyotrophic Lateral Sclerosis is often associated with cramping but the etiology of cramps in general is unknown. Movement of the painful part typically quickly diminishes and extinguishes the cramp. Although Quinine has been banned by the FDA for anything aside from the treatment of malaria because of reported fatalities, the most recent Cochrane review (59) opines that the adverse side effects are not serious in reviewed trials. The addition of Vitamin E or Theophylline may increase the effectiveness of quinine.

Tenderness

Alteration in the contractile apparatus and neurochemical milieu can produce muscle tenderness. Two common causes of persistent muscle tenderness are Fibromyalgia Syndrome (FMS) and TrPs. TrPs are tender nodules in muscle tissue and the attachment sites (55) with associated neurochemical changes that contribute to sensitization of muscle nociceptors. Peripheral sensitization causes CS and its associated phenomenon.

Examination for tenderness is generally done with digital palpation which presents two major problems:

1) The examiner may provide varying amounts of pressure, undermining the reliability of the exam. Use of pressure recording devices to precisely identify the amount of pressure needed to elicit discomfort may improve the accuracy of the examination (60-62).

2) The examination is performed on a sedentary muscle. Muscle pain most often occurs with muscle activity vs. rest. Palpation is more likely to identify areas of referred as well as primary muscle pain. Methods to replicate muscle activity to identify a specific pain generating muscle suggest that an electrical instrument theoretically utilizing the production of

a subclinical contraction could better identify the primary source(s) of muscle pain in a region of the body (63).

It is suggested that FMS tenderness is the result of CNS dysfunction; impairment of the tonic descending inhibitory pathways causes a lowered threshold for depolarization of nociceptors; however, studies have shown that successful treatment of peripheral pain generators can reduce symptoms of FMS (64).

Restricted Range of Motion

A muscle that is painful with activity will typically have restricted flexibility. Restrictions in motion may be the result of joint related dysfunction (capsule, bone, ligaments, cartilage), nerve, and/or muscle/tendon. Absent articular and nerve dysfunction, the reason may be tension and/or stiffness in related muscles. EDS patients were found to have severely diminished strength and endurance versus controls (65) with no measurable decrease in muscle mass, suggesting intrinsic muscle dysfunction (66). An eight year follow-up study (67) of strength and endurance showed progressive decrease in functionality.

Weakness

Diminished muscle strength is typically assumed in discussions of common pain syndromes such as low back pain leading to the concepts of core weakness and utility of strengthening (68) without specific standardized tests of weakness. The construct validity and treatment protocols for core strengthening have been questioned (69). Patients with hypermobility are motivated and have responded to therapeutic exercise (70); however, strengthening alone without addressing proprioception appears to produce sub-optimal results (71). Barriers to exercise include fear of injury, pain, and fatigue (72).

Tension and EMG activity

Muscle tension may occur with or without EMG activity. Hardened muscle may be the result of spasm or increased muscle tone which are both associated with increased electrical activity, whereas a hardened muscle may also result from decreases in elasticity of the fibers, without accompanying EMG activity, from stiffness, contractures, and TrPs (73). This presents a diagnostic and treatment challenge. Lacking specificity of mechanism in any one patient facilitates the current wide range of pharmacologic interventions for painful muscles with no therapeutic superiority between classes of medication (74, 75), and no clear evidence for injections and denervation procedures for back pain thought to be related to painful muscles (76).

Pain Affects Muscle Function and Patterns of Coordination

Muscle and joint pain interfere with our ability to perform tasks. Coordinated movement, maximal effort, and sustained effort are all impaired by pain. As a corollary, pain may be produced by some muscle activity. Multiple studies have demonstrated dysfunctional gait patterns in EDS thought to be related to weakness, proprioceptive challenges (77), and pain (4).

Altered muscle activity may be caused by or be the result of muscle pain

A painful muscle is inhibited from maximum voluntary contraction (MVC) (51). This occurs through inhibition in the agonist phase and increased activity in the antagonist phase. The purpose may be to diminish the load on the painful muscle, but associated effects may include recruitment of surrounding muscles inappropriate for the task, with resultant additional pain and joint instability (78).

Muscle Pain and static muscle activity

In acute experimental muscle pain, MVC is significantly lower than in controls (79-81). In fibromyalgia the mechanism appears to be different, with reduction in strength assumed to be related to impaired activation of central motor units. FMS patients had no reduced MVC of the adductor pollicis muscle with supramaximal stimulation of the ulnar nerve (82), reflecting no impairment in α-motor neuron stimulation.

Muscle pain and dynamic muscle activity

Experimental and clinical low back muscle pain affects muscle activity during gait. Muscle activity was measured while on a treadmill. In patients with myogenic low back pain, muscle activity was increased in normally electrically silent phases; and there was decreased or no electrical activity in phases where pain free subjects had strong EMG activity (83). When pain was induced in low back muscles, there was impaired activation of abdominal muscles suggesting a possible role in causing spinal instability (84). In addition to reduced MVC, muscle pain patients also demonstrated reduced endurance during submaximal contractions (26, 27).

Muscle and joint inter-action

Muscle pain can affect joint function. Gait analysis during experimental pain in the Vastus Medialis resulted in impaired knee joint function and instability (78). Impaired joint control predisposes to injury and perpetuation of musculoskeletal pain. A study of knee function in EDS children and adults (85) revealed that adults showed altered muscle activation strategies and muscle force patterns whereas children showed only altered muscle activation. This observation suggests that providing corrective rehabilitative measures to normalize gait in children with EDS could positively affect knee function in adulthood.

Pain Originating in Fascia and TrPs:

Non-specific low back pain (NSLBP) is thought to be the result of soft tissue (muscles, ligaments, and fascia) dysfunction in the low back. Muscle tissue harboring myofascial TrPs has been identified as a source of NSLBP (86), but fascia has not been extensively investigated.

The Thoracolumbar Fascia (TLF)

The TLF is the largest fascia in the lower back, it envelopes the low back muscles. It is important in the biomechanical connection of the legs and arms. It contains myofibroblasts (87) indicating that it has contractile properties. It is important in maintenance of posture.

Fascial Innervation

There have been contradictory findings concerning the sensory role of fascia. If TLF was involved in producing NSLBP, one would expect it to be densely innervated. One study found a deficiency in innervation (88); in contrast, a study in 2011 from *Siegfried Mense's laboratory* (89) found the TLF was densely innervated. Free nerve ending consistent with nociceptors, were identified as well as many sympathetic fibers. It has been speculated that the sympathetic fibers may modulate the pain sensations and explain why stress may cause an increase in NSLBP (90). *Mense's group* (91) showed that DHNs receiving sensory fibers from the TLF generally showed convergence with fibers from the Multifidus muscle and the skin, perhaps explaining why patients with NSLBP frequently complain of diffuse low back pain.

Fascial Pain Confounding the Source of Pain Sensations

The quality of pain originating in the TLF, skin and muscle, were studied by *Schilder et al.* (92). It was found that fascial and skin pain descriptors (burning, stinging) differed from muscle pain (deep ache) and may be useful descriptors in guiding physiotherapy interventions. The burning and stinging skin and fascial pain, however, may suggest neuropathic pain (e.g., spinal nerve compression) and mistakenly support nerve block treatment.

Pain due to TrPs:

Trigger points are defined as tender nodules in muscles that refer pain or discomfort to adjacent and distant muscles. Physiological studies of TrPs have supported theoretical explanations for the formation and perpetuation of TrPs, without experimental verification. The following discussion of the formation of TrPs is therefore theoretical.

Hypothesis of TrP formation

A trigger point is composed of various amounts of contraction knots in a portion of a muscle fiber, surrounded by normal tissue. Localized contraction of a part of a muscle fiber is the foundation of the TrP. It is not a true contraction; there is no electrical activity of the muscle endplate, therefore it is termed a contracture.

There are few histological studies of TrPs. A dog study (22) and one human study (93) suggest the appearance of contraction knots, but no data exists from living patients. Absent good supportive data on the initiation and evolution of TrPs, the following are only theoretical models but currently are the only ones we have.

The first stage in TrP formation is the appearance of a taut band of tissue containing a latent TrP that is tender to palpation but otherwise silent. The onset of spontaneous pain signals the evolution of an active TrP. There may be intermediate steps, however, from the initial painless muscle to painful TrPs (94).

Simons (95) postulated the *Integrated hypothesis* of TrP's, later modified by *Gerwin et al.* (96).
It is postulated that trauma to the muscle (e.g., overuse, misuse) damages the muscle endplate which causes an increase in the release of acetylcholine, causing increased release of calcium from the sarcoplasmic reticulum (the intracellular storage site for Ca^{++}). The increased (available) Ca^{++} concentration causes contraction of muscle tissue under the endplate, which produces the contraction knot, which in turn compresses the adjacent capillaries resulting in ischemia, sensitizing nociceptors, and releasing inflammatory substances. *Shah*, using a micro-dialysis needle (97), reported increased concentrations of inflammatory substances and H^+ ions in active TRPs.

Hypoxia is thought to be a significant perpetuating factor in TrP phenomena. Hypoxia results not only in sensitization of TrPs, but the reduced production of ATP. Reduced ATP impairs the calcium pump's ability to separate the actin-myosin complex in a contracted fibril, perpetuating compression of capillaries and causing ongoing hypoxia.

There are other mechanisms whereby Ca^{++} may also be released from the sarcoplasmic reticulum unrelated to the neuromuscular junction:

1. The ryanodine receptor (98) controls the release of Ca^{++} from the sarcoplasmic reticulum; dysfunction of the receptor may allow the release of excess Ca^{++}.

2. Damage to a muscle cell may result in leaks in the cell membrane and an influx of Ca^{++}.

Identification and treatment of trigger points

Identification: Inconsistencies are noted in the literature concerning physicians' ability to identify TrPs (99-104). Multiple criteria are suggested to identify TrPs with palpation, such as finding a taut band, local tenderness, patient pain recognition, pain referral, local twitch response, and a jump sign. Reviews of the literature reveal that these criteria are not applied uniformly and when they are applied, interrater identification of trigger points has been generally unreliable (105). As important is the identification of a specific muscle, rather than a TrP in a region of the body (e.g., lumbar paraspinal, erector spinae). *Simons* noted that TrPs also exist in the muscle attachment sites (55). If a specific muscle is not identified, one would not be able to determine its origin and insertion and therefore overlook possible important targets for treatment (106).

Two technologies have been suggested to image muscles thought to harbor taut bands and TrPs:

1. Magnetic resonance elastography (MRE) allows visualization of tissues with varying degrees of elasticity, allowing identification of taught bands. MRE appears to offer greater reliability than palpation in identifying taut bands (107).

2. Ultrasound has been used to identify TrPs (108, 109). These techniques offer objective identification of taut bands and TrPs but have not been clinically tested to determine if they will improve the effectiveness of treatment for putative TrP related pain.

There is no agreement on the utilization of criteria to diagnose and treat TrPs (106). Various approaches have been suggested *to treat TrP pain* including manual therapies, physical therapy and injections (110). Trigger point injections (TPIs) are done with different injectates or none (dry needling). The use of local anesthetics may be effective for two reasons: 1. diminished pain post injection (111) and 2. All Na⁺ channel blockers are myotoxic although they do not affect satellite cells; this toxicity may add to the putative effectiveness of the needle disrupting dysfunctional myofibrils. Damaged cells rarely produce clinically meaningful problems and with intact satellite cells, generally regenerate in 4-6 weeks (112, 113).

Systematic reviews of the use of Botulinum toxin and corticosteroids do not find evidence to support or reject their use (114-116). However, a Cochrane review of Botulinum toxin for neck pain found it no better than saline (117). The cost and potential risks suggest that the use of these injectates is not justified.

It is not surprising, therefore, that an evidence-based review of the effectiveness of injections for NSLBP does not rise to the level of validity (118). Head-to-head studies of varying approaches to address putative TrP pain are needed to clarify which techniques offer the most effective and longest lasting pain relief. It is suggested that injections to the entirety of a sensitized muscle, rather than to TrPs, may have longer lasting effects (119).

Low Dose Naltrexone (LDN) (120):

Naltrexone was first used to inhibit the effects of strong opioids by blocking a specific receptor in the central nervous system, the μ-receptor. A typical dose (50 mg) of naltrexone will block the effect of opioid drugs such as oxycodone, hydromorphone, fentanyl, and morphine, and produce withdrawal. However, very small doses, for example 0.1 mg - 5.0 mg which is 1/500-1/10ᵗʰ the dose, have paradoxical effects on the μ-receptor and inhibitory effects on microglia. Chronic administration of opioids shifts response of the μ opioid receptor from purely inhibitory to inhibitory and stimulatory (121), resulting in hyperalgesia and tolerance. Provision of low doses of naltrexone attenuates the stimulatory effect of the opioid receptor reversing, to some degree, the hyperalgesia and tolerance, and increasing the analgesic effect of the opioid.

LDN also acts to block TLR4 on microglia, blocking the release of pro-inflammatory cytokines and blocking TLR4 on mast cells, potentially blocking release of mast cell pro-inflammatory substances. This gives us a tool to suppress central sensitization. LDN can be given with minimal side effects in patients not taking opioids and may be given with greater caution in those on opioids as well.

The protocol at NMPI assumes that the dose of LDN is unique to each patient. Effective doses have been as low as 0.034 mg and as high as 6.0 mg/day. Increasing the dose after an effective dose is achieved may negate the effectiveness of LDN (122). Many patients successfully titrated at NMPI had prior failed trails with LDN. Some patients had improvement and by mistakenly continuing to increase their dose, subsequently found the LDN to be ineffective. When they reduced their dose to the prior effective range the effectiveness returned. Below or above the effective dose, LDN will be ineffective. Therefore, what may have appeared to be a failed trial of LDN may have only been an incorrect dose and a retrial starting low, e.g., 0.1 mg/day, and slowly increasing until a reduction in symptoms is achieved and staying at that dose, may allow an effective dose to be found.

Although anecdotal evidence suggests a possible important role for LDN based on potential effective pain reduction and mood elevation coupled with a low side effect profile (120), LDN was prescribed to only 4 of the 13,524 patients diagnosed with EDS (using the same database mentioned above).

Discussion:

Although myalgia is routinely observed in EDS and in common pain syndromes, muscle tissue is an overlooked source of pain and associated symptoms. The EDS literature does not reference intrinsic pain producing mechanisms in muscle tissue contributing to clinicians overlooking soft tissue manifestations of EDS and to the long delay in establishing a diagnosis.

Thomas Kuhn (123), explaining the evolution of new concepts in science, observes that often prior to an understanding of a challenging scientific problem, there appear a number of competing explanations to explain the puzzle. The introduction of novel information provides a linchpin to coalesce the competing explanations into a new paradigm that unifies and/or nullifies the competing theories.

Pain, weakness, stiffness, fatigue, clumsiness, poor coordination, joint pain, and social withdrawal may all be associated with muscle dysfunction. Understanding the pathophysiological mechanisms of muscle pain may allow researchers and clinicians to create more effective treatment for patients with EDS and other syndromes causing chronic pain.

Acknowledgements: Arielle Gironza BA contributed the figures of neurogenic and myogenic inflammation and performed the statistical analyses of the frequency of sensitized muscles in EDS and non-EDS patients at NMPI.

References:

1.   Scheper MC, de Vries JE, Verbunt J, Engelbert RHH. Chronic pain in hypermobility syndrome and Ehlers-Danlos syndrome (hypermobility type): it is a challenge. Journal of pain research. 2015;8:591-601. doi: 10.2147/JPR.S64251.

2.   Bénistan K, Gillas F. Pain in Ehlers-Danlos syndromes. Joint, bone, spine : revue du rhumatisme. 2020;87(3):199-201. doi: 10.1016/j.jbspin.2019.09.011.

3.   Chopra P, Tinkle B, Hamonet C, Brock I, Gompel A, Bulbena A, Francomano C. Pain management in the Ehlers–Danlos syndromes. American Journal of Medical Genetics Part C: Seminars in Medical Genetics. 2017;175(1):212-9. doi: 10.1002/ajmg.c.31554.

4.   Voermans NCMD, Knoop HP, Bleijenberg GP, van Engelen BGMDP. Pain in Ehlers-Danlos Syndrome Is Common, Severe, and Associated with Functional Impairment. Journal of pain and symptom management. 2010;40(3):370-8. doi: 10.1016/j.jpainsymman.2009.12.026.

5.   Wall P, Woolf C. Muscle but not cutaneous C-afferent input produces prolonged increases in the excitibility of the flexion reflex in the rat. J Physiol. 1984;356:443-58.

6.   Deyo R, Weinstein J. Low back pain. The New England Journal of Medicine. 2001;344(5):363-70.

7.   Rosomoff HL, Fishbain DA, Goldberg M, Santana R, Rosomoff RS. Physical findings in patients with chronic intractable benign pain of the neck and/or back. Pain. 1989;37(3):279-87. PubMed PMID: 2526943.

8.   Feleus A, Bierma-Zeinstra SMA, Miedema HS, Bernsen RMD, Verhaar JAN, Koes BW. Incidence of non-traumatic complaints of arm, neck and shoulder in general practice. Manual Therapy.13(5):426-33. PubMed PMID: 17681866.

9.   Fernández-Carnero J, AI CdlL-R, Ge H, Arendt-Nielsen L. Prevalence of and Referred Pain From Myofascial Trigger Points in the Forearm Muscles in Patients With Lateral Epicondylalgia. Clinical Journal of Pain. 2007;23(4):353-60.

10.   Jensen R, Olesen J. Initiating Mechanisms of Experimentally Induced Tension-Type Headache. Cephalalgia. 1996;16(3):175-82. doi: 10.1046/j.1468-2982.1996.1603175.x.

11.   Kumar BMD, Lenert PMDP. Joint Hypermobility Syndrome: Recognizing a Commonly Overlooked Cause of Chronic Pain. The American journal of medicine. 2017;130(6):640-7. doi: 10.1016/j.amjmed.2017.02.013.

12.   Jensen MC, Brant-Zawadzki MN, Obuchowski N, Modic MT, Malkasian D, Ross JS. Magnetic Resonance Imaging of the Lumbar Spine in People without Back Pain. The New England journal of medicine. 1994;331(2):69-73. doi: 10.1056/NEJM199407143310201.

13.   Stern CMBS, Pepin MJMA, Stoler JMMD, Kramer DEMD, Spencer SAMD, Stein CJMDMPH. Musculoskeletal Conditions in a Pediatric Population with Ehlers-Danlos Syndrome. The Journal of pediatrics. 2016;181:261-6. doi: 10.1016/j.jpeds.2016.10.078.

14.   Castori M, Morlino S, Celletti C, Ghibellini G, Bruschini M, Grammatico P, Blundo C, Camerota F. Re-writing the natural history of pain and related symptoms in the joint hypermobility syndrome/Ehlers-Danlos syndrome, hypermobility type. American journal of medical genetics Part A. 2013;161A(12):2989-3004. Epub Castori M, Morlino S, Celletti C, Ghibellini G, Bruschini M, Grammatico P, Blundo C, Camerota F. 2013. Re-writing the natural history of pain and related symptoms in the joint hypermobility syndrome/Ehlers-Danlos syndrome, hypermobility type. Am J Med Genet Part A 161A:2989-3004. doi: 10.1002/ajmg.a.36315.

15.   Koppell H, Thompson W. Peripheral Entrapment Neuropathies. Baltimore: The Williams & Wilkins Company; 1963.

16.   Marcus NJ, Mense S. Muscle Pain: Pathophysiology, Evaluation, and Treatment. In: Bajwa ZH, Wootton RJ, Warfield CA, editors. Principles and Practice of Pain Medicine. 3rd ed. New York, NY: McGraw-Hill Education; 2016.

17.   Reinert A, Kaske A, Mense S. Inflammation-induced increase in the density of neuropeptide-immunoreactive nerve endings in rat skeletal muscle. Exp Brain Res. 1998;121:174-80.

18.   Lloyd D. Neuron patterns controlling transmission of ipsilateral hind limb reflexes in cat. J Neurophysiol. 1943;6:293-315.

19.   Stacey M. Free nerve endings in skeletal muscle of the cat. J Anat. 1969;105:231-54.

20.   Mense S. Muscle nociceptors and their neurochemistry. In: Schmidt R, Willis W, editors. Encyclopedic Reference of Pain. Berlin, Heidelberg: Springer; 2007.

21.   Light AR, Hughen RW, Zhang J, Rainier J, Liu Z, Lee J. Dorsal Root Ganglion Neurons Innervating Skeletal Muscle Respond to Physiological Combinations of Protons, ATP, and Lactate Mediated by ASIC, P2X, and TRPV1. Journal of Neurophysiology. 2008;100(3):1184-201. doi: 10.1152/jn.01344.2007.

22.   Kow L, Pfaff D. Neuromodulatory Actions of Peptides. Annual Review of Pharmacology and Toxicology. 1988;28:163-88. doi: 10.1146/annurev.pa.28.040188.001115.

23.   Reeh P, Kress M. Molecular physiology of proton transduction in nociceptors. Curr Opin Pharmacol. 2001;1:45-51.

24.   Marchettini P, Simone D, Caputi G, Ochoa J. Pain from excitation of identified muscle nociceptors in humans. Brain Research. 1996;740:109-16.

25.   Liedtke W. TRPV4 plays an evolutionary conserved role in the transduction of osmotic and mechanical stimuli in live animals. J Physiol. 2005;567:53-8.

26.   Walder R, Gautam M, Wilson S, Benson C, Sluka K. Selective targeting of ASIC3 using artificial miRNAs inhibits primary and secondary hyperalgesia after muscle inflammation. Pain. 2011;152(10):2348-56.

27.   Immke D, McCleskey E. Protons open acid-sensing channels by catalyzing relief of Ca2+ blockade. Neuron. 2003;37:75-84.

28.   Stewart LC, Deslauriers R, Kupriyanov VV. Relationships Between Cytosolic [ATP], [ATP]/[ADP] and Ionic Fluxes in the Perfused Rat Heart: A 31P, 23Na and 87Rb NMR Study. Journal of Molecular and Cellular Cardiology. 1994;26(10):1377-92. doi: 10.1006/jmcc.1994.1156.

29.   Burnstock G. Physiology and pathophysiology of purinergic neurotransmission. Physiol Rev. 2007;87:659-797.

30.   Hoheisel U, Unger T, Mense S. Excitatory and modulatory effects of inflammatory cytokines and neurotrophins on mechanosensitive group IV muscle afferents in the rat. Pain. 2005;114:168-76.

31.   Caterina M, David J. Sense and specificity: a molecular identitiy for nociceptors. Curr Opin Neurobiol. 1999;9:525-30.

32.   Pezet S, McMahon S. Neurotrophins: mediators and modulators of pain. Annu Rev Neurosci. 2006;29:507-38.

33.   Perkins MN, Kelly D. Induction of bradykinin B1 receptors in vivo in a model of ultra-violet irradiation-induced thermal hyperalgesia in the rat. British journal of pharmacology. 1993;110(4):1441-4. doi: 10.1111/j.1476-5381.1993.tb13982.x.

34.   Mense S. Sensitization of group IV muscle receptors to bradykinin by 5-hydroxytryptamine and prostaglandin E2. Brain Res. 1981;225:95-105.

35.   Cairns B, Svensson P, Wang K, Castrillon E, Hupfeld S, Sessle B, Arendt-Nielsen L. Ketamine attenuates glutamate-induced mechanical sensitization of the masseter muscle in human males. Exp Brain Res. 2006;169:467-72.

36.   Cairns BE, Hu JW, Arendt-Nielsen L, Sessle BJ, Svensson P. Sex-related differences in human pain and rat afferent discharge evoked by injection of glutamate into the masseter muscle. Journal of Neurophysiology. 2001;86(2):782-91. PubMed PMID: ISI:000170322000022.

37.   Sluka KA, Kalra A, Moore SA. Unilateral intramuscular injections of acidic saline produce a bilateral, long-lasting hyperalgesia. Muscle & Nerve. 2001;24(1):37-46. PubMed PMID: ISI:000166016500005.

38.   Wall PD, Wolstencroft JH. The Presence of Ineffective Synapses and the Circumstances which Unmask Them [and Discussion]. Philosophical Transactions of the Royal Society of London Series B, Biological Sciences. 1977;278(961):361-72. doi: 10.1098/rstb.1977.0048.

39.   Mense S. Referral of muscle pain: New aspects. APS Journal. 1994;3(1):1-9.

40.   Frank MG, Fonken LK, Watkins LR, Maier SF. Microglia: Neuroimmune-sensors of stress. Seminars in cell & developmental biology. 2019;94:176-85. doi: 10.1016/j.semcdb.2019.01.001.

41.   Watkins L, Milligan E, Maier S. Spinal cord glia: new players in pain. Pain. 2001;93(3):201-5.

42.   Skaper SD, Facci L, Zusso M, Giusti P. Neuroinflammation, Mast Cells, and Glia: Dangerous Liaisons. The Neuroscientist. 2017;23(5):478-98. doi: 10.1177/1073858416687249.

43.   Valent P, Akin C, Arock M, Brockow K, Butterfield J, Carter M, Castells M, Escribano L, Hartmann K, Lieberman P, Nedoszytko B, Orfao A, Schwartz L, Sotlar K, Sperr W, Triggiani M, Valenta R, Horny H-P, Metcalf D. Definitions, Criteria and Global Classification of Mast Cell Disorders with Special Reference to Mast Cell Activation Syndromes: A Concensus Proposal. Int Arch Allergy Immunol. 2012;157:215-25

44.   Nijs J, George SZ, Clauw DJ, Fernández-de-las-Peñas C, Kosek E, Ickmans K, Fernández-Carnero J, Polli A, Kapreli E, Huysmans E, Cuesta-Vargas AI, Mani R, Lundberg M, Leysen L, Rice D, Sterling M, Curatolo M. Central sensitisation in chronic pain conditions: latest discoveries and their potential for precision medicine. The Lancet Rheumatology. 2021;3(5):e383-e92. doi: 10.1016/S2665-9913(21)00032-1.

45.   Leone CM, Celletti C, Gaudiano G, Puglisi PA, Fasolino A, Cruccu G, Camerota F, Truini A. Pain due to Ehlers-Danlos Syndrome Is Associated with Deficit of the Endogenous Pain Inhibitory Control. Pain medicine (Malden, Mass). 2020;21(9):1929-35. doi: 10.1093/pm/pnaa038.

46.   Kosek E, Ordeberg G. Lack of pressure pain modulation by heterotopic noxious conditioning stimulation in patients with painful osteoarthritis before, but not following, surgical pain relief. Pain. 2000;88(1):69-78. doi: 10.1016/s0304-3959(00)00310-9.

47.   Heymen S, Maixner W, Whitehead WE, Klatzkin RR, Mechlin B, Light KC. Central Processing of Noxious Somatic Stimuli in Patients With Irritable Bowel Syndrome Compared With Healthy Controls. The Clinical journal of pain. 2010;26(2):104-9 10.1097/AJP.0b013e3181bff800.

48.   Lannersten L, Kosek E. Dysfunction of endogenous pain inhibition during exercise with painful muscles in patients with shoulder myalgia and fibromyalgia. Pain. 2010;151(1):77-86. doi: 10.1016/j.pain.2010.06.021.

49.   Eccles JA, Thompson B, Themelis K, Amato ML, Stocks R, Pound A, Jones A-M, Cipinova Z, Shah-Goodwin L, Timeyin J, Thompson CR, Batty T, Harrison NA, Critchley HD, Davies KA. Beyond bones: The relevance of variants of connective tissue (hypermobility) to fibromyalgia, ME/CFS and controversies surrounding diagnostic classification: an observational study. Clinical medicine (London, England). 2021;21(1):53-8. doi: 10.7861/clinmed.2020-0743.

50.   Ofluoglu D, Gunduz OH, Kul-Panza E, Guven Z. Hypermobility in women with fibromyalgia syndrome. Clinical Rheumatology. 2006;25(3):291-3. doi: 10.1007/s10067-005-0040-1.

51.   Lund JP, Donga R, Widmer CG, Stohler CS. The pain-adaptation model: a discussion of the relationship between chronic musculoskeletal pain and motor activity. Canadian Journal of Physiology and Pharmacology. 1991;69(5):683-94. doi: 10.1139/y91-102.

52.   I Brock CH. Joint mobility and Ehlers-Danlos syndrome, (EDS) new data based on 232 cases. Journal of arthritis. 2015;4(2). doi: 10.4172/2167-7921.1000148.

53.   Kieschke J, Mense S, Prabhakar NR. Influence of adrenaline and hypoxia on rat muscle receptors in vitro. Progress in brain research. 1988;74:91-7.

54.   Shah J, Gilliams E. Uncovering the biochemical milieu of myofascial trigger points using in vivo microdialysis: an application of muscle pain concepts to myofascial pain syndrome. J Bodywork Movement Ther. 2008;12(4):371-84.

55.   Borg-Stein J, Simons DG. Myofascial pain. Archives of Physical Medicine and Rehabilitation. 2002;83(3, Supplement 1):S40-S7. doi: 10.1053/apmr.2002.32155.

56.   Mense S, Gerwin R. Muscle Pain: Understanding the Mechanisms. 1st ed. Heidelberg: Springer; 2010.

57.   Beighton P, Horan F. Orthopaedic aspects of the Ehlers-Danlos syndrome. Journal of bone and joint surgery British volume. 1969;51(3):444-53. doi: 10.1302/0301-620X.51B3.444.

58.   Norris FH, Gasteiger EL, Chatfield PO. An electromyographic study of induced and spontaneous muscle cramps. Electroencephalography and clinical neurophysiology. 1957;9(1):139-47.

59.   El-Tawil S, Musa TA, Valli H, Lunn M, El-Tawil T, Weber M. Quinine for muscle cramps. Journal of Evidence-Based Medicine. 2011;4(1):56.

60.   Fischer A. Pressure algometry over normal muscles. Standard values, validity and reproducibility of pressure threshold. Pain. 1987;30(1):115-26.

61.   Jensen K, Andersen HO, Olesen J, Lindblom U. Pressure-pain threshold in human temporal region. Evaluation of a new pressure algometer. Pain. 1986;25(3):313-23. PubMed PMID: 3748589.

62.   Orbach R, Crow H. Examiner expectancy effects in the measurement of pressure pain thresholds. Pain. 1988;74:163-70.

63.   Marcus NJ, Gracely EJ, Keefe KO. A comprehensive protocol to diagnose and treat pain of muscular origin may successfully and reliably decrease or eliminate pain in a chronic pain population. Pain medicine (Malden, Mass). 2010;11(1):25-34. Epub 2009/12/17. doi: 10.1111/j.1526-4637.2009.00752.x. PubMed PMID: 20002599.

64.   Affaitati G, Costantini R, Fabrizio A, Lapenna D, Tafuri E, Giamberardino MA. Effects of treatment of peripheral pain generators in fibromyalgia patients. European Journal of Pain: Ejp. 2011;15(1):61-9. PubMed PMID: 20889359.

65.   Rombaut L, Malfait F, De Wandele I, Taes Y, Thijs Y, De Paepe A, Calders P. Muscle mass, muscle strength, functional performance, and physical impairment in women with the hypermobility type of Ehlers-Danlos syndrome. Arthritis care & research (2010). 2012;64(10):1584-92. doi: 10.1002/acr.21726.

66.   Malfait F, De Paepe A. The Ehlers-Danlos Syndrome. Progress in Heritable Soft Connective Tissue Diseases. 2013;802:129-43. doi: 10.1007/978-94-007-7893-1_9.

67.   Coussens M, Calders P, Lapauw B, Celie B, Banica T, De Wandele I, Pacey V, Malfait F, Rombaut L. Does muscle strength change over time in patients with hypermobile Ehlers-Danlos syndrome/ Hypermobility Spectrum Disorder? An 8-year follow-up study. Arthritis care & research (2010). 2020. doi: 10.1002/acr.24220.

68.   Jull GA, Richardson CA. Motor control problems in patients with spinal pain: A new direction for therapeutic exercise. Journal of Manipulative and Physiological Therapeutics. 2000;23(2):115-7. doi: 10.1016/s0161-4754(00)90079-4.

69.   Lederman E. The myth of core stability. Journal of Bodywork and Movement Therapies. 2010;14(1):84-98. doi: 10.1016/j.jbmt.2009.08.001.

70.   Goldman JA. Hypermobility and deconditioning: important links to fibromyalgia/fibrositis. Southern medical journal (Birmingham, Ala). 1991;84(10):1192-6. doi: 10.1097/00007611-199110000-00008.

71.   Scheper M, Rombaut L, de Vries J, De Wandele I, van der Esch M, Visser B, Malfait F, Calders P, Engelbert R. The association between muscle strength and activity limitations in patients with the hypermobility type of Ehlers-Danlos syndrome: the impact of proprioception. Disability and rehabilitation. 2017;39(14):1391-7. doi: 10.1080/09638288.2016.1196396.

72.   Simmonds JV, Herbland A, Hakim A, Ninis N, Lever W, Aziz Q, Cairns M. Exercise beliefs and behaviours of individuals with Joint Hypermobility syndrome/Ehlers-Danlos syndrome - hypermobility type. Disability and rehabilitation. 2019;41(4):445-55. doi: 10.1080/09638288.2017.1398278.

73.   Simons DG, Mense S. Understanding and measurement of muscle tone as related to clinical muscle pain. Pain. 1998;75(1):1-17. doi: 10.1016/S0304-3959(97)00102-4.

74.   Chou R, Huffman L. Medications for Acute and Chronic Low Back Pain: A Review of the Evidence for an American Pain Society/American College of Physicians Clinical Practice Guideline. Annals of Internal Medicine. 2007;147(7):505-14.

75.   Malanga G, Wolff E. Evidence-informed management of chronic low back pain with nonsteroidal anti-inflammatory drugs, muscle relaxants, and simple analgesics. The Spine Journal. 2008;8(1):173-84.

76.   Henschke N, Kuijpers T, Rubinstein S, van Middelkoop M, Ostelo R, Verhagen A, Koes B, van Tulder M. Injection therapy and denervation procedures for chronic low-back pain: a systematic review. European Spine Journal. 2010;19(9):1425-49. doi: 10.1007/s00586-010-1411-0.

77.   Robbins SM, Cossette-Levasseur M, Kikuchi K, Sarjeant J, Shiu YG, Azar C, Hazel EM. Neuromuscular Activation Differences During Gait in Patients With Ehlers-Danlos Syndrome and Healthy Adults. Arthritis care & research (2010). 2020;72(11):1653-62. doi: 10.1002/acr.24067.

78.   Henriksen M, Alkjaer T, Lund H, Simonsen E, Graven-Nielsen T, Danneskiold-Samsoe B, Bliddal H. Experimental quadriceps muscle pain impairs knee joint control during walking. J Appl Physiol. 2007;103:132-9.

79.   Graven-Nielsen T, Lund H, Arendt-Nielsen L, Danneskiold-Samsøe B, Bliddal H. Inhibition of maximal voluntary contraction force by experimental muscle pain: a centrally mediated mechanism. Muscle Nerve. 2002;26:708-12.

80.   Graven-Nielsen T, Svensson P, Arendt-Nielsen L. Effects of experimental muscle pain on muscle activity and co-ordination during static and dynamic motor function. Electroencephalogr Clin Neurophysiol. 1997;105:156-64.

81.   Wang K, Arima T, Arendt-Nielsen L, Svensson P. EMG-force relationships are influenced by experimental jaw-muscle pain. J Oral Rehabil. 2000a;27:394-402.

82.   Bäckman E, Bengtsson A, Bengtsson M, Lennmarken C, Henriksson K. Skeletal muscle function in primary fibromyalgia. Effect of regional sympathetic blockade with guanethidine. Acta Neurol Scand. 1988;77:187-91.

83.   Arendt-Nielsen L, Graven-Nielsen T, Svarrer H, Svensson P. The influence of low back pain on muscle activity and coordination during gait: a clinical and experimental study. Pain 64:231-240. Pain. 1996;64:231-40.

550

84.   Hodges PW, Moseley GL, Gabrielsson A, Gandevia SC. Experimental muscle pain changes feedforward postural responses of the trunk muscles. Experimental Brain Research. 2003;151(2):262-71. PubMed PMID: ISI:000184579400012.

85.   Jensen BR, Olesen AT, Pedersen MT, Kristensen JH, Remvig L, Simonsen EB, Juul-Kristensen B. Effect of generalized joint hypermobility on knee function and muscle activation in children and adults. Muscle & nerve. 2013;48(5):762-9. doi: 10.1002/mus.23802.

86.   Iglesias-González JJ, Muñoz-García MT, Rodrigues-de-Souza DP, Alburquerque-Sendín F, Fernández-de-las-Peñas C. Myofascial Trigger Points, Pain, Disability, and Sleep Quality in Patients with Chronic Nonspecific Low Back Pain. Pain medicine (Malden, Mass). 2013;14(12):1964-70. doi: 10.1111/pme.12224.

87.   Schleip R, Kingler W, Lehmann-Horn F. Fascia is able to contract in a smooth muscle-like manner and thereby influence musculoskeletal mechanics. In: Findley T, Schleip R, editors. Fascia Research Basic Science and Implications for Conventional and Complementary Health Care. Munich: Urban and Fischer; 2007. p. 76-7.

88.   Bednar D, Orr F, Simon G. Observations on the pathomophology of the thoracolumbar fascia in chronic mechanical back pain. A microscopic study. Spine. 1995;20(10):1161-4.

89.   Tesarz J, Hoheisel U, Wiedenhöfer B, Mense S. Sensory innervation of the thoracolumbar fascia in rats and humans. Sensory innervation of the thoracolumbar fascia in rats and humans. Neuroscience. 2011;194:302-8.

90.   Pertovaara A. Noradrenergic pain modulation. Prog Neurobiol. 2006;80:53-83.

91.   Taguchi T, Hoheisel U, Mense S. Dorsal horn neurons having input from low back structures in rats. Pain 2008;138:119-129. Pain. 2008;138:119-29.

92.   Schilder A, Magerl W, Klein T, Treede R-D. Assessment of pain quality reveals distinct differences between nociceptive innervation of low back fascia and muscle in humans. Pain Rep. 2018;3(3):e662-e. doi: 10.1097/PR9.0000000000000662. PubMed PMID: 29922749.

93.   Reitinger A, Radner H, Tilscher H, al e. Morphologische Untersuchung an Triggerpunkten [Morphologic study of trigger points]. Man Med. 1996;34:256-62.

94.   Mense S, Gerwin R, editors. Muscle Pain: Diagnosis and Treatment. 1st ed. Heidelberg: Springer; 2010.

95.   Simons DG. Clinical and etiological update of myofascial pain from trigger points. Journal of Musculoskeletal Pain. 1996;4(1-2):93-121. (79 ref). PubMed PMID: 1997006230.

96.   Gerwin R, Dommerholt J, Shah J. An expansion of Simons' integrated hypothesis of trigger point formation. Current pain and headache reports. 2004;8:468-75.

97.   Shah JP, Phillips TM, Danoff JV, Gerber LH. An in vivo microanalytical technique for measuring the local biochemical milieu of human skeletal muscle. Journal of Applied Physiology. 2005;99(5):1977-84. PubMed PMID: ISI:000232607800046.

98.   Takeshima H, Kangawa K, Nishimura S, Numa S, Matsuo H, Matsumoto T, Ishida H, Hanaoka M, Minamino N, Ueda M, Hirose T. Primary structure and

551

expression from complementary DNA of skeletal muscle ryanodine receptor. Nature (London). 1989;339(6224):439-45. doi: 10.1038/339439a0.

99.   Christensen HW, Vach W, Manniche C, Haghfelt T, Hartvigsen L, Hoilund-Carlsen PF. Palpation for muscular tenderness in the anterior chest wall: an observer reliability study. J Manipulative Physiol Ther. 2003;26(8):469-75. PubMed PMID: 14569212.

100.   Levoska S. Manual palpation and pain threshold in female office employees with and without neck-shoulder symptoms. Clin J Pain. 1993;9(4):236-41. PubMed PMID: 8118086.

101.   Maher C, Adams R. Reliability of pain and stiffness assessments in clinical manual lumbar spine examination. Phys Ther. 1994;74(9):801-9; discussion 9-11. PubMed PMID: 8066107.

102.   Marcus N, Kraus H, Rachlin E. Comments on K.H. Njoo and E. Van der Does, PAIN, 58 (1994) 317-323. Pain. 1995;61(1):159. PubMed PMID: 7644241.

103.   Njoo KH, Van der Does E. The occurrence and inter-rater reliability of myofascial trigger points in the quadratus lumborum and gluteus medius: a prospective study in non-specific low back pain patients and controls in general practice. Pain. 1994;58(3):317-23. PubMed PMID: 7838580.

104.   Wolfe F. Stop using the American College of Rheumatology criteria in the clinic. J Rheumatol. 2003;30(8):1671-2. PubMed PMID: 12913920.

105.   Myburgh C, Larsen AH, Hartvigsen J. A Systematic, Critical Review of Manual Palpation for Identifying Myofascial Trigger Points: Evidence and Clinical Significance. Archives of Physical Medicine and Rehabilitation. 2008;89(6):1169-76. doi: 10.1016/j.apmr.2007.12.033.

106.   Marcus N, Gracely E, Keefe K. A comprehensive protocol to diagnose and treat pain of muscular origin may successfully and reliably decrease or eliminate pain in a chronic pain population. Pain Medicine. 2010;11(1):25-34.

107.   Chen Q, Basford J, An K-N. Ability of magnetic resonance elastography to assess taut bands. Clin Biomech. 2008;23(5):623-9. doi: 10.1016/j.clinbiomech.2007.12.002.

108.   Sikdar S, Shah J, Gebreab T, Yen R, Gilliams E, Danoff J, Gerber L. Novel Applications of Ultrasound Technology to Visualize and Characterize Myofascial Trigger Points and Surrounding Soft Tissue. Archives of Physical Medicine and Rehabilitation. 2009;90(11):1829-38.

109.   Park G-YMDP, Kwon DRMDP. Application of Real-Time Sonoelastography in Musculoskeletal Diseases Related to Physical Medicine and Rehabilitation. American Journal of Physical Medicine & Rehabilitation. 2011;90(11):875-86.

110.   Simons DG, Travell JG, Simons LS. Travell & Simons' myofascial pain and dysfunction : the trigger point manual. 2nd ed. Baltimore: Williams & Wilkins; 1999.

111.   Hong CZ. Lidocaine Injection Versus Dry Needling to Myofascial Trigger Point - the Importance of the Local Twitch Response. American Journal of Physical Medicine & Rehabilitation. 1994;73(4):256-63. PubMed PMID: ISI:A1994PB25400006.

112.   Zink W, Graf BM. Local anesthetic myotoxicity. Regional Anesthesia and Pain Medicine. 2004;29(4):333-40.

113.   Komorowski TE, Shepard B, Økland S, Carlson BM. An electron microscopic study of local anesthetic-induced skeletal muscle fiber degeneration and regeneration

in the monkey. Journal of Orthopaedic Research. 1990;8(4):495-503. doi: 10.1002/jor.1100080405.

114.   Waseem Z, Boulias C, Gordon A, Ismail F, Sheean G, Furlan A. Botulinum toxin injections for low-back pain and sciatica. Cochrane Database of Systematic Reviews. 2011(1). doi: 10.1002/14651858.CD008257.pub2.

115.   Staal J, Bie Rd, Vet Hd, Hildebrandt J, Nelemans P. Injection therapy for subacute and chronic low-back pain. Cochrane Database of Systematic Reviews. 2008(3). doi: 10.1002/14651858.CD001824.pub3.

116.   Soares A, Andriolo RB, Atallah ÁN, da Silva EMK, Soares A. Botulinum toxin for myofascial pain syndromes in adults. Cochrane library. 2014;2014(7):CD007533-CD. doi: 10.1002/14651858.CD007533.pub3.

117.   Peloso PM, Gross AR, Haines TA, Trinh K, Goldsmith CH, Aker P. Medicinal and injection therapies for mechanical neck disorders: a Cochrane systematic review. J Rheumatol. 2006;33(5):957-67. PubMed PMID: 16652427.

118.   van Tulder MW, Koes B, Seitsalo S, Malmivaara A. Outcome of invasive treatment modalities on back pain and sciatica: an evidence-based review. Eur Spine J. 2006;15 Suppl 1:S82-92. PubMed PMID: 16320030.

119.   Marcus NJ, Shrikhande AA, McCarberg B, Gracely E. A preliminary study to determine if a muscle pain protocol can produce long-term relief in chronic back pain patients. Pain medicine (Malden, Mass). 2013;14(8):1212-21. Epub 2013/05/23. doi: 10.1111/pme.12144. PubMed PMID: 23692059.

120.   Kim PS, Fishman MA. Low-Dose Naltrexone for Chronic Pain: Update and Systemic Review. Current pain and headache reports. 2020;24(10):64-. doi: 10.1007/s11916-020-00898-0.

121.   Largent-Milnes TM, Guo W, Wang H-Y, Burns LH, Vanderah TW. Oxycodone Plus Ultra-Low-Dose Naltrexone Attenuates Neuropathic Pain and Associated μ-Opioid Receptor–Gs Coupling. The journal of pain. 2008;9(8):700-13. doi: 10.1016/j.jpain.2008.03.005.

122.   Burns LH, Wang H-Y. Ultra-Low-Dose Naloxone or Naltrexone to Improve Opioid Analgesia: The History, the Mystery and a Novel Approach. Clinical medicine insights Therapeutics. 2010;2010(2):CMT.S4870. doi: 10.4137/CMT.S4870.

123.   Kuhn TS. The structure of scientific revolutions. [3d ed., enl.. ed. Chicago: Chicago, University of Chicago Press; 1996.

CHAPTER XIV

Cardiological and Vascular Events

By Dr. Stéphane Daens, in collaboration with:

Doctors Georges OBEID (Belgium), Kambyse SAMII (Belgium), Emmanuel TRAN-NGOC (Belgium), and Richard AMORETTI (France)

The heart is a complex organ composed of different anatomical structures. Heart disease is always distressing and stressful for patients. We will detail EDS-related breaches and give some practical steps to follow for each part.

The cardiac muscle is a striated muscle which contractions are involuntary, linked to the autonomic nervous system's activity, the endocrine system, and various chemicals. Its micro-architecture and cells are slightly different of the striated musculoskeletal muscles, which have, in contrast, a voluntary mode of contraction (except during dystonia, myoclonia, or fasciculations, etc.).

Smooth muscles, on the other hand, are in the walls of hollow organs such as the intestine, stomach, urinary tract and bladder, gallbladder, artery walls, bronchi and respiratory tract, genital organs such as the uterus and iris.

1. Damage to the internal structures of the heart.

The heart consists of two atria, two ventricles, four valves, cords, and papillary muscles. Some vessels enter in and out of cavities or chambers: the vena cava, superior and inferior, arrive in the right atrium. The pulmonary artery extends from the right ventricle. The four pulmonary veins enter the left atrium, and the aorta emerge from the left ventricle.

The two atrioventricular heart valves (tricuspid valve on the right, and mitral valve on the left) close the communication between the atria and the ventricles during systoles (the contractions of the heart muscle), but allow the flow of blood from the atria to the ventricles during diastoles (the muscular relaxation of the ventricles). These two valves are held, like boat sails, by cords which themselves are attached to particular muscles, the papillary muscles, located in the ventricles. During systoles, the ventricles contract and the papillary muscles hold the atrioventricular valves when they close.

The aortic and pulmonary valves are located at the exit of the left and right ventricles, respectively (outflow track). These valves are open during systole, allow oxygenated blood to pass from the left ventricle to the aortic artery, be distributed to the organs, and allow deoxygenated blood flow from the right ventricle to the pulmonary arteries and lungs for oxygenation.

As with all tissues, valves and strings contain collagen, which in EDS has altered properties.

The consequences can be varied:

➢ In EDS, the valves may be too loose and thus bulge towards the atria (for atrioventricular valves) or the ventricles (for aortic and pulmonary valves). In a valve insufficiency (or regurgitation), the valve is incompetent: blood may flow back from the ventricles to the atria during systoles, or from the aortic or the pulmonary arteries to the ventricles during diastoles. It is called regurgitation. Valvular insufficiencies are usually quantified by one rating out of four. In EDS, these deficiencies are most often small (1/4 or 2/4) (mostly semi-quantify as other typical echocardiograph methods can measure the exact regurgitation volume for each stroke).

➢ In the case of a valvular prolapse (affecting mostly the mitral valve), the valve leaflets and the cord that support them are or become floppy and elongated, and sometimes are partially broken: a part of the mitral valve goes back towards the atria. Mitral valve prolapse does not always lead to increase regurgitation especially in the beginning of the disease.

Abbreviations such as MI, TI, AI, and PI (for mitral, tricuspid, aortic, or pulmonary insufficiency) or MVP (mitral valve prolapse) are noted.

♦ Symptoms : Fatigue, shortness of breath, dyspnea on exertion or at rest with coughing with possible reddish sputum (hemoptoic) in severe cases. Palpitations due to arrhythmia or discomfort.

➢ Cords can partially tear, which are called micro-breaks. Exceptionally, these are completely ruptured with the result that one or more valve leaflets scallops may float freely towards the atria, hence an important increase of mitral valve regurgitation.

♦ Symptoms : Shortness of breath on exertion with decreased physical activity capacity, fatigue, chest pain, palpitations or discomfort.

➢ Cords can also be teared from the papillary muscles.

These valvular abnormalities can start at earlier age in EDS. Thus teens are to be checked by systematic screening from the age of 15 or 16, or even before if any evocative symptoms are present.

As cardiologist, Richard Amoretti points out that such valve damage is generally benign in hEDS. Valve insufficiencies of up to ¼ (or 2/4) do not require anti-Oslerian prevention (i.e., taking antibiotics before surgery or dental surgery to avoid heart valve infection -called endocarditis). Therefore, they usually do not result in surgery when they are only hEDS-related.[239]

In a recent study by *Asher SB et al. (2018)*[240] on echocardiograms of 209 patients: 6.4% had a prolapse of the mitral valve (MVP) and 1.6% dilation of the aortic root (hEDS, HSD, cEDS). No patient required surgical intervention. For *Atzinger CL et al.*

---

[239] Chango Azanza DX, Munín MA, Sánchez GA, et al. Prolapse and regurgitation of the four heart valves in a patient with Ehlers-Danlos Syndrome: a case report. Eur Heart J Case Rep. 2019;3(2):ytz052.

[240] Asher SB, Chen R, Kallish S. Mitral valve prolapse and aortic root dilatation in adults with hypermobile Ehlers-Danlos syndrome and related disorders. Am J Med Genet A. 2018;176(9):1838-1844.

(2011)[241], 6.0% patients (hEDS, cEDS) presented MVP. Other older reports gives a 11 to 33 percent aortic dilation in the hEDS *(Wenstrup et al. 2002*[242]*; Mc Donnell et al. 2006*[243]*)* and 28-67% mitral valve prolapse *(Camerota et al.*[244]*, 2014; Kozanoglu et al., 2016*[245]*)*.

Significant variations observed by transthoracic echo-cardiography are the result of the part of the subjectivity of examination. An ultrasound is by definition dynamic and depends on the clinicians experience and their knowledge of the EDS. The results are operator-dependent. Studies should be carried out by comparing, for each patient, the ultrasounds performed by two different examiners and their analysis.

Some images by transthoracic ultrasound (EDS patients):

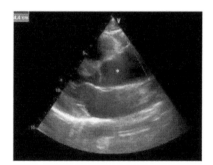 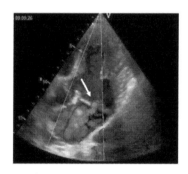

Moderate aortic dilatation (asterisk)   *Moderate MV insufficiency (arrow)*

[241] Atzinger CL, Meyer RA, Khoudry PR et al. Cross-sectional and longitudinal assessment of aortic root dilatation and valvular anomalies in hypermobile and classic Ehlers-Danlos syndrome. J Pediatr. 2011;158(5):826-830.

[242] Wenstrup RJ, Meyer RA, Lyle JS, et al. Prevalence of aortic root dilation in the Ehlers-Danlos syndrome. Genet Med. 2002;4(3):112-7.

[243] McDonnell NB, Gorman BL, Mandel KW, et al. Echocardiographic findings in classical and hypermobile Ehlers-Danlos syndromes. Am J Med Genet A. 2006;140(2):129-36.

[244] Camerota F, Castori M, Celletti C, et al. Heart rate, conduction and ultrasound abnormalities in adults with joint hypermobility syndrome/Ehlers-Danlos syndrome, hypermobility type. Clin Rheumatol. 2014;33(7):981-7.

[245] Kozanoglu E, Coskun Benlidayi I, Eker Akilli R, et al. Is there any link between joint hypermobility and mitral valve prolapse in patients with fibromyalgia syndrome? Clin Rheumatol. 2016;35(4):1041-4.

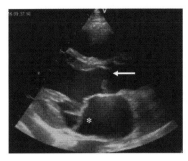 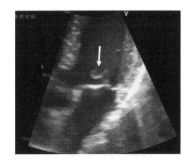

Mitral valve prolapse (asterisk)
Aortic valve (arrow)

Mitral valve cords break (arrow)

The co-morbidities for high cardiovascular risk (CVR) are severe and poorly controlled high blood pressure (HBP), diabetes, smoking, hyperlipidemia, and sedentary lifestyle. There is also alcoholism, stress, junk food—moreover, one thing inevitable: being a man.

For these patients with high CVR and high-grade valve disease (this is exceptional in EDS):

➢ In the case of isolated tricuspid insufficiency, there is dilatation of the right atrium and increased pressure in the vena cava. It is followed by hepatomegaly and edema in the lower limbs (and decubitus), an edema in the upper body (chest and neck) with turgidity of the jugular veins (this is called right side heart failure).

➢ In the case of a high-grade MI or MVP, there may be dilatation of the left atrium induced by the blood reflux, followed by left ventricular failure due to excess blood volume coming secondarily from the left atrium to the left ventricle. Eventually, the left ventricle becomes exhausted from ejecting so much blood volume into the aortic artery. Hyper pressure in the left heart chambers produces increased pressure upstream in the pulmonary veins (pulmonary arterial hypertension, PAH), followed by pulmonary oedema (this is left heart failure). The main symptoms are: breathing difficulty, shortness of breath on slight effort or even rest (dyspnea, grade III to IV), and blood pressure variations.

- Pulmonary hypertension leads to right heart decompensation (called global heart failure, left and right, including both symptoms).

- Treatments are then administered in the intensive care unit: here, water and salt restriction is necessary to relieve the heart of all this volume to be expelled during systoles. Depending on the case, diuretics, nitrates, oxygen, dobutamine, and possibly dopamine are added, intravenous antiarrhythmics, and if all goes well, valve surgery if the patient is stabilised.

Only one solution to avoid such disasters in the general population (EDS and non-EDS):

- A preventive and informative attitude among the young population regarding cardiovascular risk factors: smoking, diet, abdominal obesity, sedentary lifestyle, stress, alcohol consumption, and more.

- Regular follow-up, especially from the age of 40, or even younger in case of risk factors: a cardiac ultrasound, an electrocardiogram, a stress test, a Holter recording over 24 to 72 hours, repeated blood pressure measurements, and a blood test: diabetes, lipids, homocysteine, uric acid, and more.

Please note:

- Because EDS patients work out less than other patients, myocardial muscle is often characterized as thinned or deconditioned[246]. On the other hand, intensive sport or high blood pressure can cause a slight increase in the interventricular wall thickness.

- One should be careful to diagnose the differences between a real thin cardiac muscle and the consequence of an EDS-

---

[246] Ruiz Maya T, Fettig V, Mehta L, et al. Dysautonomia in hypermobile Ehlers-Danlos syndrome and hypermobility spectrum disorders is associated with exercise intolerance and cardiac atrophy. Am J Med Genet A. 2021;30. doi: 10.1002/ajmg.a.62446.

impaired connective tissue: both can give a decrease in total wall thickness (in millimeters) on cardiac ultrasound.

➢ Coenzyme Q10 is an essential molecule in energy production (ATP) in the mitochondria. Several articles indicate that it improves the bioavailability of nitric oxide (NO), prevents ventricular hypertrophy, and reduces left ventricular fibrosis risk[247]. It is also a potent antioxidant, improving peripheral endothelial function in patients with heart failure with reduced ventricular ejection fraction. The doses used in these cases are 300 to 400mg/day[248]. Positive effects are evident after three months of treatment.

2. Heart rhythm disorders (arrhythmias).

Palpitations are quite common in EDS. You feel your heart beating in your chest, and it is an unpleasant feeling. Sometimes you can feel your heart beating in your neck. The most frequent palpitations are extrasystoles, i.e., premature contractions in addition to systoles, which give the impression of misfiring in beats. The heart is pounding, as some patients say. Tachycardia (*Tachy* means More) can also give these symptoms.

The causes of palpitations are multiple in EDS:

➢ The ortho-parasympathetic system's activity: dysautonomia is frequent with an anarchic adaptation of the cardiac rhythm (due to the decrease of the vagal brake, for example: see Polyvagal Theory).

➢ Venous blood can accumulate in the lower limbs (venous pooling), so the heart rate increases in an attempt to send enough blood to the organs (see chapter on dysautonomia).

➢ There is also a vicious circle of bladder instability and profuse sweating. Patients will urinate very often (from 6 to more

---

[247] Sharma A et al. Coenzyme Q10 and heart failure: a state-of-the-art review. Circulation: Heart Failure 2016;9:e002639.
[248] Kawashima C et al. Ubiquinol improves endothelial function in patients with heart failure with reduced ejection fraction: a single-center, randomized double-blindplacebo-controlled crossover pilot study. Am J Cardiovasc Drugs, 2020; doi:10.1007/s40256-019-00384-y. [Epub ahead of print]

than 30 times a day). To lessen this inconvenience, they drink less. If they drink less, often urinate and sweat profusely, they will be half full (the volume of blood circulating will decrease).

- o Hypovolemic reflex tachycardia aggravates the autonomic nervous system dysfunction already present in EDS.

Note that the lower limbs' edemas are of multifactorial origin and do not always take the cup [249] (venous extravasations, chronic lymphedemas, lipedema).

Suggested treatments for palpitations:

➢ Drink enough and eat salty food if cardiac function is preserved.

- o This cannot be repeated enough in EDS, as patients usually drink too little. Salt intake is also scary, but it is unfounded.

➢ Wear compression stockings to reduce venous pooling in the lower limbs.

➢ Beta-blockers:
  - Bisoprolol 1.25mg (or Nebivolol 1.25mg) taken once or twice a day. The dose should be adapted according to blood pressure; it can be risen to 5mg/day, or even (rarely) to 10mg/day in some cases.

  - In severe asthma, Celiprolol (beta-1 blocker and partial beta-2 agonist: it is a selective modulator of adrenergic receptors) may be preferred, but it is not without side effects. Do not forget to detect and treat MCADs, which can increase bronchial reactivity. On the other hand, in EDS, they are often false-asthma, and Bisoprolol (or Nebivolol) is generally well tolerated.

---

[249] The cup sign is the thumbprint that remains embedded in the skin for a few seconds after pressure is applied; there is also the sock sign, the embedded mark of the elastic band in the edematous skin.

- If Celiprolol is used, small doses (e.g., 50mg/day) should be started, as patients with EDS may experience side effects, and the usual doses of 200mg, which is equivalent to about 10mg of Bisoprolol, are poorly tolerated.

- An alternative is Ivabradine (Procoralan® 5mg and 7.5mg per film-coated tablet) as reported by Dr. Tran-Ngoc. He has already proven himself in this subtype of tachycardia. It acts by reducing the heart rate in a particular and specific way while respecting myocardial contractility and without having the side effects of beta-blockers at the bronchial level. The doses to start with would be 5mg to 7.5mg per dose, taken twice a day.[250,251,252]

➤ If patients are going to urinate too often: the vicious circle can be broken by instituting Solifenacin treatment. (Vesicare® or Pelvicare® 5mg) at a dose of 2.5mg, once or twice a day (the doses can be increased if necessary). Its main side effect is a decrease in sweating (which satisfies patients who often heavily sweat from the upper body, hands, and feet) and maintains circulatory volume. Oxybutynin appears to work less well in the EDS, but it can be tried.

The conduction tissue of the heart is made up of a bundle that conducts the electrical activity though muscle heart to contract according to a precise succession: the atria then the ventricles. It is the bundle of His or atrioventricular bundle (*Wilhem His Jr, Swiss cardiologist, 1893*). Damage to the bundle of His may result in a blockage of more or less complete conduction: a right bundle branch block (RBB), left bundle branch block (LBB), atrioventricular block, or AVB (1st, second or 3rd degree). It does not seem common in EDS.

---

[250] Delle Donne G, Rosés Noguer F, Till J, et al. Ivabradine in Postural Orthostatic Tachycardia Syndrome: Preliminary Experience in Children. Am J Cardiovasc Drugs. 2018;18(1):59-63.

[251] Taub PR, Zadourian A, Lo HC, et al. Randomized Trial of Ivabradine in Patients With Hyperadrenergic Postural Orthostatic Tachycardia Syndrome. J Am Coll Cardiol. 2021;77(7):861-871.

[252] Ruzieh M, Sirianni N, Ammari Z, et al. Ivabradine in the treatment of postural tachycardia syndrome (POTS), a single center experience. Pacing Clin Electrophysiol. 2017;40(11):1242-1245.

There are no more aberrant pathways in the EDS. Aberrant fibers are additional conduction pathways leading to attacks of tachycardia or arrhythmias, as with the Kent bundle (causing the Wolff-Parkinson-White syndrome), the James bundle, or the Mahaïm's. To detect and treat them, stress tests, ECG recordings for several days, and then electrophysiological examinations are performed.

3. **The discomforts**.

A. **Orthostatic hypotension (OH)**:

It is defined as a drop in blood pressure of more of 20mmHg when going from lying down to standing, the patient stands up and has discomfort, a fall in blood pressure, fog in front of the eyes, feeling of empty head, sometimes a decrease or loss of consciousness. The cause is multifactorial in EDS: venous pooling in the lower limbs, the inadequate response of the sensors changes in blood pressure, low adjustment of the heart rhythm and peripheral vasoconstriction, poor contraction of the leg muscles when standing (which should help venous return to the upper body) – i.e. due to disturbances into the Krebs 'cycle.

The suggested treatment for OH:

➤ Compression stockings to limit venous pooling and restore proprioception to the legs muscles.

➤ Regular physical exercise, especially in case of myocardial deconditioning.

➤ Eat salty and take supplementation with capsules of salt (NaCl at a rate of 3 to 6 g / day) or electrolytes in water. You have to drink at least two to three liters of water per day (urine should be clear).

➤ If this fails, add Fludrocortisone (doses between 25 to 100 microgram/day, in several doses).

➤ In case of failure and contraindications, we can try Midodrine hydrochloride (Gutron®), a vasopressor, as an alpha-1 receptor agonist at the blood vessels' levels. Midodrine increases the tone of the vessels and blood pressure. It diffuses little at the blood-brain barrier and has little effect on the central nervous system. It does not act on beta-adrenergic receptors. Start treatment with a test dose (to assess tolerance) at 2.5 mg/day in the morning and rapidly increase to three doses per day (the half-life is relatively short). Increase doses according to symptoms and the patient's blood pressure. The ideal catch times are at 7:00 a.m., 12:00 p.m., and 5:00 p.m.

B. Postural tachycardia syndrome (or POTS):

It is defined as an increased heart rate (with associated clinical symptoms), with changes of position, at least 30 beats per minute in adults (over 40 in children), or a heart rate of at least 120 beats per minute, usually occurring after 10 minutes in a standing position, but this can also be immediate or delayed. Please note that in the POTS, there is no noticeable change in blood pressure (that is, a drop of less than 20mmHg in systolic or less than 10mmHg in diastolic).

Several tests can be taken in this context, including the Head-up Tilt Test: we put the patient on a rocking table, we straighten the table, and the patient's parameters are taken regularly, after certain time the table is lifted to 70°: blood pressure, heart rate, oximetry are taken all the time.[253]

POTS is sometimes a very disabling syndrome. It is accompanied by palpitations (racing heart), sweating cold, shortness of breath, and tightness feeling in the chest upon rising. Sometimes it is terribly difficult in daily life for patients.

In a recent study by *Claudia Celletti et al. (2017)*[254], evaluating cardiovascular responses of 35 patients with EDS to different tests, 48.6% of patients presented with POTS. 31.8% had an intolerance to orthostasis, and 20% of patients had a regular

---

[253] The test is not without danger and can cause, although rarely, cardiac arrest (Prof. J.F. Bravo).
[254] Celletti C, Camerota F, Castori M et al. Orthostatic intolerance and postural orthostatic tachycardia syndrome in joint hypermobility/Ehlers-Danlos syndrome, hypermobiliy Type : Neurovegetative dysregulation or autonomic failure ? Biomed Res Int. 2017;2017:9161865.

record. Only one patient presented with pure orthostatic hypotension (HOS, without tachycardia).

There is a close association between MCAD, EDS and POTS.[255,256]

The mechanism mentioned, and which confirms what we think, includes, e.g., an abnormal response of baroreceptors due to specific peculiarities of altered connective tissue in EDS.

The proposed treatment of POTS:

➢ Beta-blockers such as Bisoprolol or Nebivolol (start with 1.25mg once to twice a day, increase if necessary), or Celiprolol 50mg once to three times a day (it is a beta-selective, beta-1 antagonist but beta-2 agonist; it also seems to protect the arteries from ectasia and is not contraindicated in true asthmatics).

➢ Ivabradine (Procoralan®) may also be a reasonable indication in POTS. It is well-tolerated, alone, or in combination with a beta-blocker. This treatment appears to be more effective on symptoms during exercise or daily activity (see above).

➢ Regular physical exercise, especially in cases of myocardial deconditioning.

➢ According to the baseline blood pressure, which in this context is rarely lowered:
  • Eat salty food and take salt capsules, NaCl, from 3 to 6g/day, or add electrolytes in drink water. Drink at least 2 to 3 liters/day (urine must be clear).
  • A mineralocorticoid can then be added (Fludrocortisone at a dosage of 25 to 100 micrograms/day, in several intakes).

---

[255] Shibao C, Arzubiaga C, Roberts LJ 2nd, et al. Hyperadrenergic postural tachycardia syndrome in mast cell activation disorders. Hypertension. 2005;45(3):385-90.
[256] Bonamichi-Santos R, Yoshimi-Kanamori K, Giavina-Bianchi P, et al. Association of Postural Tachycardia Syndrome and Ehlers-Danlos Syndrome with Mast Cell Activation Disorders. Immunol Allergy Clin North Am. 2018;38(3):497-504.

- In case of failure and unless contraindicated, Midodrine hydrochloride can be taken (Gutron®), a vasopressor (an alpha-1 receptor agonist at the blood vessels' levels). It increases the tone of vessels and the blood pressure. Midodrine diffuses little at the blood-brain barrier and has little effect on the central nervous system. It does not act on beta-adrenergic receptors.

C. Vagal discomfort (VD):

It often occurs after emotion, stress, and activity. There is a drop in blood pressure, headaches, balance problems, facial flushing, malaise, sometimes loss of consciousness. In vagal discomfort, there is bradycardia (*brady* = minus) and peripheral vasodilation.

In EDS, the role of dysautonomia and hyperactivity of the autonomic nervous system is indeed fundamental in the face of an external emotion or event. Venous pooling and inadequate contractile response in the legs worsen this mechanism.

Proposed Treatment (VD):

- ➤ Put on custom-made compression stockings or support stockings.
- ➤ Drink two to three liters a day.
- ➤ Midodrine hydrochloride can be tried as a peripheral vasopressor (alpha-1 receptor agonist).
- ➤ Regular physical exercise:
  - In endurance: swimming (draining effect of orthostatic pressure in the pool), cycling, stepping, and more.
  - Gentle: Pilates type, Tai-Chi Chuan, yoga, and more.
- ➤ Relaxation and stress management: mindfulness meditation, hypnosis, self-hypnosis, acupuncture, cognitive-behavioral therapy, sophrology, and more.

Dr. Richard Amoretti, comments on what Professor J.F. Bravo previously wrote in the chapter dedicated to dysautonomia:
- ♦ The distinction between OH, POTS, and VD is challenging to make in EDS.

- In his experience, Fludrocortisone does not often have the desired effect.
- He prefers Midodrine (Gutron®), at doses of 3x 2.5mg/day up to 12 tablets, or even 16 tablets per day in some cases. He often observes a spectacular effect in patients bedridden by their dysautonomia (a "get up and walk!" effect).

4. Pericardial damage:

The pericardium is the heart's envelope—a small bag with a double sheet layer separated by a virtual cavity. In case of inflammation, infection, trauma, or autoimmune disease, the cavity may fill with fluid or blood, this is called a pericardial effusion. They are slightly more common in EDS, but they are of small importance. The altered conjunctiva properties could cause the two sheets in EDS to peel off in places, and create images of localized effusions on cardiac ultrasound.

5. Atrial or ventricular septal aneurysms, and atrial or ventricular septal aneurysms.

They appear to be more frequent than in the general population:

Maseda T, Suzuki Y, Haeno S et al. Ehlers-Danlos and congenital heart anomalies. Intern Med. 1996;35(3):200-202.

Leier CV, Call TD, Fulkerson PK et al. The spectrum of cardiac defects in the Ehlers-Danlos syndrome, types I and III. Ann Intern Med. 1980;92(2 pt1):171-178.

Rotberg T, Sanagustin MT, Salinas L et al. The Ehlers-Danlos syndrome associated with an interauricular communication, total A-V block, aortic aneurysm and growth of the left ventricle (myocardiopathy). Arch Inst Cardiol Mex. 1977;47(5):562-571.

Antani J, Srinivas HV. Ehlers-Danlos syndrome and cardiovascular abnormalities. Chest. 1973;63(2):214-217.

Amoretti R. Le cardiologue et le syndrome d'Ehlers-Danlos (SED). Journal de réadaptation médicale, 2016;36(1):28-31.

6. Arterial damages: ruptures, aneurysms and arterial dissections.

They are present in all EDS types, including hypermobile EDS (hEDS or csEDS), but they appear more frequent in specific variants, of which the vascular variant (vEDS) is the leader. It is explained that genetic mutations observed in COL3A1 promote greater fragility of the vessel wall arteries and surrounding connective tissue. They touch especially the arteries of medium and large caliber. The presence of aneurysm and dissection of the arterial walls is one complication observed, by dilation of the diameter of the artery or by tear within the arterial wall. There are also spontaneous ruptures of arteries, even in the absence of the primary elements.

Other variants of EDS are also affected by a higher risk of arterial complications: damage to the collagen 5 gene (classical EDS or cEDS) and more rarely to the collagen 1 gene, or to the PLOD-1 and FKBP22 genes of EDS kyphoscoliotic variant (or ksEDS).

I would like to emphasise that the vascular variant of EDS is, and will undoubtedly remain, rare: it concerns less than 1 case in 125,000 people. This variant remains rare, probably because most mutations are lethal: they do not result in a viable fetus (the phenotype). The embryos carrying such mutations are therefore most often eliminated by miscarriages, for example.

An aneurysm is defined as a pathological and permanent dilation of an arterial vessel of at least 50% greater than a typical homologous vessel.

In the recent classification of the International Consortium of New York, the following criteria have been established for the diagnosis of the vEDS variant:

Major criteria:

➤ A family history of vEDS, with the presence of a documented COL3A1 mutation.

➤ Arterial rupture in youth.

➤ A spontaneous perforation in the intestine, in the absence of an underlying digestive disease.

➤ A rupture of the uterus.

➤ A carotid-cavernous fistula in the absence of trauma.

Minor criteria include translucent skin, facial appearance characteristic of Madonna (a thin face, eyes that appear bulging, thin lips, narrow nose), acrogeria, hypermobility of small joints, muscle and tendon ruptures, club foot varus, early varicose veins, gum recession.

Marfan disease, Loeys-Dietz syndrome, and carotid or vertebral artery dissection syndrome (familial) should be excluded. The clinical features of these conditions may guide the diagnosis as well as specific genetic tests:

- Loeys-Dietz syndrome is caused by mutations in genes involved in the TGF-β pathway. We will note in this syndrome: hypertelorism (an increase in the distance between the two pupils, or eye orbits), tortuous arteries and aneurysms, a bifid uvula.

- For Marfan disease, which is linked to a mutation in the fibrillin 1 (FBN-1): dislocation of the lens, marfanoid characteristics (wrist sign, thumb sign, wingspan/size> 1.05, and more), joint hypermobility, aortic dilation (and/or other great arteries).

Patients' life expectancy with the vEDS variant depends on the time of diagnosis, screening for complications, and management. Indeed, at the earlier the diagnosis, the less severe complications, thanks to better screening and monitoring.

According to some studies, vEDS patients would have an average survival of 48 years, with a wide distribution of occurrence from childhood to old age, but relatively sparing adolescents. They most often die from an arterial complication or hollow organ perforation, either spontaneously or following a medical examination (*Byers* PH *et al., 2017*). [257] These perforations are mainly located in the colon but can also occur in the small intestine. It should be kept in mind that arterial complications occur most frequently after a gastrointestinal complication. [258] Therefore, this should stimulate physicians,

---

[257] Byers PH, Belmont J, Black J et al. Diagnosis, natural history, and management in vascular Ehlers-Danlos syndrome. Am J Med Genet C Semin Med Genet. 2017;175(1):40-47.
[258] Burcharth J, Rosenberg J. Gastrointestinal surgery and related complications in patients with Ehlers-Danlos syndrome: a systematic review. Dig Surg. 2012;29(4):349-357.

mainly general practitioners and gastroenterologists, to quickly diagnose EDS in a patient after a gastro-intestinal event.

Additional vascular tests should be ordered as soon as possible: Doppler arterial ultrasound of the peripheral arteries (neck, upper and lower limbs), cerebral MRI, MRI of the aortic artery and its branches. Any invasive examination should be avoided at a later stage: gastroenterological, gynecological, cardiovascular, bronchopulmonary, and urogenital examinations (except in cases of extreme necessity).

As with other genetic diseases, the variable expression of mutations and the variable protein production by different alleles will influence the phenotype. Depending on the percentage of normal collagen produced by the fibroblasts compared to the percentage of altered collagen, the phenotype may change.[259]

Keep in mind that some mutations can be either silenced or turned on, and that certain alleles of a gene can produce varying percentages of that collagen within the cell. We can thus have 1%, 10%, 25%, 50%, 75%, 90% or 99% of the cell's proteins altered. Depending on this percentage, the phenotype will vary, as will the potential complications of the mutation.

It has been noted (*Shalhub* D *et al.*, 2014[260]) that vEDS patients with high production of normal collagen had mostly aortic artery damage and delayed presentation. Patients with low production of normal collagen mainly had artery damage in the viscera and an earlier onset of the disease. Each vEDS family, or even everyone within a vEDS family, could potentially present a clinical presentation of varying severity.

---

[259] Frank M, Albuisson J, Ranque B et al. The type of variants at the COL3A1 gene associates with the phenotype and severity of vascular Ehlers-Danlos syndrome. Eur J Hum Genet. 2015 ;23(12) :1657-1664.
[260] Shalhub D, Black JH, Cecchi AC et al. Molecular diagnosis in vascular Ehlers-Danlos syndrome predicts pattern of arterial involvement and outcomes. J Vasc Surg. 2014;60(1):160-169.

Concerning the risk of the unborn child being vEDS: pregnancy in vEDS variant is not recommended, if possible, so that the child is not in turn a carrier of this potentially severe form. It is the only variant for which I recommend one or more contraception methods (oral contraceptive, tubal ligation, or IUD for women + condom for men). If a child is desired, preference will be given to oocyte donation if the woman has vEDS, or sperm donation if the man has vEDS. The goal here is to prevent the child from carrying vEDS. Prenatal screening may also be considered if the mutation(s) is known, which is not always the case (when the diagnosis is purely clinical).

Concerning the risks of obstetrical complications for the mother: if a desire for a conventional pregnancy is nevertheless present or if an unwanted pregnancy is found, an article by *Murray et al. (2012)*[261] is relatively reassuring regarding the risk of death in pregnant women with vEDS. While potentially severe complications exist, they do not affect life expectancy than those observed in vEDS women who have never had children (5.3%). However, death's risk is estimated to be 300 times higher than that observed in pregnant women not carrying vEDS (estimated at 17.8 deaths per 100,000 births in the USA). The deaths of vEDS women who have given birth are related to a risk of arterial rupture or dissection, even if the risk of uterine rupture is present. The uterine rupture is partly related to damage to the uterine arteries themselves. To avoid uterine ruptures, a preterm delivery could be proposed, which would induce less pressure on the uterine wall. The preferred mode of delivery, upper or lower route, needs to be further investigated in larger cohorts of patients. High doses of vitamin C (3 to 6 g/day) and IV Desmopressin should be considered to reduce bleeding risks drastically. Pregnancy surrogacy is also an option.

---

[261] Murray ML, Pepin M, Peterson S et al. Pregnancy-related deaths and complications in women with vascular Ehlers-Danlos syndrome. Genet Med. 2014;16(12):874-880.

Rigorous patient information and exemplary follow-up by a multidisciplinary team is extremely important (doctors, geneticists, obstetricians, anesthetists) .[262]

General precautions for manifestations of cardiovascular disease in EDS:

➤ Prohibit venous bypass surgery.

➤ Risk of bleeding from anti-aggregating drugs and anticoagulants (weigh the pros and cons).

➤ Promote endovascular treatments by an experienced surgeon, in the event of arterial complications (aneurysm, dissection).

➤ Concerning sports activities:
  • Physical endurance activities.
  • Contraindication to scuba diving if there is a history of pneumothorax.
  • Avoid sports with mechanical stress if there is a damage to the iliac artery: cycling, cross-country skiing.

---

[262] Beridze N, Frishman WH. Vascular Ehlers-Danlos syndrome: pathophysiology, diagnosis, and prevention and treatment of its complications. Cardiol Rev. 2012;20(1):4-7.

CHAPTER XV

Oxygen Therapy as Adjunctive Treatment in Ehlers-Danlos Syndrome

By Dr. Isabelle DUBOIS-BROCK, USA

1. Introduction

The Ehlers-Danlos Syndromes (EDS) are a subgroup of hereditary connective tissue disorders, with pain and fatigue as the most prominent disabling symptoms.[263,264,265,266] (See previous chapters in this book)

Oxygen therapy has been used to counteract these symptoms, but that therapy has not yet proven the remedy that its adherents propose. However, given the number of potential benefit indications, further research is a worthwhile area.

This chapter will present possible pathophysiological mechanisms that might underlie the disease process, potential oxygen therapy mechanisms in achieving optimal tissue oxygenation in EDS, and oxygen therapy's efficacy in EDS and

---

[263] Marino Lamari N. Systemic Manifestations of Ehlers-Danlos Syndrome Hypermobility Type. MOJ Cell Science & Report. 2017;4(2):9-13. doi:10.15406/mojcsr.2017.04.00080.

[264] Hakim A, de Wandele I, O'Callaghan C, Pocinki A, Rowe P. Chronic fatigue in Ehlers–Danlos syndrome—Hypermobile type. American Journal of Medical Genetics, Part C: Seminars in Medical Genetics. 2017;175(1):175-180. doi:10.1002/ajmg.c.31542.

[265] Castori M, Camerota F, Celletti C, et al. Natural history and manifestations of the hypermobility type Ehlers-Danlos syndrome: A pilot study on 21 patients. American Journal of Medical Genetics, Part A. Published online 2010. doi:10.1002/ajmg.a.33231.

[266] Chopra P, Tinkle B, Hamonet C, et al. Pain management in the Ehlers–Danlos syndromes. American Journal of Medical Genetics, Part C: Seminars in Medical Genetics. 2017;175(1):212-219. doi:10.1002/ajmg.c.31554.

its comorbidities. If oxygen therapy is proven effective in this setting, further research is also needed to determine the circumstances under which it should be prescribed.

In the meantime, *(I suggest)* oxygen therapy as an adjunct therapy while complete information is pending. There will be time to re-evaluate oxygen therapy's usefulness in EDS and its comorbidities when better treatment methods and life quality improvement are discovered in the future.

There are no specific rights set out expressly for people with disabilities. Instead, they have the same rights as everyone else, outlined in the U.N.'s Declaration of Human Rights.[267,268]

Individuals with a disability, whether visible (being in a wheelchair because of poor proprioception and lax ligaments) or invisible (like chronic pain, chronic fatigue, mental fog, and subluxations), have the same rights as healthy individuals. Adequate treatment for pain and fatigue is part of any treatment for all patients, whoever they are.

Alleviation of chronic pain is an economic good and a human right. Chronic pain creates a significant financial burden for patients, health services, and society as a whole. Even though international comparisons are difficult to make due to variations in study methods, the main point is that pain causes a considerable burden on limited healthcare resources worldwide.

The decrease in pain by 30-50% or by two points on a Likert scale, for example, decreasing pain from an 8 to a six, is considered an effective treatment and not a suitable measurement method. Any treatment that can significantly reduce pain and distress, thereby improving quality of life by aiding an individual in becoming a functioning member of the society (i.e., having enough energy to work and enjoy a social life), should be taken.

---

[267] Schulkin J. Allostasis, Homeostasis, and the Costs of Physiological Adaptation.; 2015. doi:10.1017/CBO9781316257081.

[268] Rempel D, Abrahamsson SO. The effects of reduced oxygen tension on cell proliferation and matrix synthesis in synovium and tendon explants from the rabbit carpal tunnel: An experimental study in vitro. Journal of Orthopaedic Research. 2001;19(1):143-148. doi:10.1016/S0736-0266(00)00005-X.

Chronic pain is a variable but prevalent symptom of EDS. Additional characteristics such as fatigue and mood disorders are also common and are likely to contribute to progressive and recalcitrant pain syndromes, for which many pain medications are ineffective.

Pain is not a self-contained entity. There are various types of pain, each with its underlying mechanism(s). In some instances, one set of pain can catalyst another, either additively or synergistically. As a result, pain must be approached and treated differently.[264] While we (medical professionals) are excellent at treating acute pain, many of the medications prescribed cannot significantly improve a patient's well-being in the case of chronic pain. These various types of pain will be discussed in greater detail later in the chapter. A person with EDS may exhibit one or more of these pain syndromes. Current therapies include medication, nerve blockers, electrical stimulation, and proprioceptive retraining, which provide some relief but are often ineffective. In addition, there is increasing evidence that these chronic pain syndromes have impaired tissue oxygenation and nutrient utilization. Therefore, the use of supplemental oxygen may offer an effective therapeutic option by reducing tissue stress and injury. Tissue stress and hypoxia also lead to mast cells activation, resulting in increased symptoms of various connective tissue diseases via the interaction of mast cells and their home environment, connective tissue. With chronic pain's complexity, only multimodal approaches have a chance of success.

EDS Symptoms

This book has discussed all of the signs and symptoms associated with EDS; we will thus only emphasize specific events in this chapter.

Several physicians in France reviewed 79 symptoms to obtain a comprehensive picture of the patient's condition.[269,270] In more than 70% of EDS patients, 34 of these 79 symptoms are present. In more than 70% of EDS patients. This does not mean that all EDS patients exhibit at least 34 of these symptoms. Despite this, there is a high probability of finding more than one symptom in the same patient. Some symptoms or combinations of symptoms suggest that these patients' conditions could be improved with better or optimal oxygenation.

The most significant and critical barrier between our internal and external environments is connective tissue. It is a permeable but selective barrier that allows nutrients, electrolytes, and water to be absorbed. Additionally, it is an effective barrier for regulating body temperature. Simultaneously, certain connective tissue elements promote waste product elimination while also recognizing and responding to toxic, physical, or infectious aggressions. (see MCAD chapters in this book)

Pain is triggered by a nerve's direct injury, stimulation of pain nerve endings, or an inflammatory response of specific connective tissue cells. Given the unique relationship between peripheral nerve endings and connective tissue mast cells, one chronic pain model postulates that these two elements are responsible for the metabolic injury. That activation of mast cells and nerves can occur locally or be generalized to the whole body. These interactions may be the source of chronic pain that is either nociceptive (inflammation and tissue damage), peripheral neuropathic (nerve damage or dysfunction), or central (disruption of central pain processes).[271,272]

---

[269] Hamonet, C., Brissot, R. Gompel, A. Baeza-Velasco C, Guinchat, V. Brock, I., Ducret, L., Pommeret, S., Metlaine A. Prospective Study of 853 Patients. EC Neurology. 2018;6(2018):428-439.

[270] Hamonet C, Brock I, Pommeret S, et al. Ehlers-Danlos Syndrome type III (hypermobile): Clinical somatosensory scale (SSCS-62) validation, about 626 patients. Bulletin de l'Academie Nationale de Medecine. 2017;201(1-3):405-415. doi:10.1016/S0001-4079(19)30525-4.

[271] Mense S. Muscle Pain. Dtsch Arztebl International. 2008;105(12):214-219. doi:10.3238/artzebl.2008.0214.

[272] Chang-Zern Hong. Hong_Myofascial_Pain.Pdf. Current Pain and Headches Reports. 2006;(10):345-349.

Specific treatments that address these complex interrelations provide an additional therapeutic arsenal to conventional therapies. For example, oxygen therapy has been shown to significantly reduce pain and inflammation in various painful conditions, including interstitial cystitis, fibromyalgia, migraines, and more.[273,274,275,276,277]

Pain in EDS, whether it is nociceptive (nociceptors, tissue sensors), peripheral neuropathic (free endings, for example), central (central sensitization), or even a combination of all three, is treatable. It can be attenuated or at least for the chronic pain not be present at all.

Life happens, and acute crises may occur, but pain and fatigue are not a compulsory part of life with EDS!

Quality of Life of EDS patients

EDS patients' quality of life (QoL) is reduced by multiple factors, some of which act in synergy.

A Swedish control group study specifically assessed pain, fatigue, anxiety, and depression in an EDS population compared to a general population control group. Age, fatigue, and low back pain were all associated with a higher level of anxiety.

[273] Casale R, Boccia G, Symeonidou Z, et al. Neuromuscular efficiency in fibromyalgia is improved by hyperbaric oxygen therapy: looking inside muscles by means of surface electromyography. Clinical and experimental rheumatology. 2019;37(1):75-80.

[274] Kim HR, Kim JH, Choi EJ, et al. Hyperoxygenation attenuated a murine model of atopic dermatitis through raising skin level of ROS. PLoS O.N.E. 2014;9(10). doi:10.1371/journal.pone.0109297

[275] Katznelson R, Segal SC, Clarke H. Successful treatment of lower limb complex regional pain syndrome following three weeks of hyperbaric oxygen therapy. Pain Research and Management. 2016;2016. doi:10.1155/2016/3458371

[276] Vuralkan E, Cobanoglu HB, Mirasoglu B, et al. May Hyperbaric Oxygen Therapy Play a Role in the Treatment of Allergic Rhinitis? A Double- Blind Experimental Study in Rat Model Hyperbaric Oxygen Therapy on Allergic Rhinitis. Journal of Otology & Rhinology. 2017;07(01):1-4. doi:10.4172/2324-8785.1000335

[277] Han G, Liu K, Li L, Li X, Zhao P. Effects of hyperbaric oxygen therapy on neuropathic pain via mitophagy in microglia. Molecular Pain. 2017;13:1-10. doi:10.1177/1744806917710862

Compared to the general Swedish population, patients with EDS had a lower quality of life.[273] Muscle pain (myalgia) has also been studied in terms of its effect on the quality of life (QoL). In a control study, muscle pain was reported in 87% of EDS patients.[269] Additionally, an Italian study discovered that musculoskeletal pain had a discernible negative effect on the quality of life.[274]

QoL can be decreased very early in some cases: a study of 47 children and adolescents using the Pediatric Quality of Life Inventory (PedsQL) and other scales demonstrated an early decline in QoL.[275] Additionally, we know that early therapeutic intervention, as it is with most diseases, produces the best results. It is critical in EDS because the latency to diagnosis is at best 12 years but frequently exceeds 20 years.

One of the goals of treatment is to achieve allostasis.[276,277,278,279]

Allostasis refers to the body's homeostasis at a given time. It implies that the body should be functioning optimally throughout the day. If you have a stressful day, your body needs to direct its energy toward certain tasks and away from others.

AN: Unlike homeostasis, which is the preservation of constancy (such as sodium or calcium levels), allostasis is the calibration of the body's functions in response to internal and external conditions. Allostasis that is maintained for an extended period, or is poorly regulated, results in what Mac Ewen referred to as "allostatic overload," in which immune, metabolic, or neuroendocrine responses result in chronic disease states.[280]

[278] Berglund B, Pettersson C, Pigg M, Kristiansson P. Self-reported quality of life, anxiety and depression in individuals with Ehlers-Danlos syndrome (EDS): A questionnaire study. BMC Musculoskeletal Disorders. 2015;16(1). doi:10.1186/s12891-015-0549-7

[279] Salaffi F, de Angelis R, Stancati A, et al. Health-related quality of life in multiple musculoskeletal conditions: A cross-sectional population based epidemiological study. II. The MAPPING study. Clinical and Experimental Rheumatology. 2005;23(6):829-839.

[280] McEwen BS. Stress, Adaptation, and Disease: Allostasis and Allostatic Load. Annals of the New York Academy of Sciences. Published online 1998. doi:10.1111/j.1749-6632.1998.tb09546.x

In EDS, this means returning to a time when EDS provided all its benefits without the negative consequences. Demand and supply must be balanced.

Due to the fragility of the connective tissues in EDS, the ligaments become hyperlaxed. They do not adequately hold the joints together, and the body must compensate for this increased demand. Additionally, because nutrients are not optimally distributed throughout the body, for example, the necessary supply could be decreased due to, for instance, low blood pressure. This indicates that there is increased demand concurrently with a decrease in supply. The management strategy will then consist of reducing demand (for example, by stabilizing joints and improving proprioception with compression garments) while increasing supply. Comparatively, the level of supplementation to achieve allostasis for a healthy person may not be sufficient to achieve allostasis in an EDS patient (for example, the EDS patient is probably "asking for more") as both demand is increased and supply might be decreased respectively.

2. Chronic pain and the role of oxygen treatments:

➢ **Myalgias** (see the chapter of the book). During exercise and the fatigue which may follow, central neurotransmitters, especially serotonin, dopamine, and norepinephrine, play a significant role. An energy crisis can occur when muscle oxygen requirements exceed their supply. Many precipitating factors have been suggested; their main effect is to prolong the actin-myosin bond, which causes muscle fiber contraction and increased resistance to microvascular flow in the contracted muscle. Arteriolar and capillary stress, often increased by a local vasoconstrictor reflex, leads to decreased oxygen and glucose supply to the muscle fibers and lower energy production (ATP). Concerning pain and mast cell activation, some publications demonstrate that mast cells, which live, are educated in and react in connective tissue, react when the tissue is hypoxic (that is low on oxygen). The myalgia then may diminish. So, for instance, by exercising and resolving the kinesiophobia, we can also reduce tissue hypoxia and, in consequence, attenuate mast cell activation.[281,282,283]

➢ **Cervical pain and headaches.**[283,284,285,286] (see the book chapter). In facial vascular algae, the effect of oxygen at a flow rate of 15 liters per minute is well-known (Cluster Headaches). Headaches may be caused or aggravated by a lack of oxygen to contracted occipital and cervical muscles.

➢ **MCAD** (as mast cells react in hypoxic tissue, please refer to dedicated chapters in this book). Mast cells are involved in vasodilation, vascular homeostasis, immune responses (innate and adaptive), and angiogenesis. In various conditions involving mast cells (asthma, anaphylaxis, gastrointestinal disorders, certain cancers, and more), tissues are frequently exposed to persistent or intermittent hypoxia. Some scientific data have highlighted hypoxia's influence on mast cells in their lifespan and the increase in their degranulation and cytokine release. [281,282,287]

---

[281] Steiner D.R.S., Gonzalez NC, Wood J.G. Mast cells mediate the microvascular inflammatory response to systemic hypoxia. J Appl Physiol. 2003;94:325-334. doi:10.1152/japplphysiol.00637.2002.-Systemic.

[282] Möllerherm H, Branitzki-Heinemann K, Brogden G, et al. Hypoxia modulates the response of mast cells to Staphylococcus aureus infection. Frontiers in Immunology. 2017;8(MAY). doi:10.3389/fimmu.2017.00541

[283] Henderson FC, Austin C, Benzel E, et al. Neurological and spinal manifestations of the Ehlers–Danlos syndromes. American Journal of Medical Genetics, Part C: Seminars in Medical Genetics. 2017;175(1):195-211. doi:10.1002/ajmg.c.31549

[284] Castori M, Morlino S, Ghibellini G, Celletti C, Camerota F, Grammatico P. Connective tissue, Ehlers-Danlos syndrome(s), and head and cervical pain. American Journal of Medical Genetics, Part C: Seminars in Medical Genetics. 2015;169(1):84-96. doi:10.1002/ajmg.c.31426

[285] Cook GA, Sandroni P. Management of headache and chronic pain in POTS. Autonomic Neuroscience: Basic and Clinical. 2018;215(December 2017):37-45. doi:10.1016/j.autneu.2018.06.004

[286] Puledda F, Viganò A, Celletti C, et al. A study of migraine characteristics in joint hypermobility syndrome a.k.a. Ehlers–Danlos syndrome, hypermobility type. Neurological Sciences. 2015;36(8). doi:10.1007/s10072-015-2173-6

[287] Gulliksson M, Carvalho RFS, Ulleras E et al. Mast cell survival and mediator secretion in response to hypoxia. PLoS ONE. 2010;5(8):e12360.

➢ **The CRPS**[288] **and O2** (see this chapter in the book). Tissue hypoxia and inflammation appear to play an essential role in the pathophysiology of CRPS-1 and CRPS-2.[289] In addition, a study demonstrated hyperbaric oxygen treatment's efficiency in a patient suffering from CRPS-1 for one year.[275]

Several studies in non-EDS patients demonstrate that pain decreases tissue oxygenation. Additionally, a multicenter study was conducted on EDS's comorbidities to determine whether dysautonomia, MCAD, Tethered Cord Syndrome, Chiari I malformation, and CRPS co-occur in the presence of EDS. What was demonstrated was that 80% of EDS patients also have a diagnosis of MCAD, whereas 20% of EDS patients also have a diagnosis of CRPS. However, approximately 85 % of people who have CRPS also have EDS. (Poster presentation at the ACMG conference 2021 article publication underway). Therefore the effects of oxygen therapy on other comorbidities should also be examined. Inflammation-induced hypoxia plays a significant role in the pathophysiology of CRPS. Hyperbaric oxygen is highly effective in CRPS; thus, it seems to be a problem with the tissue's oxygenation.

➢ **Dysautonomia:** Dysautonomia, POTS, or merely low blood pressure require adequate treatment, along with or before initiating oxygen therapy. Poor blood circulation (for various reasons) leads to inadequate tissue oxygenation. *A.N.: As Professor J.F. Bravo demonstrated, the patients will first have to be filled (drink, eat salty food, add salt, wear a lower limb restraint, possibly add Midodrine per os, and more.) so that the blood reaches the brain properly. Otherwise, oxygenating blood that does not reach its destination optimally will have little effect on the symptoms presented by EDS patients (see the example of the half-full bottle).*

It is possible that treating all of the underlying causes of defective tissue oxygenation (venous pooling, dysautonomia,

---

[288] Hamonet C, Brock I, Pommeret S, et al. Ehlers-Danlos Syndrome type III (hypermobile): Clinical somatosensory scale (SSCS-62) validation, about 626 patients. Bulletin de l'Academie Nationale de Medecine. 2017;201(1-3):405-415. doi:10.1016/S0001-4079(19)30525-4

[289] Koban M, Leis S, Schultze-Mosgau S et al. Tissue hypoxia in complex regional pain syndrome. Bread 2003;104(1-2):149-157)

and Krebs' cycle) is more than sufficient to improve the patient's symptomatology. Oxygen therapy will then be unnecessary.

3. Fatigue:

➢ **OSA**[290]: see the chapter on ENT events and fatigue.

4. Oxygen Therapy in EDS:

➢ The physiology of tissue oxygenation.[291,292,293,294,295]
➢ Studies concerning regular pressure oxygen therapy in EDS (NPOT).

In our 20 years of practice, we have seen over 9000 patients with EDS (Professor Claude Hamonet and collaborators). Initially, there was no treatment available for EDS. By talking with patients over the years, our team has identified treatments that have helped them, resulting in a comprehensive list of possible treatments. While many patients reported certain medications' effectiveness, we prescribed these same medications to other patients to determine if these beneficial effects were

---

[290] Jennings S v., Slee VM, Zack RM, et al. Patient Perceptions in Mast Cell Disorders. Immunology and Allergy Clinics of North America. 2018;38(3):505-525. doi:10.1016/j.iac.2018.04.006
[291] Hamilton MJ, Hornick JL, Akin C, Castells MC, Greenberger NJ. Mast cell activation syndrome: A newly recognized disorder with systemic clinical manifestations. Journal of Allergy and Clinical Immunology. 2011;128(1):147-152.e2. doi:10.1016/j.jaci.2011.04.037
[292] de Wandele I, Calders P, Peersman W, et al. Autonomic symptom burden in the hypermobility type of Ehlers-Danlos syndrome: A comparative study with two other EDS types, fibromyalgia, and healthy controls. Seminars in Arthritis and Rheumatism. 2014;44(3):353-361. doi:10.1016/j.semarthrit.2014.05.013
[293] Grigoriou E, Boris JR, Dormans JP. Postural Orthostatic Tachycardia Syndrome (POTS): Association with Ehlers-Danlos Syndrome and Orthopaedic Considerations. Clinical Orthopaedics and Related Research. Published online 2015. doi:10.1007/s11999-014-3898-x
[294] Gaisl T, Giunta C, Bratton DJ, et al. Obstructive sleep apnoea and quality of life in Ehlers-Danlos syndrome: A parallel cohort study. Thorax. 2017;72(8):729-735. doi:10.1136/thoraxjnl-2016-209560
[295] Meletis CD, Wilkesa K. The Crucial Role of Oxygen for Health. Journal of Restorative Medicine. 2019;8(1). doi:10.14200/jrm.2019.0106

reproducible. One such medication is administering low-flow oxygen through nasal cannulas.

Some patients reported that they were put on oxygen when admitted to the Emergency room for worsened pain. Independently of each other, patients not only told us their migraines had gone, but they also felt less tired and had fewer paid days after this straightforward treatment.

We then began to prescribe low-flow oxygen, administered through an oxygen concentrator (at a flow rate of 3 to 5 liters per minute, in three 20-minute sessions per day) at a fixed site and home for three months.

Their feedback on the process's effectiveness was indubitably positive. They were able to reduce their pain medication, felt less fatigued, and had fewer migraines as a result. A priori, this treatment did not affect other EDS symptoms such as proprioception or joint instability. Subjectively, their ability to concentrate and work memory improved because of the decrease in fatigue.

Over time, we noticed that the patients who benefited the most from this low-flow oxygen treatment had the following five symptoms: muscle pain, fatigue, migraines, dyspnea at very low effort, and respiratory blockages (inspiratory bradypneas).

Following that, we performed:

1. A first retrospective (subjective) study that included 100 patients. We studied the effects of different respiratory flows, fatigue, migraines, respiratory symptoms, and the possible side effects of the treatment.

2. A study that evaluated changes in quality of life (QoL).

3. Prospective studies
    a. A first short-term prospective study.
    b. A second prospective, randomized, control group study.

1/ The retrospective study 100[296]

The main adverse effect was the noise generated by the oxygen machine (hyperacusis related to EDS). However, other results still require examination.

2/ Retrospective study in collaboration with company SOS Oxygen. Quality of life (QoL) assessment (presentation at the EDS International Conference in Paris, 2018).

The study compared pre-and post-treatment changes in the Quality of Life index (QoL), flow rates used at rest and during exercise, blood oxygen saturation (with and without oxygen), and device use time in minutes per day (Table 1).

	QoL avant	QoL après	FiO2	Sat O2 sans	Sat O2 avec	L/min repos	L/min effort	Min/jour	Δ QoL
Median	0,4	0,6	96%	98%	99%	3	5	23,5	0,2
Mode	0,4	0,6	0,96	98%	99%	3	5		0
Mean	0,383333	0,6	96%	96,63636	98,52941	3,160714	4,033333	43,94425	0,273333

3/ Prospective studies - 2017 (poster presentation at EDS International Conference in Paris, 2018).

First prospective study:

The frequency of oxygen sessions.

The frequency of oxygen sessions for 30 patients was studied. 47% completed two oxygen therapy sessions per day, 17% needed only one session per day, and 17% required only half a session per day (of 10 and 15 minutes per day). 13% conducted three sessions per day, 3% conducted four sessions, and 3% required six sessions per day. The number of sessions was counted; patients were sitting with their nasal cannulas, regardless of the session's duration. Patients did not always complete a 20-minute session, depending on their occupations. They sometimes opted for shorter or longer sessions.

---

[296] Hamonet C, Vienne M, Leroux C, et al. Respiratory manifestations in Ehlers-Danlos syndrome (EDS). New treatments options. J Readapt Medicale. 2016;36(1):56-61. doi:10.1016/j.jrm.2015.11.002.

The duration of their oxygen sessions.

- 57% responded that their sessions did last 20 minutes.
- 34% were only doing a 15-minute oxygen session.
- The remaining three subgroups of patients (3% each) completed 10 minutes, 25 minutes, and 30 minutes per session, respectively.

Oxygen flow rates used (in liters/minute).

- 4 liters/minute for 25% of patients.
- 3.5 liters/minute for 21% of patients.
- 3 liters/minute for 18% of patients.
- 2.5 liters/minute for 15% of patients.
- 2 liters/minute for 12% of patients.
- 1.5 liters/minute for 9% of patients.

Oxygen flow did not change from day to day: once patients selected a flow rate, they all maintained that rate for the duration of the study.

A/ FATIGUE

We observed a decrease in fatigue equivalent to two points on a Likert scale in 73% of cases (rated between 0 and 4). In 20% of patients, a reduction of 1 point was observed. However, 7% of patients reported no improvement in the intensity of their fatigue.

B/ HEADACHES

The use of oxygen therapy is chosen for facial vascular algae (*Cluster Headaches*). We wanted to find out if there was a difference in the frequency and intensity of headaches in our EDS patients.

67% of patients reported a stable decrease in the intensity AND frequency of headaches on oxygen therapy. 33% reported a reduction in the frequency of headaches but not in their intensity. We could not determine whether this was about headaches or migraines.

C/ PAIN

Due to the subjective nature of pain, we considered the decrease in pain only when pain medication use was reduced. While some patients received only Paracetamol (also known as Acetaminophen), others received high doses of morphine derivatives.

Regardless of the baseline situation, a decrease of a single pill per day (or a decrease in the dosage of morphine derivatives) was considered evidence of a drop in overall pain intensity.

The overwhelming majority of patients, 63%, could reduce their medication by one or more tablets. This encourages us to support future studies on oxygen therapy in EDS.

D/ QUALITY of LIFE

Most patients (53%) reported a significant improvement in their quality of life, while 17% reported that their life's quality changed for the better.

For 23% of patients, their life quality would have decreased with treatment. When asked why this degradation occurred, they stated that it was primarily due to the time-consuming nature of the process without any conclusive results. 7% of patients reported that oxygen therapy had a significant detrimental effect on their life quality.

Second Prospective Study:

We enrolled 50 patients who had been on oxygen therapy for at least two months. We wanted to know if the effects on fatigue and pain observed in the first study could be confirmed or were coincidental.

Patients were surveyed using the PIPER questionnaire (*Piper fatigue scale, Piper et al. 1998*). This scale evaluates fatigue on four dimensions: behavioral/severity, emotional, sensory, and cognitive/mood. It is comprised of 22 items arranged on a numerical scale. Additionally, patients completed a multidimensional questionnaire for pain assessment.

The questionnaires were completed at the beginning of the study while patients were on oxygen therapy to establish a baseline value.

Oxygen therapy was then discontinued.

Following that, questionnaires were completed every two weeks (in the second and fourth week of the study).

At the beginning of the 5th week, four weeks after the treatment, oxygen therapy was reinstated. The questionnaires were then completed after two weeks and after four weeks of this reintroduction of treatment (i.e., at the sixth and eighth week of the study). The rest of the treatments taken by the patients were continued without any change.

If some patients developed an EDS attack upon discontinuing treatment, we asked them to resume their oxygen treatment.

Starting in January 2017, we asked each patient who had been on oxygen for at least three months to participate in the study. Patients who had another respiratory disease or were smokers were excluded from the study. By the end of January 2017, 50 patients had been enrolled in the study.

Results of the second prospective study.

Only 11 of the 50 patients who provided informed consent completed the study in its entirety; the remainder discontinued, often after only three days without oxygen therapy. Their symptoms had worsened to the point where they could no longer participate in the study.

The following is a list of comments from one patient who politely requested that the study be halted after three days: "Loss of appetite. Difficulty finishing my two very light meals. Nausea. Tiredness in fits and starts, with changes in alertness in less than 5 minutes, on several occasions, during meals. At the end of the day: nervousness, hyperacusis, just wanting to cry from exhaustion (when I had a 3-hour nap and had only prepared dinner)".

My partner's comment: "I have never seen you like this. "Uh, ... You send an email to Isabelle and get back on the oxygen. "

Patient: "I need to have my abilities to drive and think. I cannot afford to be in this state despite all my willingness for this study."

The results indicated that oxygen therapy had a beneficial effect on the quality of life, fatigue, and pain of EDS patients who were able to complete the study.

The following tables (Figure 1, Figure 2) show the results. The different columns correspond to the beginning of the study, under oxygen, O2 (1), two weeks after stopping O2 treatment (2), four weeks after stopping O2 treatment (3), and two weeks after resuming oxygen therapy (4):

Figure 1.

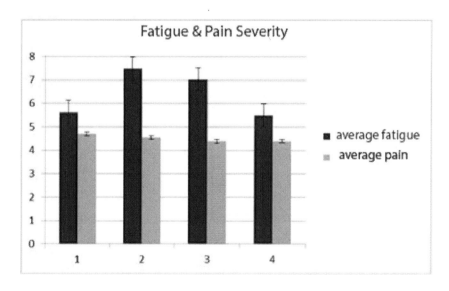

As with the first prospective study, these findings demonstrate that EDS's oxygen therapy effectively reduces fatigue (Figure 1) and migraine headache frequency (by approximately 50%, Figure 2). When oxygen therapy is discontinued, the frequency of migraine headaches increases initially and then decreases by 50% when treatment is resumed. There appears to be no effect on the intensity of migraine headaches (Figure 2).

Whether it was an actual migraine, headaches, severe headaches, or a combination of both, further studies on the effect of oxygen in EDS are necessary. Oxygen therapy is most effective in patients who experience pain, fatigue, migraines, dyspnea during exercise, and inspiratory bradypnea. It is observed in 44% of EDS patients, with 4 out of 5 symptoms in 72% of EDS patients.

Figure 2.

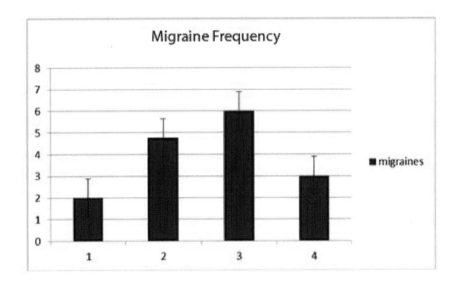

Additionally, the results confirm an increase in pain management following the cessation of oxygen therapy. The results, however, are far from conclusive. This effect on pain reduction will need to be re-evaluated in the future with additional data.

While pain scales did not decrease, medication intake decreased by 50%. (Figure 1). It seems that patients could switch between their medication and oxygen therapy (which is less toxic than pain medication).

Further studies should be conducted to determine the most appropriate rates and frequency of sessions in EDS.

4/ Ongoing studies.

A placebo-controlled study to see if oxygen therapy is more effective than placebo

It could also give us more information on when to start oxygen therapy, what patients, when it should be prescribed, and how long it should be maintained (thus when to stop it). Is there a difference between when EDS treatments are introduced, and the need for O2 treatment until other therapies take over (e.g., when the demand is no longer as high and consequently, supply needs not to be as ample)? To reiterate, the **diffusion of oxygen into the tissue** seems to be one of the problems. The perfusion index, a measure of tissue oxygenation, is often low in EDS patients, but most do not have an abnormal oxygen saturation level in the blood. However, the studies are still ongoing.

Questions: Could adequate oxygenation, for example, after relearning to breathe appropriately during rehabilitation exercises, which takes time, be sufficient to improve QoL (without sequential oxygen therapy)? Or, after correcting their breathing and thus enhancing their oxygen supply to the lungs and muscles, could a patient then stop his sequential oxygen therapy or use it only during EDS crises?

Conclusions

EDS patients are not hypoxic like COPD (chronic obstructive pulmonary disease) patients are. Therefore, the reason why there are such positive effects of oxygen therapy in a subset of EDS patients is probably different. One of the critical questions is whether the efficacy of oxygen therapy in EDS is related to oxygen's effect on mast cells. Should EDS patients that also present with MCAD be treated with oxygen directly? Sequential oxygen therapy has the potential to stabilize mast cells and increase muscle tissue oxygenation. This treatment could be tried in patients with EDS who also have mast cell activation, and the patient's clinical improvement could be assessed.

Epithelial barrier dysfunction, whether it be from EDS alone, from Mast Cell degranulation or toxic, environmental, traumatic or infectious disruption as well as dysautonomia need to be addressed.

Future studies will be needed to determine whether the current flow rate and frequency of sessions are appropriate. A study conducted on fibromyalgia patients treated with hyperbaric oxygen demonstrated that the treatment had beneficial effects on pain reduction. It may imply that patients with Ehlers-Danlos Syndrome could benefit from hyperbaric oxygen therapy or increased oxygen flow through nasal cannulas.

Additionally, studies on the pathophysiology of mitochondrial dysfunction in EDS also seem warranted. We have demonstrated that oxygen therapy can improve life quality by 0.3 points on the life quality scale. A better quality of life means that we can implement other treatments, do other things, perform exercises more easily, improve quality of life, and more. So, oxygen therapy is not the only treatment that works; rather, it is an adjunct treatment in a specific subpopulation that we have yet to identify.

As of this book's publication, current studies on oxygen therapy with EDS and its comorbidities (especially the trifecta of EDS, MCAD, dysautonomia) are still underway.

CHAPTER XVI

Nutrition in Ehlers-Danlos Syndrome

By Dr. Jessica PIZANO, DCN, CNS
Mast Cell Advanced Diagnostics
Maryland University of Integrative Health, USA

Introduction

Nutritional challenges in patients with Ehlers-Danlos Syndrome (EDS) are multi-factorial. Some are specifically related to EDS directly, but many are also consequences of co-morbid conditions such as mast cell activation (MCA) and dysautonomia. Direct EDS nutritional consequences include increased requirements for protein related to faulty collagen production and increased tissue repair requirements and decreased ability to chew secondary to jaw issues such as temporo-mandibular joint dysfunction (TMJ). Secondary challenges with nutrition include gastrointestinal challenges related to dysmotility/gastroparesis that impairs the patient's ability to consume adequate calories and a variety of food intolerance issues secondary to MCA, but also as a direct result of metabolomic consequences related both to these medical challenges and to the more typical consequences of more benign genetic single nucleotide polymorphisms (SNPs).

Ehlers-Danlos Syndrome, Mast Cell Activation, and Nutrition. The intersection of EDS and MCA can cause a large number of nutritional issues in patients. Many have difficulty tolerating a wide variety of foods which can cause severe ramifications for nutritional status. Metabolomics studies can be crucial in determining what food constituents may trigger a patient's reactions. Histamine intolerance is a common occurrence in this population, but anti-nutrients such as salicylates and oxalates, used as a plant-defense mechanism, can also become a problem.

Nutrigenomic issues such as upregulation of cystathionine-beta-synthase (CBS C699T) can cause not only intolerance to foods high in dietary sulfur such as eggs, garlic, onions, and cruciferous vegetables, but can also impact the patient's ability to synthesize the endogenous antioxidant glutathione. It is often necessary to use supplemental micronutrients either orally or via intravenous infusions to help patients overcome their unique biochemistry. Dietarily, it is important to assess the patient for likely intolerance and then correct the faulty biochemistry in order to be able to overcome the sensitivities and gradually reintroduces these dietary constituents.

The more limited a diet a patient has, the more important it is to assess for frank deficiency states. Regular evaluation of metabolomics (organic acids, amino acids, fatty acids, etc.) and more standard laboratory assessments, including a complete blood count to rule out anemias, comprehensive metabolic panel, anion gap, 25(OH) vitamin D, total iron and ferritin, and red blood cell mineral levels, should be take into account.

Histamine

While not all EDS patients have MCA, the fact that mast cells are present within connective tissue, where they are in close proximity to blood vessels and act as sentinel cells important in the defense against potential pathogens, greatly increases the risk for MCA. Histamine itself has a host of roles in the body and is released upon mast cell degranulation. Not only involved in allergic reactions, histamine is also a major neurotransmitter that acts on 4 distinct receptor sites (H1R-H4R).

H1R are found throughout the body and nervous system, and are associated with the typical allergic symptoms such as mucus production, sneezing, hives, etc. In the nervous system, H1R plays a role in feeding rhythms, energy metabolism, sleep, and pain and neuroinflammation. Typical antihistamines such as diphenhydramine, levocetirizine, loratadine, fexofenadine, and cetirizine all act to block the H1 receptor site.

H2R are found throughout the gastrointestinal tract and, along with the hormone gastrin, allow for production of hydrochloric acid in the stomach. In the nervous system, H2R is involved in learning and memory consolidation, pain and neuroinflammation, and help to regulate neuronal physiology and plasticity. First generation antacid medications such as famotidine and cimetidine act on H2R.

H3R is involved in involved in numerous central nervous system functions such as cognition, emotion, learning and memory. When H3R function is lost, it can cause problems with behavior, decreased movement ability, metabolic syndrome marked by hyperphagia, obesity, increased insulin and leptin levels, and increased severity of neuroinflammatory diseases.

There is a great deal of similarities between H4R with H3R with the differences being that H4R is expressed in peripheral cells and tissues more so than the brain (*Haas, H.L., Sergeeva, O.A. and Selbach, O., 2008*).

While not found in all patients with EDS or even all patients with MCA, histamine intolerance can be an issue that can lead to symptoms ranging from asthma and congestion to gastrointestinal reflux and diarrhea. Food highest in histamine can be a problem for these patients. These foods include those found in Table 1. Histamine intolerance is most commonly related to single nucleotide polymorphisms (SNPs) to the enzyme diamine oxidase (DAO). This FAD [297] -dependent enzyme is found both in the intracellular and extracellular histamine catabolism pathway (*Figure 1*). Relevant variants include rs2070586 (risk allele A), rs2111902 (risk allele G), rs3741775 (risk allele C).

While some recommend porcine DAO supplements, I find that the use of 40 to 80 mg of riboflavin-5-phosphate per day is typically a better solution for histamine intolerant patients. DAO supplements can be effective, but the compounding may be problematic for some patients and the cost prohibitive. It is also a short-term solution rather than a more permanent fix for histamine intolerance.

---

[297] FAD: flavin adenin dinucleotide, redox-active coenzyme associated with various proteins, which are involved with several enzymatic reactions.

While SNPs may account for a portion of histamine intolerance in patients, those who have elevation of either plasma histamine or 24-hour urinary N-methylhistamine often slowly deplete nutrients required for histamine catabolism including riboflavin. Further, a second enzyme, monoamine oxidase (MAO) is used in the intracellular histamine catabolism pathway and is also FAD/riboflavin dependent. This typically creates an excessive drain on riboflavin, that is nearly impossible to obtain through the typical diet, and even more problematic in those with a more limited diet due to intolerance. To best assess riboflavin status the urinary organic glutaric acid may be assessed. This marker elevates when there is a riboflavin insufficiency. Secondarily, one may also assess beta-oxidation via the organic acid markers adipate and suberate which elevate when there are deficiencies in either riboflavin and/or carnitine.

Figure 1. Histamine Pathways

Histamine Extracellular Pathway

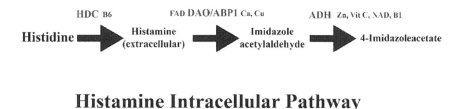

Histamine Intracellular Pathway

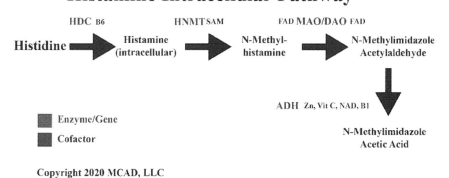

598

Table 1. Histamine in Foods

Moderate	High
Avocado	Citrus fruits (oranges, lemons, limes, pineapple, tangerine, grapefruit, kiwi)
Grapes	Papaya
Strawberries	Tomatoes
Sesame seeds/tahini	Eggplant
Raw egg whites	Peppers (bell, chili, red pepper flakes)
Ground meats	Tree nuts (walnuts, hazelnuts, pecans, Brazil nuts, filberts)
Frozen/fresh fish	Pumpkin seeds
Yeast	Anything fermented or microbially ripened (alcohol, vinegar, bacteria, pickled foods)
Cocoa/chocolate	Canned fish and meats
Cinnamon	Turmeric
Leftover poultry and meats (longer than 36 hours)	Ginger
	Chili powder/peppers, paprika
	Mature, processed, age, or hard cheese
	Yogurt
	Canned, cured, dried, marinated, smoked or preserved meat; dry-aged meat, most sausages, skin of poultry)
	Shellfish
	Wheat/gluten
	Additives (benzoate, sulfites, nitrites, glutamate, food dyes)
	Black and green tea

The histamine pathway begins with the conversion of the amino acid histidine to histamine, via histamine decarboxylase, a vitamin B6-dependent enzyme. While not particularly polymorphic, the sheer over use of this enzyme in those with increased histamine often leads to depletion in vitamin B6 which can have widespread ramifications for biochemistry.

Elevations of the organic acids xanthurenate or kynurenate are indicative of B6 insufficiency. An even more sensitive marker is increased levels of essential amino acids which require B6 for transamination. Similarly, assessment for low alanine aminotransferase (ALT) and/or aspartate transaminase (AST) in a comprehensive metabolic panel will also indicate B6 deficiency. Please note that serum B6 is not a good indicator of actual B6 status. Plasma pyridoxal-5-phosphate (P5P) is the most commonly used biomarker of vitamin B6 status. But, plasma P5P can vary due to albumin concentration, alkaline phosphate (ALP) activity, alcohol consumption, drug usage (hydralazine, penicillamine, isoniazid, phenelzine, cycloserine, thiamphenicol, L-dopa, progabide, and theophylline), inflammation, diabetes, and pregnancy. In these cases, measuring plasma pyridoxal (PL) can be useful as it shows a strong correlation with P5P, and total B6 aldehyde (P5P+PL) has been suggested to be the most useful direct marker of B6 status in patients with increased ALP activity (i.e. those who are diabetic or pregnant). PL increases markedly in serum, even in the absence of supplementation, and serum PL is therefore not a useful tool for determining B6 status (*Ueland et al., 2015*).

After production of histamine, catabolism depends on whether the extracellular or intracellular pathway is being used. Extracellular catabolism is typically related to H2R and occurs primarily in the gastrointestinal tract. Histamine undergoes degradation first by DAO (discussed above) as well as the calcium and copper dependent amiloride binding protein 1 (ABP1) to create imidazole acetaldehyde. Further catabolism is dependent on alcohol dehydrogenase (ADH) which requires zinc, vitamin C, NAD (nicotinamide adenine dinucleotide), and thiamine as co-factors. This accounts for why those who are histamine intolerant do not tolerate alcoholic beverages. The intracellular pathway which degrades histamine that typically triggers H1R receptors and accounts for more typical allergy symptoms including sinus symptoms and hives, begins with conversion of histamine to N-methylhistamine via histamine methyltransferase (HNMT). Like all methyltransferases, this enzyme is dependent on S-adenosylmethionine (SAM) our universal methyl donor.

Assessing vitamin B12, B6 and folate status via the organic acids methylmalonic acid (MMA), xanthurenic acid/kynurenic acid and formiminoglutamate (FIGLU), respectively, is important for determining the capacity of this enzyme. N-methylhistamine undergoes further degradation to N-methylimidazole acetaldehyde via the FAD-dependent enzymes DAO and MAO. Finally, conversion to N-methylimidazole acetic acid occurs via ADH, again requiring zinc, vitamin C, NAD, and thiamine as co-factors. Assessment and support of all of these micronutrients is crucial for histamine breakdown.

Salicylates

Salicylates are an anti-nutrient found in many plant foods. They are also found in analgesic and anti-inflammatory medications such as aspirin and willow bark, the botanical that aspirin was originally derived from. These non-steroidal anti-inflammatory drugs (NSAIDs) are used to help with pain and inflammation and work by inhibiting the cyclooxygenase pathway to decrease prostaglandin synthesis. Even in those without EDS and the associated MCA, salicylate sensitivity appears to be similar to an allergy but lacks an immunologic response. While not a true immunoglobulin E (IgE) reaction to aspirin, affected individuals appear to have an activation of basophils, eosinophils, macrophages, mast cells, platelets, and lymphocytes. This leads to symptoms of pseudoallergy (*Baenkler, 2008*).

These patients can have symptoms involving the respiratory tract, skin, and gastrointestinal tract including nasal polyps, bronchial asthma, polyps with asthma, rhinitis, chronic intestinal inflammation, urticaria/Quincke edema, and even anaphylaxis in those with MCA. Diagnosis is typically based on clinical symptoms or a provocation test. Provocation testing is only effective if the patient has immediate symptoms such as asthma. During this test, acetyl-salicylic acid may be given orally or nasally to elicit a response. Caution should be taken as the individual may have a rapid and emergent response requiring immediate medical attention. Biopsy and fine tissue studies may also be undergone to determine presence of eosinophilia in the respiratory and gastrointestinal tracts and skin (*Baenkler, 2008*).

Additionally, since salicylates are largely detoxified via glycine conjugation, insufficiencies of either glycine and/or pantothenic acid will cause a functional salicylate sensitivity. Given that collagen requires glycine, proline, and hydroxyproline for formation, glycine deficiency is quite common in those with EDS. Glycine conjugation may be assessed via organic acids and/or amino acids. In organic acids, 2-methylhippurate is a sensitive marker for glycine conjugation issues. This marker increases when there is exposure to xylene which must be detoxified via glycine conjugation. Additionally, conversion of benzoic acid to hippuric acid, generated from microbial degradation of polyphenols, also requires glycine conjugation. Therefore, elevation of benzoic acid with low hippuric acid is also a good indicator of glycine conjugation difficulties. Finally, on an amino acid test one may assess directly for glycine deficiency.

Use of approximately 500 to 1000 mg of glycine in combination with 500 mg of pantothenic acid may be used to help improve glycine conjugation and therefore salicylate intolerance (*Lord and Bralley, 2012*).

After a patient has been confirmed to have salicylate sensitivity, it is important to avoid salicylate containing medications such as aspirin, botanical medicines which are all high in salicylates, and begin a low salicylate diet (*see table 2*).

Once glycine and pantothenic acid levels have been normalized, a gradual introduction of moderate to high salicylate foods may occur.

It is also important to note that the use of oral contraceptives will increase salicylate clearance by 41% as they induce glycine conjugation, and therefore improve the clearance of salicylic acid (*Miners et al., 1986*).

Table 2. Salicylate Content in Food

Low Salicylate Foods

Fruits: Banana, canned pear, lime, pear (ripe and peeled), apple-golden delicious, Nashi pears, papaya, paw paw, tamarillo.

Vegetables: Bamboo shoots, cabbage, celery, iceberg lettuce, dried peas, potato (white), rutabaga, bean sprouts, Brussels sprouts, cauliflower, chives, choko, asparagus, green beans, green peas, leeks, mung bean sprouts, onion, shallots.

Herbs/Spices: Golden syrup, malt vinegar, maple syrup, salt, apple butter, chives, fennel (dried), garlic, parsley, saffron, shallots, soy sauce.

Nuts & Seeds: poppy seeds, cashews, hazelnuts, pecan, sunflower seeds.

Beans & Legumes: Beans, green split peas, lentils, dried peas, yellow split peas, chickpeas.

Grains: rice flour, rye flour, wheat flour, corn starch, barley, buckwheat, millet, oats, rice, rice cereals.

Oils & Fats: Butter, canola oil, margarine, safflower oil, soy oil, sunflower oil, ghee.

Dairy/Dairy Substitutes: butter, cream, cheese (not blue vein), milk, yogurt, ice cream, rice milk, goat milk, soymilk, tofu.

Meat: Beef, chicken, eggs, fish, lamb, organ meats, rabbit, sausage casing, scallops, tripe, veal, liver, prawns, shellfish.

Other: Arrowroot, golden syrup, malt extract, sago, soy flour, sugar, tapioca, carob, cocoa, caramel, maple syrup, plain potato chips.

Moderate Salicylate Foods

Fruits: Apple-red delicious, canned or dried fig, canned pear, custard apple, lemon, loquat, mango, passion fruit, pear (with peel), persimmon pomegranate, rhubarb, apple chips.

Vegetables: Canned asparagus, eggplant, beet, black olives, carrot, fresh tomato, frozen spinach, lettuce (other than iceberg), marrow, mushrooms, parsnips, potato (new and red), pumpkin, snow peas, sprout, sweet corn, turnip.

Herbs/Spices: Coriander (fresh), horseradish, mayonnaise.

Nuts & Seeds: desiccated coconut, peanut butter, pumpkin seeds, sesame seeds, walnuts.

Dairy: Blue vein cheese.

Oils & Fats: Almond oil, corn oil, peanut oil.

Meat: canned fish (with high salicylate oil or seasonings), processed lunch meats, seasoned meats (salami, sausages, hot dogs, etc.).

Other: molasses, raw sugar.

High Salicylate Foods

Fruits: Apple-all other varieties, canned morello cherries, cantaloupe, grapefruit, kiwi, lychee, mandarin, melons, mulberry, nectarine, peach, sugar banana, watermelon, all dried fruits, apricot, avocado, blackberry, blackcurrant, blueberry, boysenberry, cherries-all other kinds, cranberry, currant, date, grape, guava, loganberry, orange, pineapple, plum, prune, raisin, raspberry, redcurrant, rock melon, strawberry, sultana, tangelo, tangerine, youngberry.

Vegetables: Alfalfa sprouts, artichoke, eggplant (with peel), broad bean, broccoli, canned black olive, cucumber, fresh spinach, okra, radish, sweet potato, water chestnut, watercress, zucchini, green olives, chicory, chili peppers, summer squash, endive, gherkin, hot peppers, bell peppers, radish, tomato products.

Herbs & Spices: All spice, bay leaf, caraway, cardamom, cinnamon, cloves, coriander (dried), ginger, mixed herbs, mustard, pimento, aniseed, basil, black pepper, cayenne, celery powder, chili flakes, cider vinegar, commercial gravies and sauces, cumin, curry, dill, fenugreek, pastes (fish, meat and tomato), garam masala, mace, marmite, mint, mustard, nutmeg, oregano, paprika, peppermint, rosemary, sage,

tobacco, tarragon, thyme, turmeric, vegemite, yeast extracts, white pepper, wine vinegar, Worcester sauce.
Nuts & Seeds: Brazil nuts, macadamia nuts, pine nuts, pistachio, almond, peanuts with skins on.

Oils & Fats: Copha, sesame oil, walnut oil, coconut oil, olive oil.

Grains: Breakfast cereals that include fruit, nuts, honey or coconut; corn cereals, cornmeal, flavored breakfast cereals, maize, polenta, popcorn.

Other: Corn Syrup, chewing gum, fruit flavors (candy, gelato, ices, popsicles, sherbet, sorbet, sweets), honey, jam (except pear), licorice, mint (peppermint, wintergreen, spearmint), pickles (and anything pickled).

As mentioned above, salicylates are primarily detoxified via glycine conjugation. Secondarily, they may also move via glucuronidation, or through the phase I cytochrome P450 enzymes (CYP). Metabolism of salicylic acid may be influenced by gender, while aspirin/salicylate metabolism is influenced by additional factors such as alcohol intake, urinary pH, ethnicity, and genetic variants in UGT enzymes (UGT = uridine-diphosphate-glucuronosyltransferase). Diet may also influence salicylate metabolism by increasing total salicylate load and/or providing insufficient glycine, pantothenic acid and/or sulfur. Genetic polymorphism to the glycine N-acetyltransferase (GLYAT) gene may also influence salicylate metabolism. When adequate glycine is present, glycine conjugation is the preferred method of salicylate catabolism. This is a non-enzymatic reaction which takes acetylsalicylic acid (aspirin) and produces salicylic acid. This is then conjugated with glycine, forming 2-hydroxyhippurate and acetate. Salicylic acid may also move through conjugation, via glucuronidation, where it will produce salicyl phenolic glucuronide and salicyl acyl glucuronide, as well as the oxidation product gentisic acid. Following this process, these products must undergo further glycination to form salicyluric acid (*Miners et al., 1986*).

Salicylates may also move via glucuronidation. In this pathway, several UNP-glucuronosyltransferases (UGTs) enzymes are used. The UGT1A6*2 variant demonstrated *"a 2-fold lower salicylic acid glucuronidation compared with UGT1A6*1"* (*Kuehl et al., 2006*). This study further showed that *"results suggest that all UGTs except for 1A4, 2B15, and 2B17 might be involved in the glucuronidation of salicylic acid in vivo"* . Of all UGT enzymes, UGT1A9 does appear to have the highest rate of salicylic acid glucuronidation, though UGT1A6 is also required.

UGT enzymes are induced by dietary constituents (i.e. quercetin found in citrus fruits, isothiocyanates and indoles found in cruciferous vegetable and genistein found in soy. Such phytonutrients upregulate glucuronidation via *"interaction with the cytoplasmic-anchoring protein Keap1 (Kelch-like ECH-associated protein 1) and the human transcription factor Nfe2l2 (nuclear factor erythroid-derived related-factor 2-like 2; also known as Nrf2) via the antioxidant response element"* (*Navarro et al., 2011*). Increased intake of vegetables (especially cruciferous) (more than 2.5 servings/day) can improve glycine conjugation. Certain cruciferous vegetables (cabbage, cauliflower, and Brussels sprouts) all have negligible to low levels of salicylates, meaning increased intake may help improve salicylate tolerance.

Oxalates

Oxalates are naturally occurring substances found in a wide variety of foods. In plants, oxalates help to bind calcium, a required nutrient for plant's growth and development.

Unfortunately, this same process also occurs in animals. When a high oxalate plant is consumed, it binds minerals in the individual. When these oxalates bind to minerals or calcium in the body, they accumulate in the tissues causing inflammation. Oxalate crystals are known to solidify in and impact the muscles, eyes, gastrointestinal tract, urinary tract, and kidneys. In most patients with EDS and MCA, the issue with oxalates comes from a narrow diet that forces the individual to consume a high oxalate diet rather than presence of a genetic hyperoxaluria which is relatively rare. Some symptoms of oxalate sensitivity may include kidney stones, calcium deposits, irritable bladder, vulvodynia, tinnitus, chronic fatigue, depression, "fibromyalgia", rashes, headaches, and panic attacks. Lowering dietary intake of oxalates to more moderate levels may help to reduce symptoms.

Table 3. Oxalate Content in Food

Low Oxalate Foods - 0 points per serving

Fruits: Apples-Golden Delicious, Granny Smith, Jonathan, Red Delicious, Apricots-Fresh, Avocados, Casaba (Melon), Cherries-Fresh, Grapes-Green, Grapes-Red, Honeydew, Huckleberries, Kumquats, Lemon Juice, Lemons, Lime Juice, Lychees, Mangos, Passion Fruit, Peaches, Pears-Peeled, Pineapple, Plums, Raisins, Watermelon.

Vegetables: Acorn Squash, Asparagus, Bok Choy, Broccoli-Boiled, Brussel Sprouts-Boiled, Green Cabbage-Boiled or Raw, Cauliflower-Boiled, Steamed or Raw, Collard Greens-Raw, Cucumbers, Green Beans, Kohlrabi, Lettuce, Mushrooms, Onions, Peas, Red Peppers, Pickles (Dill), Pumpkin, Radishes-Red or White, Turnip (Swede), Water Chestnuts, Watercress, Zucchini.

Herbs/Spices: Chives, Cilantro, Ginger, Mustard (Spice), Nutmeg, Parsley, Pepper, White (spice), Rosemary, Sage, Tarragon, Thyme, Vanilla, Vanillin.

Nuts & Seeds: Chestnuts, Flax.

Beans & Legumes: Blacked-Eyed Peas.

Grains: Barley, Corn, White rice.

Oils & Fats: Butter, Canola Oil, Olive Oil, Soy Lecithin, Soybean Oil, Coconut oil.

Dairy: Cheddar Cheese, Ghee, Parmesan Cheese, Swiss Cheese, Port Wine, Yogurt (commercial).

Meat: Bacon, Beef, Eggs, Fish, Ham, Lamb, Meats, Pork, Poultry, Shellfish.

Other: Apple Cider Vinegar, Ketchup, Mayonnaise, Baking Powder, Baking Soda, Cream of Tartar, Evaporated Cane Juice, Honey, Maple Syrup, Sugar, Turbinado Sugar.

Moderate Oxalate Foods – 1 point per serving

Fruits: Bananas, Limes, Mandarin Oranges, Papayas, Pears-Unpeeled.

Vegetables: Artichokes (French), Broccoli-Raw, Brussel Sprouts-Raw, Green Cabbage-Steamed, Carrots-Boiled, Celeriac-Canned, Collard Greens-Boiled, Eggplant, Leek, Green Peppers, Red Potatoes-Peeled, Sauerkraut, String Beans, Tomatoes-Fresh.

Herbs/Spices: Basil.

Nuts & Seeds: Mung Beans, Pumpkin Seeds, Sunflower seeds (1 oz).

Beans & Legumes: Chick Peas, Garbanzo Beans, Lentils -Boiled, Lima Beans, Split Peas-Green, Tofu.

Grains: Cornstarch, Oats, Rice-Brown.

High Oxalate Foods – 3 points per serving

Fruits: Blackberries, Currants-Red & Black, Dewberries, Figs-Dried & Fresh, Gooseberries, Kiwi fruit, Lemon Peel, Lime Peel, Orange Peel, Oranges, Persimmons, Raspberries-Red & Black, Star Fruit.

Vegetables: Beets, Broccoli-Steamed, Brussel Sprouts-Steamed, Carrots-Raw, Carrots-Steamed, Celery-Raw, Chard, Chili Peppers, Collard Greens-Steamed, Dandelion Greens, Okra, Olives, Black, Olives, Green, Potatoes-Peeled, Potatoes-Unpeeled, Rhubarb, Sorrel, Spinach -Fresh, Spinach-Frozen, Sweet Potatoes, Tomato Paste-Canned, Tomato Purée-Canned, Tomato Sauce-Canned, Yellow Dock.

Herbs & Spices: Cinnamon, Oregano, Black Pepper, Peppercorn, Turmeric.

Nuts & Seeds: Almonds, Cashews, Hazelnuts, Macadamia Nuts, Pecans, Pine Nuts, Pistachio Nuts, Sesame Seeds, Walnuts.

Oils & Fats: Sesame Oil.

Beans & Legumes: Black Beans, Kidney Beans, Navy Beans, Peanuts,

608

Soy.

Grains: Amaranth, Buckwheat, Durum Flour, Wheat Flour, Kamut, Millet, Rye.

Other: Date Sugar, Stevia, Chocolate, Cocoa Powder, Milk Thistle.

Gastrointestinal Symptoms, Gastroparesis, and Dysmotility

Those with EDS commonly suffer from a variety of gastrointestinal symptoms. In a 10-year retrospective study by *Alomari et al.,(2020)*, they looked at 218 hEDS patients of which 62.3% had at least gastrointestinal symptoms. Gastric motility was a common problem in this group with 42 patients in the cohort having been tested for motility resulting in 11.9% with esophageal dysmotility, 42.8% with gastroparesis, 22.9% having small bowel/colon dysmotility, and an additional 9.5% that had global dysmotility. Abdominal pain (49.8%), nausea (49.5%), and constipation (45.5%), impacted nearly half of the study's participants. Gastrointestinal reflux disease (GERD) was also quite common and can be caused by both dysmotility and/or MCA.

Gastroparesis

Gastroparesis is a condition that affects the ability of the stomach muscles to contract and move food through your digestive tract. This condition is also sometimes referred to as delayed gastric emptying. Slower than normal motility (or contractions of the stomach muscles) results in the stomach not being able to empty properly. This results in food staying longer in the stomach than it should. The symptoms vary person to person and may include stomach pain, constipation (often severe), bloating, gastrointestinal reflux disease (GERD), anorexia, nausea, vomiting, blood sugar imbalances, early satiety, weight loss, and malnutrition. Medical interventions may include metoclopramide, gastric electrical stimulation, and anti-emetics. These, unfortunately, rarely fully alleviate gastroparesis.

Symptom relief is often a mainstay of the traditional medical response and may use off-label use of medications such as domperidone, erythromycin (short term), and centrally acting antidepressants (*Camilleri et al., 2013*). It is also common to use either partial or full enteric feeding via a jejunal tube. This should be the last resort as it typically can still cause symptoms if small intestinal and colonic motility is involved.

For those with gastroparesis it can be extremely difficult to get in adequate nutrition. In my experience, most tend to avoid eating to prevent the resultant pain that occurs. Many patients will fast for prolonged periods as eating can cause moderate to severe pain. This fast is then followed by eating a larger meal. Most would benefit, however, from eating smaller meals more frequently. It is often helpful to separate macronutrients. By eating a serving of carbohydrate first, gastric emptying is allowed to occur relatively normally. An hour or two after this, most are able to eat a lower fat protein option such as egg whites, white meat poultry, or white fish along with a serving of vegetables. Often, blending fruits and vegetables into purees and soups can be helpful in allowing gastric emptying to be more rapid. It is especially important to avoid large, heavy meals especially at night. High fiber foods should be cooked well and not eaten raw. Examples of some high fiber foods include beans, squash, peas, broccoli, collard greens, sweet potatoes, carrots, oats, quinoa, etc. In times of high gastroparesis symptoms, it can be helpful to consume a largely liquid diet with the focus on smoothies, soups, and purees. Mashed/pureed vegetables are also easier to digest. Consider mashed cauliflower, potatoes, sweet potato, parsnip, carrot, etc.

Fluid intake is important for those with gastroparesis as it typically occurs concurrently with dysautonomia. Use of electrolyte powders or capsules is quite helpful in allowing better absorption of water. However, with delayed gastric emptying fluids can also prevent patients from being able to eat and obtain sufficient calories. For this reason, it is important to separate consumption of liquids from meals. For those who have difficulty drinking sufficient liquids soups and smoothies frequently are a good way to provide fluids in the context of a meal.

Nutritional supplementation is often necessary for those with gastroparesis to meet caloric, macronutrient, and micronutrient needs. Use of formulas is often helpful either supplementally to a normal diet or may also be required as the complete diet. Enteral or partially enteral feeding is often recommended by gastroenterologists for those with gastroparesis. This should be the last resort as it is difficult to transition patients back to a more normal diet. Dietary supplements such as multivitamins may help bridge the gap and prevent nutritional deficiencies. However, these are not always well tolerated between the impact of supplements on gastrointestinal emptying and concurrent mast cell issues in this patient population. In those with either severe gastroparesis and/or severe intolerance issues may require IV nutrition. In those with iron deficiency anemia and gastroparesis, the use of iron IVs can help prevent the severe constipation issues that iron supplementation can cause. More balanced formulas such as a Meyer's cocktail or multivitamin and mineral infusion typically are easier to manage that individual nutrients. However, in the case of frank deficiency it may be necessary to use isolated nutrient IVs for repletion purposes.

While gastroparesis is defined as slow gastric emptying, many with EDS suffer from gastrointestinal dysmotility that may impact any portion or the entirety of the digestive tract. Combating constipation and/or obstipation is quite important as patients often experience anorexia the more dysmotility is impacting them. Smaller, more frequent meals may stimulate peristalsis as can a blended diet. However, most will require various aids for their dysmotility. While prescription medication can sometimes benefit patients, starting with more benign supplements is often better tolerated.

Triphala, an Ayurvedic botanical preparation comprised of dried fruits in equal amounts of *Terminalia chebula* (black myrobalan), *Terminalia bellerica* (bastard myrobalan), and *Phyllantus emblica* (emblic myrobalan or Indian gooseberry). *Terminalia chebula* is used medicinally for constipation, hemorrhoids, skin disease, asthma, dysentery, uterine debility, anemia, diabetes, leukoderma, tumors, and heart disease. *Terminalia bellerica* is traditionally used for cough, asthma, anorexia, vomiting, arthritis, fever, epilepsy, splenomegaly, piles, diarrhea, leprosy, as a brain tonic, and as a laxative. *Phyllanthus embilica* is used in Ayurvedic tradition for diabetes, hysteria, jaundice, eczema, piles, diarrhea, menorrhagia, scurvy, to rebuild and maintain new tissues, and to increase red blood cell counts. Phytochemical constituents of triphala include gallic acid, which is helpful for the prevention of neuronal death, and has anticancer properties; chebulic acid scavenges free radicals; chebulic acid is an anti-inflammatory agent and inhibits vascular endothelial growth factor-a mediated angiogenesis; ellagic acid is neuroprotective; tannic acid is an astringent and an anti-toxin; epicatechin serves as an antioxidant, prevents cisplatin-induced apoptosis, production of intracellular reactive oxygen species, and mitochondrial dysfunction; syringic acid is an antioxidant and antibacterial agent; and ascorbic acid (vitamin C) is an antioxidant (*Tarasiuk et al., 2018*).

The therapeutic benefits of triphala for gastroparesis seem to occur through its roles as an antimicrobial, an antioxidant, and immunomodulation. Slower peristalsis can cause overgrowths of opportunistic bacteria. Triphala is an effective antibacterial agent against many Gram-positive and Gram-negative bacteria including *Helibocater pylori.* In addition, triphala also is antiviral and is considered effective against swine glue, HSV-1, HIV-1, cytomegalovirus, and hepatitis B virus-surface antigen. As an antioxidant, Triphala appears to increase the activity of superoxide dismutase, catalase, and glutathione peroxidase. It may also be an effective chelating agent as they impede the oxidative cascades caused by heavy metals. The antioxidant properties of triphala also inhibit lipid peroxidation by modulating the mRNA expression of pro-inflammatory cytokines IL-2, IL-10, and TNFα. This immunomodulatory effect is combined with the improvement of natural killer cell viability and antibody-dependent cellular cytotoxicity. Further, research has shown that triphala also decreases nuclear factor kappa B (NF- κB) and therefore serves as an anti-inflammatory substance (*Tarasiuk et al., 2018*).

In terms of constipation, a study by *Munshi et al.* showed an increased bowel frequency after one week of treatment by 64.4% and after two weeks this had further improved by 79.5%. After 7 days, the mean number of bowel movements was also 18% higher than baseline (*Munshi et al., 2008*). *T. chebula,* a component of triphala, is thought to improve digestion, decrease constipation, and reduce cramping. Despite helping with constipation, triphala is also effective against diarrhea which makes it ideal for preventing the diarrhea we find with osmotic laxatives (*Tarsiuk et al., 2018*). However, for more extreme cases of dysmotility it is often helpful to combine triphala with an osmotic laxative such as magnesium in the citrate, oxide, or sulfate form.

Ehlers-Danlos Syndrome, Neurology, and Nutrition

Neurological ramifications of EDS can range from headaches and migraines, to dysautonomia and small fiber neuropathy. Neck pain and headache is particularly prevalent in EDS, with a 1996 study by *Spranger et al.*, showing that this occurs in 30-40% of cases. Patients may have various types of challenges including migraines with or without aura and tension-type headaches. These can be from neck issues directly, can be a symptom of temporomandibular joint dysfunction, and may also result as a symptom of mast cell activation. Neuropathies, including small fiber neuropathy, autonomic neuropathy, and compression mononeuropathies are also prevalent in the EDS population (*Castori et al., 2014*).

Dysautonomia is common in EDS. In a 2020 observational retrospective by *Celletti et al.* study of 102 patients with hEDS or hypermobility spectrum disorder (HSD), the authors found that 48% of patients had postural orthostatic tachycardia syndrome (POTS), 25.5% had orthostatic intolerance, and an additional 3.9% had hypotension. The percentage of patients in the *Celletti et al.* 2020 study was similar to that found in a smaller 2017 study by the same author where 48.6% of patients had POTS (*Celletti et al. 2017*). POTS is defined as a heart rate increase of 30 beats per minute or more for adults and 40 beats per minute or more for individuals ages 12 to 19 years, within 10 minutes of standing or on a head-up tilt in the absence of orthostatic hypotension. Commonly, in those with POTS their standing heart rate is 120 beats per minute or more. Pathophysiologic mechanisms involved in POTS include volume dysregulation, hyperadrenergic response, increased or impaired sympathetic response that may cause vasoconstriction in the lower extremities, and physical deconditioning. Patients may experience symptoms including dizziness, pre-syncope/syncope, palpitations, tachycardia, dysmotility and abdominal pain, fatigue, sleep issues, migraines, orthostatic headaches, and cognition issues (*Grigoriou et al., 2015*).

A 2016 study by *De Wandele et al. 2016* investigated whether orthostatic intolerance was a good predictor of fatigue in hEDS. The study looked at 80 patients with hEDS and 52 controls. Subjects took a series of questionnaires including the Checklist Individual Strength (CIS) to assess fatigue, Autonomic Symptom Profile (ASP) to assess orthostatic intolerance, habitual physical activity, affective distress (Hospital Anxiety and Depression Scale—HADS), pain, medication use and generalized hypermobility. Additionally, 39 patients and 35 controls were also tested with a 20-minute head-up tilt (70°) while heart rate and blood pressure were monitored. Fatigue was assessed using a numerical rating scale both before and after the tilt table test.

The study did in fact show that orthostatic intolerance was a good predictor of fatigue in hEDS versus controls. Additional factors appear to include pain, affective distress, decreased physical activity and sedative use (*De Wandele et al., 2016*).

The authors also felt that cerebral hypoperfusion is a likely link between fatigue and orthostatic intolerance found in POTS. "During tilt, patients showed a significantly lower TPR (NA: Total Peripheral Resistance) compared with controls (AN: and a higher heart rate), which reflects insufficient peripheral vasoconstriction, and could be attributed to several possible factors, including partial sympathetic neuropathy; medication use with a sympathetic influence or a direct influence on the vascular diameter/blood volume; and an increased vascular distensibility based on altered connective tissue. Each of these factors contributes to peripheral blood pooling, which is normally counteracted by sympathetically mediated vasoconstriction" (*De Wandele et al., 2016*).

Further, in hEDS the issue may be that there is a limit for constrictive capacity within the sympathetic nervous system. This is called vasoconstrictor reserve. When the dilatory tendency is greater than the vasoconstrictor reserve and/or because of damage to sympathetic nerve fibers, that causes decreased capacity. As a result, venous pooling occurs since there is insufficient venous return. As a result, heart rate is increased significantly by the sympathetic nervous system in an attempt to maintain system systolic blood pressure, but this is not always enough to allow for adequate brain perfusion. This may result in blurred vision, decreased concentration, drowsiness and fatigue (*De Wandele et al., 2016*).

In terms of modulating these conditions with nutrition it has been postulated that thiamine deficiency, loss of oxidative efficiency, excessive renal sodium loss and high calorie malnutrition may be etiologies of dysautonomia (*Lonsdale, 2009*). Hypovolemia is a common finding in those with POTS, thus increasing water and salt intake can be helpful in expanding plasma volume (*Low et al., 2009*).

Patients with hypovolemic POTS should aim for a salt intake of between 150-250 mEq of sodium which is equivalent to 10 to 20 grams of salt per day (*Low et al., 2009*). Further, some patients may be more or less sensitive to salt and the exact amount of intake should be fine-tuned to their personalized requirements. Fluid intake may be optimized to their needs based on body weight. Typical calculations for water intake are half of the body weight in ounces of water per day. An easy recommendation for patients can simply be to consume at least one large glass of water with each meal, and at least one large glass at least twice more during the day. This should allow for 2 to 2.5 liters of water per day (*Low et al., 2009*). Caution is advised for those that have congestive heart failure or daily IV saline injections in addition to POTS, as the excess water may complicate the condition. For those who have difficulty consuming adequate water per day related to gastroparesis and/or dysmotility issues use of IV fluids is often helpful. This may be given one or more times per week to aid in appropriate hydration.

Neuropathic conditions are often noted in those with EDS. While biomechanical and immune mediated neuropathies may be present, it is also helpful to evaluate for micronutrients deficiencies that may cause neuropathy, including thiamine (B1), vitamin B6, vitamin B12, vitamin E, and copper. Given the frequency of malnutrition in the EDS patient population secondary to mast cell activation, gastroparesis and dysmotility, and gastrointestinal issues such as chronic diarrhea, it is absolutely essential to assess nutritional status at a regular interval.

Thiamine deficiency, often overlooked by many nutrition and medical professionals, is typically thought to be associated with alcoholism, but is also often found in EDS patients. Signs and symptoms of thiamine deficiency (also known as beriberi) include: Poor memory, irritability, sleep disturbance, loss of appetite, weakness, pain in the limbs, shortness of breath, and swollen feet or legs (*Osiezagha, K., 2013*). There are three distinct types of beriberi including dry, wet and acute. Dry beriberi results from chronic low intake of thiamine, often found in conjunction with high carbohydrate intake. It is characterized by muscle weakness and cramping, peripheral neuropathy often with symmetrical sensory and motor nerve conduction issues that mostly affect distal parts of the extremities that can progress up the extremities. Asymmetrical foot or wrist drop with calf muscle tenderness and paresthesia is often also found. Wet beriberi involves more cardiovascular problems and is characterized by tachycardia, cardiomegaly, right-side heart failure that may include lung involvement, and peripheral edema. Acute beriberi is less common in EDS and is typically found in breastfed infants when the mother is either deficient or insufficient. Acute beriberi symptoms may include nausea, anorexia, vomiting, cardiomegaly, tachycardia, and lactic acidosis (*Groper and Smith, 2013*).

Found in whole grains, nuts, legumes, meats (especially lean pork), and yeast, along with enriched cereals and other enriched foods. Thiamine in foods can be destroyed by heat and there is risk of vitamin loss when cooking thiamine-rich foods in water. Thiamine deficiency can easily be deduced by observing an elevated anion gap (7-13 mEq/L) and is best supplemented in the fat-soluble form of benfotiamine. Benfotiamine is converted directly to thiamine in the body and is very readily absorbed at a rate up to 3.6 times more than water-soluble forms of thiamine. This results in significantly increased levels of metabolically active thiamine diphosphate and higher bioavailability of thiamine than other forms. It is also thought to penetrate the nerves much more effectively given its lipid solubility (*Gropper and Smith, 2013*). A typical dosage of benfotiamine is 300-600 mg per day in divided dosages with meals.

Figure 2. Anion Gap Calculation:
Anion Gap = Na-(CL + HCO3)

In the nervous system thiamine regulates sodium channels and permeability. It is also important for maintaining fixed negative charge on the surface of the inner membrane of the cell. Thiamine provides phosphate as TTP (thiamine pyrophosphate) for phosphorylation of synaptic proteins, and for activation of chloride transport. In energy production in the brain, thiamine is required for the conversion of pyruvate to acetyl-CoA (coenzyme A); and is also required for the production of the neurotransmitter acetylcholine, essential for proper cognition and memory. Finally, thiamine is required for conduction of nerve impulses via acetyl-CoQ-dependent myelin (*Gropper and Smith, 2013*).

Interestingly, vitamin B6 can cause neuropathy both in excess and in deficiency states. Deficiency is a known cause of seizures and can also cause numbness, paresthesias, or burning pain in the feet that may eventually progress to impact the legs and even the hands (*Hammond et al., 2003*). Vitamin B6 is found in beef, chicken, turkey, salmon, tuna, whole grains, potatoes, bananas, nuts, chickpeas, and fortified cereals. Processing foods containing B6 can deplete this vitamin. Vitamin B6 must undergo dephosphorylation via the zinc-dependent enzyme zinc phosphatase (or other intestinal phosphatases) to be absorbed. For this reason, zinc deficiency may contribute to and/or exacerbate B6 deficiency (*Gropper and Smith, 2013*).

In supplements, B6 is found in either the pyridoxine or pyridoxal-5-phosphate (P5P) forms. Pyridoxine is a synthetic form of B6, whereas P5P is an active, phosphorylated form of vitamin B6. For this reason, supplementation of the P5P form is typically preferable at a dosage of between 50 and 100 mg per day.

Excessive supplementation with vitamin B6 is a known, albeit rare, cause of neuropathy. Pyridoxine supplementation at 500-1000+ mg/day for several months is required to cause neuropathy. At 1-6 grams per day of pyridoxine for 12-40 months can cause severe and progressive sensory neuropathy characterized by ataxia, areflexia, and impaired cutaneous sensation (*Hammond et al., 2013*). Symptoms will typically resolve if supplementation is discontinued as soon as neurological symptoms present. Pyridoxine supplementation competitively inhibits the active P5P and may therefore result in neurological symptoms. Long-term supplementation of pyridoxine at less than 200 mg per day has, however, not been associated with neuropathy. While toxicity is possible via pyridoxine supplementation, this does not occur when B6 is obtained from food sources or from P5P supplementation (*Vrolijk et al., 2017*).

Assessment of B6 status can be problematic when using traditional lab values. Plasma P5P is the most commonly used biomarker of vitamin B6 status. However, it can vary due to albumin concentration, alkaline phosphatase activity, alcohol consumption, medication use (hydralazine, penicillamine, isoniazid, phenelzine, cycloserine, thiamphenicol, L-dopa, progabide, and theophylline), inflammation, diabetes and pregnancy. In these cases, measure plasma pyridoxal (PL) can be useful as it shows a strong correlation with P5P, and total B6 aldehyde (P5P +PL) has been suggested to be the most useful direct marker of B6 status in patients with increased alkaline phosphatase activity (i.e. those who are diabetic or pregnant). PL increases markedly in the serum, even in the absence of supplementation, and serum PL is therefore not a useful tool for determining B6 status (*Ueland et al., 2015*). Therefore, the best means of assessing vitamin B6 status is via metabolomic markers. Xanthurenate is an organic acid that elevates when there is a lack of P5P. The organic acid marker kynurenate will also elevate in B6 deficiency. The kynurenine pathway in the liver is used as a means of regulating plasma tryptophan levels. It uses excess dietary tryptophan not required for protein synthesis and concerts it into nicotinate (vitamin B3). Since the enzyme kynureninase is required to convert 3-hydroxykynurenine into 3-hydroxyanthranilate is P5P-dependent, B6 deficiency causes and accumulation of 3-hydroxykynurenine which is converted into kynurenine and then ultimately into xanthurenate and kynurenate (*Lord and Bralley, 2012*).

Vitamin B12 deficiency is a well-known cause of neuropathy. Vitamin B12 is exclusively found in animal proteins and dairy products, though it may also be synthesized by certain microorganisms (*Hammond et al., 2013*). Therefore, those with a vegan diet are at high risk for vitamin B12 deficiency. It can take up to three to five years for a serum B12 deficiency to develop. This is related to the fact that two to four milligrams of vitamin B12 is stored in the body with half being stored in the liver. Adenosylcobalamin is the primary form (70%) of stored B12, whereas methylcobalamin is the main form found in the blood (60% to 80%) with the remainder as adenosylcobalamin (*Gropper and Smith, 2013*). By this means, serum B12 is actually a more accurate representation of methylation capacity than B12 status. Hydroxocobalamin and methylcobalamin are stored in small amounts in muscle, bone, kidney, heart, brain, and spleen.

Even those eating a diet that provides adequate protein from animal sources, various genetic SNPs may influence vitamin B12 needs. Methionine synthase (MTR) and methionine synthase reductase (MTRR) are found in the methylation pathway. MTR (rs1805087 A>G) is a vitamin B12-dependent enzyme that catalyzes the transfer of a methyl group from 5-methyltetrahydrofolate to homocysteine, to produce methionine and tetrahydrofolate. It is important for maintaining adequate intracellular methionine required for production S-adenosyl methionine (SAM), the universal methyl donor.

MTR is also responsible for maintaining sufficient intracellular folate pools and regulating homocysteine levels. MTRR (rs1801394 (A>G), rs1802059 (G>A), rs162036 (A>G) is responsible for maintaining sufficient levels of methyl B12 required for homocysteine remethylation to methionine (*Zhi et al, 2016*). SNPs related to vitamin B12 transport are also highly polymorphic and can represent another genomic cause of increase B12 requirements. Transcobalamin 1 (TCN1 rs526934 C>G) is required for up to 80% of vitamin B12 transport and is thought to function as a circulating storage form that can prevent bacterial use of the vitamin (*Gropper and Smith, 2013*). The hydroxocobalamin form bypasses TCN1 SNPs. However, this form of vitamin B12 is contraindicated for use in those with hypertension. Transcobalamin 2 (TCN2 rs1801198 G>A,C) is a major part of the secondary granules found in neutrophils and facilitates the transport of cobalamin to the liver. TCN2 is responsible for 20% to 30% of all cobalamin transport (*Gropper and Smith, 2013*). To bypass TCN2 SNPs, the adenosylcobalamin form of vitamin B12 may be used.

Figure 3. The Intersections of One Carbon Metabolism, Methylation, and Transsulfuration

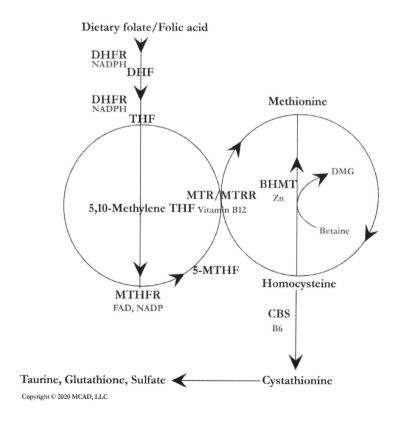

Measuring vitamin B12 status via serum B12 is a sensitive marker of frank deficiency, but elevation is never a sign of toxicity, as there is no known toxicity symptoms with even very large doses of B12. For this reason, there is no Tolerable Upper Intake Level established for vitamin B12 (*Gropper and Smith, 2013*). Typical laboratory ranges for serum B12 are 190 to 914 ng/L. Given that vitamin B12 is a water-soluble vitamin, recent intake and supplementation can cause elevation. Additionally, TCN1 and TCN2 SNPs may cause an increase in serum vitamin B12 even without supplementation. The organic acid marker, methylmalonic acid (MMA) is a functional marker that elevates when there is vitamin B12 insufficiency (including when caused by TCN1 or TCN2 polymorphism). Methylmalonyl-CoA is a byproduct of the catabolism of the amino acids isoleucine, valine, methionine, and threonine, as well as the catabolism of odd-chain fatty acids. MMA is converted into succinic acid via methylmalonyl-CoA mutase which requires B12 as its cofactor. MMA will also inhibit malate in the citric acid cycle making it another functional marker for B12 deficiency.

Supplementation with vitamin B12 to replete deficiency may take anywhere from 2000 to 8000 mcg of vitamin B12 per day. It is best absorbed in sublingual form, though the use of flavoring agents and sugar replacers can be problematic in those who have sensitivities secondary to mast cell activation. Injectable and intravenous B12, may be required for some with more severe deficiency or with pernicious anemia. It should be noted that since methyl donors may increase production of the catecholamines (dopamine, norepinephrine, and epinephrine) that the methylcobalamin form of B12 should be used sparingly. Use of hydroxocobalamin and adenosylcobalamin in supplementation is therefore preferred.

While vitamin E is found in animal fat, nuts, vegetable oils, and grains, it is difficult to consume sufficient vitamin E for many who struggle with gastroparesis and dysmotility as dietary fat may further slow the digestive process. Deficiency of vitamin E may cause ataxia, hyporeflexia, loss of proprioception and vibration, dysarthria, nystagmus, opthalmoparesis, retinopathy, head titubation, decreased sensation, and proximal muscle weakness (*Hammond et al., 2013*). Those with vitamin E deficiency, that have undergone nerve conduction studies, show the presence of sensory predominant axonal neuropathy, with nerve biopsy showing large fiber neuropathy. Electromyography, however, is frequently normal though can show mild denervation. Overall, vitamin E deficiency will cause swelling and damage to the large myelinated axons in the posterior columns, peripheral nerves, and sensory roots (*Hammond et al., 2013*). Repletion with 400 IU of vitamin E twice per day is appropriate.

Unlike with water soluble vitamins, fat soluble vitamins, such as vitamin E, may be measured accurately in the serum when a patient is supplementing with vitamin E. Typically, alpha-tocopherol will be used to assess status, however, serum levels can be a poor assessment of status. The dietary peptide product 1-methylhistamine may be a more sensitive marker of vitamin E status. It is derived mainly from the hydrolysis of anserine in dietary meat and, more specifically, poultry. Carnosinase splits anserine into beta-alanine and 1-methylhistidine. Low levels are therefore found in individuals consuming a vegetarian or vegan diet. High levels of 1-methylhistidine are associated with vitamin E deficiency from the increased oxidative effects in skeletal muscle (*Lord and Bralley, 2012*).

Copper deficiency may also cause peripheral neuropathy. Copper is found in meats, shellfish, nuts, seeds, legumes, dried fruits, potatoes, whole grains, and cocoa. Since copper and zinc share a transporter, supplementing with high doses of zinc (40 mg or more per day) may cause a copper deficiency (and vice-versa). Symptoms of deficiency include microcytic anemia, leukopenia/neutropenia, hypopigmentation of skin and hair, impaired immune function, bone abnormalities, altered cholesterol metabolism, and cardiovascular and pulmonary dysfunction (*Gropper and Smith, 2013*). Repletion dosing is typically only 1-2 mg per day with 10 mg being the Tolerable Upper Intake Level. Copper assessment may include the use of serum copper and ceruloplasmin (<20 mg/dL). Red blood cell copper is another viable means of assessing copper status.

Neurological ramification of copper deficiency includes changes in gait due to lower limb paresthesias. Additional signs and symptoms of deficiency may include decreased proprioception and vibration related to loss of dorsal column dysfunction and sensory ataxia. Bladder dysfunction, brisk knee jerks, and extensor plantar reflexes may show problems with upper motor neurons (*Hammond et al., 2013*).

Macronutrients and Ehlers-Danlos Syndrome

While there are no specific dietary guidelines for either EDS or connective tissue disease in general, one of the chronic health challenges in this population are constant subluxations, dislocations, and joint injuries. Some of these injuries, as well as challenges such as craniocervical instability and Chiari malformation, require surgery causing even more need for nutrition to help with repair and protein to sarcopenia during the period of convalescence. For this reason, one can draw upon knowledge from what we know about nutrition and injury, which has been studied extensively in sports nutrition as a source for new dietary guidelines in those with EDS.

The various minor to major injuries sustained in EDS patients create a hypermetabolic state during the injury-healing process that can increase macro- and micronutrient needs. Additionally, during any injury there are a variety of inflammatory, immune, and metabolic responses (*Smith-Ryan et al., 2020*). While in the general population this is an infrequent occurrence, this occurs constantly in those with connective tissue disease. Further, following injury, individuals typically will decrease activity to allow for immobilization of the impacted joint, which results in further muscle loss. According to *Smith-Ryan et al., 2020*, even at 36 hours of this decreased activity muscle tissue is lost with changes in global gene expression occurring 48 hours, and a more significant loss of muscle within five days of inactivity. When longer term immobilization occurs, this can be even more problematic causing muscle disuse atrophy that occurs at a rate of 0.5% per day. This will also result in muscle protein synthesis declining by approximately 50%. This causes a further decline of strength in the individual. Further, this process will cause an increase in atrophy-inducing cytokines, a loss of bone calcium that may contribute to osteopenia/osteoporosis risk, decreased metabolic rate, risk for insulin resistance, and increased adipose tissue (*Popadopoulou, 2020*).

Given all of this, dietary goals should be to optimize muscle and prevent loss of lean body mass. Further, decreasing inflammatory and immune responses that may occur during the injury cycle become a constant concern in EDS, and may impact blood glucose levels and insulin sensitivity. This is typically related to the initiation of the stress response and increasing cortisol and catecholamine levels related to this stress. The increased cortisol is important for the upregulation of the utilization of amino acids and proteins in an attempt to prevent muscle catabolism. While helpful in short-term injury, in those with connective tissue disease, this can lead to chronically elevated cortisol and stress response that can have cardiometabolic consequences as well as cause increased sympathetic tone.

The injury cycle and resultant inactivity in EDS patients can also cause a decreased capacity to produce energy. This occurs secondary to muscle loss which then causes a downregulation of mitochondrial protein transcription, decreases the biogenesis of mitochondria within the cell, and decreases the enzymatic reactions occurring within mitochondria. These changes can occur as soon as 48 hours after inactivity begins (*Tipton, 2015*). Further, this inactivity and the resultant decrease in the production and activity of mitochondria may contribute to decreased insulin sensitivity.

Caloric intake in EDS patients can become problematic. Between dysmotility issues and food sensitivity reactions intake is often much lower than required. This is very problematic as recovery from injury, as well as injury prevention requires adequate caloric intake. Caloric needs for remodeling of tissues are higher than that of healthy individuals, so this must be considered when providing dietary guidance for this population. Calculating resting metabolic rate (RMR) and then using either an activity level or stress level is important for calculating appropriate caloric intake. RMR may be calculated using either, the Harris Benedict Equation of the Cunningham formula. I have found for those with lower muscle mass, the Cunningham formula is more accurate as it considers fat-free mass. However, measuring body fat for each patient is not always practical. Overall caloric needs may be expressed as Total Daily Energy Requirements = RMR X Stress Factor X Activity Multiplier (*Smith-Ryan et al., 2020*). While many with connective tissue issues are fairly inactive either due to energy or fear of injury, a negative energy balance is likely to further deplete strength levels, increase muscle loss, and lead to further injuries. When caloric intake becomes problematic, it is essential to increase dietary protein to about 2.0 g/kg/day to prevent sarcopenia (*Papadopoulou, 2020*).

Figure 4. Basal Metabolic Rate Calculation

Harris Benedict
- Men: RMR = 66 + (13.7 X wt [kg]) + (5 X ht [cm]) – (6.8 X age [y])
- Women: RMR = 655 + (9.6 X wt [kg]) + (1.8 X ht [cm]) – (4.7 X age [y])

Fat-Free Mass (Cunningham, 1980)
- RMR = 370 + (21.6 X FFM [kg])

Figure 5. Activity Multipliers

- Sedentary: 1.2 (little or no exercise, desk job)
- Lightly active: 1.375 (light exercise/sports 1-3 d/wk)
- Moderately active: 1.55 (moderate exercise/ sports 6-7 d/wk)
- Very active: 1.725 (hard exercise every day, or exercising 2X/d)
- Extra active: 1.9 (hard exercise 2+ times/day; training for long endurance event)

Figure 6. Injury/Stress Factors

- Minor injury (ankle sprain dislocation), minor surgery, clean wound, bone fracture: 1.2
- Infected wound: 1.5
- Major trauma (anterior cruciate ligament surgery): 1.5
- Severe burn: 1.5

Macronutrient guidelines in those recovering from injury are often far higher in protein content than for the general population.

The RDA (Recommended Dietary Allowance) for protein intake is 0.8 g/kg which may prove to be too low for patients with EDS. Given that injury-induced stress can increase protein requirements by about 80%, athletes recovering from injury are typically guided to consume 1.4 to 2.0 g/kg/day of protein in order to maintain muscle mass. Increased protein intake therefore stands as a means of maintaining a net protein balance even when there is injury. In particular, appropriate intake of the essential amino acids which must be taken in through the diet are key, with the branched chain amino acid leucine being a means of stimulating anabolism of muscle when consumed at 3 g per serving of protein (*Smith-Ryan et al., 2020*). The complete proteins found in animal proteins are typically higher in leucine content, and are important for maintaining muscle mass in those with connective tissue disease. Intake of adequate protein per meal is important, often with a need for more frequent meals to achieve appropriate protein intake and to allow for a constant influx of amino acids required in the remodeling process. Intake of approximately 20 to 25 g or (0.25 to 0.30 g/kg) per meal of protein helps to maximize the response of muscle protein synthesis (*Tilton, 2015*). For those looking to use vegetarian protein options, these are often lower in essential amino acids and particularly leucine. Pea protein is a higher quality option than other vegetarian proteins and may be used to augment protein intake in those needing or wanting to consume vegetarian proteins.

Given the higher need for protein, a slight reduction of carbohydrate intake to approximately 40% of calories will be needed to not create an energy deficit. This will allow for about a 2:1 ratio of carbohydrate to protein. Timing of carbohydrate to prior to physical therapy and exercise is quite important to provide appropriate energy. Carbohydrate intake should be focused on the complex carbohydrates found in whole grains, fruits, and vegetables.

Fat intake should be kept to no more than 20% to 25% of caloric intake. This is for the dual purpose of not further decreasing gastric emptying, but also to prevent creating a caloric excess. Fats are particularly important for the body with polyunsaturated and monounsaturated fatty acids required for appropriate cell membrane creation. Saturated fatty acid consumption should be kept in moderation to prevent cardiometabolic consequences. It is also important to take in sufficient essential fatty acids with a focus on omega-3 fatty acids which are highly anti-inflammatory and are found in fish, flax, nuts, seeds, and avocado. Intake of 4 g of omega-3 fatty acids through diet and or supplementation can help with inflammation, enhances anabolic sensitivity to amino acids (*Papadopoulou, 2015*). Care should be taken to choose wild rather than farm-raised fish to insure adequate presence of omega-3 fatty acids. Fish should be very fresh as well to keep histamine exposure to a minimum. However, keeping these in balance with omega-6 fatty acids is still important (*Smith-Ryan et al., 2020*).

Works Cited:

Haas, H.L., Sergeeva, O.A. and Selbach, O. (2008) Histamine in the Nervous System. Physiol Rev. 88, 1183-1241.

Ueland PM, Ulvik A, Rios-Avila L, Midttun Ø, Gregory JF. (2015) Direct and Functional Biomarkers of Vitamin B6 Status. Annu Rev Nutr. 35:33-70. doi:10.1146/annurev-nutr-071714-034330

Baenkler, H.W. (2008) Salicylate Intolerance. Dtsch Arztebl Int. 105(8), 137-42.

Miners, J.O., Grgurinovich, N., Whitehead, A.G., Robson, R.A. and Birkett, D.J. (1986) Influence of gender and oral contraceptive steroids on the metabolism of salicylic acid and acetylsalicylic acid. Br. J. clin Pharmac. 22, 135-142.

Lord, R.S. and Bralley, J.A. (2012) Laboratory Evaluations for Integrative and Functional Medicine. Revised 2nd Edition. Duluth, GA: Metametrix Institute.

Kuehl, G.E., Bigler, J., Potter, J.D. and Lampe, JW. (2006) Glucuronidation of the Aspirin Metabolite Salicylic Acid by Expressed UDP-Glucuronosyltranserases and Human Liver Microsomes. Drug Metabolism and Disposition. 34(2), 199-202.

Navarro, S.L., Saracino, M.R., Makar, K.W., Thomas, S.S., Li, L., Zheng, Y. . . . Lampe, J.W. (2011) Determinants of Aspirin Metabolism in Healthy Men and Women: Effects of Dietary Inducers of UDP-Glucuronosyltransferases. Journal of Nutrigenetics and Nutrigenomics. 4, 110-118.

Tarasiuk, A., Mosinska, P., and Fichna, J. (2018) Triphala: current applications and new perspectives on the treatment of functional gastrointestinal disorders. Chinese Medicine. 13:39.

Munshi R, Bhalerao S, Rathi P, Kuber VV, Nipanikar SU, Kadbhane KP. (2008) An open-label, prospective clinical study to evaluate the efficacy and safety of TLPL/AY/01/2008 in the management of functional constipation. J Ayurveda Integr Med. 2011;2:144–52.

Alomari, M., Hitawala, A., Chadalavada, P., et al. (2020) Prevalence and Predictors of Gastrointestinal Dysmotility in Patients with Hypermobile Ehlers-Danlos Syndrome: A Tertiary Care Center Experience. Cureus. 12(4): e7781.

Camilleri, M., Parkman, H.P., Shafi, M.A, Abell, T.L., and Gerson, L. (2014) Clinical Guideline: Management of Gastroparesis. Am J Gastroenterol. 108(1): 18-38.

Spranger, S., Spranger, M., Kirchhof, K. Steinmann, B. (1996) Ehlers-Danlos Syndrome type VIII and leukodystrophy. Am J Med Genet. 66(2):239-40.

Castori, M. and Voermans, N.C. (2014) Neurological Manifestations of Ehlers-Danlos syndrome(s): A Review. Iran J Neurol. 13(4):190-208.

Celletti, C., Borsellino, B., Castori, M., Censi, F., Calcagnini, G., Camerota, F. and Strano, S. (2020) A new insight on postural tachycardia syndrome in 102 adults with hypermobile Ehlers-Danlos Syndrome/hypermobility spectrum Disorder. Mondaldi Atchives for Chest disease. 90:1286.

Celletti, C., Camerota, F., Castori, M, Censi, F., Gioffré, L., Calcagnini, G., and Strano, S. (2017) Orthostatic Intolerance and Postural Orthostatic Tachycardia Syndrome in Joint Hypermobility Syndrome/Ehlers-Danlos Syndrome, Hypermobility Type: Neurovegetative Dysregulation or Autonomic Failure? BioMed Research International. Epub 2017 Feb 12.

Grigoriou, E., Boris, J.R. and Dormans, J.P. (2015) Postural Orthostatic Tachycardia Syndrome (POTS): Association with Ehlers-Danlos Syndrome and Orthopaedic Considerations. Clin Orthop Relat Res. 473:722-728.

Lonsdale, D. (2009). Dysautonomia, A Heuristic Approach to a Revised Model for Etiology of Disease. Evidence-Based Complementary and Alternative Medicine: eCAM, 6(1), 3–10. http://doi.org/10.1093/ecam/nem064

Low, P.A., Sandroni, P., Joyner, M. and Shen, W.K. (2009) Postural Tachycardia Syndrome
(POTS). J Cardiovasc Electrophysiol. 20(3), 352-358.

Osiezagha, K., Ali, S., Freeman, C., Barker, N. C., Jabeen, S., Maitra, S., ... Bailey, R. K. (2013). Thiamine Deficiency and Delirium. Innovations in Clinical Neuroscience, 10(4), 26–32.

De Wandele, I., Rombaut, L., De Backer, T., Peersman, W., Da Silva, H., De Mits, S. . . . Malfait, F. (2016) Orthostatic intolerance and fatigue in the hypermobility type of Ehlers-Danlos Syndrome. Rheumatology. 55, 1412-1420.

Gropper, S. and Smith, J. (2013) Advanced Nutrition and Human Metabolism. 6th Edition. CA: Wadsworth.

Vrolijk MF, Opperhuizen A, Jansen EHJM, Hageman GJ, Bast A, Haenen GRMM. The vitamin B6 paradox: Supplementation with high concentrations of pyridoxine leads to decreased vitamin B6 function. Toxicol Vitro Int J Publ Assoc BIBRA. 2017;44:206-212. doi:10.1016/j.tiv.2017.07.009

Hammond, N., Wang, Y., Dimachkie, M. and Barohn, R. (2013) Nutritional Neuropathies. Neurol. Clin. 31(2):477-489.

Ueland PM, Ulvik A, Rios-Avila L, Midttun Ø, Gregory JF. Direct and Functional Biomarkers of Vitamin B6 Status. Annu Rev Nutr. 2015;35:33-70. doi:10.1146/annurev-nutr-071714-034330

Zhi, X., Yankg, B., Fan, S., Wang, Y., Wei, J., Zheng, Q. and Sun, G. (2016) Gender-specific interactions of MTHFR C677T and MTRR A66G polymorphism with overweight/obesity on serum lipid levels in a Chinese Han populations. Lipids in Health and Disease. 15, 185.

Smith-Ryan, A. E., Hirsch, K.R., Saylor, H.E., Gould, L.M. and Blue, M.N.M. (2020) Nutritional Considerations and Strategies to Facilitate Injury Recovery and Rehabilitation. Journal of Athletic Training. 55(9):918-930.

Papadopoulou, S.K. (2020) Rehabilitation Nutrition for Injury Recovery of Athletes: The Role of Macronutrient Intake. Nutrients. 12:2449.

Tipton, K.D. (2015) Nutritional Support for Exercise-Induced Injuries. Sports Med. 45 (Suppl 1):S93-S104.

CHAPTER XVII

Physical Therapy Management of Hypermobile Ehlers-Danlos Syndrome (hEDS) and Hypermobility Spectrum Disorders (HSD)

By Dr. Michael P. Healy, PT, DPT, DOMTP, IOMT, MBA
East Providence, Rhode Island, USA
&
Prof. David Levine, PT, PhD, DPT, CCRP, Cert. DN, FAPTA
Chattanooga, TN, USA

As part of a multidisciplinary team, physical therapists/ physiotherapists (PT's) focus on interventions such as manual therapy, therapeutic exercise prescription, pain management, energy conservation, orthotics (braces), environmental modifications, activity & task modifications, adaptive equipment, and sleep hygiene. These interventions can be implemented to improve function and quality of life, as well as decrease pain. When a multidisciplinary team is utilized with hypermobile Ehlers-Danlos Syndrome (hEDS) or Hypermobility Spectrum Disorders (HSD), patient care is managed more effectively and holistically (*Ericson & Wolman, 2017*). Within this multidisciplinary team; physical therapy plays a critical role in the evaluation, treatment and management of individuals with hypermobility syndromes (*Simmonds and Keer, 2007; Grahame and Hakim, 2008; Scheper et al., 2013, 2016*). Recent research has indicated that many physical therapists and other healthcare providers are not familiar with the diagnostic criteria, prevalence, or common clinical presentation of individuals with hEDS/HSD (*Billings et al., 2015; Lyell et al., 2016; Russek et al., 2016*). This chapter outlines the various physical therapy interventions utilized in the management of hEDS/HSD.

The clinical presentation in children and adults with hEDS/HSD appears to be similar, with pain being the most frequent complaint. This musculoskeletal pain has been hypothesized to be a localized biomechanical overload during activity, with a high risk of repetitive trauma. The resulting generalized joint instability may cause micro-traumas in the joint surfaces, causing compensations and adaptations in movement patterns; therefore, causing overloading of the musculoskeletal system (*Ferrel et al., 2004*). Pain exacerbated by activity is a distinguishing feature of hEDS/HSD (*Adib et al., 2005*). Hypersensitivity to painful stimuli is another characteristic of individuals with hEDS/HSD. The presence of generalized hyperalgesia (GHA) may indicate involvement of the central nervous system in the development of chronic pain and may not only provide insights as to the phenotype of general joint hypermobility (GJH) related disorders, but also indicates diagnostic qualities that may be useful in clinical practice (*Scheper et al., 2016c*).

Dysfunction in hEDS/HSD can be the results of chronic pain, the involvement of multiple systems, or psychological distress and related disabilities (*Engelbert et al., 2017*). Another important factor within the biomechanical pathway in hEDS/HSD patients may be reduced proprioceptive activity, which has been suggested to be important for the occurrence of gait abnormalities and musculoskeletal pain (*Smith et al., 2013*). Decreased muscle strength is also associated with activity limitations in hEDS/HSD patients. Joint proprioception has been found to influence this association and should be considered in the development of new treatment strategies for patients with hEDS/HSD (*Scheper et al., 2016a*). Hypermobility, especially with associated soft tissue damage, may contribute to proprioceptive deficits and limitations in physical activity. In addition, pain may impair proprioception. Impaired proprioception may lead to injuries such falls but can be improved with rehabilitation. (*Clayton et al. 2015, Aydin E. et al. 2017, Uzunkulaoğlu and Çetin, 2019*).

Individuals with hEDS/HSD usually have a decreased tolerance to exercise and physical activity. This may be due to exercise and physical activity frequently increasing their pain. These individuals are usually less physically active and tend to have decreased aerobic capacity, decreased strength, and decreased core stability. Hypermobility in babies can present as "*Floppy Infant*" Syndrome. Individuals with hEDS/HSD can have a lack of body awareness, balance and coordination as well as feel they are clumsy and/or falling more than their non-hypermobile counter parts. In children, decreased gross motor control can lead to developmental delays, including learning to walk at a later age. Similarly, decreased fine motor control can result in difficulty with handwriting as children develop. (*Engelbert et al., 2017*).

Fatigue is another major complaint of individuals with hEDS/HSD and is sometimes more disabling than pain. Psychological symptoms such as anxiety, depression, and panic disorders are also common. Problems can be seen with the autonomic nervous system where the sympathetic nervous system's "fight or flight" is over stimulated causing tachycardia, or the patient's heart to race in their chest. Gastrointestinal issues may include, but are not limited to, nausea, vomiting, constipation, diarrhea, gastroesophageal reflux disease (GERD), gastroparesis, intestinal permeability (leaky gut syndrome), poor motility and abdominal pain. The patient's skin may be velvety, overly stretchy, present with striae or stretch marks, abnormal scarring (atrophic, keloid, etc.), easy bruising, and have slower wound healing. (*Engelbert et al., 2017*).

The combination of pain, fatigue, poor coordination, and other systemic symptoms can ultimately lead to a decreased ability to perform normal, daily tasks at home, school, or work. This, in turn, can result in a significant decrease in quality of life, self-image and social function for people with hEDS/HSD. (*Engelbert et al., 2017*). It is important that PT's performs a comprehensive physical therapy evaluation to determine the patient's functional, biomechanical and soft tissue deficits. Key to this evaluation is utilizing that information in conjunction with the patient's goals and creating a successful treatment plan that is realistic and appropriate for that individual patient's wants and needs. The patient must be an active part of this process. The patient must feel that he or she has been heard, validated, and that you are actively listening to them. More often than not, our hEDS/HSD patients know more of what is going on with them than their own physicians or therapists. Patient's will do their own research and they will test you to see if you have knowledge or are willing to gain knowledge regarding their dysfunction and related co-morbidities.

As physical therapy professionals, this comprehensive evaluation is also important to rule out other move serious connective tissue disorders, such as; other forms of EDS, Loeys-Dietz Syndrome, Marfan's Syndrome, Osteogenesis Imperfecta, etc. If any of these conditions are suspected then the patient should be immediately referred to a Geneticist or Rheumatologist for evaluation. However, if any other conditions, such as Craniocervical Instability (CCI), Atlantoaxial Instability (AAI), Chiari Malformation, Cerebrospinal Fluid Leak (CSF), Postural Orthostatic Tachycardia Syndrome (POTS), Orthostatic Intolerance (OI), Kinesiophobia (fear of movement), etc. are suspected, these patients should be referred to the appropriate medical specialist for evaluation and care.

Things to think about when performing your PT evaluation:

➢ If you accidently knock something out of alignment you must re-align it.
➢ While the BEIGHTON Score is helpful in determining if the patient has hypermobility; the BEIGHTON tests, especially the thumb extension, can be quite painful and cause an injury. Be mindful of this when asking your patients to perform the test.
➢ Our hEDS/HSD patients can do "party tricks" and they are often willing to show them to you; however, again be mindful of this, because some of these positions can injure the patient.

After a thorough physical therapy evaluation has been performed and you have determined if the patient is an appropriate candidate for physical therapy, then a treatment plan needs to be set up. The important thing here is to talk with the patient and find out what their goals are and what level of functionality are they interested in and if that goal is realistic. If their goals are not realistic or attainable, then a separate conversation must be had. There needs to be open two-way active communication and listening occurring. It is important you as the healthcare provider, as well as the patient, know that currently there is no cure for hEDS or HSD, so ultimately our goal is to manage their healthcare and keep them as independent and functional as possible. It is important to note, that hEDS or HSD will require physical therapy intermittently throughout their life cycle. They need to know that they are welcome back when it is appropriate. As a healthcare provider, you must remember that hEDS and HSD patients tend to heal slowly, and they do not progress as rapidly as non-connective-tissue-disorder patients. Once you have an agreement then you can proceed with your treatment plan. Many hEDS/HSD patients have failed Physical Therapy, Chiropractic Care and Osteopathic Manipulative Therapy (OMT) in the past. These patients usually had negative experiences with significantly increased pain levels and significantly decreased functional abilities that have lasted weeks, months, and even years after incorrect treatment, often due to a lack of active listening on the healthcare provider's side. This is where you have a chance to make a huge difference and get the patient to buy-in to this new treatment plan. You just have to get out of your own way and actively listen to the patient.

Many patients with hEDS have pain levels that average 5 to 6/10; where #5 is moderate pain via a visual analog scale (VAS). Using this VAS helps educate patients on pain levels post treatment and how to distinguish between Home Exercise Program (HEP) pain vs injury pain. The goal is to improve the patient's soft tissue and structural alignment, so the patient's body is working at a mechanical advantage with little to no pain. Then we initiate functional therapeutic exercises; however, the patient's tissues or fascia have a memory of their old position and the tissues become confused. This confusion causes the tissues and joints or spinal segments to go back and forth between their old position and their new position, requiring a therapeutic adaptation period for success. This adaption will take up to 3 days or so while the body releases histamine to assist in the healing process. This release can potentially cause a Mast Cell Activation (MCAS, *AN: or MCAD*) flare up. The patient's pain level should only go up 1 or 2 points from their baseline at the time of the exercise or hands on treatment. This pain level should drop back down to its prior level (at the start of therapy) within a few hours. This is normal post treatment soreness or pain. If the patient's pain lasts greater than 3 days and the pain level has significantly increased, then we have done too much or inappropriate exercises. These physical responses need to be well instructed to the patient and the patient's family. By taking this important step, the patient and the patient's family will have a buy-in on their HEP.

A number of cohort/uncontrolled clinical studies of hEDS/HSD in children and adults report positive effects of strength, core stability, and endurance training combined with education in pain management (*Bathen et al., 2013*), as opposed to different intensity of resistive training alone (*Ferrel et al., 2004; Moller et al., 2014*), or education in pain management alone (*Rahman et al., 2014*). However, these reports need to be further evidenced with more rigorous research designs. Existing consensus-based hospital and UK pediatric rheumatology guidelines may also offer helpful advice and treatment strategies to clinicians (*The British Society for Pediatric and Adolescent Rheumatology, 2013; Cincinnati Children's Hospital Medical Center, 2014*). Qualitative interviews of 28 families with children with hEDS/HSD (5-17 years) on prerequisites for the best adherence to exercise is reported to be parental motivation adapting family routines, making exercise a family activity and seeing the benefit (*Birt et al., 2014*). On the other hand, there are factors for non-adherence to exercise for these children, including lower levels of parental supervision, not understanding the treatment, not seeing the benefit, and not having specific time to dedicate for doing exercises (*Birt et al., 2014*).

Education, reassurance, manual therapy, exercise, taping, hydrotherapy and relaxation training are used by PTs (*Lyell et al., 2015; Palmer et al., 2015, Rombaut et al., 2011b, 2015b; Billings et al., 2015*) and clinical experts recommend these strategies (*Russek, 2000; Simmonds and Keer, 20007; Keer and Simmonds, 2011*) based on clinical experience and some evidence of their efficacy with other patient groups. Therapies should be individualized (*Simmonds and Keer, 2007, 2008; Simmonds et al., 2016a*) and applied carefully to avoid exacerbation of pain, as peripheral and central sensitization is commonly observed (*Rombaut et al., 2011b*).

Cardiovascular, musculoskeletal and physical fitness training parameters should be encouraged in both children and adults according to the criteria of the *National Strength and Conditioning Association* (NSCA) and the *American College of Sports Medicine* (ACSM) (*Faigenbaum et al., 2009; Faigenbaum and Myer, 2010; Garber et al., 2011*). In general, specialists recommend a carefully graduated exercise training prescription underpinned by motor learning theory (*Smith et al., 2014b*) to avoid injury and overtraining, as this may lead to loss of confidence in the physical therapist. Pain, fatigue, and fear of injury are commonly reported barriers to exercise (*Simmonds et al., 2016b*). Graduated returns to higher levels of sports or dance are recommended, and training loads should be observed to ensure adequate recovery.

Patients with hEDS/HSD have numerous complaints and an impaired functional status that strongly determine their rate of treatment consumption. The outcome of surgical and physical therapy treatment is largely disappointing, which illustrates the need for a stronger evidence base (*Rombaut et al., 2011a*). Education for health professionals (*Billings et al., 2015; Rombaut et al., 2015b; Terry et al., 2015; Lyell et al., 2016; Russek et al., 2016*) is paramount in order to optimize physical therapy provision. Physical Therapists play an important role in management, education, and treatment of these connective tissue disorders.

An example of a typical physical therapy evaluation session is discussed here. Greet the patient in the waiting room and introduce yourself as you move to a private treatment room. Start your evaluation at this meet and greet. Patients don't care how much you know unless they know how much you care. Notice the patient's gait, movement, and sitting posture. Do you notice any obvious abnormalities in their biomechanical or soft tissue structures, or in their functional abilities? The patient at this point does not know that you are evaluating them. This is a good time to see the patient's natural habits and natural functional limitations. They believe the evaluation starts in the evaluation room and at this point the patient might change from their natural habits to their evaluation habits. Be mindful of this and compare the two. The *Hawthorne effect* (an alteration of behavior by the subjects awareness of being observed) can be minimized by watching them before the evaluation begins.

Once we get to the evaluation room, sit down at the patient's eye level and sit directly in front of the patient so they do not have to turn their heads or move their eyes, which can flare up their neck pain, cervical instability, or dysautonomia symptoms. By sitting at the patient's eye level and directly in front of the patient it immediately calms the patient, shows the patient that you understand their disorder, and that you respect them. The patients usually have 100s of pages of medical records and numerous diagnostic tests to review. If the patient attempts to hand you all this information, ask them to please hold onto their medical records and tell them you will be happy to review them after the evaluation. If they ask me why you do not want them first, simply answer, "I do not treat medical records or diagnostic imaging. I treat patients. If I look at your medical records and imaging first, my evaluation of you will become biased to those medical records and diagnostic test results, causing me to potentially miss something." Patients appreciate the honesty and open communications. Let the patient know that you want first-hand knowledge of their journey not second hand opinions.

After the physical therapy evaluation (discussed later in this chapter), review your findings, especially the biomechanical findings, with the patient and let them know this is the reason why they cannot do certain physical or functional activities that they mentioned to you earlier in the evaluation. Now the patient knows you are actively listening to them and that they have been heard. You can also mention that their diagnostic testing might have revealed this, and this is why from a biomechanical standpoint you cannot do this or that specific activity. Usually at this time the patient goes "wow you just told me what the diagnostic testing said without even looking at it." The patient now feels validated, understood, not crazy or that their symptoms are just in their head, and respected. At this point, review the medical records and diagnostic testing results to correlate the findings. You need to explain what their primary, secondary, tertiary, etc. issues are, and what their treatment plan is going to look like. You need to discuss the step by step approach of what we are going to attempt to do to help manage their symptoms and how we are going to get them to their realistic functional goals that we discussed earlier. This mapped out treatment approach gives the patient realistic hope of making functional improvements while managing their symptoms. We would also discuss the appropriate outside assistance that they might require, from peer support groups to other appropriate medical providers, etc.

Now the patient is ready to be treated. They feel like a person, not a number. It is critical to get patient buy-in or therapeutic alliance, so we as healthcare providers can help our patients help themselves. Every patient with hEDS/HSD must be treated as a unique individual, because even though they have the same diagnoses it doesn't mean they are experiencing the same issues or have the same complaints. Everyone reacts differently; therefore, you must treat them as a unique patient.

Therapeutic Exercise

Exercise is the cornerstone of treatment and there are several high-quality research trials in both children and adults which provide the evidence for this. However, prior to exercising our patients with hEDS/HSD the patients need to understand the difference between normal post exercise soreness and pain vs pain related to an injury from over exercising. Post exercise soreness and pain is commonly diffuse in nature and presents as bilateral soreness or pain that is located in the muscles used during that exercise session and can last up to 3 days post exercise treatment session. Conversely, pain related to an injury is usually sharp in nature and localized pain in the affected joint or spinal segment. It can be attributed to a specific exercise movement or a sudden event. It causes edema (swelling) and generates heat or warmth around the injured joint or spinal segment. The patient's pain level will commonly be greater than 5/10 on the numeric rating scale.

Prior to attempting any treatment, the PT and the patient must understand how the patient's co-morbidities might affect the patient's treatment plan, positioning, and progress. First, we must remember that our connective tissue patients (hEDS/HSD) tend to bruise easily and heal slowly. This needs to be taken into account when initiating any PT treatment plan. Set clear boundaries on what they should feel, how the treatment is going to progress, and what they should expect out of that treatment session. The patient has the right to stop that treatment at any point for any reason. This gives the patient some control and the knowledge that you are attempting to help them instead of accidentally injuring them. When progressing hEDS/HSD patients it must be done slowly, taking into consideration their slower than normal healing time and understanding their recovery from each visit might take longer compared to our non–connective tissue patients. Progression of treatment is also dependent on the patient's co-morbidities such as POTS, Tethered Cord, Chiari Malformation, CCI, AAI, MCAS (*AN: or MCAD*), Complex Regional Pain Syndrome (CRPS), Dysautonomia, etc., or if weather patterns have flared up their condition.

Our patients need to be treated as a whole person, not just a body part that is flared up for that treatment session. That flared up body part can cause structural compensations throughout the body, causing the patient's body to function at a decreased mechanical advantage. Therefore, we need to treat the whole patient at every visit. Most if not all of our hEDS/HSD patients arrive to the PT Clinic in sympathetic overload of their autonomic nervous system. They are in "fight or flight" mode, and jumping right into therapeutic exercises most likely will flare their sympathetic system up more, causing the PT treatment session to fail. Secondly, if the patient arrives to the PT Clinic with alignment issues in any body part, or throughout the body, jumping right into therapeutic exercises will cause increased joint pain from the mechanoreceptors within the joint(s) or spinal segment(s) to compress on each other; causing additional wear and tear on the joint(s) or spinal segment(s). Prolonged joint or spinal segment surfaces grinding on each other will lead to early onset of joint osteoarthritis and/or degenerative disc disease of the spine; thus causing the bad post treatment pain that we discussed earlier.

When the patient arrives at the clinic the patient must be assessed prior to each treatment session. Prior to starting any therapeutic exercises the patient's entire body needs to be aligned and their sympathetic nervous relaxed. This is where manual therapy is paramount. If the patient is in sympathetic overload or "fight or flight", have the patient lay on the treatment table in the Yoga corpse position while performing diaphragmatic (relaxation) breathing. Then get the patient's permission to do hands on treatment. Getting permission to palpate or touch the patient is extremely important. It builds trust and respect. Some hEDS patients have Post Traumatic Stress Disorder (PTSD) from sexual assaults and if you palpate or touch the patient without their permission this could lead the patient into a full-blown PTSD episode, significantly increasing their sympathetic overload, or "fight or flight" response. This then causes the patient to shutdown physically and emotionally; decreasing their trust in you as their healthcare provider and resulting in a wasted treatment session.

Once you have the patient's permission to palpate or touch them, you might start the treatment with gentle myofascial release (MFR) and/or a craniosacral release (CST) from T-1 to L-2, secondary to this is where the patient's sympathetic nervous system is located. Once the patient is relaxed and out of "fight or flight" then you would treat the base of the occiput or skull, and the sacrum, with MFR and CST to improve the parasympathetic nervous system and to maintain homeostatic balance of the autonomic nervous system. Some patients benefit from modalities such as heat, interferential current, or other modalities such as therapeutic laser to calm the ANS. Once this has been completed then treat any structural dysfunctions throughout the patient's body with manual techniques. Kinesiology taping can help maintain the joint in position and one tape (Thrive) has been designed for the skin of EDS patients. A side note, many EDS patients have skin sensitivity to the adhesive of tape or Band-Aids. A trick to try when patients have skin sensitivity is to first apply Milk of Magnesia to the skin, let it dry then apply the kinesiology tape. This tends to significantly decrease their skin sensitivity.

Once the patient is aligned, begin gentle therapeutic exercises. Start supine (lying on the back), as this position helps maintain the patient's alignment while they are strengthening their deep core stabilizers. Once deep-core stabilizers are strengthened, progress to superficial muscle groups. If the patient has CCI, AAI or cervical instability, have the patient don or wear their rigid cervical brace (thick or short neck Aspen Visa and long thin necks or children Miami J, seem to work well as a general rule). This supine position potentially limits any issues the patient may have with POTS, OI, MCAS (*AN: or MCAD*), CCI, AAI, cervical, thoracic or lumbar, SIJ, ISJ instabilities. It is important that the patient is in pelvic neutral prior to doing any exercises. This will help decrease pain and allow for greater core stability.

Many patients do not understand pelvic neutral and have decreased proprioceptive awareness of their pelvic girdle muscles. If your patient is having difficult performing pelvic neutral; there are tricks that seem to help. First, have them place their fingers gently on their pelvic muscles then have them say "Ha, Ha, Ha." The correct pelvic neutral muscles will contract and the patient will be able to palpate or feel those muscles contract. Second, you can utilize a blood pressure cuff bladder and pump it up to 40mm while it is under the patient's lower back and have the patient gently tighten their pelvic floor muscles causing their back to compress into the blood pressure cuff bladder causing the reading to increase. As an example, patients can hold the compression at 60mm for 6 seconds then release and repeat. Both methods utilize some form of biofeedback to the patient. The third example would be to have the patient gently tighten their buttock thus in turn contracting the lower abdominals. Have the patient palpate or feel the lower abdominals while the contraction is occurring. At the initial visit the patient is instructed in proper log rolling transfer going from supine to sit and proper sit to standing while maintaining joint and spinal segment alignment. This protects the patient's spinal alignment and decreases or prevents their Dysautonomia symptoms from flaring up.

When appropriate, progress the patient to hook lying position with their head and upper trunk elevated for exercising. This hook lying position adds some gravity-based resistance to their muscles and helps control and gently challenge their Dysautonomia issues such as POTS, OI and head pressure. When appropriate the patients are progressed to prone (lying on the stomach) positions with pillow support at the hips and towel support at the forehead. When appropriate, progress to side lying, then quadruped (hands and knees); however, many times this position needs to be modified with a treatment box or step where the patient is on their knees and resting on their forearms. Do not push this position if the patient has shoulder, wrist, hand, hip, knee, patellar (knee cap) or ankle issues. When appropriate the patient is progressed to standing exercises and once stable enough they are progressed to coordination, balance and proprioception activities.

The key to successful exercise is maintaining alignment during exercise. The progress is slow. It is better to do one repetition correctly then to force 10 repetitions incorrectly. Once the patient is able to master 10 repetitions x 3 sets with a 6 second hold then the patient is ready to be progressed to the next level of that exercise. It is important to remember that the patient might require kinesiology taping, bracing, or compression garments when they are exercising. This will add extra proprioceptive awareness and improve the joint quality of motion and stability. If a patient has POTS, orthostatic intolerance (OI), or lymphedema, compressive garments can be a game changer. These can assist in maintaining their blood pressure levels and decrease their edema or swelling. Recent studies have found that abdominal and upper thigh compression was more effective than lower limb compression in patients with POTS (*Bourne et. al, 2021, Miller and Bourne, 2020*).

Table 1. General exercise guidelines are as follows:

1. Generalized exercise protocols should be avoided.

2. Exercise programs need to be individualized based on your patient's evaluation and re-assessment findings and tied to the patient's goals.

3. The patient and the patient's family need to understand why they are exercising and how it is going to help achieve their desired goals.

4. The patient's hypermobility has been assessed by a qualified physical therapist prior to the prescription of exercises.

5. Exercises prescribed and instructed/supervised by a qualified physical therapist.

6. The exercises themselves are engaging to the patient.

7. The exercises are convenient for the patient to perform.

8. Exercises are prescribed with the respect of the patient's experiences and preferences.

9. The exercises are modified to the patient's individual abilities.

10. Exercises are performed where the patient has neuromuscular control within their range of motion (ROM).

11. Exercises are focused on postural re-education, endurance, strength and core stability.

12. Initial exercises are focused on recruitment of deep stabilizers rather than large superficial muscle groups.

13. Poor posture and body mechanics need to be corrected prior to exercising to prevent excessive pain or injury.

14. Poor structural alignment of joints and spinal segments need to be corrected prior to exercising to prevent excessive pain or injury.

15. The patient must understand the difference between post exercise soreness and pain vs injury.

16. The level and quality of exercise supervision needs to be appropriate to prevent excessive pain or injury.

17. Appropriate proprioceptive feedback and joint/spinal segment support is provided (i.e., taping, compression garments, braces or therapist tactile support).

18. The patient needs to understand correct pacing of their exercise program to prevent excessive pain or injury.

19. The patient's co-morbidities must be controlled and managed prior to exercising.

20. Initial exercise dosage and progression of exercise dosage needs to be gradual and to the patient's tolerance not the therapist's or insurance company's. It is about quality of motion not quantity.

21. Daily cardiovascular or aerobic exercise should be undertaken.

22. Exercises need to be undertaken for life to manage symptoms.

23. Ideally exercises should be undertaken 3 to 4 times per week.

24. Ideally exercises should be undertaken for 150 minute per week at a moderate intensity, but to the patient's tolerance.

Table 2. Progression of functional therapeutic exercises should involve the following:

1. Exercise progression is undertaken slowly in negotiation with the patient.

2. Exercise progression is initiated once the patient can maintain joint stability and spinal segmental alignment with current exercise program.

3. The patient understands the difference between post exercise soreness vs pain related to an injury.

4. The current exercises have not exacerbated the patient's pain, co-morbidities, functional abilities, and fatigue or injured the patient.

5. Progression from individualized exercises to more generic exercise program.

6. Progression from joint specific exercises to whole-body exercises.

7. Progression from single joint movement to more complex functional movements.

8. Progression from single joint stability to whole-body stability.

9. Progression from recruiting deep stabilizing muscles to more superficial movement muscles.

10. Progression from closed to open chain exercises.

11. Progression from short-level to long-level exercises.

12. Increasing the exercise repetitions and/or time of exercises.

13. Increasing the weight, load or resistance of the exercises.

14. Increasing the exercise session frequency.

15. Reducing the rest between each exercise.

16. Reducing the level of professional supervision and feedback.

Table 3. The following functional therapeutic exercise programs may be beneficial to patients with hEDS/HSD:

1. Postural Re-Education Exercises.
2. Hydrotherapy.
3. Muscle specific stretching secondary to tightness, trigger points, tender points, spasms or facilitated segments.
4. Strength, Toning and Resistance Training.
5. Core Stabilization.
6. Whole Body Training.
7. Pilates.
8. Motor Control Training.
9. Aerobic Exercising; recumbent bike, stationary bike, bicycle, treadmill and/or elliptical.
10. Walking Program.
11. Swimming Program must have shoulder stability.
12. Balance, Coordination and Proprioceptive Training.
13. Team and Individual Sports.
14. Competitive Sports.
15. Non-Contact or Low-Impact Sports.
16. Exergaming.
17. Inspiratory Muscle Strengthening.
18. Functional Task Training.
19. Qigong Training.
20. Tai Chi Training.
21. Other Mindfulness Training that would be appropriate for the patient's exercise tolerance.
22. 90-90 positioning with relaxation breathing (diaphragmatic breathing).
23. Yoga corpse position with relaxation breathing (diaphragmatic breathing).

Benefits of functional therapeutic exercise for individuals with EDS and HSD are as follows:
1. Decreased pain
2. Decreased anxiety and depression
3. Decreased fatigue
4. Improved sleep
5. Improved deep to superficial core strength and stability
6. Improved proximal to distal core strength and stability
7. Improved cardiovascular endurance
8. Improve flexibility
9. Improved balance, coordination and proprioception
10. Improve joint and spinal segmental protection
11. Improved psychological well being
12. Increased motor control
13. Improved posture
14. Improved self-efficacy
15. Improve static and dynamic postural stability
16. Increased independence
17. A sense of self control over their pain and their disabilities
18. Improved social interaction

Manual Therapy

Manual therapy can be defined as any intervention that uses the practitioners' hands. This can include joint mobilization, thrust manipulation, soft tissue mobilization, massage, craniosacral therapy, myofascial release, and others. A multimodal approach that incorporates manual therapy can be beneficial for this patient population (*Pennetti, 2018*). While the description of the plethora of manual therapy techniques is important in this patient population it is beyond the scope of this chapter to discuss them all, however certain precautions must be understood (Table 4).

Table 4. Precautions for Manual Therapy Techniques (Physical Therapy, Chiropractic, and Osteopathic)
1. Joint Protection; we must protect the patient's joints and spinal segments so they are not getting excessive wear

and tear on their joint surfaces or spinal segments. This will decrease pain, keep their joints and spinal segments healthy and prevent early onset of arthritic changes. In turn, the patient will be compliant with their home exercise program (HEP) which the review of the literature indicates will allow the patient to maintain their independence.

2. No Cervical Spine Manipulations [Grade 5 or High Velocity, Low Amplitude Manipulations (HVLA)] secondary to significant risk of Transient Ischemic Attack (TIA) or Mini Stroke, Cerebrovascular Accident (CVA), Myocardial Infarction (MI), Respiratory Arrest, Quadriplegia, Paraplegia, Fracture, Severe Spinal Cord Injury or Death. Remember EDS have collagen abnormalities; therefore, the potential for weakened blood vessels, aneurysms, and weakened ligaments potentially causing CCI and AAI or aneurysms or blood vessels to rupture.

3. If the patient has Vascular EDS (vEDS) or aneurysms, no spinal manipulations [Grade 5 or High Velocity, Low Amplitude Manipulations (HVLA)] should be performed. See above # 2 for risks.

4. Exercises or activities where the patient may perform a Valsalva can increase intrathoracic pressure and cause aneurysms to rupture. These should always be avoided.

5. Getting the patient to understand pain vs injury especially post treatment and while the patient is performing their HEP. This is where having a baseline pain level at rest and with activity is crucial. Most healthcare providers dislike asking this question with our hEDS/HSD patients, because their pain levels are so variable as well as these patients tends to dwell on their pain and take minutes giving an answer which takes time away from the patient's visit. The patients themselves don't like answering this question either, because their symptoms are so variable minute to minute While the importance of establishing a base-line

pain level at rest and with activity shows progress to the insurance company and the patient, in the treatment itself it is more valuable.

Fatigue and Sleep

Individuals with hEDS commonly reported fatigue and sleep disturbances (*Domany, et. al, 2018, Voermans et. al, 2011*). The prevalence of fatigue in individuals with hEDS was reported in one study as 79.5% (*Krahe et. al, 2018*). Fatigue ultimately affects normal daily activities by impeding energy levels and decreasing activity (*Rich et. al, 2020*). Physical therapy can help reduce fatigue by implementing interventions through energy conservation techniques, pacing, and environmental modifications.

In clients with hEDS, sleep interventions such as proper joint positioning (pregnancy pillows are common), proper mattress support, ambient room temperature, avoiding alcohol, caffeine, and large meals before bedtime, relaxation exercises and/or apps, heating pads or blankets, and weighted blankets can all be utilized. If sleep is not addressed, it may exacerbate the symptoms of hEDS (*Muriello et. al, 2018*). This may include increased pain, decreased physical performance, increased likelihood for mental health complications, and a decrease in overall quality of life (*Domany, et. al, 2018*).

Energy Conservation and Activity Pacing

Patients with chronic pain may push themselves to do lots of physical activity or work when they are having a "good" day. Unfortunately, later the pain is usually increased and they may have to rest for a long time to recover. Activity pacing is a strategy that is frequently implemented to modify activities among patients with long-term conditions such as hEDS/HSD. The aims of activity pacing include reducing this overactivity–underactivity, cycling in order to improve overall function, and reduce the likelihood of exacerbating symptoms (*Antcliff, 2018*).

649

Energy conservation involves changing an activity or the environment to decrease the level of energy required to complete a task. The use of these techniques can include interventions ranging from rest breaks to task prioritization to workspace organization to simplify tasks (*Vatwani and Margonis, 2019*). Clients have reported that energy conservation helped them not only function throughout the day, but also may prevent flare ups which may impair function for days (*Krahe et. al, 2018, Rich et. al, 2020*). By utilizing energy conservation and activity pacing techniques, clients may be able to re-establish a sense of control over their symptoms and improve their functional levels.

20 Clinical Pearls
1. The patient must feel that he or she has been heard, validated, and that you are actively listening to them.
2. It is important that physical therapists perform a comprehensive physical therapy evaluation to determine the patient's functional, biomechanical, and soft tissue deficits, but the key to this evaluation is taking that information in conjunction with the patient's co-morbidities, goals and making a successful treatment plan that is realistic and appropriate for that individual patient's wants and needs. The patient must be an active part of this process.
3. It is important you as the healthcare provider and patient know that currently there is no cure of hEDS or HSD, so ultimately our goal as a healthcare provider is to manage their healthcare and keep them as independent and functional as possible.
4. As a healthcare provider you must remember that hEDS and HSD patients tend to heal slowly and they do not progress like our non-connective tissue patients. So physical therapy rehabilitation will take longer.
5. Prior to treating our patients, especially those with hEDS/HSD, the patient needs to understand the difference between normal post exercise soreness and pain vs pain related to an injury from over exercising. Post exercise soreness and pain is diffuse in nature, it is

	bilateral soreness or pain that is located in the muscles used during that exercise session and can last up to 3 days post exercise treatment session. Conversely, pain related to an injury is usually sharp in nature, localized pain in the affected joint or spinal segment. It can be attributed to a specific exercise movement or a sudden event. It causes edema (swelling) and heat or warmth around the joint or spinal segment. The patient's pain level will be greater than 5/10 on the NRS Scale.
6.	When the patient arrives to the PT Clinic the patient must be assessed prior to each treatment session. Prior to starting any therapeutic exercises, the patient's entire body needs to be aligned and their sympathetic nervous relaxed. This is where manual therapy is key.
7.	Generalized exercise protocols should be avoided.
8.	Exercises are performed where the patient has control within their range of motion (ROM).
9.	Initial exercises are focused on recruitment of deep stabilizers rather than large superficial muscle groups.
10.	Poor musculoskeletal alignment, posture and body mechanics need to be corrected prior to exercising to prevent excessive pain or injury.
11.	Initial exercise dosage and progression of exercise dosage needs to be gradual and to the patient's tolerance not the therapist's or insurance companies. It is about quality of motion not quantity.
12.	Joint Protection: we must protect the patient's joints and spinal segments so they are not getting excessive wear and tear on their joint surfaces or spinal segments. This will decrease pain, keep their joints and spinal segments healthy, and prevent early onset of arthritic changes. In turn, the patient will be compliant with their home exercise program (HEP) which the review of the literature indicates will allow the patient to maintain their independence.
13.	No Cervical Spine Manipulations [Grade 5 or High Velocity, Low Amplitude Manipulations (HVLA)] secondary to significant risk of TIA, CVA, MI, Respiratory Arrest, Quadriplegia, Paraplegia, Fracture, Severe Spinal Cord Injury or Death. Remember EDS have weakened collagen; therefore, the potential for

	weakened blood vessels, aneurysms, and weakened ligaments potentially causing CCI, AAI or aneurysms or blood vessels to rupture. If the patient has vEDS or aneurysms No Spinal Manipulations [Grade 5 or High Velocity, Low Amplitude Manipulations (HVLA)] anywhere on their body.
14.	The body is a unit (*Still AT, 1977*). When treating hEDS/HSD or any patient for that matter. Look at the whole patient and how their injury, dysfunction, or disorder is impacting their entire body and all the systems of their body. Treat all of their adaptations and compensations. Don't just treat the joint they were referred for. Just treating the joint they were referred for and not treating all of the compensations and adaptations throughout the patient's body is limited thinking and this is one of the reasons why physical therapy treatments drastically fail, because you are treating symptoms and not their dysfunctions.
15.	Structure governs Function (*Still AT, 1977*). If a joint of spinal segment is hypermobile and it is painful or if that joint or spinal segment has subluxed or dislocated then function of that joint or spinal segment will be limited or non-existent.
16.	Somatic Component of Disease (*Still AT, 1977*). Having a working knowledge of your patient's disease process and their co-morbidities will allow you as the healthcare provider to make better informed decisions and decrease the chance of injuring the patient.
17.	Healing Power of the Body (*Still AT, 1977*). The body possesses its own mechanism for repairing and restoring health. Once we have done our job as healthcare providers, we just have to get out of our own way and let the patient's body do what it is supposed to do.
18.	The use of Manual Therapy or Osteopathic Manipulative Therapy (OMT) (*Still AT, 1977*). Manual Therapy or OMT are a hands-on approach to treating patients. The human body wants other human touch. Gentle, hands-on, manual therapy is a great way to begin a professional relationship that will foster trust and belief that the patient's barriers, both physical and

	emotional, will be respected. Remember to ask and get the patient's permission first before touching or palpating a patient.
19.	These patients will require physical therapy intermittently throughout their life cycles. They need to know that they are welcome back when appropriate.
20.	Exercises, self-corrections and functional activities will be undertaken for the patient's life cycle, 3 to 4 times per week, for up to 150 minutes per week, at a moderate intensity, but always to the patient's tolerance.

Overview for the practitioner

It is possible for patients to respond in ways that differ from the textbook responses that we would normally expect to find as healthcare providers. This happens more frequently with hEDS/HSD patients than non-connective tissue patient populations. These patients' reactions are unique to them, just as all individuals are unique to themselves; therefore, we must view our patients holistically in concert with their specific conditions and co-morbidities as specific to that individual.

A patient that experiences POTS, Dysautonomia, MCAS (*AN: or MCAD*), PTSD, Anxiety, Depression, Fibromyalgia and Hypothyroidism in the presence of hEDS, will manifest differently than one who has a different set of symptom constellation.

Preconceived notions, lack of communication, and provider biases, can do a great disservice to our patients. A patient's physical, emotional, mental and physiological health are all inextricably tied to one another, and must be taken into account if an accurate assessment of their condition is going to be achieved.

These aspects are intertwined, and all are invaluable to compiling an understanding of the patient as a complete individual, rather than viewing them as a singular and myopic diagnosis.

When treating patients, the Five Philosophies of A.T. Still, MD, DO the Father of Osteopathic Medicine are important to remember (*Still AT, 1977*):

I. **The body is a unit**. When treating hEDS/HSD or any patient for that matter, look at the whole patient and how their injury, dysfunction or disorder is impacting their entire body and all the systems of their body. Treat all of the adaptations and compensations, not just the joint they were referred for. Just treating the joint they were referred for and not treating all of the compensations and adaptations throughout the patient's body is limited thinking and this is one of the reasons why physical therapy treatments drastically fail.

II. **Structure governs Function**. If a joint or spinal segment is hypermobile and it is painful, or if that joint or spinal segment has subluxed or dislocated, then function of that joint and/or spinal segment will be limited or non-existent.

III. **Somatic Component of Disease**. Having a working knowledge of your patient's disease process and their co-morbidities will allow you as the healthcare provider to make better informed decisions and decrease the chance of injuring the patient.

IV. **Healing Power of the Body**. The body possesses its own mechanism for repair and to restore health. Once we have done our job as a healthcare provider, we just have to get out of our own way and let the patient's body do what it is supposed to do.

V. **The use of Manual Therapy**. Manual Therapy is a hands-on approach to treating patients. The human body wants other human touch. Gentle hands-on manual therapy is a great way to begin a professional relationship that will foster trust that the patient's barriers, both physical and emotional, will be respected. Remember to ask and get the patient's permission first before touching or palpating a patient.

Example of a Physical Therapy Evaluation

According to the American Physical Therapy Associate, APTA, all physical therapy evaluations should have the following sections:

Medical Diagnosis.

This is the diagnosis or diagnoses given by MD, DO, DDS, DMD, DC, NP and/or PA.

Patient Information.

This information will detail:

Date of Birth.
Age of Patient.
Gender of Patient:.
Primary Language of Patient.

Past Medical History.

This section is extremely important as treatment secondary to these co-morbidities will influence your treatment plan and how you will progress your patient. For example, if your patient has Mitochondrial Disorder your progress of exercise repetitions will be less than someone who does not have Mitochondrial Disorder. The mitochondria function to synthesis ATP which allows for the release of energy to fuel our body's cells. When there is a breakdown in this function our bodies become fatigued, have muscle weakness, low muscle tone and the patient experiences exercise intolerance. Progressing an EDS patient with Mitochondrial Disorder too quickly will cause the treatment plan to fail and the patient will experience increased muscle pain.

Another good example would be Arnold-Chiari Malformation co-morbidity in an EDS patient. Care must be taken to ensure that the patient is breathing correctly while exercising or during an exertion activity to prevent increased intrathoracic pressure and intracranial pressures. The patient must understand that they are not allowed to perform a Valsalva (a forceful attempt at expiration while the nostrils are closed and the mouth is shut) while exercising or while they are performing exertional activities.

Another example is Autonomic Nervous System Dysfunction (Dysautonomia, POTS or OI); when the patient is exercising they begin to sweat and/or have irregular heartbeats or irregular breathing. It is not that the patient is exercising or working too hard; the patient may be having symptoms of one of these disorders. The Borg scale of perceived exertion may be useful to examine how their objective measures such as heart rate correlates to perceived exertion, thus allowing a secondary or tertiary measurement for safety.

Stress tests in this population may induce hyperventilation which is not true hyperventilation but caused by dysautonomia. When the test is adjusted and progressed more gradually they may be able to complete the test by giving the body time to accommodate.

History of Present Illness.

Medication List:

Having a working knowledge of the patient's medication would be helpful.

Allergies.

Medications, Environmental and Chemical: Having a working knowledge of the patient's medications are helpful if that patient is having a flare up and which medication(s) would be beneficial to get the patient out of that flare up. The important thing to understand is that all EDS patients do not necessarily metabolize their medications well, so understanding the side effects of those medications can save your patient's life. Environmental and chemical allergens in your office can cause your EDS patient to flare their symptoms, so be aware of those allergens to allow for a better overall treatment.

Precautions.

All treatment goals should take into consideration joint protection, no cervical manipulations secondary to the potential of TIA, CVA, MI, Quadriplegia, severely injuring the patient's cervical spine or death. Remember our EDS have a tendency for instability and if the patient has a CCI or AAI you could seriously injury the patient. No manipulations (HVLA) if the patient has vEDS.

Pain Assessment.

Having a good understanding of the patient's baseline pain levels are important especially when you start to exercise or progress exercises or any new activity with the patient. For example, if their average pain level is # 5/10; VAS; however, after exercising it increases to # 8/10 and does not abate after 3 days then this is an issue; however, if the pain level decreases back down to # 5/10 within 3 days then the patient just had some post treatment inflammation. That pain level increase was significant for that patient, therefore having a good understanding of the patient's pain level is key to progressing a patient. This ensures your patient does not have a panic attack or go into "fight or flight" when their pain level increases.

Objective Findings.

Gait:

Looking for symmetry vs asymmetry?
Toe walking
Heel Walking
Tandem walking

Posture:

Standing and sitting; observe from the front, back, right and left sides of the patient, so you can have a complete picture of the patient's postural deficits.
Looking for symmetry vs asymmetry?
Forward head posture?
Increased or decreased spinal curves?
Scoliosis?
Kyphosis?
Kyphoscoliosis?
Collapsed Arches vs Pes Planus? (Flat Feet)
Soft Tissue asymmetries?
Structural or Boney Landmark asymmetries?

AROM.

Looking of hypermobility vs hypomobility?

STRENGTH/MMT.

Assessing deep vs superficial, proximal vs distal vs core weakness?
Determining if weakness is pain vs neurological?

Sensation.

Determining Dermatomal or Sensory deficits.

Balance.

Determining balance, proprioceptive, coordination and fall risk potential? Remember Dysautonomia, POTS and Orthostatic Intolerance patients for fall precautions.

Palpation.

Assessing for soft tissue tightness, tender points, trigger points, muscle spasms, hypertonicity vs hypotonicity? Assessing bony structural landmarks in neutral for asymmetries?

Skin.

Does the patient bruise easy?
Does the patient have poor wound healing?
Understanding the answer to the above two questions will assist you in setting up your treatment plan taking into consideration these two issues.
Velvety Skin, Stretchy Skin, Stretch marks?
Atrophic Scarring and/or Keloid Scarring?

Structural Integrity and Joint Mobility.

Test joints and spinal segments actively and passively and look for asymmetries?

Special Testing.

Assessing all special testing for the specific issues that the patient has to determine a physical therapy diagnoses and to correlate subjective complaints from the patient and tying together the objective findings.

Beighton Score: /9

Testing of C-T-L-S spine for facet pathologies vs instabilities?

Testing of TMJ?

Testing of any and all joints that have subluxed and/or dislocated?

Functional Scores.

Numerous functional scales are applicable e.g., Oswestry Neck and Back, Shoulder Pain and Disability Index (SPADI), Quick DASH, Lower Extremity Functional Scale (LEFS), pain scales, sleep and fatigue scales, etc.

Physical Therapy Deficits commonly seen in hEDS/HSD:

1. Ligament laxity.
2. Joint, bone and spinal segment instability.
3. Muscle weakness from underuse.
4. Muscle weakness from muscle spasms.
5. Core stability weakness.
6. Lack of proprioceptive input.
7. Poor cardiovascular and musculoskeletal Endurance.
8. Decreased Functional Abilities.

An optimal program should consist of:

1. Manual Therapy or Osteopathic Manipulative Therapy.
2. Therapeutic Postural Re-education Exercises.
3. Specific Stretching Exercises.
4. Therapeutic Core Stabilization Exercises.
5. Therapeutic Joint Stabilization Exercises.
6. Coordination, Balance and Proprioceptive Exercises.
7. Cardiovascular and Musculoskeletal Endurance Exercises.

There are Four Steps to a Good Physical Therapy Program:

1. Control, Decrease and/or Eliminate Pain.
2. Improve, Increase, Normalize or Control Range of Motion (ROM).
3. Improve, Increase and Normalize Strength and Core Stability.
4. Improve, Increase and Normalize Mobility and Functional Activities.

There are numerous treatment techniques that consist of Manual Physical Therapy and/or Osteopathic Manipulative Therapy (OMT); however, below are the most commonly used.

Structural Manual Therapy Consists of:

1. Myofascial Releases (MFR)
2. Soft Tissue Mobilization (STM)
3. Jones Strain/Counter strain (JSCS)
4. Cranial Therapy
5. Craniosacral Therapy (CST)
6. Visceral Manipulation/Mobilization (VM)
7. Manual Lymph Drainage
8. Dry Needling
9. Zero Balancing

Finding the Right Physical Therapist (PT)
1. PT has a working knowledge of your diagnoses and co-morbidities.
2. PT is willing to work with you and your team of medical care providers.
3. PT has good manual therapy or OMT skills combined with a good working knowledge of therapeutic exercises and appropriate progression with individuals with connective tissue disorders or willing to learn.
4. PT needs to work one-on-one with their patient in a hand on approach in a private quiet treatment room.

5.	PT must understand that your progression is Rehab is going to be slower and different than their typical patient population.
6.	You need to find a PT Clinic that will treat you in a private quiet treatment room especially during manual therapy sessions and not in an open noisy well light gym.
7.	The PT Clinic should use no or low fragrances cleaners.
8.	The PT and staff must adhere to no fragrance, deodorant and detergents, etc.
9.	The PT Clinic must provide low sensory sensitivity; no or low talking, appropriate heating and cooling, lighting, sound and safe cleaning products.

References.

Abonia JP, Wen T, Stucke EM, Grotjan T, Griffith MS, Kemme KA, Collins MH, Putnam PE, Franciosi JP, von Tiehl KF, Tinkle BT, Marsolo KA, Martin LJ, Ware SM, Rothenberg ME. 2013. High prevalence of eosinophilic esophagitis in patients with inherited connective tissue disorders. J Allergy Clin Immunol 132: 378–386.

Adib N, Davies K, Grahame R, Woo P, Murray KJ. 2005. Joint hypermobility syndrome in childhood. A not so benign multisystem disorder? Rheumatol 44:744–750.

Antcliff D, Keeley P, Campbell M, Woby S, Keenan AM, McGowan L. Activity pacing: moving beyond taking breaks and slowing down. Qual Life Res. 2018;27(7):1933-1935. doi:10.1007/s11136-018-1794-7.
Atkinson HL, Nixon-Cave K. 2011. A tool for clinical reasoning and reflection using the international classification of functioning, disability and health (ICF) framework and patient management model. Phys Ther 91:416–430.

Aydın E, Metin Tellioğlu A, Kurt Ömürlü İ, Polat G, Turan Y. 2017. Postural balance control in women with generalized joint laxity. Turk J Phys Med Rehabil. 2017;63(3):259-265.

Balshem H, Helfand M, Schunemann HJ, € Oxman AD, Kunz R, Brozek J, Vist GE, Falck-Ytter Y, Meerpohl J, Norris S, Guyatt GH. 2011. GRADE guidelines: 3. Rating the quality of evidence. J Clin Epidemiol 64:401–406.

Bathen T, Hångmann AB, Hoff M, Andersenand L, Rand-Hendriksen S. 2013. Multidisciplinary treatment of disability in Ehlers-Danlos Syndrome hypermobility type/hypermobility syndrome: A pilot study using a combination of physical and cognitive-behavioral therapy on 12 women. Am J Med Genet Part A 161A:3005–3011.

Beighton P, Solomon L, Soskolne CL. 1973. Articular mobility in an African population. Ann Rheumatic Dis 32:413–418. Beighton P, De Paepe A, Steinmann B, Tsipourasand P, Wenstrup RJ. 1998. Ehlers-Danlos syndromes: Revised nosology, villefranche, 1997. Ehlers-Danlos National Foundation (USA) and Ehlers-Danlos Support Group (UK). Am J Med Genet 77:31–37.

Billings S, Deane JA, Bartholomew J, Simmonds JV. 2015. Knowledge and perceptions of joint hypermobility syndrome amongst pediatric physiotherapists. J Physiother Pract Res 36:33–51.

Birt L, Pfeil M, MacGregor A, Armon K, Poland F. 2014. Adherence to home physiotherapy treatment in children and young people with joint hypermobility: A qualitative report of family perspectives on acceptability and efficacy. Musculoskel Care 12:56–61.

Bourne, K. M., Sheldon, R. S., Hall, J., Lloyd, M., Kogut, K., Sheikh, N., Jorge, J., Ng, J., Exner, D. V., Tyberg, J. V., & Raj, S. R. (2021). Compression Garment Reduces Orthostatic Tachycardia and Symptoms in Patients With Postural Orthostatic Tachycardia Syndrome. *J Am Coll Cardiol*, 77(3), 285-296.

Carbone L, Tylavsky FA, Bush AJ, Koo W, Orwoll E, Cheng S. 2000. Bone density in Ehlers Danlos Syndrome. Osteoporos Int 11:388–392.

Cederlof M, Larsson H, Lichtenstein P, Almqvist € C, Serlachius E, Ludvigsson JF. 2016. Nationwide population-based cohort study of psychiatric disorders in individuals with Ehlers-Danlos syndrome or hypermobility syndrome and their siblings. BMC Psychiatry 16:207.

Clark C, Khattab A, Carr E. 2014. Chronic widespread pain and neurophysiological symptoms in Joint Hypermobility Syndrome. Int J Ther Rehab 21:60–68. Clarke C, Simmonds JV. 2011. An exploration of the prevalence of hypermobility syndrome in Omani women attending an outpatient department. Musculoskel Care 9:1–10.

Clayton HA, Jones SAH, Henriques DYP. 2015. Proprioceptive precision is impaired in Ehlers–Danlos syndrome. SpringerPlus 7;4:323.

Connelly E, Hakim A, Davenport HS, Simmonds JV. 2015. A Study exploring the prevalence of Hypermobility Syndrome in a musculoskeletal triage clinic. Physiother Res Pract 36:43–53.

De Kort LM, Verhulst JA, Engelbert RH, Uiterwaal CS, de Jong TP. 2003. Lower urinary tract dysfunction in children with generalized hypermobility of joints. J Urol 170:1971–1974.

De Paepe A, Malfait F. 2012. The Ehlers-Danlos syndrome, a disorder with many faces. Clin Genet 82:1–11.

De Wandele I, Rombaut L, Leybaert L, Van de Borne P, De Backer T, Malfait F, De Paepe A, Calders P. 2014. Dysautonomia and its underlying mechanisms in the hypermobility type of Ehlers—Danlos syndrome. Semin Arthritis Rheum 44:93–100.

Domany, K. A., Hantragool, S., Smith, D. F., Xu, Y., Hossain, M., & Simakajornboon, N. (2018). Sleep Disorders and Their Management in Children With Ehlers-Danlos Syndrome Referred to Sleep Clinics. *J Clin Sleep Med*, 14(4), 623-629.

El-Metwally A, Salminen JJ, Auvinen A, Kautiainen H, Mikkelsson M. 2005. Lower limb pain in a preadolescent population: Prognosis and risk factors for chronicity—A prospective 1- and 4-year follow-up study. Pediatrics 116:673–681.

Engelbert RH, Bank RA, Sakkers RJ, Helders PJ, Beemer FA, Uiterwaal CS. 2003. Pediatric generalized joint hypermobility with and without musculoskeletal complaints: A localized or systemic disorder? Pediatrics 111: e248–e254.

Engelbert RH, van Bergen M, Henneken T, Helders PJ, Takken T. 2006. Exercise tolerance in children and adolescents with musculoskeletal pain in joint hypermobility and joint hypomobility syndrome. Pediatrics 118:e690–e696.

Evans AM, Rome K. 2011. A Cochrane review of the evidence for non-surgical interventions for flexible pediatric flat feet. Eur J Phys Rehabil Med 47:69–89.

Evidence based Care Guideline for Management of Pediatric Joint Hypermobility Guideline Copyright © 2014. Cincinnati Children's Hospital Medical Center, James M. Anderson Center for Health Systems Excellence Evidence Based Care Guideline Identification and management of Pediatric Joint Hypermobility In children and adolescents aged 4 to 21 years old Publication Date: October 21, 2014.

Faigenbaum AD, Kraemer WJ, Blimkie CJ, Jeffreys I, Micheli LJ, Nitka M, Rowland TW. 2009. Youth resistance training: Updated position statement paper from the national strength and conditioning association. J Strength Cond Res 23:S60–S79.

Faigenbaum AD, Myer GD. 2010. Resistance training among young athletes: Safety, efficacy and injury prevention effects. Br J Sports Med 44:56–63.

Falkerslev S, Baagø C, Alkjær T, Remvig L, Halkjær-Kristensen J, Larsen PK, JuulKristensen B, Simonsen EB. 2013. Dynamic balance during gait in children and adults with Generalized Joint Hypermobility. Clin Biomech (Bristol Avon) 28:318–324.

Fatoye F, Palmer S, Macmillan F, Rowe PP, van der Linden M. 2009. Proprioception and muscle torque deficits in children with hypermobility syndrome. Rheumatol 48:52–57.

Fatoye FA, Palmer S, van der Linden ML, Rowe PJ, Macmillan F. 2011. Gait kinematics and passive knee joint range of motion in children with hypermobility syndrome. Gait Post 33:447–451.

Ferrell WR, Tennant N, Baxendale RH, Kusel M, Sturrock RD. 2007. Musculoskeletal reflex function in the joint hypermobility syndrome. Arthr Care and Res 57:1329–1333.

Ferrell WR, Tennant N, Sturrock RD. 2004. Amelioration of symptoms by enhancement of proprioception in patients with joint hypermobility syndrome. Arthr Rheum 50:3323–3328.

Garber CE, Blissmer B, Deschenes MR, Franklin BA, Lamonte MJ, Lee IM, Nieman DC, Swain DP. 2011. American College of Sports Medicine position stand. Quantity and quality of exercise for developing and maintaining cardiorespiratory, musculoskeletal, and neuromotor fitness in apparently healthy adults: Guidance for prescribing exercise. Med Sci Sports Exerc 43:1334–1359.

Grahame R, Hakim AJ. 2008. Hypermobility. Curr Opin Rheumatol 20:106–110.

Grahame R, Bird HA, Child A. 2000. The revised (Brighton 1998) criteria for the diagnosis of benign joint hypermobility syndrome (BHSD). J Rheumatol 27:1777–1779.

Guidelines for Management of Joint Hypermobility Syndrome in Children and Young People. 2013. The British Society for Pediatric and Adolescent Rheumatology. Available online https://www.google.co.uk/gws_rd¼ssl#q¼bsparþforþhypermobility. Publication Date: 20. 6.2013.

Hanewinkel-van Kleef YB, Helders PJ, Takken T, Engelbert RH. 2009. Motor performance in children with generalized hypermobility: The influence of muscle strength and exercise capacity. Pediatr Phys Ther 21:194–200.

Jansson A, Saartok T, Werner S, Renstrom P. 2004. General joint laxity in 1845 Swedish school children of different ages: Age- and genderspecific distributions. Acta Pardiatr 93:1202–1206.

Juul-Kristensen B, Schmedling K, Rombaut L, Lund H, Engelbert RH. 2017. Measurement properties of clinical assessment methods for diagnosing generalized joint hypermobility—A systematic review. Am J Med Genet part C submitted, in press.

Keer R, Simmonds JV. 2011. Joint protection and physical rehabilitation of the adult with hypermobility syndrome. Cur Opinions Rheumatol 23:131–136.

Kemp S, Roberts I, Gamble C, Wilkinson S, Davidson JE, Baildam EM, Cleary AG, McCann LJ, Beresford MW. 2010. A randomized comparative trial of generalized vs targeted physiotherapy in the management of childhood hypermobility. Rheumatol (Oxford) 49:315–325.

Kirby A, Davies R. 2007. Developmental coordination disorder and joint hypermobility syndrome—Overlapping disorders? implications for research and clinical practice. Child Care Health Dev 33:513–519.
Kirby A, Davies R, Bryant A. 2005. Hypermobility syndrome and developmental coordination disorder: Similarities and features. Int J Ther Rehabil 12:431–443.

Krahe, A. M., Adams, R. D., & Nicholson, L. L. (2018). Features that exacerbate fatigue severity in joint hypermobility syndrome/Ehlers-Danlos syndrome - hypermobility type. *Disabil Rehabil*, 40(17), 1989-1996.

Lyell M, Simmonds JV, Deane J. 2015. Physiotherapists' knowledge and management of adults with hypermobility and joint hypermobility syndrome in the UK; A nationwide survey. Poster, WCPT May, Singapore. Physiotherapy 101:e919.

Lyell M, Simmonds JV, Deane JA. 2016. Future of education in hypermobility and hypermobility syndrome. J Physiother Pract and Res 37:101–109.

Mastoroudes H, Giarenis I, Cardozo L, Srikrishna S, Vella M, Robinson D, Kazkazand H, Grahame R. 2013. Lower urinary tract symptoms in women with benign joint hypermobility syndrome: A case-control study. Int Urogynecol J 24:1553–1558.

Miller, A. J., & Bourne, K. M. (2020). Abdominal Compression as a Treatment for Postural Tachycardia Syndrome. J Am Heart Assoc, 9(14), e017610.

Mintz-Itkin R, Lerman-Sagie T, Zuk L, ItkinWebman T, Davidovitch M. 2009. Does physical therapy improve outcome in infants with joint hypermobility and benign hypotonia? J Child Neurol 24:714–719.

Morrison SC, Ferrari J, Smillie S. 2013. Assessment of gait characteristics and orthotic management in children with Developmental Coordination Disorder: Preliminary findings to inform multidisciplinary care. Res Dev Disabil 34:3197–3201.

Møller MB, Kjær M, Svensson RB, Andersen JL, Magnusson SP, Nielsen RH. 2014. Functional adaptation of tendon and skeletal muscle to resistance training in three patients with genetically verified classic Ehlers Danlos Syndrome. Muscles Ligaments Tendons J 4:315–323.

Muriello, M., Clemens, J. L., Mu, W., Tran, P. T., Rowe, P. C., Smith, C. H., Francomano, C., Bodurtha, J., & Kline, A. D. (2018). Pain and sleep quality in children with non-vascular Ehlers-Danlos syndromes. *Am J Med Genet A, 176*(9), 1858-1864.

Murray KJ. 2006. Hypermobility disorders in children and adolescents. Best Pract Res Clin Rheumatol 20:329–351.

Nijs J, Van Essche E, De Munck M, Dequeker J. 2000. Ultrasonographic, axial, and peripheral measurements in female patients with benign hypermobility syndrome. Calcif Tissue Int 67:37–40.

Pacey V, Nicholson L, Adams R, Munn J, Munns C. 2010. Generalised joint hypermobility and injury risk of lower limb injury during sport. Am J Sports Med 38:1487–1497.

Pacey V. 2014. PhD thesis: Joint Hypermobility Syndrome in Children, University of Sydney, Sydney, Australia. Pacey V, Adams RD, Tofts L, Munns CF, Nicholson LL. 2015a. Joint hypermobility syndrome subclassification in pediatrics: A factor analytic approach. Arch Dis Child 100:8–13.

Pacey V, Tofts L, Adams RD, Munns CF, Nicholson LL. 2015b. Quality of life prediction in children with joint hypermobility syndrome. J Paediatr Child Health 51:689–695.

Pacey V, Tofts L, Adams RD, Munns CF, Nicholson LL. 2013. Exercise in children with joint hypermobility syndrome and knee pain: A randomized controlled trial comparing exercise into hypermobile versus neutral knee extension. Pediatr Rheumatol Online J11:30.

Palmer S, Bailey S, Barker L, Barney L, Elliott A. 2014. The effectiveness of therapeutic exercise for joint hypermobility syndrome: A systematic review. Physiotherapy 100:220–227.

Palmer S, Cramp F, Lewis R, Shahid M, Clark E. 2015. Diagnosis, management and assessment of adults with joint hypermobility syndrome: A UK-Wide survey of physiotherapy practice. Musculoskeletal Care 13:101–111.

Palmer S, Terry R, Rimes KA, Clark C, Simmonds J, Horwood J. 2016a. 166 AMERICAN JOURNAL OF MEDICAL GENETICS PART C (SEMINARS IN MEDICAL GENETICS) ARTICLE Physiotherapy management of joint hypermobility syndrome—A focus group study of patient and health professional perspectives. Physiother 102:93–102.

Palmer S, Cramp F, Clark E, Lewis R, Brookes S, Hollingworth W, Welton N, Thom N, Terry R, Rimes KA, Horwood J. 2016b. The feasibility of a randomized controlled trial of physiotherapy for adults with joint hypermobility syndrome. Health Technol Assess 20:1–264.

Pennetti A. A multimodal physical therapy approach utilizing the Maitland concept in the management of a patient with cervical and lumbar radiculitis and Ehlers-Danlos syndrome-hypermobility type: A case report. Physiother Theory Pract. 2018 Jul;34(7):559-568.

Rahman A, Daniel C, Grahame R. 2014. Efficacy of an out-patient pain management program for people with joint hypermobility syndrome. Clin Rheumatol 33:1665–1669.

Remvig L, Jensen DV, Ward C. 2007. Are diagnostic criteria for general joint hypermobility and benign joint hypermobility syndrome based on reproducible and valid tests? A review of the literature. J Rheumatol 34:798–803.

Remvig L, Engelbert RH, Berglund B, Bulbena A, Byers PH, Grahame R, Juul-Kristensen B, Lindgren KA, Uitto J, Wekre LL. 2011. Need for a consensus on the methods by which to measure joint mobility and the definition of norms for hypermobility that reflect age, gender and ethnic-dependent variation: Is revision of criteria for joint hypermobility syndrome and Ehlers-Danlos syndrome hypermobility type indicated? Rheumatol 50:1169–1171.

Rich, E. M., Vas, A., Boyette, V., & Hollingsworth, C. (2020). Daily Life Experiences: Challenges, Strategies, and Implications for Therapy in Postural Tachycardia Syndrome (POTS). *Occup Ther Health Care*, 1-18.

Rombaut L, Scheper M, De Wandele I, De Vries J, Meeus M, Malfait F, Engelbert RH, Calders P. 2015a. Chronic pain in patients with the hypermobility type of Ehlers-Danlos syndrome: Evidence for generalized hyperalgesia. Clin Rheumatol 34:1121–1129.

Rombaut L, Deane J, Simmonds J, De Wandele I, De Paepe A, Malfait F, Calders P. 2015b. Knowledge, assessment, and management of adults with joint hypermobility syndrome/ Ehlers-Danlos syndrome hypermobility type among Flemish physiotherapists. Am J Med Genet C Semin Med Genet 169C:76–83.

Rombaut L, Malfait F, De Wandele I, Taes Y, Thijs Y, De Paepe A, Calders P. 2012. Muscle mass, muscle strength, functional performance, and physical impairment in women with the hypermobility type of EhlersDanlos syndrome. Arthritis Care Res (Hoboken) 64:1584–1592.

Rombaut L, Malfait F, De Wandele I, Thijs Y, Palmans T, De Paepe A, Calders P. 2011a. Balance, gait, falls, and fear of falling in women with the hypermobility type of Ehlers-Danlos syndrome. Arthr Care Res (Hoboken) 63:1432–1439.

Rombaut L, Malfait F, De Wandele I, Cools A, Thijs Y, De Paepe A, Calders P. 2011b. Medication, surgery, and physiotherapy among patients with the hypermobility type of Ehlers-Danlos syndrome. Arch Phys Med Rehabil 92:1106–1112.

Russek L. 2000. Examination and treatment of a patient with hypermobility syndrome. Phys Ther 80:386–398.

Russek LN, LaShomb EA, Ware AM, Wesner SM, Westcott V. 2016. United States physical therapists' knowledge about joint hypermobility syndrome compared with fibromyalgia and rheumatoid arthritis. Physiother Res Int 21:22–35.

Sahin N, Baskent A, Cakmak A, Salli A, Ugurlu H, Berker E. 2008. Evaluation of knee proprioception and effects of proprioception exercise in patients with benign joint hypermobility syndrome. Rheumatol Int 28:995–1000.

Scheper MC, Engelbert RH, Rameckers EA, Verbunt J, Remvig L, Juul-Kristensen B. 2013. Children with generalised joint hypermobility and musculoskeletal complaints: State of the art on diagnostics, clinical characteristics, and treatment. Biomed Res Int 2013:121054.

Scheper MC, de Vries JE, Verbunt J, Engelbert RH. 2015. Chronic pain in hypermobility syndrome and Ehlers—Danlos syndrome (hypermobility type): It is a challenge. J Pain Res 20:591–601.

Scheper MC, Juul-Kristensen B, Rombaut L, Rameckers EA, Verbunt J, Engelbert RH. 2016a. Disability in adolescents and adults diagnosed with hypermobility related disorders: A meta-analysis. Arch Phys Med Rehabil 97:2174–2187.

Scheper MC, Pacey V, Rombaut L, Adams RD, Tofts L, Calders P, Nicholson LL, Engelbert RH. 2016b. Generalized Hyperalgesia in children and adults diagnosed with Hypermobility Syndrome and Ehlers-Danlos Hypermobility type: A discriminative analysis. Arthr Care Res 15:1–7.

Scheper MC, Rombaut LL, de Vries JE, de Wandele I, Esch van M, Calders P, Engelbert RH. 2016c. Factors of activity impairment in adult patients with Ehlers Danlos Syndrome hypermobility type): Muscle strength and proprioception. Disabil Rehabil 24:1–7.

Simmonds JV, Keer RJ. 2007. Hypermobility and the hypermobility syndrome. Masterclass Man Ther 12:298–309. Simmonds JV, Keer RJ. 2008. Hypermobility and the hypermobility syndrome. Masterclass. Illustrated via case studies, part II. Man Ther 13:e1–e11.

Simmonds J, Herbland A, Hakim A, Ninis N, Lever W, Aziz Q, Cairns M. 2016a. Attitudes, beliefs and behaviors towards exercise amongst individuals with joint hypermobility syndrome/Ehlers Danlos syndrome— hypermobility type IFOMPT Proceedings. Man Ther 25:335336.

Simmonds JV, Pacey V, Keer RJ, Castori MM. 2016b. Advancing practice in hypermobility Syndrome/Ehlers Danlos syndrome— hypermobility type focused symposium. IFOMPT, Glasgow, UK. Man Ther 25: e21–e22.

Simmonds JV, Herbland A, Hakim A, Ninis N, Lever W, Aziz Q, Cairns M. 2016c. Attitudes, beliefs and behaviours towards exercise amongst individuals with joint hypermobility syndrome/Ehlers Danlos syndrome— hypermobility type IFOMPT, Glasgow, UK. Man Ther 25:e35–e36.

Smith TO, Jerman E, Easton V, Bacon H, Armon K, Poland F, Macgregor AJ. 2013. Do people with benign joint hypermobility syndrome (BHSD) have reduced joint proprioception? A systematic review and meta-analysis. Rheumatol Int 33:2709–2716.

Smith TO, Easton V, Bacon H, Jerman E, Armon K, Poland F, Macgregor AJ. 2014a. The relationship between benign joint hypermobility syndrome and psychological distress: A systematic review and meta-analysis. Rheumatol (Oxford) 53:114–122.

Smith TO, Bacon H, Jerman E, Easton V, Armon K, Poland F, Macgregor AJ. 2014b. Physiotherapy and occupational therapy interventions for people with benign joint hypermobility syndrome: A systematic review of clinical trials. Disabil Rehabil 36:797–803.

Still A.T. 1977. Philosophy of osteopathy. (Reprinted, The American Academy of Osteopathy, Colorado Springs, Colorado, Originally published, Kirksville, Missouri: Self-Published by A. T. Still; 1899. p. 28, 146, 197).

Terry RH, Palmer ST, Rimes KA, Clark CJ, Simmonds JV, Horwood JP. 2015. Living with joint hypermobility syndrome: Patient experiences of diagnosis, referral and selfcare. Fam Pract 32:354–358.

Tinkle BT, Bird HA, Grahame R, Lavallee M, Levy HP, Sillence D. 2009. The lack of clinical distinction between the hypermobility type of Ehlers-Danlos syndrome and the joint hypermobility syndrome (a.k.a. hypermobility syndrome). Am J Med Genet Part A 149A:2368–2370.

Uzunkulaoğlu A, Çetin N. 2019. Hypermobility Syndrome and Proprioception In Patients With Knee Ligament Injury, East J Med 24(1): 38-41.

Vatwani, A., & Margonis, R. (2019). Energy Conservation Techniques to Decrease Fatigue. *Arch Phys Med Rehabil*, *100*(6), 1193-1196.

Voermans NC, Knoop H. 2011. Both pain and fatigue are important possible determinants of disability in patients with the EhlersDanlos syndrome hypermobility type. Disabil Rehabil 33:706–707.

World Health Organization. 2015. International Classification for Functioning Disability and Health. http://www.who.int/classifications/ icf/en/ [Accessed April 2016].

Zarate N, Farmer AD, Grahame R, Mohammed SD, Knowles CH, Scott SM, Aziz Q. 2010. Unexplained gastrointestinal symptoms and joint hypermobility: Is connective tissue the missing link? Neurogastroenterol Motil 22:252–278.

CHAPTER XVIII

Precautions for Invasive Examinations and Surgeries

By Dr. Stéphane Daens

The unique properties of the connective tissue in EDS make it more fragile and brittle. As a result, complications can be potentially severe or life-threatening during technical procedures, surgery, or childbirth.

It is vital to inform caregivers of an individual's EDS status and show them the *Emergency and Care card* issued by your doctor or patient association. Similarly, all caregivers (general practitioners, surgeons, anesthetists, gynecologist-obstetricians, dentists, and stomatologists) must always consider Ehlers-Danlos Syndrome. Surgery is associated with a higher risk of complications in all EDS variants, and each surgery type requires specific precautions. It is also true for screening procedures such as gastroscopies, colonoscopies, hysteroscopies, bronchoscopies, arteriographies, and more.

Let us break down the main precautions for better results of any actions taken and ease eventual stress.

1. The tendency to bleed:

Franciska Malfait and Anne De Paepe (2009) [298] described the bleeding tendency and bruising associated with all EDS variants, including the so-called hypermobile form, which is the most prevalent.

---

[298] Malfait F, De Paepe A. Bleeding in the heritable connective tissue disorders: mechanisms, diagnosis and treatment. Blood Rev. 2009;23(5):191-197.

In a recent study by *Artoni A et al. (2018)*[299], which looked at the risk of bleeding in 141 patients with EDS (mainly hEDS and cEDS), an assessment of bleeding tendency (*Bleeding Assessment Tool of the ISTH or BAT-ISTH*) and a bleeding severity score (*Bleeding Severity Score or BSS*) were performed.

Coagulation tests used for this study:

♦ Dosing of PTT and APTT.
♦ Determination of hemoglobin and creatinine clearance (renal function).
♦ Determination of coagulation factors VII, VIII, IX, XI, and XII, when PTT or APTT were prolonged.
♦ Determination of factors V and X and fibrinogen level, in case of prolongation of PTT and APTT.
♦ The von Willebrand factor has also been studied (*VWF antigen and VWF/RCo*).
♦ Evaluation of Endogenous Thrombin (*Endogenous Thrombin Potential, FTE*).
♦ Evaluation of platelet function (aggregation and secretion by stimulation with ADP).

Results:

♦ BSS is abnormal in 42% of patients.
♦ Platelet counts and fibrinogen levels are normal for everyone.
♦ Clotting factor levels do not appear to be affected by EDS.
♦ Platelet function is impaired in 83% of patients:
  • 56.7% of patients have a disorder in platelet aggregation.
  • 78.7% had an abnormality in the secretion of platelet factors.
  • 42.6% of patients had a problem with aggregation and secretion.

The authors conclude that the altered vessel wall, through collagen damage, may be the basis for platelets' lower reactivity to various stimulants (such as adenosine diphosphate or ADP).

---

[299] Artoni A, Bassotti A, Abbattista M et al. Hemostatic abnormalities in patients with Ehlers-Danlos syndrome. J Thromb Haemost. 2018;16:2425-2431.

Additionally, they emphasize that all types, or variants, of EDSs are at risk of bleeding (not just the vascular variant, or vEDS).

According to *Jesudas R et al. (2019)*[300], collagen damage results in the fragility of tissues and vessel walls. Also, they emphasize that alteration of the subendothelial collagen can disrupt its interaction with platelets and Von Willebrand factor, resulting in bleeding. Mast cell activation syndrome is observed in many patients with EDS and is also associated with bleeding. The two phenomena combine where appropriate. Again, they talk about Ehlers-Danlos syndrome in general rather than specifically to vEDS.

When I was a young doctor, it was easy to appreciate the bleeding time at the patient's bedside: a small cut was made in the earlobe, a small compress was placed beneath, and time was counted until the bleeding ceased. Although it is considered somewhat barbaric, this simple test is allowed for the global estimation of coagulation in consultation (like the resulting from coagulation factors, platelet count, platelet function, tissue, and capillary fragility, and more). Furthermore, I have observed that when skin biopsies are performed, the bleeding time and abundance of bleeding are significantly increased in EDS.

It is recommended to take tranexamic acid (Exacyl®) at a rate of 3 x 1g/day in drinkable ampoules starting the day before the operation in the morning and to continue for several days afterward (time varies according to the type of operation and its importance).

Also, it is necessary to increase daily vitamin C intake to 3x1g, for example, from D-15 to D+15 (empirical), as it reduces intraoperative and postoperative bleeding. 1 to 2g of vitamin C per day is recommended as a daily dose, excluding surgical or bloody operations.

---

[300] Jesudas R, Chaudhury A, Laukaitis CM. An update on the new classification of Ehlers-Danlos syndrome and review of the causes of bleeding in this population. Haemophilia. 2019;25(4):558-566.

Intravenous Desmopressin is indicated one hour prior to surgery in patients undergoing potentially bloody surgery (arterial vascular surgery, major thoracic or abdominal surgery) or when the patient has a history of significant bleeding.

Desmopressin (or 1-Deamino-8-D-Arginine Vasopressin), often abbreviated to DDAVP, is a derivative of the antidiuretic hormone (ADH). It has been used in hemophilia-A and von Willebrand Disease since 1977. It promotes increased plasma levels of factor VIII and von Willebrand factor. It does not influence the number of blood platelets or their aggregation function, but it increases platelets' adhesion to the vessel wall. It decreases APTT and bleeding time. On DDAVP, the sodium level should be monitored and may fall in the blood (hyponatremia). Commonly used doses of DDAVP: 0.3µg/kg body weight (b.wt) in 30 minutes.

Some authors (Bolton-Maggs PHB et al., 2004[301] and Faber P et al., 2007[302]) have also administered recombinant activated factor VII (NovoSeven®), which is produced by genetic engineering and activated during the purification process. It was administered intravenously at doses of 90 or 120µg/kg b.wt (variable doses between 60 and 150µg/kg b.wt, half-life 2-3 hours).

2. The fragility of tissues and capillaries:

It also plays an essential role in the risk of bleeding and vessel rupture in EDS, even more so in the vascular variant (or vEDS).

3. The anesthetics:

Anesthetics are not always effective in EDS. Either it is ineffective in local anesthesia (dental anesthesia, wound edge anesthesia, and more), loco-regional anesthesia (nerve block,

---

[301] Bolton-Maggs PH, Perry DJ, Chalmers EA, et al. The rare coagulation disorders--review with guidelines for management from the United Kingdom Haemophilia Centre Doctors' Organisation. Haemophilia. 2004;10(5):593-628.
[302] Faber P, Craig WL, Duncan JL, et al. The successful use of recombinant factor VIIa in a patient with vascular-type Ehlers-Danlos syndrome. Acta Anaesthesiol Scand. 2007;51(9):1277-9.

epidurals during childbirth), or general anesthesia (the patient wakes up too early, sometimes in the middle of the operation, or later, with a legitimate concern of relatives and nursing staff).

Several causes could explain these phenomena:

- During local dental anesthesia (especially the posterior and lower teeth), the dentist puts a dose of anesthetic around the dental nerve. However, due to the loose fabrics, the product leaks forward. As a result, several doses of anesthetic are required to saturate space in the oral mucosa and reach the dental nerve.

- In epidurals (for vaginal deliveries, Caesarean sections, or other lower limb procedures), the phenomenon could be the same; the product sneaks in where it should not go. During epidurals, let us keep in mind that there is a risk of meningeal breaches (persistent headaches, cerebrospinal fluid discharge, and more) and hematomas. The possibility of using a meningeal *Blood-patch*, if necessary, should be anticipated. Epidurals either do not work at all, work only partially (e.g., with only one of the two limbs being anesthetized), or have a short-term effect (with an early reawakening of sensitivity intraoperatively).

4. Difficulties and complications during endotracheal intubation:

- The fragility of the connective tissue (especially in the classical variant EDS) can make intubation difficult (hypotonia of the pharynx and larynx, laryngotracheomalacia, hypermobility of the structures of the upper airways and bronchial tree, exacerbated cough reflex, and more) and make it potentially risky (tracheal or bronchial rupture or perforation, laryngeal lesions, heavy bleeding, and more).
- Dislocation of the temporomandibular joints is also possible: the mouth should open gradually and gently.
- The endotracheal tubes should be as small in diameter as possible to reduce the risk of injury to the tracheobronchial tree.

- Craniocervical instability can further complicate the picture by creating dislocations.
- Airway pressure during controlled ventilation should be as low as possible to avoid pneumothorax.
- It is perhaps even more difficult during laparoscopy (laparoscopy in a patient who has been intubated and ventilated) with insufflation of CO_2 into the peritoneal cavity: in this case, the pressure in the airways must combat the peritoneal pressure for inspiration, and there is, admittedly very rarely, a risk of capnothorax (because of the CO_2).

5. Complications of monitoring of patients with EDS:

- Blood pressure measurement through a cuff can cause bruising, sometimes severe.
- Invasive blood pressure monitoring (e.g., catheter in the radial artery) can lead to ruptures or dissections of walls: it is not recommendable.
- The same applies to venous catheters in the jugular (risk of tearing) or in the subclavian (tear, pneumothorax).
- Bladder catheters can cause urethral or bladder damage.

6. Patient positioning during surgery:

- Patient handling and positioning should be done carefully to avoid joint subluxations or dislocations and brachial plexus injury.
- The eyes must be protected, and excessive pressure on the eyeballs must be avoided (risk of detachment of the retina or rupture of the eyeball).
- During handling, the skin must be protected from tears or abrasions.
- Be cautious of overly sticky dressings that may pull the skin off from the patient or cause allergic reactions, especially in the context of MCAD. The same applies to the electrodes used for continuous or discontinuous heart rate monitoring.

7. Delayed healing:

- It results from damage to connective tissue and small vessels, and of platelet function disorders (aggregation and secretion). These have a more significant influence on the bleeding time.
- Sutures should be removed at a rate of two to three times the time that a non-EDS patient.
- Non-absorbable threads must always be used, both indoors and outdoors. As the absorbable sutures are composed of sugars, they are digested faster than the time it takes for the scar to develop. The sutures, in unsuitable conditions, loosen, and the scars become large and unsightly.
- Stitches or staples should be removed gradually: every second stitch or staple should be removed at first, and the progress of healing should be checked. In case of incomplete healing, suture removal should be delayed by one week.

8. Dysautonomia:

It can induce blood pressure disturbances and arrhythmias during surgery. Hence, vasopressors, antiarrhythmics, solutions to increase circulating volume are sometimes necessary. There may also be POTS and HOS post-operatively (see chapters on dysautonomia and cardiovascular events).

9. The risk of algoneurodystrophy (CRPS-1):

Preventive treatment of algoneurodystrophy or CRPS type 1 is recommended for orthopedic surgery. Vigilance is required in the presence of mast cell activation disorders associated with EDS (or EDS/MCA). The causes and preventive or curative treatments of CRPS-1 have been explained above.

10. Functional orthopedic interventions:

They are rarely indicated, especially in the knees and shoulders. They do not work very well in the long term. The anterior shoulder stops with iliac bone graft and screws eventually melt. Usually, only the screw is found on follow-up x-rays.

Regarding vaccinations:

➤ Annual influenza vaccination is recommended in EDS.
➤ Consider pneumococcal vaccination in chronic respiratory problems (asthma, COPD, active smoking, MCADs, and more).
➤ Vaccination against covid-19 (SARS-CoV-2).

Regarding antibiotics:

Fluoroquinolones are not recommendable for EDS and other hereditary connective tissue diseases (HCTD). A Canadian study (*N. Daneman et al., 2015*[303]), involving 657,950 patients who took fluoroquinolones as antibiotics showed: a significant increase in the risk of tendon rupture (adjusted risk x 2.4) and aortic aneurysm (adjusted risk x 2.24). Since the risk is already much higher in the general population studied, it could be worse in EDS.

Arendt-Nielsen L, Kaalund S, Bjeering P et al. Insufficient effect of local analgesics in Ehlers Danlos type III patients (connective tissue disorders). Acta Anaestesiol Scand. 1990;34:358-361.

Castori M. Surgical recommendations in Ehlers-Danlos syndrome(s) need patient classifications : the example of Ehlers-Danlos syndrome hypermobility (a.k.A. Joint hypermobility syndrome). Dig Surg. 2012;29:453-455.

Malfait F, De Paepe A. Bleeding in the heritable connective tissue disorders: mechanisms, diagnosis and treatment. Blood Rev. 2009;23:191-197.

Hakim AJ, Grahame R, Norris P et al. Local anaesthetic failure in joint hypermobility syndrome. J R Soc Med. 2005 ;98:84-85.

Wiesman T, Castori M, Malfait F et al. Recommendations for anesthesia and perioperative management in patients with Ehlers-Danlos syndrome(s). Orphanet Journal of Rare Disease. 2014;9:109

Hamonet C, Bahloul H, Ducret L. Anesthesia and Ehlers-Danlos syndrome (EDS). J Anesth Pain Med. 2018;3(1):1-4.

---

[303] Daneman N, Lu H et Redelmeier DA. Fluoroquinolones and collagen associated severe adverse events: a longitudinal cohort study. BMJ, 2015;5:e010077. Doi:10.1136/bmjopen-2015-010077.

CHAPTER XIX

Psychopathological Correlates of Ehlers-Danlos Syndromes

By Professor Antonio Bulbena-Vilarrasa, Psychiatry (Spain) [6,7],
Professor Carolina Baeza-Velasco, Psychology (France) [1-3]
& Professor Andrea Bulbena-Cabré, Psychiatry (Spain) [4,5]

[1]*Université de Paris, Laboratoire de Psychopathologie et Processus de Santé, France.*
[2]*Department of Emergency Psychiatry and Acute Care, CHU Montpellier, France.*
[3]*Institute of Functional Genomics, University of Montpellier, CNRS, INSERM, France.* [4]*Icahn School of Medicine at Mount Sinai, NY, USA.* [5]*Metropolitan Hospital, New York City Health and Hospitals, NY, USA.* [6]*Institut Neuropsychiatry and Addictions. Parc Salut Mar. Hospital del Mar, Spain.* [7]*Department Psychiatry and Forensic Medicine. Universitat Autònoma Barcelona, Spain.*

Introduction

In addition to the plethora of physical symptoms affecting people with Ehlers-Danlos syndromes (EDS), psychological and psychiatric alterations are common in these patients as highlighted recent research (e.g., Bulbena et al., 2017; Cederlöf et al., 2016). However, unfortunately it is not uncommon to find reluctance among physicians and patients to recognize them and give to the mental area the importance required. At least three explanations can be evoked. Firstly, the trivialization of mental symptoms that are mainly subjective (i.e., perceptible only to the patient) and without an identifiable organic origin. Secondly, the fear of stigmatization related to mental conditions, and maybe even more, the fear that the recognition of mental difficulties in the context of EDS might reinforce the widespread disbelief in this pathology (especially hypermobile EDS) as a somatic condition arguing instead for a mental cause (Baeza-Velasco et al., 2018a). Indeed, as Hamonet et al., (2018) stated, many physicians who are unaware of the EDS clinical picture, attribute somatic complaints of patients to psychological problems ("You are depressed, your MRI is normal, it's in your head", "It's a mood disorder", "go see a psychiatrist or psychologist"). These misconceptions should be surpassed in order to avoid neglecting a possible psychiatric comorbidity which adds to the suffering to patients, and so that the management of EDS is carried out with a true biopsychosocial approach. Thus, it is important to disseminate knowledge about EDS among the medical community to promote early diagnosis. It is also necesary to understand that mental conditions are frequent in the general population and even more in people suffering from chronic somatic conditions (Dudek and Sobański, 2012). Thus psychopathology in EDS should be explored and treated. Indeed, several studies have put in evidence a large psychopathological burden as well as frequent atypical neurodevelopmental attributes among people in the hypermobility spectrum disorders (HSD) and EDS such as anxiety and mood disorders, eating disordered behaviors, personality disorders, suicidal behaviors, autism, attention deficit and hyperactivity disorder, among others.

In this chapter, we present a state of the art concerning the psychiatric correlates of EDS.

Anxiety and anxiety disorders

Anxiety is probably the psychopathological dimension that has been most studied in the context of hypermobility-related disorders. The finding of an excess of anxiety disorders in people with joint hypermobility (JHM) published in 1988 by Bulbena et al. inaugurates a new line of research interested in the psychopathology related to collagen conditions that contribute to understanding of mind-body relationships or psychosomatic. Since then, several researchers have confirmed that people with joint hypermobility (JHM), joint hypermobility syndrome (JHS) and EDS display more anxiety as well as anxiety disorders than those without these collagen altered conditions (Bulbena et al., 2017). This association that have been studied mainly in adult populations, has been recently confirmed in children and in the elderly. Indeed, Ezpeleta et al. (2018) found greater hypermobility scores associated with greater anxiety symptoms

In pediatric populations, while Parvaneh et al. (2020) also found a greater prevalence of hypermobility scores in children with anxiety symptomatology. In the same line, Bulbena-Cabre et al. (2019) observed that children with JHS have higher frequency of anxiety disorders and greater intensity of physiological anxiety and somatic complaints. Authors suggested that JHS might be considered a marker for this anxiety phenotype in youngsters. More recently, de Vries et al. (2021) reported a high co-occurrence between JHM and anxiety among adolescents and young adults. For their part, Bulbena-Cabré et al. (2018) observed that the association between JHS/EDS and anxiety is preserved in the elderly.

Similarly to depression, pathological anxiety could be understood as secondary to the burden of a chronic disease. As an adaptive response to threat, anxiety can be reactive to the constant danger of injury experienced by people with EDS, in whom tissue fragility leads to an inherent propensity for trauma. Nevertheless, the available data rather suggest a primary connection. Thus, biological hypotheses have been formulated to explain such an association (Bulbena et al., 2017; Smith et al., 2014; Sinibaldi et al., 2015; Lumley et al., 1994; Baeza-Velasco et al., 2015). For instance, a common genetic milieu (Gratacos et al., 2001), alterations in the body awareness (Baeza-Velasco et al., 2011; Mallorqui-Bagué et al., 2015), dysautonomia (Bulbena et al., 2017) and structural brain differences in emotion regulation areas (Eccles et al., 2012) are clues to understand the vulnerability of anxiety in EDS patients.

Taking together, these data highlight the importance to screen for pathological anxiety in patients with hypermobility-related disorders. In this regard, in 2018 we reported that people with hEDS and high level of anxiety presented a poorer social functioning and general health than those with low levels of anxiety (Baeza-Velasco et al., 2018a). Concordantly, de Vries et al. (2021) reported that anxiety has a disabling role in young people with JHM since the combination of JHM and anxiety is associated with decreased physical and psychosocial functioning, decreased workload, increased fatigue, and pain catastrophizing. Thus, anxiety in EDS patients should not be neglected.

Affective disorders

Studies evaluating a variety of psychiatric aspects in hEDS (Cederlof et al., 2016; Hershenfeld et al., 2016; Smith et al., 2014) converge on the relationship between depressive states and JHS/hEDS. In addition, bipolar disorder has also been associated with JHS and EDS (Cederlof et al., 2016). Interestingly, according to Bulbena-Cabre et al. (2017) patients with bipolar disorder and comorbid anxiety have a specific phenotype characterized by JHM, somatosensory amplification and increased body perception.

Suicidal behaviors

Although few systematic studies (n=3) have explored suicidal behaviors in the context of hypermobility-related disorders, all agree on an excess of suicide attempt among patients with EDS. Indeed, Cederlöf et al. (2016) in a large cohort of patients with EDS and JHS in Sweden observed an increased risk of attempted suicide in this population as well as in their siblings. In France, Benistan and Martinez (2019) reported a high rate of suicide attempts (22%) among young hEDS patients. Concordantly, Baeza-Velasco et al., (2021a) found that 11 out of 35 (31.4%) female patients with hEDS had antecedents of suicide attempt. Factors related to suicide attempt in this study were age, personality disturbances specially depressive, avoidant, antisocial and borderline traits, mania/hypomanic episodes and anxiety disorders.

Eating disorders

Several characteristics of EDS such as gastrointestinal symptoms, dental problems, chemosensory alterations, food allergies, temporomandibular disturbances and fragility of oral mucosa may negatively impact eating behaviors, weight and nutrition (Baeza-Velasco et al., 2016). In addition, some studies have reported that abnormal body mass index (BMI) is overrepresented in people with JHM and EDS (e.g., Baeza-Velasco et al., 2018a; Sanjay et al., 2013). Thus, increased interest has raised in last years in the exploration of an eventual link between eating disorders and JHM, HSD and EDS. Goh et al.

(2013) reported that JHM was significantly more common among anorexic subjects (63%) than in the relative (34%) and the healthy control group (13%). Moreover, Eccles (2016) although in few subjects observed similar results. That is a higher proportion of people with eating disorders among psychiatric patients with JHM compared to those non-hypermobile. Bulbena-Cabré et al. (2017) compared scores on bulimia and anorexia between non-hypermobile and hypermobile non-clinical youngsters. The last group had significantly higher scores than their counterpart. Recently, we published results of an observation study aimed to compare gastrointestinal symptoms, disordered eating, and BMI between EDS patients and healthy controls, and to explore the link between these variables in EDS patients. Results showed that patients with EDS had a higher prevalence of gastrointestinal symptoms, antecedents of eating disorders and current risk of eating disorder as well as lower BMI than healthy subjects. In addition, the risk of current eating disorder was associated with gastrointestinal symptoms in the EDS group (Baeza-Velasco et al. 2021b). Coyado et al. (submitted) explored JHS/hEDS in children with the newly described "Avoidant/restrictive food intake disorder (ARFID)", which is characterized by a persistent failure to meet appropriate nutritional and/or energy needs, which can result in significant weight loss or nutritional deficiency, dependence on enteral feeding or nutritional supplements, and/or a marked interference in psychosocial functioning (American Psychiatric Association, 2013). Results showed that children with ARFID have greater JHS/hEDS features including somatosensory amplification compared to controls.

Personality disorders

Very few studies in patients with HSD and EDS have explored personality disorders. Espiridion et al. (2018), who published a case of a young female suffering from EDS, borderline personality disorders and major depression, stated that EDS patients may be at increased risk of being diagnosed with a personality disorder such as borderline. To the best of our knowledge, only Pasquini et al. (2014) have reported data of a systematic study in this domain. In this study, patients with JHS presented an increased risk of obsessive-compulsive personality disorder. According to these authors, on the one hand, the lack of recognition of JHS by health professionals may promote perfectionism in those affected, and, on the other hand, motor instability may favor behaviors of hyper control. For our part, we assessed altered personality traits in hEDS patients and we observed that these were related to suicidal behaviors as mentioned before (Baeza-Velasco et al., 2021b). Subsequently, we compared personality disturbances between patients with hEDS, rheumatoid arthritis and healthy subjects. Results showed that hEDS patients presented significantly higher scores on personality disturbance than healthy controls. However no difference was observed with rheumatoid arthritis patients on this variable (Kalisch et al., submitted). This is consistent with literature which shows that personality disorders are more prevalent in the pain population compared to the general population (Weisberg et al., 2000).

Neurodevelopmental disorders

Among neurodevelopmental disorders, attention deficit hyperactivity disorder (ADHD) has been the most studied in the context of HSD and EDS. Koldas Dogan et al. (2011) and Shiari et al. (2013) observed an increased prevalence of JHM in children with ADHD. Csecs et al. (2020) confirmed the association between JHM and ADHD in adults. Concerning symptomatic JHM, authors such as Cederlöf et al. (2016), Castori et al. (2014), Celletti et al. (2015), Piedimonte et al. (2018) and Kindgren et al. (2021) highlighted a high frequency of ADHD in patients with HSD/EDS. Although the link between JHM, HSD, EDS and ADHD is poor understood, impaired coordination and proprioception, fatigue, chronic pain, and dysautonomia have been identified as potential bridges between these conditions (Baeza-Velasco et al., 2018b).

Autism has also been linked to JHM and EDS. Descriptions of autism include hypotonia, clumsiness, apraxia, and toe walking as common finding. These characteristics as many other overlap with those of hEDS (Baeza-Velasco et al., 2016b). The scarce systematic research existing in this field suggests that autism and JHM, HSD and EDS co-occur more often than expected by chance. Shetreat-Klein et al. (2014) was the first to compare JHM between children with and without autism observing that this somatic characteristic was more prevalent among autistic children. Concerning HSD and EDS, the study by Cederlöf et al. (2016) reported an increased risk of autism spectrum disorders in people with these syndromes. Explanatory hypotheses about the overlap/comorbidity between autism and collagen altered conditions includes brain heterotopias, immune, endocrine and metabolic alterations have been proposed to understand the comorbidity with autism (Baeza-Velasco et al., 2018c; Casanova et al., 2018, 2019, 2020; Skalny et al., 2020).

From a clinical point of view, these results are important implications. Increase awareness on this association may contribute to identifying autistic individuals susceptible to suffer from pain, which is very challenging due to communication difficulties (Baeza-Velasco et al., 2018b). The therapeutic approach of these complex mixed cases (i.e., autism comorbid with HSD/EDS) is also challenging. In this sense, the work by Guinchat et al. (2020) deserve attention. This group explored the benefits of compression garments on control posture and challenging behaviors in children and adolescents with autism and severe proprioceptive dysfunction including individuals with JHS/hEDS. It is worth remembering that considering the expressive particularities in people with autism, aberrant behaviors may underlie pain (Dubois et al., 2010). Compression garments in this study were well accepted by participants and a reduction of aberrant behaviors as well as benefits in terms of postural control and motor performance were observed. These encouraging results should be replicated by further research.

Other neurodevelopmental conditions such as learning disorders (e.g., Adib et al., 2005; Celletti et al., 2015), communication disorders (e.g., Adib et al., 2005; Hunter et al., 1998), tic disorders such as Tourette syndrome (Csecs et al., 2020), and motor developmental disorder (Kirby et al., 2005; Celletti et al., 2015) are frequently seen in patients with HSD and EDS. Since the comorbidity between neurodevelopmental disorders is the rule rather than the exception, patients with HSD and EDS should be screening at early age for these conditions that add to the burden of the disease.

Other psychiatric conditions

To the best of our knowledge, there is no evidence so far concerning an increased prevalence of psychotic disorders in HSD or EDS. However, it is worth mentioning the study by Bulbena-Cabré and Bulbena (2018) in which they demonstrated that anxiety was a frequent comorbidity in patients with schizophrenia (30%) and that those with these conditions experienced greater JHS. Indeed, the presence of JHM and symptomatic JHM justify its exploration of psychiatric conditions such as pathological anxiety since solid evidence confirm this association.

Although few studies have focused on substance misuse, there are some data of interest. An association between JHM and alcoholism in females was reported by Carlsson and Rundgren (1980). In the same vein, we reported that the rate of at-risk drinkers and smokers was significantly higher among females with JHM than among those without it (Baeza-Velasco et al., 2015). Finally, Lumley et al. (1994), who explored the psychosocial status of patients with EDS, reported that 12% out of 42 patients had antecedents of alcohol dependence and illicit drug consumption.

Conversion disorders renamed as neurological functional disorders is another condition of interest in the context of HSD and EDS since it is not uncommon to diagnose (wrongly) conversion disorder in patients with atypical symptoms presentations. This clinical situation was illustrated in a case report published by Barnum (2014) in which medical providers diagnosed conversion disorder in a girl with EDS who was suspected to purposely dislocating her joints, alter her gait and demonstrating atypical spasmodic tremors. Thus, disseminate knowledge about altered collagen conditions and comorbidities will contribute with diagnosis accuracy and adapted therapeutic proposition to patients.

Conclusion

As EDS itself, the psychological and psychiatric area in the context of this disease has been neglected for many years.

Fortunately, a growing body of research emerges highlighting how mental problems are common in these patients and the significant burden that mental comorbidities add to those affected. Several mental conditions (e.g., anxiety disorders, depression) are susceptible to be treated until remission. Other are chronic (e.g., autism). However, with an adapted approach we can improve the quality of life of patients suffering from these mixed clinical pictures. Overcoming misconceptions (e.g., stigma) concerning mental disorders is the first step to advance in this area. HSD and EDS illustrate very well body-mind connections. Its management, requiring a veritable holistic approach, contributes to relativizing the outdate Cartesian dualism still present in the medical culture. Models of psychopathology integrating mental and somatic features, which are lacking in the current psychiatric nosology, are necessary to better reflect the reality of patients. Some interesting contributions in this sense have been made. For instance, the Neuroconnective Phenotype by Bulbena et al. (2015) which describes five components (behavioral pattens, somatic illnesses, psychopathology, somatosensory symptoms and signs and somatic symptoms and signs) surrounding the core anxiety – collagen laxity. The ALPIM syndrome by Coplan et al. (2015) which describes a spectrum disorder that has a core of anxiety with clusters of comorbid disorders within each of the following domains: joint laxity, chronic pain, autoimmune conditions, and mood disorders. Other models integrating somatic and neurobehavioral conditions have been proposed to understand eating disorders (Baeza-Velasco et al., 2016a) and neurodevelopmental conditions in HSD and EDS (Baeza-Velasco et al., 2018b).

We hope that these conceptualizations and the research in this field will reach clinicians so that we can collaboratively improve the living conditions of patients.

References

Adib, N., Davies, K., Grahame, R., Woo, P., & Murray, KJ. (2005) Joint hypermobility syndrome in childhood. A not so benign multisystem disorder? *Rheumathology (Oxford)* 44(6):744-50.

American Psychiatric Association. (2013). Diagnostic and Statistical Manual of Mental Disorders. (5th Edition). Washington, DC.

Baeza-Velasco, C., Bourdon, C., Montalescot, L., de Cazotte, C., Pailhez, G., Bulbena, A., & Hamonet, C. (2018a). Low- and high-anxious hypermobile Ehlers-Danlos syndrome patients: comparison of psychosocial and health variables. *Rheumatol Int, 38*(5), 871-878. https://doi.org/10.1007/s00296-018-4003-7

Baeza-Velasco, C., Cohen, D., Hamonet, C., Vlamynck, E., Diaz, L., Cravero, C., Cappe, E., & Guinchat, V. (2018c). Autism, Joint Hypermobility-Related Disorders and Pain. *Front Psychiatry, 9*, 656. https://doi.org/10.3389/fpsyt.2018.00656

Baeza-Velasco, C., Stoebner-Delbarre, A., Cousson-Gelie, F. *et al.* (2015). Increased tobacco and alcohol use among women with joint hypermobility: A way to cope with anxiety? *Rheumatology International* 35:177-181.

Baeza-Velasco, C., Hamonet, C., Montalescot, L., & Courtet, P. (2021b). Suicidal Behaviors in Women With the Hypermobile Ehlers-Danlos Syndrome. *Arch Suicide Res*, 1-13. https://doi.org/10.1080/13811118.2021.1885538

Baeza-Velasco, C., Lorente, S., Tasa-Vinyals, E., Guillaume, S., Mora, M. S., & Espinoza, P. (2021a). Gastrointestinal and eating problems in women with Ehlers-Danlos syndromes. *Eat Weight Disord*. https://doi.org/10.1007/s40519-021-01146-z

Baeza-Velasco, C., Sinibaldi, L., & Castori, M. (2018b). Attention-deficit/hyperactivity disorder, joint hypermobility-related disorders and pain: expanding body-mind connections to the developmental age. *Atten Defic Hyperact Disord, 10*(3), 163-175. https://doi.org/10.1007/s12402-018-0252-2

Baeza-Velasco, C., Van den Bossche, T., Grossin, D., & Hamonet, C. (2016a). Difficulty eating and significant weight loss in joint hypermobility syndrome/Ehlers-Danlos syndrome, hypermobility type. *Eat Weight Disord, 21*(2), 175-183. https://doi.org/10.1007/s40519-015-0232-x

Baeza-Velasco, C., Hamonet, C., Baghdadli, A., & Brissot, R. (2016b). Autism Spectrum Disorders and Ehlers-Danlos Syndrome Hypermobility-Type: Similarities in clinical presentation. *Cuadernos de Medicina Psicosomática y Psiquiatría de Enlace 118*:49-58.

Barnum R (2014) problems with diagnosig Conversion Disorder in response to variable and usual symptoms. Adolescent Health, Medicine and Therapeutics. April. Dove Press.

Benistan, K., & Martinez, V. (2019, Jul). Pain in hypermobile Ehlers-Danlos syndrome: New insights using new criteria. *Am J Med Genet A, 179*(7), 1226-1234. https://doi.org/10.1002/ajmg.a.61175

Bulbena A, Pailhez G, Bulbena-Cabré A, Mallorqui-Bagué N, Baeza-Velasco C (2015) Joint hypermobility, anxiety and psychosomatics: two and a half decades of progress toward a new phenotype. Adv Psychosom Med 34:143–157

Bulbena, A., Baeza-Velasco, C., Bulbena-Cabre, A., Pailhez, G., Critchley, H., Chopra, P., Mallorqui-Bague, N., Frank, C., & Porges, S. (2017, Mar). Psychiatric and psychological aspects in the Ehlers-Danlos syndromes. *Am J Med Genet C Semin Med Genet, 175*(1), 237-245. https://doi.org/10.1002/ajmg.c.31544

Bulbena A, Duro JC, Porta M, Vallejo J. (1988) Joint hypermobility syndrome and anxiety disorders. *The Lancet* 332(8612),694.

Bulbena-Cabre, A., Duno, L., Almeda, S., Batlle, S., Camprodon-Rosanas, E., Martin-Lopez, L. M., & Bulbena, A. (2019). Joint hypermobility is a marker for anxiety in children. *Rev Psiquiatr Salud Ment, 12*(2), 68-76. https://doi.org/10.1016/j.rpsm.2019.01.004 (La hiperlaxitud articular como marcador de ansiedad en ninos.)

Bulbena-Cabré, A., Pailhez, G., Cabrera, A., Baeza-Velasco, C., Porges, S., & Bulbena, A. (2017). Body perception in a sample of nonclinical youngsters with joint hypermobility. *Ansiedad y Estrés, 23*(2-3), 99-103.

Bulbena-Cabre, A., Rojo, C., Pailhez, G., Buron Maso, E., Martin-Lopez, L. M., & Bulbena, A. (2018, Jan). Joint hypermobility is also associated with anxiety disorders in the elderly population. *Int J Geriatr Psychiatry, 33*(1), e113-e119. https://doi.org/10.1002/gps.4733

Bulbena-Cabre, A., Salgado, P., Rodriguez, A., & Bulbena, A. (2017). Joint hypermobility: A potential biomarker for anxiety disorders in bipolar patients. *J Psychosom Res, 97*, 141.

Bulbena-Cabre A, Bulbena A. Schizophrenia and anxiety: yes, they are relatives not just neighbours. Br J Psychiatry. 2018 Aug;213(2):498. doi: 10.1192/bjp.2018.126. PMID: 30027877.

Carlsson C, Rundgren A. (1980) Hypermobility of the joints in women alcoholics. *J Stud Alcohol*
41:78–81.

Casanova, E. L., Baeza-Velasco, C., Buchanan, C. B., & Casanova, M. F. (2020). The Relationship between Autism and Ehlers-Danlos Syndromes/Hypermobility Spectrum Disorders. *J Pers Med, 10*(4). https://doi.org/10.3390/jpm10040260

Casanova, E. L., Sharp, J. L., Edelson, S. M., Kelly, D. P., & Casanova, M. F. (2018, Mar 17). A Cohort Study Comparing Women with Autism Spectrum Disorder with and without Generalized Joint Hypermobility. *Behav Sci (Basel), 8*(3). https://doi.org/10.3390/bs8030035

Casanova, E. L., Sharp, J. L., Edelson, S. M., Kelly, D. P., Sokhadze, E. M., & Casanova, M. F. (2019). Immune, autonomic, and endocrine dysregulation in autism and Ehlers-Danlos syndrome/hypermobility spectrum disorders versus unaffected controls. *bioRxiv*, 670661.

Castori, M., Dordoni, C., Valiante, M., Sperduti, I., Ritelli, M., Morlino, S., Chiarelli, N., Celletti, C., Venturini, M., Camerota, F., Calzavara-Pinton, P., Grammatico, P., Colombi, M. (2014) Nosology and inheritance pattern(s) of joint hypermobility syndrome and Ehlers-Danlos hypermobility type: A study of intrafamilial and interfamilial variability in 23 Italian pedigrees. *American Journal of Medical Genetics A* 164A:3010–3020.

Cederlof, M., Larsson, H., Lichtenstein, P., Almqvist, C., Serlachius, E., & Ludvigsson, J. F. (2016, Jul 4). Nationwide population-based cohort study of psychiatric disorders in individuals with Ehlers-Danlos syndrome or hypermobility syndrome and their siblings. *BMC Psychiatry, 16*, 207. https://doi.org/10.1186/s12888-016-0922-6

Coplan, J., Singh, D., Gopinath, S., Mathew, S. J., & Bulbena, A. (2015). A Novel Anxiety and Affective Spectrum Disorder of Mind and Body-The ALPIM (Anxiety-Laxity-Pain-Immune-Mood) Syndrome: A Preliminary Report. *J Neuropsychiatry Clin Neurosci, 27*(2), 93-103. https://doi.org/10.1176/appi.neuropsych.14060132

Csecs, J. L., Iodice, V., Rae, C. L., Brooke, A., Simmons, R., Dowell, N. G., Prowse, F., Themelis, K., Critchley, H. D., & Eccles, J. A. (2020). Increased rate of joint hypermobility in autism and related neurodevelopmental conditions is linked to dysautonomia and pain. *medRxiv.*

De Vries J, Verbunt J, Stubbe J, Visser B, Ramaekers S, Calders P, Engelberg R. (2021) Generalized joint hypermobliity and anxiety in adolescents and young adults, the impact on physical and psychosocial functionig. *Healthcare 9,525.*

Dubois A, Rattaz C, Pry R, Baghdadli A. Autism and Pain—A literature review. Pain Res Manage. (2010) 15:245–53. doi: 10.1155/2010/749275

Duder D, Sobański JA. (2012) Mental disorders in somatic diseases: psychopathology and treatment. Polskie Archiwum Medycyny Wewnętrznj 122(12):624-629.

Eccles JA, Beacher FD, Gray MA, Jones CL, Minati L, Harrison NA, Critchley HD (2012) Brain structure and joint hypermobility: relevance to the expression of psychiatric symptoms. B J Psychiatry 200:508Y9.

Espiridion, E. D., Daniel, A., & Van Allen, J. R. (2018, Dec 21). Recurrent Depression and Borderline Personality Disorder in a Patient with Ehlers-Danlos Syndrome. *Cureus, 10*(12), e3760. https://doi.org/10.7759/cureus.3760

691

Ezpeleta, L., Navarro, J. B., Osa, N., Penelo, E., & Bulbena, A. (2018, Jul/Aug). Joint Hypermobility Classes in 9-Year-Old Children from the General Population and Anxiety Symptoms. *J Dev Behav Pediatr, 39*(6), 481-488. https://doi.org/10.1097/DBP.0000000000000577

Goh Min, Olver J, Huang CH, Millard M, O'Callaghan CH. Prevalence and familial patterns of gastrointestinal symptoms, joint hypermobility and diurnal blood pressure variations in patients with anorexia nervosa. J Eat Disord. 2013; 1(Suppl 1): O45.

Gratacòs M, Nadal M,Martín-Santos R, PujanaMA, Gago J, Peral B, et al. A polymorphic genomic duplication on human chromosome 15 is a susceptibility factor for panic and phobic disorders. Cell 2001;10(106):367–79.

Guinchat, V., Vlamynck, E., Diaz, L., Chambon, C., Pouzenc, J., Cravero, C., Baeza-Velasco, C., Hamonet, C., Xavier, J., & Cohen, D. (2020, Jul 13). Compressive Garments in Individuals with Autism and Severe Proprioceptive Dysfunction: A Retrospective Exploratory Case Series. *Children (Basel), 7*(7). https://doi.org/10.3390/children7070077

Hamonet C, Schatz P-M, Bezire P, Ducret L, Brissot R. (2018) Cognitive and psychopathological aspects of Ehlers-Danlos syndrome - Experience in a specialized medical consultation. Res Adv Brain Disord Ther

Hershenfeld, S. A., Wasim, S., McNiven, V., Parikh, M., Majewski, P., Faghfoury, H., & So, J. (2016, Mar). Psychiatric disorders in Ehlers-Danlos syndrome are frequent, diverse and strongly associated with pain. *Rheumatol Int, 36*(3), 341-348. https://doi.org/10.1007/s00296-015-3375-1

Hunter, A., Morgan, AW, & Bird, HA. (1998). A Survey of Ehlers–Danlos Syndrome: Hearing, Voice, A Survey of Ehlers–Danlos Syndrome: Hearing, Voice, Speech and Swallowing Difficulties. Is There an underlying relationship ? *British Journal of Rheumatology* 37,803–804.

Kindgren, E., Perez, A. Q., & Knez, R. (2021). Prevalence of ADHD and Autism Spectrum Disorder in Children with Hypermobility Spectrum

Disorders or Hypermobile Ehlers-Danlos Syndrome: A Retrospective Study. *Neuropsychiatric Disease and Treatment, 17,* 379.

Kirby, A., Bryan, A., & Davies, R. (2005) Hypermobility syndrome and developmental co-ordination disorder: similarities and features. *International Journal of Therapy Rehabilitation 12,*431–437.

Koldas Dogan, S., Taner, Y., Evcik, D. (2011) Benign joint hypermobility syndrome in patients with attention deficit/hyperactivity disorders. *Turkish Journal of Rheumatology 26,*187–192

Lumley MA, Jordan M, Rubenstein R, Tsipouras P, Evans MI. (1994) Psychosocial functioning in the Ehlers–Danlos syndrome. Am J Med Genet 53:149–52.

Mallorqui-Bagué N, Bulbena A, Roe-Vellve N, Hoekzema E, Carmona S, Barba-Muller E, Fauquet J, Pailhez G, Vilarroya O (2015) Emotion processing in joint hypermobility: a potential link to the neural bases of anxiety and related somatic symptoms in collagen anomalies. Eur Psychiatry 30:454–458.

Piedimonte, C., Penge, R., Morlino, S., Sperdutti, I., Trzani, A., Giannini, MT,...& Castori, M. (2018) Exploring relationships between joint hypermobility and neurodevelopment in children (4–13 years) with hereditary connective tissue disorders and developmental coordination disorder. *American Journal of Medical Genetics B 177*(6),546-556.

Shetreat-Klein, M., Shinnar, S., & Rapin, I. (2014). Abnormalities of joint mobility and gait in children with autism spectrum disorders. *Brain & Development 36:*91–6

Shiari, R., Saeidifard, F., & Zahed, G. (2013) Evaluation of the prevalence of joint laxity in children with attention deficit/hyperactivity disorder. *Annals of Paediatric Rheumatolology 3,*78–80

Sinibaldi L, Ursini G, Castori M (2015) Psychopathological manifestations of joint hypermobility and joint hypermobility syndrome/Ehlers–Danlos syndrome, hypermobility type: the link between connective tissue and psychological distress revised. Am J Med Genet 169C:97–106. https://doi.org/10.1002/ajmg.c.31430

Smith, T. O., Easton, V., Bacon, H., Jerman, E., Armon, K., Poland, F., & Macgregor, A. J. (2014, Jan). The relationship between benign joint hypermobility syndrome and psychological distress: a systematic review and meta-analysis. *Rheumatology (Oxford), 53*(1), 114-122. https://doi.org/10.1093/rheumatology/ket317

Weisberg JN (2000) Personality and personality disorders in chronic pain. *Current Review of Pain 4,60-70.*

CHAPTER XX

Psychological Care in EDS

Mrs. Dominique Weil, Graduate in Psychological Sciences, Belgium
&
Doctor Daniel Grossin, General Practitioner, France

Psychological follow-up as part of global management of Ehlers-Danlos Syndrome

Text by Mrs. Dominique WEIL, Licentiate in Psychological Sciences (clinical orientation), Systematicist and Psychotherapist in Bioenergetic Analysis.

- **Introduction**

Let me present my way of managing pathologies related to chronic pain and EDS, the Ehlers Danlos Syndrome.

Practical therapeutic approaches are quite different from one person to another. Nevertheless, I will select those from my *toolbox* that will help the individual move forward on the path to Ehlers-Danlos Syndrome. There are, among others, cognitive-behavioral therapies, relaxation, coaching, and more. My practice, as an EDS care provider, is mainly focused on systemic psychotherapy and bioenergetic analysis. Systemic therapy is a type of therapy that takes the subject's relationship with his or her environment into consideration. The bioenergetic analysis takes into consideration the individual's psychic and physical aspects.

There are several complementary treatments, such as hypnosis. One of the hypnosis practices is that of Milton H. Erickson, the

E.M.D.R *(Eye Movement Desensitization and Reprocessing)* or T.R.E. *(Tension and Trauma Releasing Exercises)*.
In some cases, depending on the patient's history of chronic pain syndrome, consultation with another practitioner who specializes in other areas may be recommended.

Additionally, when performed in collaboration with the doctors(s), this type of multidisciplinary management produces excellent results in all cases of chronic pain syndromes.

- **The importance of the patient's personal history**

When a person presents for consultation, the psychotherapist must listen attentively and empathetically to the patient. His/her story is fundamental. Sometimes the person brings a perspective that Medicine cannot assess. Indeed, the caregiver must dig into the patient's history. Patient experience cannot be measured scientifically. He *"speaks to himself"*. The origin of the pain will often nestle in the nooks and crannies of his/her memory. For example, in cases of abuse and mistreatment, in various forms of psychological and physical violence, or in cases of family genetic inheritance.

It is easy to understand that the practitioner cannot afford to make any value judgments about pain, which is, by definition, unique for everyone. With time, I realized that regardless of the *tool* used, the quality of the connection between the patient and the therapist, regardless of the therapist's orientation, is the most important thing.

- **Interviewing the patient in the past and present**

In my practice, the patient is listened to according to the biopsychosocial model. It is represented according to a 3-dimensional Venn diagram. It is three circles with several intersections.

1. **The biological circle**

The biological part concerns the patient's medical history. The doctors and the practitioners of the various disciplines, he met. I quote: general practitioners, rheumatologists, algologists, orthopedic surgeons, osteopaths, physiotherapists, acupuncturists, nutritionists, Phyto therapists, energy therapists, masseurs, and so forth. Sometimes the person in pain meets an astrologer, numerologist, tarologist, and more. No longer knowing where to turn, the person meets all the possibilities offered to him. The hope of being finally heard and understood is a genuine quest to stop suffering.

Listening to the patient, one quickly realizes that it is a fighter's journey before that person finally meets the EDS practitioner and finally receives the proper diagnosis. It often takes many years between the first complaints (the onset of symptoms) and the diagnosis of EDS.

From the time of diagnosis, the psychotherapist accompanies the patient during the continuation of his treatment. The psychologist's ideal is to be in contact with the various people the person meets. The goal is to help the person to get better and manage their daily pain and treatment.

2. The psychological circle

The consequences of years of stabbing and permanent pain are exhausting. As a result, some patients develop severe depression. Accompaniment by a practitioner who understands the concept of *Pain* is essential. Every pain is different and is conceived differently. It has repercussions in all areas of a patient's life. Physical pain results in decreased movement or activity. Sometimes, the person is forced and coerced to stop working. Consider people who work in the cleaning industry, for example. It is a daily Hell!

So far, EDS patients I have met have exhibited a much more courageous personality than the average. Mostly, they find it hard to assess their physical limitations. Full of goodwill, these people will gorge themselves on pain medication, sold freely in pharmacies, to keep them going. It is advisable to keep in mind that these people have frequently heard: *"It is in your head, it is psychological, go see a psychologist!"* When the limit is exceeded and work stoppage is necessary, withdrawal, low self-esteem, lack of confidence, and self-image become more pronounced. Phrases such as "*I cannot even do it anymore*" are regularly uttered. Some patients experience stopping work as a loss of their autonomy. When they can no longer drive their vehicle and do things by themselves, it increases the concept of dependence, an intolerable notion for a combative psychological profile! However, a period of downtime is essential. Once accepted by the patient, this can lead to other consequences that I will discuss in the social circle.

Also, many of these patients have incredibly active brains. Their brain is always active, and none of them symbolically find the ON/OFF button. It leads to a consistent form of rumination.

Moreover, by observing his patients' functioning, the psychotherapist quickly realizes their ability *to give the change*. In psychologic language, this is called *the False Self*. For example, if the person is in considerable Pain (what shows on their facial expressions), they will give a vague "*I am fine*" answer when asked how they are doing. Sometimes a vague "*so-so*", but always accompanied by a broad smile. Body language is not compatible with what the patient says. It can be confusing for doctors or others who are not familiar with this behavior.

3. The social circle

The social consequences are very significant. As mentioned above, withdrawal due to pain and difficulty moving will discourage the person from exercising (kinesiophobia). The slightest movement hurts him/her. It takes time for the patient to realize how critical it is to move in order to prevent the body from becoming *frozen*. It is also part of psychological care.

Absences from work end up having a significant financial impact. Sometimes the person is fired for presenting many medical certificates.

The family and the couple's consequences are often disastrous, as those around them cannot understand the level of Pain, fatigue, exhaustion, withdrawal, and depression. Many patients report moments of psychological abuse. Remarks such as: "*You are useless, you are lazy, you are getting fat, you are becoming a larva, you look like a whale, you are useless, you complain all the time, we cannot do anything because of you, get by"* are legion, and unfortunately not exhaustive.

As Jacques Salomé says: the "You, Kills"! (*Le « Tu », « Tue » ! in French*)

Meetings with friends, family, and acquaintances are sometimes canceled at the last minute. Eventually, friends stop inviting them over. Once again, some friends understand the situation very well and do not take offense.

While the desire to participate is present for the person experiencing pain, their body does not necessarily follow suit. This situation leads to the development of a significant level of guilt. Some patients no longer dare to accept an invitation for fear of not keeping their appointment that day.

Fortunately, a few families, spouses, and friends are interested and informed on the subject. In that case, the person will have benevolence around them. Frequently, the entourage adapts to the Pain and fatigue of the moment and becomes a pro at improvisation: *"How do you feel? Are you all right? A small movie theater? A walk? Come on, let us enjoy it, and let us go! Too tired today? It is okay, another day when you feel better."*

How to explain to a boss that an employee wishes to work but can no longer perform specific work movements? A friend of mine, an EDS-suffering laboratory technician, reported that she had started working part-time again. At first, her boss assigned her administrative tasks, which she considered adequate. She was required to return to the lab very quickly and sometimes stay in the same position for several hours to perform a manipulation. What she goes through daily is a real torture! The choice can be summed up as follows: either she agrees to go back to the laboratory, or she receives her notice! There is no in-between.

When the patient obtains disability status, the boss sometimes adapts the work to accommodate the person in Pain, allowing them to set their own hours, take regular breaks, and work remotely. Although one might believe that disability status would protect the patient, this has yet to be determined in practice.

- **EDS or the paradox disease**

EDS is *a paradoxical disease* that changes rapidly. In the morning, the patient is in a wheelchair, and in the afternoon, he walks his dog, like most people. The pain fluctuates in intensity, and there is only a moment, sometimes short, between needing the chair and walking.

The energy level is also of incomprehensible variability for his relatives. For some, mornings are a time for thorough cleaning because they have the energy. DIY in a workshop and jogging for others. However, after a while, the battery runs down to the point where they stay in place - there is no way to return home or do anything else.

EDS or the "*I am fine but*"... or the *False Self* disease, as I explained above. It is understandable that for the companions it is very disturbing. Fit in the morning, exhausted the next moment.

- **Conclusions**

Reorienting his life: the "*AND*" in power.

Therapeutic management aims to empower patients to manage their Pain and exhaustion. To discover one's rhythm, even if it requires technological assistance. Spend 15 minutes on the move, program on your phone, and then take a break afterward. Use a stopwatch or hourglass. Sometimes the dishes will be done in several times, painting a wall will take several days. One must learn to listen to themselves. It is not a simple task. The patient must be taught self-discipline and self-regulation in order to cope with his painful body and intense exhaustion. Relaxation and micro-naps are particularly beneficial.

All this learning inevitably involves mourning between "*who I was before*" and "*who I am today*." It takes time to achieve this acceptance. Usually, people with EDS get there long before the outside world does.

The goal is to take it easy *and* move at the same time.

Find out more:

➢ Systemic therapy: definition.
  • A Systemic Psychologist is a person who specializes in the engineering of complex systems of interacting elements. The systematist tries to understand how the symptom came into the system (family, couple) and what is its function into.

➢ Psychotherapy in Bioenergetic Analysis. The Sobab: Belgian Society for Bioenergetic Analysis. For more information, see the Sobab website: https://www.sobab.org, and https://usabp.org

➢ Milton H. Erickson Institute of Belgium (IMHEB):
  • https://www.imheb.be ; https://erickson-foundation.org

➢ EMDR (*Eye Movement Desensitization and Reprocessing*) "is a revolutionary method based on scientific studies that treat psychological problems in depth. When processing in EMDR, the causes of the complaints are researched beforehand. Each complaint is treated with a scientifically validated approach. This technique uses eye movements while ensuring patient safety".
  • https://emdr-belgium.be/fr/ or https://emdr.com

➢ TRE stands for "*Tension and Trauma Releasing Exercises*". *David Berceli*, the founder of this method, is an international traumatologist. The TRE is a body method designed to be practiced autonomously, with prior initiation from a certified practitioner. Simple muscular exercises activate a natural reaction of the body: the slackening tremors.
  • https://tre-belgium.com/fr/cest-quoi-le-tre/ or https://tre-usa.org

Parallel worlds between EDS and non-EDS patients

By Dr. Daniel Grossin, General Practitioner, Acupuncturist, graduate of DU Ehlers-Danlos Syndrome.

EDS patients live next to other people, but in a different, parallel world, without necessarily being aware of these differences. As the reverse is possible!

Couples can live out their daily lives for decades without having fully perceived, grasped, or apprehended all the different perceptions of his partner's world, his feelings, and experiences.

The proprioception is different, but also the sensoriality, the emotionality, and all other perceptions including Pain, fatigue, orientation, experience, or merely the fact of preferring to take a shower in the evening!

These dimensions are as poorly understood on the non-EDS side as on the EDS side.

What is the real World? The one with the most people.

Despite my familiarity with the subject and my commitment to these concepts, I came close to making a mistake during a consultation with a young girl, Clotilde, a brilliant student despite having a severely disabling EDS and whom I had been following for several years. I explained to her what the condition, MCAD, she was suffering from and all the new concepts and treatments around it. Clotilde looked at the paintings on the room's walls with acuity during my speech and moved from one to the next with sustained attention, demonstrating great interest. Seeing this, and no doubt offended, I immediately stopped talking. Then she looked at me and immediately began questioning me. I almost made her think about her lack of interest in my speech, but I managed to gather myself in time:

- "You see, Clotilde, it is fortunate that I am familiar with EDS, and that I am confident you would listen to me with the same attention you gave to the paintings. However, you must understand that we, the non-EDSs, cannot fathom your ability to pay such close attention to two or even three things at the same time. You risk getting pushed aside and alienating people if you do not consider the fact that non-EDSs see your incomprehensible ability to give the impression that you are not listening to a discussion as a disinterest."

To illustrate this discordance of perception or its relativity, here below is another example.

When we try to screen for hyperacusis in an EDS patient, we are led to ask:

- "Can you hear well? "
- " ? " Skeptical and questioning air.
- "Better than the others? "
- "?" The same air of incomprehension.
- "Is one of your parents watching television with a too high volume? "
 - "Oh, yes, Daddy! We always ask him, with Mom and my sister Clotilde, to turn it down! "

It is the great classic of the *deaf father* in an EDS family that he is not affected by.

This relativity must be always sought during interrogation. It is not perceived as a singularity, but as normalcy in an EDS family.

To the question:

- "Are you chilly? "

The same *deaf* father, present at the consultation, might answer:

- "You should see the three of them, wrapped in fleeces when they watch television together with a low volume when it is more than 20°C in the room! "

Another example of this relativity, to the question:

- "Are you constipated? "

The answer:

- "No."

Always be clear:

- "How many days can you go without a bowel movement? "
- "Four or five days."

In an EDS family, this can be normal, like Clotilde and her mom.

Yet another example of this relativity and these disjointed, separate worlds:

- "Do you smell well? "
- "? "
- "Are the perfumes sometimes too strong and bother you? "
- "Yes, in a supermarket, I cannot stay too long, and I avoid the perfume shelf. The scent is too strong! "
- "And that can give you a headache or a migraine? "
- "Of course! "

These differences in perception could be amusing if they did not cause embarrassment or even disabling symptoms. Thus, for an EDS patient, odors can cause headaches or migraines, just as loud sounds or bright lights can. The hubbub can deafen an EDS who is unable to respond to questions due to his inability to hear them, as in a so-called *normal* relationship, despite having hyperacusis. Then, EDS patients may exhibit an avoidance reaction and withdraw from these too noisy meetings, leading to the beginning of desocialization.

These parallel worlds can remain unsuspected, even within a couple.

During a meeting for patients and, to explain a possible MCAD, often associated with EDS, we developed a questionnaire, including the very telling *Shower' sign*:

- "Do you have a rash or itching after showering? "
- "Are you tired after the shower? Do you have to rest after the shower? "
- "For these reasons, do you shower at night? "

Furthermore, in the room, a husband exclaims to his wife:

- "Oh, is that why you shower at night? Moreover, does that help you sleep?"
- "And the reason you take it in the morning, it wakes you up," she replied.

This couple had just understood, live, their differences, their worlds, their different experiences for decades through external and medical explanations.

Another skit:

We were with a doctor friend and EDS patient in training on the particular aspects of proprioceptive disorders. I told him that I did not understand the phrase: "EDS patients very often bumping into a door."

- "Well, bumping into a door! Do not ever walk into a door? Have you never bumped into a door frame before? "
- " Uh no, when there is a door, I go through the middle! If I hit myself, I have been pushed! "

Each of us had our own world experience . Since she was a little girl, she has always bumped into the doors, like her mother and sister.

- "So, it is not customary to bump into doors? " She says to me.

A little girl explained in a consultation:

- "Doctor, my room is down the hall, on the right (showing me as usual in EDS... the left!). Well, every time I turn around, I turn around too short! "

Proprioceptive disorders are rarely mentioned in EDS patient complaints. Their clumsiness amuses both themselves and others.

- "I am a Leslie Nielsen! I am a Miss or Mister Disaster! I am clumsy! I am dropping everything. If there is an obstacle in the street, a pole, a banana peel, a garbage can, a rock... it is for me!"
- "Be careful," my father keeps telling me.
- "But I'm careful! "

However, proprioception disorders are among the significant causes of fatigue (one must always, even unconsciously, be very careful and clumsiness hurts!) and pain, if only by promoting sprains and dislocations. It is essential to treat these proprioceptive disorders properly.

EDS patient is most often to minimize his symptoms, his pain. He does not want to complain or be seen as, at least, a hindrance. He will then eventually say that he has a bit of a headache when it is a big headache, or will not say anything, used to having Pain (probably like everyone else!). He will eventually force himself to go for a walk to make an excellent impression to not be seen as an irritating, annoying, in a word: a real "Pain in the ass".

However, he will pay a high price for this effort the next day, with an exacerbation of his pain, fatigue, and difficulties in living free of his omnipresent EDS. "Breathing, even Living, can be painful."

On the other hand, hyper-emotivity can be considered minor or originality of emotion when EDS patients laugh out loud when reading a book or cry big tears, closing it slowly and painfully. I even met a patient who always starts reading books at the end, to avoid being taken aback by an overly dramatic and upsetting outcome!

While some symptoms can be apprehended by non-EDSs, hyperesthesia can be a source of guilt and frustration, which can be the bedrock of deep disagreement if not addressed calmly, immediately, or remotely.

Two sketches:
- "Ouch, you hurt me! "
- "But I just grabbed your arm. "
- "No, you pinched me hard! "
- "You are exaggerating; I assure you I just took your arm gently."
- "I know how I feel anyway! You pinched me, and you're brutal!"

If it stops there, it is like one is planning an explosion at the slightest opportunity. For example, on the one who did not properly close the toothpaste tube. Since we want this to end well for this couple, we are going to continue the dialogue…

For example:

- "I am sorry if I hurt you, I did not mean to, and I had no intention of pinching you."
- "I am also sorry I overreacted. Nevertheless, in this syndrome, the pain may also be surprisingly sharp and dazzling. It is not your fault, my love."

Next episode:

- "Stop caressing me like that; it pisses me off! "
- "But, my darling, it is just little caresses as you like them, and I do too."
- "Stop it, it is infuriating, it is terrible, it is annoying, it is irritating, it is titillating! "

It is up to you to complete this dialogue if you want to defuse the future overflow in this couple.

We realize that the frustrations and guilt are tremendous, and on both sides. There is a difficulty in understanding the world felt and experienced by the other. It must then be explained in order to defuse the bed of a possible future conflict. A mutual explanation is required to understand the other's world and live more harmoniously together.

Auditory, olfactory, taste, and visual sensory perceptions are often exacerbated, and are often oriented toward higher artistic sensibilities. Similarly, memory skills may be above normal levels when attention can be maintained without severe pain and fatigue. Lessons can then be recorded directly on your hard disk as soon as you listen to them! These are still two advantages over the experience of non-EDSs.

To illustrate these different worlds, this phrase is often used by patients trying on compression garments and insoles for the first time:

- "I am in another world! "

And then a final word on the psychological signs of EDS. I, for one, find that there are none or very few.

I find that EDSs have to put up with the unbearable pain and fatigue, the injustices of not knowing about the syndrome, the medical wandering, the psychiatric diagnoses they are given, the difficulties in getting themselves known and recognized by doctors, sometimes by their own families, and the difficulties in accessing treatment, and more.

For all these reasons, there would be cause for depression, but EDSs resist, do not give up, and, surprisingly, most of the time, maintain a positive attitude. Indeed, I would be incapable of enduring even a tenth of this journey, which is strewn with successive pitfalls and injustices.

CHAPTER XXI

EDSian Building:
5 Pillars and 10 Cornerstones

According to S. Daens, 2021©

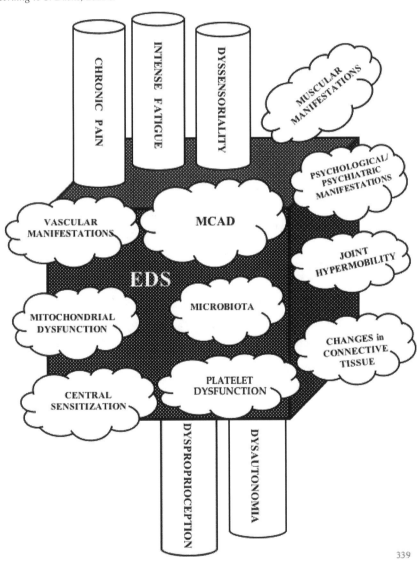

Here is a diagram of my own that synthesizes the main signs and symptoms encountered in Ehlers-Danlos Syndrome and, on the other hand, finally highlights the complexity of the clinical pictures that can be found in our patients.

I called it *EDSian Building*, in reference and in memory of the philosophy course given in the final year of high school by one of my teachers, Professor Paul Ronflette, abbot of his state. This brilliant teacher, who has since died, was the bearer of three doctorates (history, philosophy, and theology) and completed the School of Saint Thomas Aquinas (see Thomism, Catholic University of Louvain - UCL). In philosophy classes, he often spoke to us about the *Kantian building* concerning the thoughts of the German philosopher Emmanuel Kant (Königsberg, East Prussia: 1724 - 1804), founder of transcendental idealism. The complexity of Kant's thought, summarized by this brilliant teacher as a building, a temple of the mind composed of successive layers, all constituting something stable and coherent.

In my EDSian Building, I have retained five main Pillars, which are like the load-bearing walls of the clinic for patients with EDS (a little wink to my daddy, an architect, who disappeared too soon):

➢ Chronic Pain (1).
➢ Intense Fatigue (2).
➢ Dysproprioception (3).
➢ Dyssensoriality (4).
➢ Dysautonomia (5).

From experience, all EDS patients are affected by the Five Pillars at the same time. To put it simply, they are tired, and they are in pain, they are clumsy, they have disturbances of the autonomic nervous system and sense organs. Alongside these five fundamental Pillars, there are ten Cornerstones which add to the clinical picture.

Selected items:

➢ Joint hypermobility (1).
➢ The MCAD associated with EDS (MCA/EDS) (2).

- Changes in connective tissue (3).
- Muscular manifestations (4).
- Dysbiosis, the vital role of the microbiota (5).
- Mitochondrial dysfunction (Krebs' cycle) (6).
- Vascular manifestations (arterial and venous) (7).
- Psychological/Psychiatric manifestations (8).
- Platelet dysfunction (9).
- Central sensitization (10).

These ten Cornerstones are not what some call co-morbidities; many colleagues worldwide have the same opinion. These signs and symptoms are not just in the background; they are sometimes prevalent and can lead to severe disability, false accusations of child abuse (due to bruises, hematomas, and fractures), or abusive psychiatrization. These Cornerstones often remain heavy to drag and move.

Some will be tempted to say that illnesses such as gastrointestinal, gynecological, or respiratory manifestations are not on this diagram. The Pillars and Cornerstones are the most important things to remember every day. I consider that the other attacks, not taken up individually by the Pillars or Cornerstones, result from a compilation of certain Pillars and Cornerstones. On the other hand, some Cornerstones overlap at first glance (such as connective tissue changes and vascular damage), but it seemed easier to me to categorize them in this way to express the full diversity of signs and symptoms presented by patients. They can be more readily associated with a particular clinical situation.

Explanations:

Let us take the example of some breathing difficulties in EDS; they could be a compilation of the following types: connective tissue changes + dysproprioception + muscle damage + MCAD.

For specific gastrointestinal manifestations, it could be changing in connective tissue + dysautonomia + dysproprioception + alteration of the microbiota + MCAD.

For certain gynecological disorders: changes in connective tissue + platelet dysfunction + alteration of the vaginal microbiota + MCAD + dysproprioception + dyssensoriality.

For algoneurodystrophy: connective tissue changes + MCAD + central sensitization + dysautonomia.

Etc.

This scheme allows for all possible associations to explain most signs and symptoms in EDS.

So, remember:

5 Fundamental Pillars and 10 Cornerstones.

Chapter XXII

EDS Treatments:
Ad Causas et Consecutiones

By Dr. Stéphane Daens

Continuing my Greco-Roman and philosophical analogy, inspired by ancient texts, the title can call out: *Ad Causas et Consecutiones (about the causes and consequences).*

Many doctors and caregivers sometimes make desperate attempts to treat the consequences of an illness rather than the causes. They only relieve the patient's signs and symptoms, but not their origin, their starting point. This approach has the potential to result in fundamental care errors.

Two examples:

➢ An undiagnosed EDS patient consults his family physician or specialist for recurrent tendonitis. Without a further examination of the patient, the doctor performs a peritendinous infiltration with cortisone derivatives. He may have to see this patient repeatedly, and each time he may opt for the same local treatment.

Rather than treating the patient with infiltration from the outset, it would have been preferable to look for joint hypermobility, dysproprioception, or even EDS. However, the doctor has chosen to treat the consequence (recurrent tendonitis) and not the cause (hypermobility, dysproprioception).

However, joint hypermobility and proprioceptive disorders have resulted in chronic tendon inflammation. A tendon generally straddles a joint. If it moves too much in the presence of a hypermobile and unstable joint, it will become inflamed over time.

To treat the causes: the problematic joint(s) should have been stabilized, and proprioception restored. A stabilizing brace and compression garment could have been prescribed. After two weeks of this treatment, corticosteroid injections could have been considered only at that time. There is, in this exemplary case, at least one Pillar (dysproprioception) and two Cornerstones (connective tissue changes and joint hypermobility).

> ➤ A woman consults after experiencing syncopal-like discomfort, migraines, palpitations, and drops in blood pressure (mainly when standing or sitting for long periods without moving her extremities). Additionally, she suffers from severe fatigue, allergic rashes, irritable bowel, and interstitial cystitis. She is afraid to leave her house and is anxious.

She saw her family doctor and then a cardiologist. She was prescribed beta-blockers (bisoprolol) for palpitations and migraines, or even topiramate (it is an antiepileptic, prescribed as an adjunct against migraines). Exercise and a salt-free healthy diet were recommended. She was naturally encouraged to manage stress and consult a psychologist. Caregivers recommended an anti-anxiety medication.

Ah! Stress, the root cause of all of our society's ills! The consequences are addressed, but the causes are ignored. It is a fallacious reasoning here. Palpitations, malaise, migraine headaches, digestive disorders, stress, and anxiety were considered separately.

However, why does she not walk anymore? Why doesn't she go out anymore?

She is no longer walking because she is afraid of fainting or feeling worse.

Unfortunately, the treatments instituted by these doctors could exacerbate these symptoms:

- The non-selective β-blockers (bisoprolol) could decrease cardiac contractility.
- The salt-free diet could exacerbate the decrease in circulating blood volume (these first two elements could worsen discomfort and blood pressure disorders).
- Potential side effects could develop under topiramate.
- And, the icing on the cake, this patient could be abusively psychiatrized (prescription of anxiolytics, offer consultation in psychology or psychiatry).

These side effects are those of treating the consequences.

In this case, the causes would be dysautonomia + connective tissue changes + vascular damage (venous pooling) + MCAD + microbiota alteration. That is at least one Pillar and four Cornerstones.

Therefore, the cause's treatment consists, in the absence of contraindications such as severe hypertension, renal failure, and cardiac decompensation:

- Encourage drinking at least two liters of fluids per day.
- Eating salty food or adding 3 to 6g of salt per day (in capsules) or/and drinkable electrolytes supplements.
- Exercising regularly, moving her extremities.
- Wear compressive garments.
- Adding Midodrine or Fludrocortisone, if necessary.
- For MCAD, prescribing antihistamines, Cromoglycate, and vitamin C, for example.
- Taking suitable probiotics to improve intestinal microbiota.

It is the treatment of the causes rather than the treatment of the consequences.

In both cases, the must would have been to evoke an EDS by thoroughly questioning, examining, and believing these patients.

Caregivers always have to consider the causes rather than the consequences. Moreover, This approach should be applied to all areas of medicine.

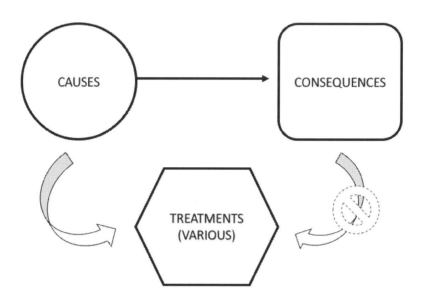

The management of EDS patients should be a step-by-step process

EDS patients need to be listened to and relieved quickly. They require encouragement and an broader perspective to get better.

Therefore treatment must be initiated during the first consultation. The latter will need to provide some measure of relief and help patients in developing a positive perspective for the future. This treatment should not discourage them, but rather motivate them to persevere and continue their care.

Therefore, there is a hierarchy of therapeutic priorities.

It is not essential to wish to fix everything during the initial consultation. That would be an illusion! At first glance, what irritates patients the most is intense fatigue and chronic pain. Two particularly disabling symptoms, each of which is multifactorial in origin.

Above all, it is necessary to keep in mind that:

> *Too many treatments kill treatments!*
>   o The lack of patient compliance with the mass of pills to be ingested is evident.

> *To want to treat everything, we drown the fish!*
>   o It will not be possible to treat everything right away; what works well and the eventual side effects of each treatment would be unknown.

> *Treatments are expensive!*
>   o Medications for people with hereditary illnesses that cause disability are often costly, significantly if several members of the same family are affected.

Therefore, when dealing with a patient with chronic pain, disabling fatigue and other very varied problems, the advice here is to manage the signs and symptoms along different axes and in a preferential order:

1. Dysautonomia - Microbiota – MCAD.
2. Dysproprioception – Joint Hypermobility - Muscular manifestations.
3. Central sensitization.
4. Dyssensoriality.
5. Psychological / Psychiatric manifestations.
6. Residual clinical signs and symptoms.

Let us call this a Casuistic approach. Casuistry is a method of solving problems through concrete action, based on general principles on the one hand and the study of specific cases experienced on the other.

It is a fundamental approach in Ehlers-Danlos Syndrome, unknown by some (most) caregivers.

The first two axes are generally taken care of at the first consultation.

It is crucial to understand that the average wait time between two appointments for a specialized consultation for Ehlers-Danlos Syndrome is more than a year.

Chapter XXIII

GENERAL CONCLUSIONS

By Dr. Stéphane Daens

> « *It is done. It is a performative verb.*
> *It must be said — as it must be said in the*
> *absolute sense of the verb — and it is done.* »
>
> Amélie Nothomb, *Soif (Thirst)*, 2019

The **Ehlers-Danlos Syndrome** is a complex, confusing to the layman, polymorphic and fluctuating condition. It is gradually coming out of oblivion, largely thanks to the hard work of Professor Claude Hamonet (author of: *"Ehlers-Danlos: La Maladie oubliée par la Médecine"*, i.e. the *Disease forgotten by Medicine*, in English), but also to many doctors, paramedics, and patient associations throughout the world.

EDS is neither a rare disease nor an orphan disease: many treatments exist to improve patients' quality of life and their reintegration into this increasingly dehumanized society.

Let us remember that rheumatoid arthritis affects between 0.5 and 1% of the population and spondyloarthropathies 1%. Duchenne muscular dystrophy would affect 1/4000 people.

Every doctor knows about these diseases.

When you type *Ehlers-Danlos* in the "*American National Bookstore of Medicine - PubMed*" search engine (pubmeb.nbci.nlm.nih.gov), you will find more than 4480 references of articles on EDS, including more than 1715 in the last ten years, or 38% of the publications on the subject. The oldest dates from 1936, written by *Frederik Parkes Weber*.

Surprisingly, this disease, which generates situations of disability, sometimes significant, is not, or very little, taught in medical schools throughout the world. Doctors mainly retain a too elastic skin (comparing patients to one of the Fantastic 4) and hallucinating generalized hypermobility (worthy of a circus contortionist of the Roaring Twenties). Neither of these two clinical features is constant or peremptory for a diagnosis of EDS.

The term "*Ehlers-Danlos*" itself is misleading: even though *Edvard Lauritz Ehlers* did describe a single case of this disease at the end of the 19th century, *Alexandre Danlos* was mistaken and, despite himself, caused more than 100 years of confusion in the minds of doctors. All this is because of one mislabeling error, one misclassification.

Unfortunately, the damage was done!

The photos of his clinical case, one of the first in everyday medicine, have been shown all over the Universities and the World, misleading teachers, researchers, and students.

The damage was done!

It only took a second confusion to lead EDS into the abyss of oblivion, that of the systematic labeling of painful and misunderstood patients in the Fibromyalgia and Psychiatry boxes.

Fragmented and piecemeal Medicine, worthy of the predictions of Charlie Chaplin's film, *Modern Times (1936)*, has finished the pernicious work already begun: we no longer listen to patients, we no longer examine them, we no longer believe in the clinic, we only believe in imaging and biological examinations.

Health professionals no longer talk to each other; they no longer exchange. From multidisciplinarity, We have moved on to the *Modern Times* of *Every Man for Himself, No One for the Patient*.

It is unacceptable and intolerable mistreatment, and this is the most serious, of patients who are often in great physical pain and, as if that were not enough, mistreatment by some colleagues of doctors who diagnose and follow up patients with Ehlers-Danlos Syndrome.

In an e-mail received in March 2020, a lady talks about a meeting with a Belgian rheumatologist, a few years older than me. She first tells about her signs and symptoms, as well as those of her two daughters, which she explained to the rheumatologist in question: joint hyperlaxity, congenital hip dysplasia, cracked and dislocated joints, Arnold-Chiari syndrome, scoliosis, retraction of the hamstrings, repeated sprains, tachycardia, hyperacusis, bruxism, and so forth.

It is a very evocative picture of Ehlers-Danlos Syndrome, not to say "a textbook case".

She then wrote that the rheumatologist did not want to consider that all these signs and symptoms were related and that he would have told her: "*If you want to be diagnosed with EDS, go to Dr. Daens, I studied with him, and he would find EDS even in a cat! And in any case, skin biopsies prove nothing since hyperlaxity modifies collagen*".

I would retort to this confrere, but I will not, that the Doctor *Lucie Chevallier*, Senior Lecturer in Molecular and Medical Genetics at the *Alfort National Veterinary School* (EVNA), whom I had the pleasure of meeting at the last Colloquium organized by *Professor Claude Hamonet*, would be delighted to explain to him that animals do indeed suffer from EDS. EDS would affect certain breeds of horses, calves, and dogs, but probably also cats. These adorable animals suffer from joint and digestive complications. Nor will I remind him that the Code of Ethics forbids him to criticize another colleague by name in front of a patient. Finally, I will say that it is the modified collagen that induces hyperlaxity and not the other way around.

No, I think this colleague is a lost cause for EDS. However, this case is exemplary. I have accumulated dozens of these testimonials that may at first glance seem tiring and despairing.

"Man is a victim of the conditioning of souls, of sanctions and of permissions," said Charlie Chaplin.

This sentence particularly echoes the current management of Dysautonomia, POTS, MCAD, and, as far as we are concerned, Ehlers-Danlos Syndrome.

I will try to explain why this mistreatment persists thanks to a theorem invented by C. K. Prahalad and G. Hamel to illustrate their book on Business and Management: *"Competing for the Future,"* a Bestseller published by *Harvard Business Review Press* in 1996.

They explained this:

> ➢ Take five monkeys and put them in a cage. In this cage, hang a banana in a corner with a small ladder to reach it. Shortly afterward, a monkey decides to climb the ladder to catch this banana. Then, spray the other monkeys, who are still down there, with cold water. They will not look too happy. When a second monkey tries to take the banana, respray the other monkeys. After a few failed attempts with such a cold shower, no more monkeys in the cage trying to climb the ladder to take the hanging fruit.

> ➢ Then take one of the monkeys out of the cage and replace it with a monkey that has not seen or heard anything from the previous little merry-go-round or sprayed water. After a short time, this new monkey, seeing the banana, rushes towards the ladder. Before he can catch the coveted fruit, the other four monkeys jump on him and beat him, preventing them from being sprayed with cold water.

> ➢ Then, replace one of the four monkeys at the start with a second new monkey. When he tries to go up the ladder, again, the other monkeys in the cage, including the first new monkey, rush to hit him.

> ➢ Follow that process until new ones replace all the first monkeys.

> ➢ None of the new monkeys will try to get the banana at the end. Even though none of them have been sprayed on, they will avoid the banana!

Prahalad and Hamel's lesson was: "*Precedents, enacted into policy manuals, corporate processes, and training programs often outlive the particular industry context that created them.*"

Thus: "Precedents survive the context that created them."

In other words, it is about the "continuity of myths" through "social culture," without any questioning, whether it is societal culture, corporate culture, family culture, or, as far as we are concerned, medical culture.

For these reasons, when our patients go to the emergency department, they have turned away with hysteria diagnoses, Münchhausen, depression, anxiety, and more.

Doctors do not know why they misdiagnose patients with EDS, MCAD, POTS, or Dysautonomia, but they do... Because that is the way it is always done with these patients!

Medicine is on the move, and it is evolving. A caregiver cannot afford to be complacent about what is learned by graduation time! Mine goes back more than 25 years. There was no internet or cell phone then. Yes, telephone booths were enthroned around every corner! We had to go to the library to read scientific articles, go to medical meetings, talk to each other, write letters, exchange ideas. At that time, not so long ago, it was understandable that EDS was forgotten and not studied as it should have been. We could, in the past, only rely on our teachers' teachings, and not everyone was curious about everything.

With all the information sources available to us, in a few "clicks," we cannot fail to evolve and learn.

It is our role as caregivers, and it is our responsibility to patients to become better. EDS patients are in great pain. Our job and vocation are to welcome them, listen to them, and even refer them to another specialist when our medical limits are reached. It is our responsibility to (in)train ourselves to be able to carry out their medical follow-up, in order to relieve them as well as possible, to give them back their confidence in this piecemeal and inhuman Medicine, to give them back confidence in themselves and us.

This book aims to:

Bring to light the founding mechanisms of EDS based on connective tissue's altered properties, dysproprioception, dysautonomia, and the interactions between our body and mind; the brain-body concept (the Porges' Theory), dyssensoriality. The microbiota's crucial role, the genetic and epigenetic theories that influence the evolution and transmission of the disease, central sensitization, pain pathways, MCAD, mitochondrial and platelet dysfunction, muscle and cardiovascular damage are also part of the presentation.

It all makes sense, and this book must be seen as a Global Vision to Tame the Ehlers-Danlos Syndrome in its complexity.

What I retain from this Third Part

The GERSED Belgium

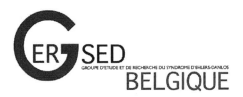

GERSED Belgium (non-profit association) is the Study and Research Group on Ehlers-Danlos Syndrome (Belgium), created in October 2017 by health professionals (specialists, general practitioners, and paramedics) involved in Ehlers-Danlos Syndrome. It is recognized as an EDS Experts Network by the ORPHANET portal since February 2020.

Website : www.gersedbelgique.com.
Email : Contact@gersedbelgique.com

The purpose of this association of health professionals is:

♦ The exchange of knowledge and experience on the diagnosis and treatment of Ehlers-Danlos Syndrome (EDS) and Hypermobility Spectrum Disorders (HSD).
♦ Bibliographic information.
♦ The organization of epidemiological investigations.
♦ The enrichment of the semiological knowledge of EDS.
♦ Therapeutic perspective and evaluation of treatments.
♦ The organization of training courses for health professionals and social actors.
♦ The organization of clinical and therapeutic education sessions for patients and their families.
♦ The production of scientific work on EDS.
♦ The publication of books on EDS.
♦ To have the social and therapeutic rights of EDS patients recognized.

Composition of the Board

Chairman:
Doctor Stéphane DAENS, *MD, DATC, Internal Medicine & Rheumatology, Dilbeek, Belgium*

Secretary:
Mrs. Patricia HERLANT, *Special educator, Tournai, Belgium.*

Treasurer:
Mrs. Tamara SADIGHI, *Ortho-Bandagist, Brussels, Belgium.*

Honorary Presidents

Professor Claude HAMONET, *MD, PhD, M.D. Physical and Rehabilitation Medicine, Paris, France.*

Professor Rodney GRAHAME, *MD, PhD, Rheumatologist, London, UK.*

Professor Stephen W. PORGES, *PhD, Neuroscience, North Carolina, USA.*

Professor Jaime F. BRAVO, *MD, Rheumatologist, Santiago de Chile, and Denver USA.*

Professor Antonio BULBENA, *MD, PhD, MSc, Psychiatrist, Barcelona, Spain.*

Professor Andràs PALDI, *MSc, PhD, Geneticist and Epigeneticist, Paris, France.*

Professor Michel VERVOORT, *MSc, PhD, Geneticist, Paris, France.*

Professor Marco CASTORI, *MD, PhD, Medical Genetics, Milano, Italy.*

Doctor Pradeep CHOPRA, *MD, MHCM, Algologist, Brown Medical School, RI, USA.*

Doctor Trinh HERMANNS-LE, *MD, PhD, Dermatologist, Verviers, Belgium.*

Doctor Kambyse SAMII, *MD, Internal Medicine & Cardiology, Brussels, Belgium.*

Doctor Georges OBEID, *MD, Internal Medicine & Cardiology, Brussels, Belgium.*

Honorary members

Doctor **Isabelle DUBOIS-BROCK**, *MD, Clinical Researcher, New York, USA.* Chairman of GERSED France.

Doctor Katja KOVACIC, *MD, Pediatric Gastroenterology, Wisconsin, USA.*

Association recognized by:

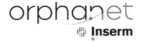

The Author and Co-authors
of the Book

Doctor Stéphane DAENS, *MD, DATC*
Main Author
Internal Medicine & Rheumatology (Belgium)

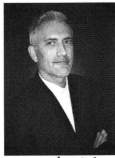

Stéphane Daens holds a doctorate in Medicine, Surgery, and Childbirth (1995), and a specialization diploma in Internal Medicine & Rheumatology, from the Université Libre de Bruxelles (ULB) in Belgium. He finished his Residency and Fellowship at the Brugmann University Hospital (Brussels). He is graduated in Traditional Chinese Acupuncture (DATC), and trained in musculoskeletal ultrasound, neuro-physiological examinations, electromyography, needle-arthroscopic synovial biopsy, radiation protection and bone densitometry (by DEXA and ultrasound). In 2017, he founded the GERSED Belgium with other health professionals. He is the chairman of this group. Dr. Stéphane Daens is particularly interested in the complex interactions between mast cells, microbiota, and autonomic nervous system in EDS. He designed the concept of Global Vision of EDS, and developed the potential role of Epigenetics in order to explain the clinical differences that exist between patients, as well as the evolution of the disease over time. In 2020, he wrote his first book in French, with other international co-authors: *Apprivoiser le Syndrome d'Ehlers-Danlos*.

Doctor Isabelle DUBOIS - BROCK, *MD*
Main Co-author
EDS Clinical Research (USA)

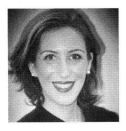

Dr. Isabelle Brock holds a degree in medicine from Windsor University School of Medicine, a certification in diagnosis and treatment for Ehlers-Danlos Syndrome (EDS) from Paris Est Créteil University in Paris, France, and a certification in Ayurvedic medicine for medical professionals from the Institute of Ayurveda &

Alternative Medicine, University of Ruhuna, Sri Lanka. Dr. Brock currently serves as President for the Research & Study Group for EDS (GERSED) in France and is a member of the Belgian GERSED. Her efforts in the support of EDS research have led to her to founding President and CEO of the medical research company, QoLify (Quality of Life Improvements for You) as well as co-founding Clinical Paradigms and 3- Pillars Therapeutics for seeing EDS patients regularly. She is a visiting scientist at Indiana University in the Department of Medical & Molecular Genetics, and the Health Center for EDS. In addition to service as the Chief Scientific Officer at the EDS Initiative – Deutschland, Dr. Brock holds memberships to the Allergy, Immunology & Pain Management Working Groups of the International Consortium on EDS and its Comorbidities as well as in the AHEAD Coalition and the 'Breaking Down Barriers' Initiative of the EDS Society. As the Global Coordinator for Centers and Networks of Excellence for the EDS society she aims to establish networks around the globe to give patients with EDS better access to care. She is a member of the scientific committee of the Foundation for Research & Advocacy in Muscle Pain Education (FRAME) and formerly held positions as Lead Scientist at the Hospital Hotel Dieu de Paris, and at Ellasanté, Paris. Further accomplishments include her having co-created and taught tele-courses on EDS for medical professionals and spearheaded the establishing of two clinics dedicated to helping patients with EDS and its comorbidities. Before her medical studies she obtained a bachelor's degree in philology from the University of Stockholm, Sweden, and is fluent in English, French, German, Italian and Swedish.

Professor Claude HAMONET, MD, PhD
Physical Medicine and Rehabilitation (France)

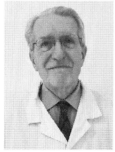

Claude Hamonet is a former gold medal intern at the Paris Hospitals, a specialist in Physical Medicine and Rehabilitation (European Board of Physical Medicine and Rehabilitation), Doctor in Social Anthropology (Université de Paris V Descartes) and University Professor (Université Paris 12, Université Paris-Est-Créteil - UPEC). He is a former Head of the Department of the Paris Hospitals, former Director of the Faculty of Communication and Insertion in the Society (UPEC) and former international disability expert at the WHO, he was also Adjunct Professor of Anthropology at the University of Kansas (USA), disability expert at the FRSQ, and co-project leader (*Assistive devices for paralyzed persons*) at the Commission de Recherche en Génie Biomédical auprès de la CEE (D.G. XII) in Brussels. He is a member of the Ehlers-Danlos Society and the International Society of Medical Ethics. He has gained experience through the follow-up of an international cohort of nearly 6,000 Ehlers-Danlos patients at the University Hospital Center in Paris, then in specialized EDS consultations at the ELLAsanté Medical Center for Diagnosis and Prevention in Paris, as well as in Boulogne Billancourt at the Medical Centre *Integrative Systemic Medicine*. He was the creator, along with Professor Jean-Michel Graciès, from the University Diploma *Ehlers Danlos Syndrome* (2014) at UPEC. He is the author of the book: *Ehlers-Danlos, la maladie oubliée par la Médecine* (*Éditions L'Harmattan 2018, 2019*). He organized five international university symposia, held in Paris, on diagnosis, treatment, and EDS screening. He is heavily invested in preventing the abusive removal of children, on suspicion of parental violence, due to the non-diagnosis of Ehlers-Danlos disease. By applying his experience in PMR, he has been able to put in place a set of effective treatments that have changed the defeatist view of this disease.

Professor Jaime F. BRAVO, *MD*
Rheumatology (Chile and USA)

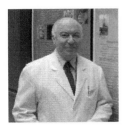

A doctor specializing in Rheumatology graduated from the University of Chile Medical School (1954 - 1961). He was awarded the title of Professor of Medicine and Rheumatology at the University of Colorado in 1998. He teaches students in various hospitals and also works in private practice in Denver, USA. He is a member of *Arthritis Foundation* for more than 34 years. He returned to Chile in 1998 and became interested in EDS and dysautonomia. He is a professor at the University of Chile and works at the Hospital San Juan de Dios in Santiago. He is one of the emblematic figures, throughout the world, of Dysautonomia in EDS.

Professor Michel VERVOORT, MSc, PhD
Genetics (France)

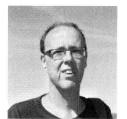

After his Master in Zoological Sciences at the Université Libre de Bruxelles in 1992 (ULB), Michel Vervoort obtained a Doctorate in Zoological Sciences. He then completed a Post-Doctorate in Genetics at the Université de Montpellier II (France). His scientific research activity is very prolific and international (ULB, University of Heidelberg, Montpellier II, Toulouse III, Paris-Sud, Centre of Molecular Genetics - UPR CNRS 2143, Institut Jacques Monod- UMR 7592). He is in charge of the "Stem Cells, Development and Evolution" team. His favorite subjects are the Developmental Genetics, Comparative Genomics, and Neurogenesis, Phylogeny, and Stem Cells. He is a professor of first-class universities since 2013 (Université Paris Diderot, Paris 7, France) and an Honorary Member of the *Institut Universitaire de France*. He has also participated in the writing of several books.

Professor Andràs PALDI, MSc, PhD
Genetics and Epigenetics (France)

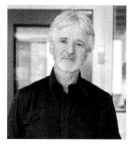

Born in Budapest, Andràs Paldi graduated in biochemistry and holds a Doctor of Science from the Eötvös L. University in Budapest, obtained in 1983 and 1988, respectively. He has carried out numerous research activities in molecular genetics, genomic fingerprinting, and epigenetics. He worked for INSERM (Institut Jacques Monod, Institut Cochin of molecular genetics, 1988 - 2003). He has been Director of the Molecular Genetics Laboratory at the *École Pratique des Hautes Études* (EPHE), Life and Earth Sciences Section, since 1995 (Paris, France). He has been working at the GENETHON (home laboratory) since 2004. He published numerous international articles and is the author of *"L'épigénétique ou la nouvelle ère de l'Hérédité"* (Éditions Le Pommier 2009; 2018).

Professor Anne MAITLAND, *MD, PhD*
Internal Medicine, Allergy and Immunology (USA)

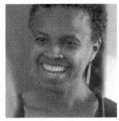

Dr. Maitland was named one of New York Times 2011 Super Doctors and one of America's Top 21 Women's Doctors by Lifescript.com in 2009. She is a Fellow of the American College of Allergy, Asthma and Immunology and a member of the American Academy of Allergy, Asthma and Immunology. Dr. Maitland is very active in local societies and the surrounding communities, to increase awareness of immune mediated disorders. She is also involved with research to continually improve the treatments of allergies, asthma and recurrent infections. Her clinical focus includes the diagnosis and treatment of allergic skin disorders, allergic rhinitis (hayfever), drug allergies, food allergies/sensitivities, asthma and recurrent infections. Education: MD, PhD from the University of Pennsylvania in Philadelphia, PA. Residency - Internal Medicine at the Brigham and Women's Hospital in Boston, MA. Fellowship - Allergy & Immunology at the Brigham and Women's Hospital and Mount Sinai Hospital in New York, NY. Certifications: American Board of Allergy & Immunology, American Board of Internal Medicine.

Dr. Pradeep CHOPRA, *MD, MHCM*
Pain Medicine (USA)

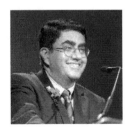

Pradeep Chopra completed his Anesthesia residency from Harvard Medical School. He then went on to complete his Fellowship in Pain Management, also from Harvard Medical School. Dr. Chopra is double Board Certified in Pain Management and Anesthesiology by the American Board of Anesthesiology. He holds the prestigious appointment of Assistant Professor (Clinical), Department of Medicine, Brown Medical School, Division of Biology and Medicine and Assistant Professor of Anesthesiology (Adjunct), Boston University School of Medicine. Dr. Chopra has a keen interest in both Acute and Chronic Pain Management. His areas of interest are Back Pain, Neck Pain, Joint Pain, Arthritis, and Muscle Pains. He has an extensive experience in complex Pain states, Headaches, Neuropathic Pain and most chronic pain conditions. His approach to treatment of Chronic and Complex Pain states is multi-disciplinary and multi-modality, including Interventional Pain Management, Physical Therapy, Relaxation Techniques, Biofeedback and Psychological Approach. His approach for Chronic Pain patients is to get them to a point to allow them to do the things they want to do and not let Pain take over their lives. He has a very 'out of the box' approach to treating complex and refractory conditions. He has a special interest in managing complex pain conditions such as Complex regional Pain Syndrome (CRPS), Reflex Sympathetic Dystrophy (RSD), Collagen disorders such as Ehlers Danlos Syndrome (EDS).

Professor Stephen W. PORGES, PhD
Behavioral Neuroscience (USA)

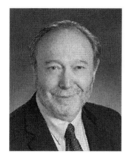

Professor Stephen Porges is a *Distinguished University Scientist* of the Kinsey Institute (Indiana University). He is a Professor in the Department of Psychiatry at the University of North Carolina and Professor Emeritus at the University of Illinois and the University of Maryland (USA). In 1994, he conceived the Polyvagal Theory that deals with the parasympathetic nervous system's dual aspect. This theory stresses the importance of the interaction between physiological state and behavioral regulation. He has written more than 300 scientific articles and several books.

Dr. Katja KOVACIC, MD, PhD
Pediatric Gastroenterology (USA)

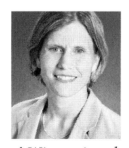

Katja Kovacic is an Assistant Professor of Pediatric Gastroenterology at Medical College of Wisconsin (USA). Graduated from Dartmouth-Brown Medical School, she completed her training in Gastroenterology at the Medical College of Wisconsin. She is the Director of the "Motility and Cyclic Vomiting Syndrome Programs" at the Children's Hospital of Wisconsin where she specializes in functional gastrointestinal and motility disorders. She has published numerous articles relating to pediatric functional gastrointestinal disorders including the association with joint hypermobility. She is working on evaluating different forms of non-invasive neuromodulation therapies in hypermobile EDS patients (auricular neurostimulation of the vagus nerve, for example).

Dr. Jacek KOLACZ, *PhD*
Assistant Research Scientist (USA)

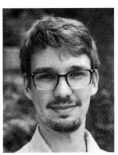

Jacek Kolacz is a research associate at the Kinsey Institute, Indiana University, Bloomington (USA). He is a member of the Socioneural Physiology Laboratory and the Traumatic Stress Research Laboratory. It studies how life experiences shape biological systems, psychological well-being, and physical health over time. It examines the bio-behavioral factors that promote danger and resilience to trauma, their effects on psychological well-being and physical health, and their influences on relationships, social interactions, and sexual health.

Dr. Norman MARCUS, *MD, DABPM*
Pain Medicine (USA)

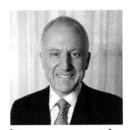

Dr. Marcus is the Director of Clinical Muscle Pain Research at Weill-Cornell Medicine in the Departments of Anesthesiology and Neurological Surgery. He is a member of the Ehlers Danlos Syndrome International Consortium and serves on the Pain Committee. He has focused on the study of pain throughout his career, with a special interest in muscle pain. He is a past president of the American Academy of Pain Medicine and is currently on the BOD of the American Board of Pain Medicine. He is President of the Foundation for Research and Advocacy for Muscle Pain Education (FRAME). He started and co-directed the first pain center in New York City at Montefiore Hospital from 1978-1984, then established and directed the Lenox Hill Hospital Inpatient Pain Center from 1984-1998. From 1995-1998, he directed the Princess Margaret Pain Treatment and Functional Restoration Center in Windsor, UK. He has authored numerous papers, textbook chapters, and lay books on the etiology and treatment of muscle pain and on the evaluation of pain treatment outcomes. He received a $500,000 grant from Medtronic to study outcomes at pain centers for the American Academy of Pain Medicine in 1990. He has 3 patents on his approach to evaluate and treat muscle pain and is currently working on producing an instrument that will allow most clinicians to identify and treat specific muscles that are the source of common back, neck, and shoulder pains.

Professor Antonio BULBENA, MD, MSc, PhD
Psychiatry (Spain)

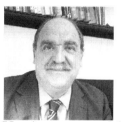 Antonio Bulbena, MD, PhD, MSc (Cantab) is professor and Chairman of Psychiatry at the Department of Psychiatry and Forensic Medicine in the Universitat Autonoma Barcelona, and Research Director of the Institute of Neuropsychiatry and Addictions Hospital del Mar Barcelona. He did his medical training at the U. Autonoma Medical School, and obtained his MD at the University of Barcelona. He spent three years in the Department of Psychiatry (Prof M Roth) at the University of Cambridge, Addenbrookes and Fulbourn Hospital, training in clinical research in Psychiatry, obtaining a MSc under Prof G Berrios and Prof. E.Miller. Dr. Bulbena has been doing extensively teaching in several medical schools in Spain for the last 25 years. He has also carried out an active career in management, either as director of the hospital and also creating networks of services including general hospital, psychiatric hospital, community care, inpatient and outpatient adult and child psychiatry, mobile teams, inpatient and outpatient addiction psychiatry. His research includes topics like dementia and pseudodementia, psychiatric emergencies, memory and depression, chocolate and carbohydrates, clinical measurement in psychiatry, phobias, seasonality and biometeorology. More recently he has carried out international comparisons on attitudes towards psychiatry among medical students and also advanced research in neuroimaging. His most prominent line of research is the relationship between anxiety disorders and somatic conditions as he observed and originally described in 1988 the strong link between several anxiety disorders and joint laxity (a benign hereditary collagen). This strong partnership has extensively researched by his group in the last 25 years. He has put forward a

new model of anxiety disorders based on the relationship between the connective tissue and the autonomic nervous system.

Professor Carolina BAEZA-VELASCO, *MSc, PhD*
Clinical Psychology (France)

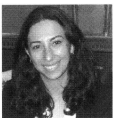

Carolina Baeza-Velasco is Associate Professor on Psychopathology at Université Paris Descartes – Sorbonne Paris Cité, and researcher at the Department of Emergency Psychiatry and Post-Acute Care of the University Hospital of Montpellier in France. She is clinical psychologist (University Andres Bello, Chile) with a master degree and a PhD in psychopathology by the Autonomous University of Barcelona. Her PhD thesis focused on the psychopathology associated to the Joint Hypermobility Syndrome under the direction of Prof. Antonio Bulbena. Dr. Baeza-Velasco subsequently obtained her Habilitation for Research Training at the University Paris Descartes. Her professional background includes clinical and research experiences in several health institutions in France, Spain, and Chile. Her main research interests are the psychopathology and neurodevelopmental problems associated to joint hypermobility and hypermobility related disorders as well as the psychosocial factors associated to pain and disability in chronic painful conditions.

Dr. Andrea BULBENA-CABRE, *MD, MSc, PhD*
Psychiatry (Spain, USA)

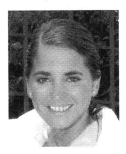

Andrea Bulbena-Cabré, MD, PhD, MSc is a research fellow at the Icahn School of Medicine at Mount Sinai/Bronx VAMC (Mental Illness research, Education and Clinical Center). She obtained her MD at the University Autonoma of Barcelona and completed her psychiatry residency training at Yale University. Prior to this, she also trained at New York Medical College and participated in exchange programs at NYU and at the University of Monterrey (Mexico). She has worked as co- investigator in several clinical trials at the Barcelona Biomedical Institute (Spain) and her interest in research led her to complete a Master's Degree in Clinical Research methodology and a PhD at the University Autonoma of Barcelona. Her main line of research involves the study and understanding of the interface between somatic and mental illness, and particularly between new somatic biomarkers, anxiety disorders and related conditions. She has studied the anxiety-joint hypermobility phenomena in bipolar disorder and other major mental illnesses as part of her PhD program at the University Autonoma of Barcelona. Throughout the course her career, she has received academic and research awards and has been particularly involved in studying the psychiatric aspects of the hypermobile Ehlers-Danlos syndrome.

Ms. Dominique WEIL, *MPsych*
Psychology (Belgium)

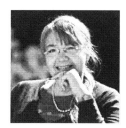

She holds a degree in Psychological Sciences from the Université Catholique de Louvain (UCL) and works as a clinical psychologist and psychotherapist. She has a systemic approach (family, couple, or individual) and a psycho-corporal approach (bio-energetic analysis). She manages patients with chronic pain, including Ehlers-Danlos Syndrome and algoneurodystrophy.

Dr. Michael P. HEALY, *PT, DPT, DOMTP, IOMT, MBA*
Physical therapist, Osteopathy, Sports Medicine (USA)

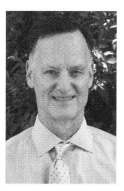

Dr. Michael Healy is the Owner, President, and CEO of Healy Physical Therapy & Sports Medicine. He opened his physical therapy practice in 2003, in his home state of Rhode Island (USA). In 1986, Dr. Healy graduated from the University of New England (USA) with a Bachelor of Science in Physical Therapy. In 2008, he received his Diplomate in Osteopathic Manipulative Theory & Practice, from The Osteopathic College of Ontario (Canada). In 2012, Dr. Healy earned his Doctorate of Physical Therapy, from Simmons College (USA). Dr. Healy is also a certified Integrated Osteopathic Manual Therapist, personal trainer, and sports nutritionist. Dr. Healy specializes in advanced manual therapy. He is highly regarded for his experience with treating patients diagnosed with connective tissue disorders such as Ehlers-Danlos Syndrome, Loeys-Dietz Syndrome, and Marfan Syndrome.

Professor David LEVINE, *PT, PhD, DPT, CCRP, Cert. DN, FAPTA*
Physical therapist, Orthopedist (USA)

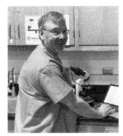

Dr. Levine is a Professor and the Walter M. Cline Chair of Excellence in Physical Therapy at the University of Tennessee at Chattanooga. In addition, he is board certified as a specialist in orthopedics by the American Board of Physical Therapy Specialties and is also certified in dry needling. Dr. Levine has been working and conducting research in many fields including gait analysis since the early 1990's. He continues to practice in physical therapy in addition to his University position. He has presented at over 100 conferences, and has lectured in more than a dozen countries. Dr. Levine has published in numerous peer-reviewed journals and conference proceedings with over 100 publications. His latest research focuses on control of clinical infectious disease as a founding member of the Clinical Infectious Disease Control Unit at UTC, chronic pain, animal assisted therapy, and rehabilitative interventions for individuals with Ehlers-Danlos Syndrome.

Dr. Jessica PIZANO, *DCN, CNS*
Clinical Nutrition (USA)

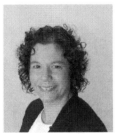

Dr. Jessica Pizano graduated with honors from the University of Bridgeport's functional nutrition master's program. She continued her education at Maryland University of Integrative Health where she graduated with a Doctor of Clinical Nutrition. The owner of Mast Cell Advanced Diagnostics and co-owner of Clinical Paradigms, Dr. Pizano uses nutrition, nutritional genomics, and metabolomics to help improve clinical outcome in those with mast cell activation disorders, Ehlers-Danlos Syndrome, dysautonomias, and other related conditions. She has developed course work at the master's and post-graduate level at MUIH in nutritional genomics, has published a series of peer-reviewed journal articles on the microbiome, and contributed two chapters on nutritional genomics in a graduate level nutrition textbook.

Dr. Trinh HERMANNS-LÊ, *MD, PhD*
Dermatology & Dermatopathology (Belgium)

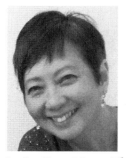

Specialist in Dermatology and Venereology at the Université de Liège in Belgium (1981), his doctoral thesis was entitled: Dendrocytes and pathophysiology of the dermis structure (2003). Much of this thesis focused on EDS. Specialized in transmission electron microscopy (TEM), she was a lecturer at the Université de Liège from 2003 to 2017. She is the author of more than 129 publications referenced on the PubMed portal, including 30 on Ehlers-Danlos Syndrome.

Mr. Olivier HOUGRAND
Electron microscopy (Belgium)

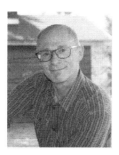

His interest in ultrastructural studies began in the early 2000s. Research into muscular pathologies has undoubtedly given him a taste for the infinitely small. Over time, other tissues and pathologies were added to his observations. Dr. Trinh Hermanns-Lê, he says, taught him all about the intricacies of connective tissue. He works at the Electron Microscopy Laboratory, Department of Dermatopathology, CHU de Liège (Belgium).

Dr. Daniel GROSSIN, *MD, DATC*
General Medicine (France)

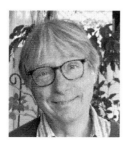

General Medicine's specialist and Acupuncturist, Daniel Grossin, trained in Ehlers-Danlos Syndrome with Professor Claude Hamonet in Paris. Holder of a university graduate of EDS, Université de Paris-Est Créteil (UPEC), he regularly consults at the ELLAsanté medical center. He leads numerous meetings and conferences throughout France about EDS.

Doctor Richard AMORETTI, *MD*
Cardiology (France)

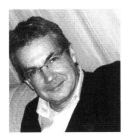

Richard Amoretti is medical doctor, specialist in cardiology and sports medicine. Formerly teaching director in Sports Cardiology at the Pitié-Salpêtrière Faculty of Medicine in Paris, he specialized in Ehlers-Danlos Syndrome. It ensures the diagnosis, follow-up, and cardiological assessment of patients with EDS. He consults at the ELLAsanté Centre in Paris and at the ISM Medical Centre in Boulogne-Billancourt.

Doctor Kambyse SAMII, *MD*
Internal Medicine & Cardiology (Belgium)

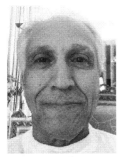

Doctor of Medicine, graduated from the Université de Paris V and the Université Libre de Bruxelles (ULB), Kambyse Samii is specialized in Internal Medicine and Cardiology. His favorite subject is the epidemiological study and management of hypertension (he is one of the founding members of the Belgian Committee for the Control of Hypertension).

Doctor Georges OBEID, *MD*
Internal Medicine & Cardiology (Belgium)

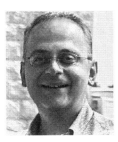

He is a Clinical Cardiologist. He is particularly interested in cardiac ultrasound, tissue deformation, and the impact of scuba diving on the heart. Cardiology's new integrative vision, including myocardial, valvular, or vascular tissue damage, combined with a nutritional approach, fascinates him at the highest level. He takes care of also pacemakers as well as the preventive development of sportsmen and women.

Doctor Emmanuel TRAN-NGOC, PT, *MD*
Internal Medicine & Cardiology (Belgium)

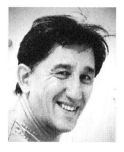

He graduated in physiotherapy in 1983 and became a Doctor of Medicine at the Université Libre de Bruxelles (ULB) in 1994. He obtained his specialization diploma in Cardiology, then in coronary angiography and coronary angioplasty. He is currently working at EPICURA Mons, Belgium. His preferred activities are general cardiology, interventional cardiology, Pacemaker implantation, ultrasound, transthoracic and transesophageal cardiac, stress testing, Pacemaker control, and internal defibrillator.

Doctor Michel HORGUE, *MD, DATC*
General and Thermal Medicine (France)

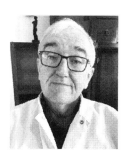

Michel Horgue graduated in 1985 from the Université de Bordeaux II in France. He also holds a DU in Sports Medicine, Acupuncture, and EDS. He also holds a University Certificate of Capacity in Hydrology and Medical Climatology and a diploma in Osteopathy. He practices at the DAX Thermal Hospital, where he specializes in the care of, among others thermal baths, patients with Ehlers-Danlos Syndrome.

Mr. David LEROY, *D.O.*
Physiotherapy, Osteopathy, Posturology (Belgium)

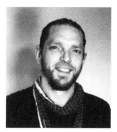

He developed his first professional experiences as a physiotherapist and radiology scanner technician in a hospital environment. He then opened his physio-therapy practice. He is also a specialist in osteopathy and posturology. Sensitive to the benefits of teamwork, he created his paramedical center, which now includes a dozen therapists specialized in physiotherapy, osteopathy, posturology, micro-physiotherapy, and psychology. He is a member of GERSED Belgium.

Mr. Dominique OUHAB, *PT*
Physiotherapy (France)

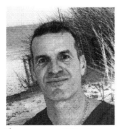

Graduated in 1986, Dominique Ouhab worked for several years in top-level sport within the French Gymnastics Federation. At the same time, he practiced in the hospital sector with children while maintaining a private practice in Paris. He is specialized in sports and preventive physiotherapy, as well as pediatric physiotherapy. He is very invested in the management of patients with EDS. Currently, EDS patients make up 80% of his patient load.

Doctor Georges VEROUGSTRAETE, *MD*
Ears, Nose and Throat (Belgium)

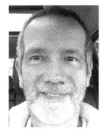

Doctor of Medicine from the Université Libre de Bruxelles (ULB) specialized in general, pediatric, and oncological otorhinolaryngology (ENT). He also practices ear surgery and maxillofacial surgery. He has a general practice in Brussels, Belgium.

Websites to Visit

GERSED Belgium: http://www.gersedbelgique.com
GERSED (France): http://www.gersed.com

Author et co-authors of the book "Transforming Ehlers-Danlos Syndrome":

Dr. Stéphane Daens: www.docteurdaens.be
Dr Isabelle Dubois-Brock: www.qolify.org ; www.ctissues.net; www.clinicalparadigms.com; www.3-pillars-therapeutics.com; www.gersed.com.
Prof. Claude Hamonet: www.claude.hamonet.free.fr/fr/sed.htm
Prof. Jaime F. Bravo: www.reumatologia-dr-bravo.cl
Prof. Stephen W. Porges: https://www.stephenporges.com
Dr. Pradeep Chopra: www.painri.com

EDS Patient associations:

SED1+ Association: http://www.assosed1plus.com
Ehlers-Danlos Syndrome Canada: https://www.ehlers-danlossyndromecanada.org
Hypermobility Syndromes Association (UK): http://www.hypermobility.com
Ehlers-Danlos Society : http://www.ehlers-danlos.org

Rare Diseases and Orphan Drugs Portal:
https://www.orpha.net

Social Networks

GERSED Belgium: https://www.facebook.com/GERSED.Belgique/
Instagram: gersed_belgique

Stéphane Daens auteur (main author):
https://www.facebook.com/stephanedaensauteur/
docteurdaens@hotmail.com

Isabelle Brock (main co-author): IBrock@qolify.org

GERSED (France): https://www.facebook.com/gersedfrance/

RAAL (cover artwork): raal.painter@gmail.com

Books to Discover

Claude Hamonet : "*Ehlers-Danlos - La maladie oubliée par la médecine*", L'Harmattan, 2018.

Andràs Pàldi: "*L'épigénétique ou la nouvelle ère de l'hérédité*", Éditions Le Pommier, 2018.

Stephen W. Porges: "*The Polyvagal Theory – Neurophysiological foundations of emotions, attachment, communication, and self-regulation*", W. W. Norton & Company, 2011.

Stephen W. Porges: "*Clinical insights from the Polyvagal Theory – The transformative power of feeling safe*", W. W. Norton & Company, 2013.

Stanley Rosenberg: "*Accessing the healing power of the vagus nerve*", North Atlantic Book – Berkeley, California, 2017 (French Edition, 2020).

Deb Dana: "*Polyvagal exercises for safety and connection*", W. W. Norton & Company, 2020.

Éric Marlien: "*Le système nerveux autonome. De la théorie polyvagale au développement psychosomatique*", Éditions Sully, 2018.

Navaz Habib: "*Activate your vagus nerve*", Ulysse Press, 2019.

Florian Ismail & Benoît Martin: "*En quête d'équilibre – Vers une stratégie de prise en charge de l'hypermobilité et de l'hypersensibilité*", 2021.

Céline Huillet: "*Et si … je devenais Pétronille*", Art et Caractère, 2019.

Lucille Sergent, Samuel Pouvereau: "*Petit guide de survie des patients face à la blouse blanche*", Éditions First, 2019.

Virginie Burner-Lehner: "*La Dame en bleu*", L'Harmattan, 2016.

Isabelle Delbarre Grossemy: "*Goniométrie – Manuel d'évaluation des amplitudes articulaires des membres et du rachis*", Éditions Masson, 2008.

Joshua Clelang, Shane Koppenhaver: "*Netter's orthopaedic clinical examination: an evicence-Based approach*", Saunders, 2011.

Gabriel Perlemuter: "*Stress, hypersensibilité, depression… Et si la solution venait de nos bactéries?* " Éditions Flammarion/Versilio, 2020.

Joël de Rosnay: "*La symphonie du vivant*", LLL éditions, 2018.

Ariane Giacobino: "*Peut-on se libérer de ses gènes ? L'épigénétique.* ", Editions Stock, 2018.

Joël de Rosnay, Dean Ornish, Claudine Julien, David Khayat, Pierre-Henri Gouyon: "*La révolution épigénétique*", Editions Albin Michel, 2018.

Diana Jovin et al. Disjointed – Navigating the diagnosis and management of Hypermobile Ehlers-Danlos Syndrome and Hypermobility Spectrum Disorders. Hidden Stripes Publications, Inc. 2020.

INDEX

C

D

750

E

F

G

H

N

O

P

U

V